Secondary and Functional Rhinoplasty
The Difficult Nose

Secondary and Functional Rhinoplasty
The Difficult Nose

Rodolphe Meyer
F.M.H. Plastic, Reconstructive, and Aesthetic Surgery
Postgraduate Professor ISAPS (IPRS)
Centre de Chirurgie Plastique
Former Associate Professor
University Clinic
Lausanne, Switzerland

G&S

Grune & Stratton, Inc.

Harcourt Brace Jovanovich, Publishers
Orlando New York San Diego London
San Francisco Tokyo Sydney Toronto

Grune & Stratton, Inc.
Orlando, Florida 32887

Distributed in the United Kingdom by
Grune & Stratton, Ltd.
24/28 Oval Road, London NW 1
Printed in Hong Kong

Library of Congress Catalog Number 87-072357
International Standard Book Number 0-8089-1879-6
Printed in Hong Kong
87 88 89 90 10 9 8 7 6 5 4 3 2 1

To My Wife Liliane,
My Beloved Secondary Case

Contents

Foreword

In the entire specialty of aesthetic and reconstructive surgery of the nose, there are only a few surgeons in the world who can match the skill, imagination, originality, and the wealth of experience of Rodolphe Meyer, known affectionately to many of his colleagues as "Rudi." Whenever a major symposium on corrective nasal surgery is held anywhere in the world, one would literally find it surprising if Rudi were not a member of the symposium's panel of distinguished senior surgeons. With the publishing of this book, *Secondary and Functional Rhinoplasty,* a second book has now appeared under his authorship which is as outstanding if not more so than the first book.

In 1967, a book on corrective and reconstructive rhinoplasty was published, whose authors were Hans Joachim Denecke of Heidelberg and a younger Rodolphe Meyer of Lausanne. This book is still a remarkable collection of chapters with extremely handsome illustrations describing a multitude of various aspects of reconstructive nasal surgery, as well as primary corrective or "aesthetic" surgery of the nose. In this 1967 publication, however, there is very little written about secondary nasoplastic operations as we know them today in the year 1987, 20 years later.

In writing the Foreword to Denecke and Meyer's book, the late highly respected Gustavo Sanvenero-Rosselli of Milan, accurately described it as follows:

> . . . At last a book of splendid format has been published in which the authors, although they are very talented surgeons, almost everywhere abstain from displaying their ability through photographic reproduction and instead, with a modesty comparable to that of the classic poet, expose every most obscure detail of basic and lesser known procedures using meticulously accurate illustrations which are of unsurpassed artistic efficacy. This work is destined to find its place and retain it because it deserves the rare praise of being truly a tool to which many surgeons will have cause to resort in order to refine their own experience, in the same manner in which Horace thought his works should be used.

In contrast to what Sanvenero-Rosselli wrote in his Foreword to Dr. Meyer's first book, this present book, *Secondary Rhinoplasty,* is entirely different, especially since it is such a photographic pleasure for the eyes of any serious surgeon and clinician, containing for the first time a wealth of pre- and postoperative photographs, as well as excellent accompanying illustrations of the corrective surgical procedures employed by Dr. Meyer and his colleagues. This book, therefore, is an outstanding major treatise describing every conceivable sort of problem that can face the surgeon who performs secondary rhinoplasty with its clearly demonstrable logical solution.

With the appearance of this book, one might conceivably say that this is truly the first major book devoted almost entirely to secondary rhinoplasty. Dr. Meyer's name is one of the very few that dominates the field of secondary rhinoplasty today, and this is certainly understandable to any of us in the specialty who are familiar with the skill and refinement of his work and have heard him give one of his many colorful and instructive lectures on this subject.

Dr. Meyer's interest in secondary rhinoplasty has been historically one of the earliest in the modern post World War II era of the development of plastic and reconstructive surgery. Incredibly, today, there are still only a minimal amount of papers describing secondary nasoplasty in the medical literature compared not only to the huge volume of corrective nasoplasties which are performed daily throughout the world, and to the greater number of articles written about primary nasoplasty as well. The first book that dealt to any extent whatsoever with secondary nasoplasties was that published by James Barrett Brown and Frank McDowell in 1951, in which only ten pages at the end of the book presented the reader with cases requiring secondary nasal correction. In the 1950s, 1960s, and up to the middle of the 1970s only a very few authors had confined themselves to reporting the specific problems of secondary nasoplasty and their correction, including Brown and McDowell (1951), O'Connor and McGregor (1955), Denecke and Meyer (1967), Rogers 1967; 1972), Millard (1969), Rees and Wood-Smith (1970), Meyer 1974–1977, etc.), and finally Sheen (1975–1976, etc.).

A mere referral to the extensive bibliography in this book will give the reader a very good idea of the number of important secondary nasoplasty articles dealing with highly difficult cases that were written by Dr. Meyer from 1974 up to the present.

As a young man with training in both otolaryngology and plastic surgery techniques, Dr. Meyer had already shown an interest in plastic surgery of the nose in his very first paper on nasoplasty published in 1951, as well as a paper discussing the treatment of septal perforations. From 1956 onward, numerous papers by Dr. Meyer appeared up to and including the publication of his book in 1967 dealing with primary and secondary correction of problems of the harelip nose.

This present book by Meyer contains so many fascinating case histories and the means by which to treat them that it would be redundant here to discuss any one of them. One of the most valuable portions of this book, however, is Chapter 2 in which Meyer describes in detail the many factors that have brought about the current need for performing skillful secondary nasal surgery by properly trained and experienced plastic surgeons. Meyer emphasizes in Chapter 2:

> . . . A certain number of rhinoplasties become imperfect and unsatisfactory for the patient, or perhaps only for the operator, even if the result on the operating room table was perfect. Thus, no rhinoplastic surgeon will ever be free from cases requiring secondary intervention, which will occur in about 5 percent of the cases seen by an experienced operator and reaching probably up to 15 percent of all rhinoplasties. Artistic judgment is an intangible concept and postoperative healing is unpredictable. No matter how well trained, experienced, careful, artistic, or lucky a surgeon may be, there will still be some secondary deformities.

With the quotation of these few lines of sage advice and understanding that demonstrate Dr. Meyer's humility, it should merely be further emphasized that secondary nasoplasties are being performed with greater frequency with each passing year. Unfortunately, many of these would be unnecessary if the surgeons who performed the primary rhinoplasty either had previously obtained better training in rhinoplastic procedures, or, at least, knew their limitations. It goes without saying, therefore, because of the difficulty in performing secondary rhinoplasties, it would probably be wise for the novice plastic surgeon to refer any postrhinoplastic deformities as a result of surgery by himself or others to senior surgeons such as Meyer who are known throughout the world for having the necessary expertise in performing highly successful secondary nasoplastic surgery.

With this having been said, I shall bring this Foreword to an end at this point, and let the reader hear directly in the next 23 chapters from the master himself—Rodolphe "Rudi" Meyer!

Blair Rogers, M.D., F.A.C.S.
Professor of Clinical Surgery (Plastic Surgery)
New York University Medical Center
Attending Surgeon
Department of Plastic Surgery
Manhattan Eye, Ear and Throat Hospital
New York, New York

Foreword

It is not surprising that Dr. Rodolphe Meyer has written this splendid book on *Secondary Rhinoplasty*. His entire professional life is a rich compilation of experience and success as a surgeon, medical philosopher, and master craftsman. He, more than anyone, has the ability to analyze a difficult problem and then proceed with the appropriate surgical technique to correct it. It is easy for me to remember the facial surgical seminars held in Würzburg, under the aegis of the late Professor Horst Wüllstein, when Dr. Meyer accepted some of the most difficult problems requiring rehabilitative surgery about the nose, lips, and eyelids. He carried off his teaching responsibilities in an innovative and creative series of surgical procedures with the highest professional skill.

Everything that Dr. Meyer does has his unique stamp of excellence. Few surgeons are able to gain so much expertise from surgical involvement. He has been able not only to sustain these high levels of performance for decades, but actually is constantly improving upon that level. It is therefore noteworthy that he should state his experience in the science and art of secondary rhinoplasty.

Dr. Meyer has organized this book in a very logical way that makes his subject very broad, understandably human, and artistic. Simultaneously, he has established the criteria for successful management within this framework. The main substance of the book is a tour de force of photographic documentation of the patients' nasal problems and the methods used to correct these problems. This is complemented by an impressive set of drawings that are graphic, uncluttered, and detail a specific part of the technique. This imagery is supported by a rich text that embraces the historical development, psychological aspects, motivations, social determinants and medico-legal responsibilities pertaining to this subject.

The fundamental subject of this book relates to the abnormalities that make secondary rhinoplasty necessary and challenging. Secondary rhinoplasty is certainly recognized by the experienced surgeon in this field to be forever challenging and somewhat elusive. It begins with the basic anatomy of the nose that often predetermines what technique is possible and what technique is realistic. Each region of the nose and its particular anatomy is analyzed and explained as a specific unit and as part of the total aspect of management. Biologic deteriorations, tumors, the effects of aging, and associated congenital abnormalities are also realistically dealt with. Nothing of substance has been left out, and yet the primary value of this text is the presentation of the most optimal surgical methods of correction.

This book has overlapping values for both the younger surgeon who is trying to sort out all of these difficulties, and the advanced craftsman who has struggled with them and has partially solved them. Otolaryngologists—Head and Neck surgeons, plastic surgeons, maxillofacial surgeons, and academicians will find this book essential as a text, as a source of reference, and as an instructional facility.

John Conley, M.D.
Professor Emeritus
St. Vincent's Medical Center
Columbia Presbyterian Medical Center
Department of Head and Neck Surgery
New York, New York

Acknowledgments

The author gratefully acknowledges the beautiful artwork of Kathy Sisson-Schlesser, the expert assistance of Louis O. Boileau, M.D., Camille B. Williams, M.D., Dominique M. Rheims, M.D., and Jeffrey M. Israel, M.D., and the secretarial help.

Secondary and Functional Rhinoplasty
The Difficult Nose

1

History

Reconstructive surgery of the nose dates back more than 4000 years according to ancient Indian writings, continuing through the Middle Ages as witnessed in Sicily, Italy, and Germany. The true corrective rhinoplasty appeared only in the last two decades of the last century.

Ingals ushered in modern septal surgery in 1882 by removing a small triangular piece of cartilage. In 1886, Trendelenburg reported on corrections of deflected noses in Germany. Kreig (1889) removed most of the septal cartilage and, when he felt it necessary, included the perpendicular plate of the ethmoid and vomer. In 1891 Asch described the use of through and through cruciate incisions. He claimed that, if the segments were completely broken at the bases, deviations could not occur because the resiliency of the cartilage was destroyed. In 1901, Goodale described repositioning laterally displaced nasal bones in the U.S.A.

Credit for developing the submucous resection belongs to Freer (1902) and Killian (1905). Basically the approach of both surgeons was to incise the cephalic to the caudal end of the septum on the convex side. After elevating the septal membrane and incising through the cartilage on this side a flap was elevated on the opposite side and the deviated portions were removed. The procedures used today are modifications of their techniques. Killian (1908) suggested resecting of the cartilaginous and bony septums with restoration of a centimeter of cartilaginous and bony septums with restoration of a centimeter of cartilage just beneath the dorsum to safeguard against saddling, as well as retaining of the caudal end of the septum to prevent any retraction of the columella.

Dieffenbach in Germany performed the first aesthetic corrections of the nose in 1845 through external incisions and by means of fractures of the nasal bones. Using these techniques he reduced excessively large noses and straightened crooked noses. The distinction of having performed the first rhinoplasty through intranasal incisions goes to John Orlando Roe of Rochester, who presented in 1887 three cases of "pug" noses corrected by transmucous cartilaginous tailoring. In 1891, he presented four cases of intranasal hump reduction by osteotomy using a chisel with pre- and postoperative photographs to document the operative results. These interventions were possible with the advent of cocaine topical anesthesia, which was first advocated by Moreno and Maij (1890). In 1892 the intranasal correction of a crooked nose by osteotomies and transnasal steel fixation of the nasal bones was described by Robert Fulton Weir of New York.

It is important in detailing the history of secondary rhinoplasty to note that Weir was the first to describe a nasal revision in a patient operated on three times previously and who was never satisfied. In this same patient he performed for the first time the crescent-shaped wedge resection at the lower lateral base for lower lateral reduction, which still today bears his name. We give credit to the same author for being the first to attempt to correct a saddle nose by insertion of a heterotopic bone graft for dorsal augmentation followed by its extrusion. It was contained in a subcutaneous pocket of the dorsum. The rejection occurred 7 weeks later. In 1886, Trendelenburg reported on corrections of deflected noses in Germany and in 1901 Goodale described repositioning laterally displaced nasal bones in the USA.

The real popularizer of modern aesthetic rhinoplasty, however, was Jacques Joseph of Berlin who described the basis of today's actual methods in his famous book *Nasenplastik und sonstige Gesichtsplastik* (1932). He accomplished his first reduction of the nasal pyramid by external access with cutaneous, cartilaginous, and bony mucosal excisions in the shape of a reverse V in 1898. He described his rhinoplastic technique in detail, but he never mentioned complications, pitfalls, and secondary procedures. Joseph, after Roe, was the second surgeon to use preoperative and postoperative photographs to document the operative results. His pupils, Aufricht (1934, 1943, 1944, 1958, 1961, 1969), Safian (1935, 1953, 1956, 1970, 1973), and Rode (1938), continued his eminent work in aesthetic rhinoplasty in New York and Berlin.

Sheehan (1925), another famous rhinoplastic surgeon in New York, Sanvenero-Rosselli (1931), in Milano, and Eitner (1935) in Vienna wrote important books on rhinoplasty with technical innovations. All three did not touch the delicate problems of revision rhinoplasty.

The principles in rhinoplasty worked out in the first half of this century were then refined in the second half. Among these additions was the important contribution made by Eitner (1934) who proposed the method of access to the bony structures and to the whole septum through a mucoperichondrial dissection gained by freeing the upper lateral cartilage at its septal insertion. This method was also used by Fomon (1960), Meyer (1964), and Anderson (1966) and introduced as a routine method for rhinoplasties by Robin (1970), Pollet (1970), and Jost (1972) who called it "the extramucosal method." Another procedure advocated in the last few decades by Cottle (1960) was the method of nasal bone "push-down" and "push-up" for bony contour correction. This method of handling the nasal bones has been adopted by many rhinoplastic surgeons. Actually the technique, not being versatile enough for the whole spectrum of sophisticated corrections, is used by plastic surgeons only in exceptional cases.

In the last decades, an enormous variety of contributions to the perfections of this surgical treatment have appeared. Among the most important books published since 1900 are:

1900—Keegan
1904—Nelation and Ombredanne
1926—Sheehan
1926—Dufourmjentel L.
1932—Joseph
1932—Eitner
1935—Safian
1936—Sheehan
1947—Maliniac
1949—Seltzer
1950—Galtier
1951—Brown and McDowell
1952—Fruehwald
1957—Aubry and Giroud
1964/1967—Denecke and Meyer
1965—Farina
1966—Walter
1968—Bozzi et al. (Denecke-Meyer)
1971—Hinderer
1973—Rees
1973—Lewis
1975—Jost
1978—Sheen
1984—Peck
1985—Micheli-Pellegrini

In textbooks on plastic surgery and rhinoplasty, there is relatively little written about the dangers of secondary rhinoplasty. Joseph (1932) mentioned very little about the complications. Nowhere did he mention that it is sometimes necessary to operate on the nose two or three times. Later on, some contributions concerning mistakes and pitfalls in rhinoplasty and their corrections were made by Berson (1948), Maliniac

(1949), Sarnoff (1950), Berndorfer, (1950), Silver (1952), Wexler (1952), Seltzer (1953), Dufourmentel (1954), Safian (1953), Cohen (1956), McGregor, O'Connor, and Saffier (1958), Levignac (1958), Aufricht (1961), Grignon (1963), Converse (1964), Denecke and Meyer (1964–1967), Champion (1966), Rogers (1967 and 1972), Millard (1969), Rees et al (1970), Micheli-Pellegrini (1975), Meyer (1971 and 1981), Sénéchal (1976), Hellmich (1979), Flemming (1979), Juri (1979), Bruck (1981), Lawson, Kessler, and Biller (1983), and others.

The history of septal surgery in children began with the nineteenth century.

- In 1890—Dent reported on the septal correction and removal of hypertrophic bone of the inferior turbinate in a 7-year-old child.
- 1895—Czerny corrected a saddle nose with lateral bone and cartilaginous structures.
- 1899—Boenninghaus resected the lower half of the septal cartilage and a part of the vomer in a 9-year-old child and published in 1899 five further resections in 6–13-year-old children.
- 1899—Donnelan performed a septal resection in a 6-year-old child for traumatic deviation.
- 1900—Mangoldt undertook a correction on a syphilitic saddle nose in a 15-year-old boy with autogenous rib cartilage.
- 1902—Freer published his method of submucous septal resection that was also used in children.
- 1908—Killian reported good results with submucous septal resection in 9 children.

Freer's and Killian's procedure was later used in children by Hayton (1916), Metzenbaum (1929), White (1930), Ombredanne (1942), Jennes (1964), Sénéchal (1965), Reidy (1968), Bloom (1970), and others.

Metzenbaum's technique for septal corrections in children was the most structured and was then followed and partially modified by surgeons such as Carter (1923), Cottle (1939, 1948, 1951, 1958), Salinger (1939), Cohen (1947), Fomon (1948), de Vido (1953), Wexler (1955), Goldman (1956), Jennes (1964), Peska-Luskowska (1967), Witwicka (1968), Stocksted (1969), Masing (1974), and others.

Nowadays septal corrections, called septoplasties, are accomplished using more sophisticated techniques, removing, scoring, crosshatching, and morcelizing strips of cartilage as advocated by Converse (1950), Becker (1952), Dingman (1956), Denecke and Meyer (1964, 1967), and others.

2

General Considerations

Corrective rhinoplasty, the most fascinating and also the most exacting of all corrective operations on the facial features, has become a very common operation all over the world and is in increasing demand. But like all surgery, corrective rhinoplasty has its dangers.

Textbooks and monographs on this subject sometimes give the impression that the best results can be obtained with the first attempt. The experienced surgeon knows that touch-ups are often necessary and must be done carefully and with long consideration. Thus, there is not a single rhinologic surgeon having practiced for any appreciable length of time who does not have a certain number of unfavorable results.

Dealing with rhinoplasties, the surgeon has to face some unpredictable secondary deformities. In other surgeries, the complications are determined by the character of the disease; while in plastic surgery, especially rhinoplasty, the patients are usually in good health and the complications sustained reflect the ability of the surgeon and the condition of the inherent tissues. Thus, complications occur and can not be avoided even with the greatest caution and the best skill of the operator.

Public awareness of the fact that the nose is one of the most important elements in facial aesthetics and the emphasis on beauty in our modern society make rhinoplasty the most commonly requested aesthetic operation. Thanks to the increasing popularity, a great demand is placed on aesthetic rhinoplasty. Often the patient expects too much from the corrective operation. It can happen that an operation does not attain the desired and expected results. It is then important for the surgeon to determine the cause of the inadequacy.

A certain number of rhinoplasties become imperfect and unsatisfactory for the patient, or perhaps only for the operator, even if the result on the operating room table was perfect. Thus, no rhinoplastic surgeon will ever be free from cases requiring secondary intervention, which will occur in about 5 percent of the cases seen by an experienced operator and reaching probably up to 15 percent of all rhinoplasties. Artistic judgment is an intangible concept and postoperative healing is unpredictable. No matter how well-trained, experienced, careful, artistic, or lucky a surgeon may be, there will still be some secondary deformities.

Dissatisfaction with unfavorable results after primary rhinoplasty brings more and more patients to the rhinoplastic surgeon every year seeking to achieve the desired appearance. In rare cases, a secondary imperfection can even be predictable preoperatively or intraoperatively because of technical difficulties encountered. The most important factor for obtaining good results is that the surgeon has to be extremely self-critical, constantly analyze operative results, and be ready to learn from previous problems and complications. In general, the young surgeon is well advised to be conservative. To err by not doing enough is better evil than doing excess.

Surgeons should never impose their own ideals in addition to what the patients request. We must consider the potential conflict that may arise in the patient with a deformity: what are his subjective ideas of perfection and what can actually be achieved through surgery? One has to know the limitation of the patient's desire to get rid of the deformity. Surgeons should, if possible, take care of the undesirable sequelae of their own patients. However, in an increasing number of cases operated on by novice surgeons this is not possible due to the lack of skill and experience of the surgeon. Indeed, the result required often surpasses the capability of the operator. Thus, the experienced surgeon is solicited more and more often to perform a difficult and sometimes unappreciated secondary corrective rhinoplasty.

Rhinoplasty, in fact, is still practiced by too many inadequately trained operators and specifically by too many so called "aesthetic surgeons" without thorough knowledge and training in plastic and reconstructive surgery who may have observed some skilled operators for a short time, and who believe they are able to succeed in this delicate and dangerous field. The source of this audacity lies in the fact that in the hands of experienced operators, rhinoplasty seems to be a very easy intervention. This is the principal reason why we see more and more badly operated noses that require a secondary correction.

The larger proportion of perfect results obtained by the experienced surgeon is attributable to more skill in the operating technique, to the care taken in the selection of cases, to an ability to adapt particular operative methods to the preoperative shape of the nose, and to obtain the new desired shape, ensuring the durability of the achieved result.

The nose is the most important aesthetic feature of the face since it is the most prominent one. Leonardo da Vinci used to say that a nose is there to manifest the character of a face. The same opinions were expressed by Dürer and Lavater, who was the inventor of the physiognomic doctrine. Schopenhauer, in the late 18th century, went so far as to say that the fate of many women depends on the curvature of their nose. Bertillon (1853), the criminologist, regarded noses as being the characterologic key, par excellence. According to the studies of Micheli-Pellegrini (1975, 1979), Aristotle, Avicenna, Kant, Rousseau, and many others regarded the nose as an indispensable feature of the physiognomy and the index of the mind. Besides the well-known character of Cyrano de Bergerac, there are innumerable other characters described in literature with distinguishing nasal features, indicating that writers throughout different ages and in different countries have paid attention to the characterologic, emotional, and sociologic influence that the nose has had in the history of man.

Concerning the motivational and psychological implications of rhinoplasty, Linn and Goldman (1949) described a "psychiatric syndrome" in patients undergoing rhinoplasty that included cases of minor neurotic reaction and cases showing actual psychosis. Patients with these disorders believe that others look at them noting the size and shape of their noses. They are anxious and avoid showing their profiles. As they are incapable of using all their powers of concentration, they appear absent-minded, and those who associate with them, regard them as being incapable of making friends. This "prominence" of the nose in the wider complexity of the "body image" is even more manifest in patients who have already undergone an aesthetic rhinoplasty. They may not be completely satisfied or not know if the surgery has been done in the ideal way. They may wonder if there is still a further possibility of perfection.

In 1950 Mill and Silver studied a series of patients who wished to have their noses changed. All of them wanted to avoid changes that would make it impossible for them to be recognized by their own friends. All wanted to improve their body image, which seems to be of utmost importance in adolescence. Mill and Silver (1964) emphasized the fact that much of an adolescent's psychic energy is spent in establishing identity. In this respect, they pointed out the mistakes made by those surgeons who gave a Roman nose to a patient with Semitic features.

Ten years ago we operated on an Algerian adolescent with an Assyrian nose who wanted a Caucasian one. We transplanted the hump into his chin. The young man seemed to be quite satisfied with his superb new nose, but at home some weeks later he was not accepted by his family. His parents wanted him to change again his new European nose back into the characteristic nose of the family. So we had to retransplant the hump from the chin back into the dorsum of the nose. Fortunately the secondary rhinoplasty was as successful as the first one. Nowadays this race-born mentality is decreasing all over the world, revealing a world that wants to become more and more homogenous. Many noncaucasian people want to lose the characteristics of their race.

McGregor and Schaffner (1950) investigated patient motivation with pre and postoperative interviews. Their patients generally talked about having difficulties in breathing and complained of nose bleeds. Some requested rhinoplasty saying that it would help them in their jobs. Many reluctantly admitted to having suffered misery and humiliation because of their ugly noses. In our experience this latter reason is a very frequent presenting complaint in the motivation for a secondary procedure after an unsuccessful primary rhinoplasty.

The analysis made by these two investigators demonstrates how important it is for a person to have attractive features in order to win social approval. The inner build-up of an individual's desire's sometimes grows to such an extent that any disapproval experienced, whether real or imaginary, may cause severe psychological disturbances. The operation thus comes to be regarded as the only means for removing the basis of the patient's undesirability to society. McGregor and Schaffner (1950) describe the following important factors that characterize the patient who requests rhinoplasty: (1) a wish to get rid of the malformation, as it is a social and economic drawback; (2) a wish to reach a standard of beauty; (3) a wish to change personality by changing looks; (4) a wish to appear brave; (5) rejection of familiar features; (6) ascribing personal failures to the malformation.

In secondary surgery our findings agree largely with theirs. McGregor and Schaffner say that a patient who is mostly seeking social approval through the operation but who fails to achieve this aim may take it out on the surgeon and even come to hate the surgeon. For this reason the surgeon should if possible try to improve this sad situation by undertaking the revisionary surgery.

In 1938 Smith and De Kleine pointed out that for certain personalities, a physical defect may give rise to abnormal psychological attitudes. Therefore, it would be extremely logical and sensible to correct the morphologic defect before severe personality changes could develop.

Barsky (1950) divides patients into "two basic neurotics," one in whom a physical defect covers a more significant inner disturbance and the second, the situational neurotic. In the former a corrective operation is of no use as the neurosis is simply redirected toward another symptom. The latter, the situational neurotics, are disturbed and anxious people; surgery is definitely indicated as their physiological condition is a direct consequence of their physical defect. In this second category the patient would certainly insist on having a secondary rhinoplasty if the first did not give the desired result. In these cases the patients need our help until the corrective operation has attained the final goal. For that to occur, it is extremely important for the surgeon to find out what the essential wishes of the patient are. Generally, after a primary intervention the residual defects are only small and may even be appreciated only subjectively. They can however cause more unhappiness than the largely visible primary defect because now after the first intervention the patient is fixed on the imperfection of his nose. For Reich (1984) the dissatisfaction reflects psychological disturbances that are also dependent on the opinion of others, especially when the aesthetic result of the first operation is good.

Mayer (1964), one of the many psychiatrists dealing with the relationship between cosmetic surgery and psychology and the problems that may arise as the two meet, said that in no field of surgery other than plastic surgery, and especially the corrective arena of surgery, are physicians faced with so many important psychological, social, and ethical problems. He attaches great importance to social background and stresses the importance of the family's attitude as one of the strongest social drives in action.

Bittle (1975) made a survey of the more frequent complications following cosmetic surgery. Of great importance is the possible deterioration of psychotic conditions and the increased display of abnormal personality traits. Bittle (1975) lists the following personality types as susceptible to the following potential psychological disorders: (1) Hysterical personality (histrionic, seductive, highly emotional behavior tending to involve others in an underhand sort of way to assure their continuous affection and attention; altered sexual functions), (2) Depressed females going through the menopause, (3) Paranoid personality.

Anderson (1974) regards rhinoplasty as a psychological operation and proposes a list of operations as a premise for good psychological selection of patients. He points out some of the psychological danger signs in a series of 24 observations, among which the following stand out; the person who is seeking perfection; the one who keeps moving his or her hands (hysterical personality), and finally the one whose family is against the operation.

Secondary deformities are mostly the result of incomplete correction of the original deformity or the result of over-zealous resections. The preoperative planning and assessment is very important in order to avoid results that are good as regards a technical performance but not in harmony with the surrounding features of the face and therefore unsuitable for the patient's general appearance.

The appreciation of a rhinoplastic result is not always the same for the surgeon as for the patient. Many times the patient is dissatisfied with the primary surgery and seeks a revision although the result appears satisfactory to the surgeon. Occasionally the patient is happy although an imperfection is evident to the surgeon.

It is important that we not fall into the trap of the polydysmorphophobic patients going from specialist to specialist in the search for perfect certain facial features, which can never be attained, since the best results possible in our eyes can only be imperfect in their eyes.

We have to consider the viewpoints of the patient concerning the details to be corrected and his or her appreciation of what is beautiful, which may not always correspond to those of the surgeon. Sometimes a compromise has to be made and for this reason the design of a detailed morphological representation of the nasal deformities can be helpful in detecting, establishing, and evaluating the incongruence of opinions.

If the patient suffers from dysmorphophobia it will be difficult for the rhinoplastic surgeon to reveal the real deformity to be corrected and subsequently to manage the correction. The surgeon will know what the average size of the nasofrontal and nasolabial angles and the ideal measurements of the nasal profile in comparison with the size of the other facial features should be, but only the surgeon's experience and artistic feeling can help in finding the particular ideal shape of the nose suitable for the patient's general appearance, staying in harmony with the rest of the face. A desirable end result should conform not only to the patient's aesthetic preference, but also maintain the patient's nasofrontal, nasomaxillary, nasooral, and nasomandibular relationships. A surgeon's failure to consider facial balance or imbalance may lead to a poor result.

The choice of special technique and a certain flexibility on the part of the surgeon in performing his or her personal method, and also frequent preoperative and intraoperative evaluations of specific characteristics of the nasal structures requiring particular attention, are important factors in preventing mistakes, failures, and complications in rhinoplasty.

The spectrum of postoperative deformities after primary surgery range from minor irregularities of the dorsum, indentations in the tip area, insufficient osteotomies to saddle-nose deformities, and, in extreme cases, a mutilation of the nose with stenosis of the nares, the so called crucified noses. Far more problems and complications arise from conservative corrections. Inappropriate techniques applied persistently without regard for the existing anatomy creates frequent complications. Over the last 30 years I have had to revise a number of my own cases. Fortunately, in cases where I misjudged what the passage of time was going to do to my primary work the case almost always involved my being too cautious in not resecting quite enough in the original operation. In studying those cases referred for secondary rhinoplasty we get the impression that unskilled and inexperienced surgeons have a tendency to fail by being too cautious and conservative in their techniques more than by being excessive and over-zealous. In general, more significant complications occur when too much tissue is removed as opposed to a failure to remove enough. Excessive removal is often associated with pinching, scarring, and restriction of nasal breathing. More importantly, deformities related to excessive tissue removal are generally more difficult to restore. Rhinoplasty should be approached as an anatomic dissection of the nasal structures requiring alteration. These elements should be conservatively shaped and repositioned.

Natural sculpturing of the nose during the

primary rhinoplasty is the common goal of every rhinoplastic surgeon: For this, rhinoplasty is still the most challenging of all aesthetic operations since no two procedures are quite identical. Each patient's nasal configuration and structure requires individual operative planning. Therefore, no single technique, no matter how well mastered, will prepare the surgeon for the various anatomic patterns encountered. It is essential to regard rhinoplasty as an operation planned to reconstitute and shape the anatomic features of the nose into a new more pleasing relationship to one another and the surrounding facial features without altering the physiologic function of the nose, except perhaps for a possible amelioration of that physiologic function.

Much more than in primary rhinoplasty, individual planning is of paramount importance from case to case in secondary surgery. Revisionary surgery cannot follow the usual rules and use the usual methods. In many cases it is reconstructive in nature and therefore more difficult technically and the results are generally less predictable and more likely to fall short of expectation. The need for aesthetic surgical judgment is more important than in primary surgery and it is more difficult for the surgeon to understand the healing dynamics at play on these operated noses. Finally, the greatest difficulty with any revision is to avoid the appearance of an "operated" or "surgical" nose, giving back to the secondary nose a natural appearance.

It is a matter of surgical philosophy whether a surgeon wants to deal with difficult problems. There are many rhino surgeons who will not accept secondary cases operated on primarily by other colleagues, probably because they want to have surgical material with a minimum of problems and with a minimum of medico-legal risks, which is a factor of increasing importance and because this surgery can easily be a reputation destroyer. Nowadays, the philosophy is to undertake only a correction where little modifications are indicated and requested. This is encountered in every field of plastic surgery but especially in rhinoplasty. In our mind, one has to be able to deal with difficult problems in this field too.

A very delicate problem is presented in cases where there is no evidence of deformity or deranged function. Anderson (1974) recommends not to consider operating on the patient who simply wants a modification to the shape of an already properly structured nose. He states: "The fact that the operation did not quite accomplish what the patient had in mind should not sway one's resolve." There are, however, cases where we have decided to accept the patient for surgery, because they knew they could improve the shape of the nose and to meet the special ideas of the patient, even if these ideas are uncommon and because they can still make them happy.

Occasionally, we are consulted to correct minor secondary deformities such as a slight irregularity of the dorsum, which requires but a little rasping or a hanging columella, where a small piece of columellar skin needs to be excised, or where a tiny marginal resection is needed. But there are also deformities that although they appear minor to the patient are very difficult to correct, even for the very experienced surgeon, as, for instance, is a dimple or a furrow in the tip-ala complex.

We agree with the thoughts of Anderson (1974), who says that young surgeons should probably not accept revisions early in their careers. Before undertaking secondary procedures, the surgeon should at least have a few years of experience. The revision of a whole nose should only be undertaken by a really experienced rhinosurgeon.

In rhinoplasty, experience is more important than in other fields of plastic surgery. The results obtained by the same surgeon using the same technique improve with time with refinement in technical maneuvers permitting better adaptation of these maneuvers to the procedures, as mentioned by Gonzales Ulloa and Stevens (1964).

For our own primary patients we like to add, as an out-patient procedure, a little secondary correction, when we are able to improve the result without too much downside risk. On many occasions we don't hesitate to suggest minor corrections to the patient who, in most cases, agrees, trusting our efforts in seeking perfection.

3

Sociology

Reich (1983) found that in follow-up, patients usually attributed dissatisfaction with their rhinoplasties to postoperative reactions of families, close friends, or casual acquaintances. Negative reactions from significant others may elicit disappointment, self attributions of vanity and blame, and feelings of guilt, anxiety, or depression or, alternatively, may lead to suspicion of surgical error and feeling of anger toward the surgeon.

We live in a world in which one's physical appearance influences one's psychological development, social interactions, self-esteem, self-consciousness, and body-image. While some people are able to cope with or compensate for physical features that are personally or socially unattractive, others cannot transcend the effect of such features. In increasing numbers, people who once felt they had no choice except to live with their fate now consult plastic surgeons in the hope of alleviating their feelings of unattractiveness (Cash and Horton, 1983).

In a social psychological approach to facial aesthetic corrective problems, Kalick (1978) conducted an experiment in which subjects viewed either preoperative or postoperative photographs of female aesthetic surgical patients and rated them on a variety of dimensions. In concordance with our own experience, his results indicated that the patient's postoperative photographs were seen not only as more physically attractive, but that the patients were judged, especially by male subjects, also to have more desirable personalities, to be better potential marital partners, to be happier, and more likable. Many times after a corrective rhinoplasty the whole face changes, not only in attractiveness, but also adopting an expression of self-confidence and positive self-esteem.

Goldwyn (1972) says that "ideally the doctor should listen more than talk with an unhappy patient." We believe one has to listen even if one does not agree with a patient's viewpoint because sensitive interaction evolves from observing and by responding on a human plane.

M. R. Wright (1980) states that when a complication does occur, the patient's confidence in the value of aesthetic surgery and his right to have had surgery must be reestablished before a secondary procedure is discussed. The surgeon should bear in mind that a secondary procedure should always be initiated and followed through in the same enthusiastic spirit as in the initial procedure. In our experience this is unfortunately not always true. Too often the patient's psychic pain and feeling of disappointment can only be diminished with a new surgeon, and the new surgeon-patient relationship achieved should be through reasonable discussion so that the patient can be prepared for any secondary procedure with as little emotionality as possible.

4

Jurisprudence

It has to be clear for the beginner that there is always risk that is bound to an operation. There is always the possibility of pitfalls and undesired secondary sequelae and especially of unsatisfactory results. The latter is possible even if the surgeon pays attention using all of his or her skill in performing the operation. It is important to explain this fact to the patient with regards to the present legal situation the doctor finds himself in, which is very critical in countries like the United States, West Germany, France, Italy, England, and Switzerland.

If an operation fails and the grievance is carried through the legal system, then it becomes the duty of the court to decide whether the surgeon has failed in his or her responsibility. The injured patient seeks indemnification as proof of the causal relationship between the unsatisfactory result and the alleged failure of the surgeon. In the current litigious atmosphere where many rhinosurgeons must practice, informed consent, with the laying out of options, alternative methods of treatment and risks, is imperative.

The preoperative patient consultation should discuss in a comprehensible manner the operative plan. In many countries (e.g., Germany) the surgeon obtains written consent of the operative plan. In other countries, such as Switzerland, a written consent is legally unimportant. In the United States and in Germany it can be a mistake to make a preoperative sketch of the projected outcome, as this might be misconstructed as being a guarantee or a contract. The legal nature of the medical service is very important in plastic surgery, especially in rhinoplasty since the patient sometimes wants a true guarantee concerning the postoperative shape of the nose. On the other hand, it is mandatory to document the preoperative situation complete with photographs in order to be protected from unjustified claims.

5

Anatomy

The nose projects from the face as an irregular three-sided pyramid. It consists of a framework of bone and cartilage covered by muscles, subcutaneous tissue, and skin. Externally we distinguish (a) the dorsum or bridge and (b) the side walls (composed of the nasal bones and the upper lateral cartilages), which form the upper immobile part of the nose, and (c) the tip, the alae, and columella (composed of the lower lateral cartilages and the sesamoid cartilages), which form the lower mobile part of the nose.

The overlying skin is of considerable importance. Its thickness and characteristics vary over different areas of the nose and with aging. Its elasticity determines its ability to drape properly over the underlying framework. It must be handled with care during surgical intervention to avoid excessive scar tissue formation.

The anterior lining of the nose is of vestibular skin and that of the cavity is mucosa which covers the cartilage and bone of the nasal septum and bone of the turbinates.

BONES

The bony skeleton of the nose is formed by the maxilla, the nasal bones, and in part by the frontal bone. The nasal bones meet in a suture along the dorsum of the upper bridge. There is a similar junction with the frontal bones, at the glabella, and laterally with the maxilla, just anterior to the medial rim of the orbit.

The nasal bones may vary in size, or be completely absent congenitally or as the result of injury or surgery. Cephalically they are closely-spaced and thicker; caudally they diverge and are thinner, making them easier to be cut through with the osteotome. In the caucasian adult, the nasal bones extend caudally beyond the ventral junction with the ethmoid plate; in young persons and in individuals of Asian descent, the plate extends beyond the nasal bones.

The periosteum of the nasal bones extends into the median suture. That is why it can not be elevated in the midline of the dorsum without being torn.

The angle formed by the nasal bones and frontal bone is a transition from an almost straight line, as in the Greek ideal, to sharp angling. In the region of the nasion, i.e., of the intersection of the midline with the nasofrontal suture, we usually find thick compact bone.

The maxillary crest and vomer are located in a separate compartment off from the septal cartilage. The latter is wrapped in its perichondrium and the bone is in its periosteal envelope and these are fused at the septal-cartilage maxillo-vomerine junction. There is no such compartmentalization posteriorly between the vomer and the ethmoid as both are bone and covered by periosteum.

The vomer develops bilaterally posterior and inferior to the septum with an ossification center in each side, both of which usually become fused. A critical site for future growth and projection is in the area of the vomeronasal organ of Jacobson and the paraseptal cartilages. The suture line between the vomer and premaxilla (prevomerine bone) is an important area of growth potential and an important consideration in the management of the protruding premaxilla in cases of bilateral cleft lip.

Since its size and strength vary widely, the nasal spine may offer considerable resistance to infracture.

CARTILAGES

The upper lateral cartilages form the side-walls as well as a portion of the bridge from the nasal bones down to the lower lateral or alar cartilages. They are firmly attached along the free oblique line of the nasal bones cranially with fibrous tissue connecting them to the upper edge of the lower lateral cartilage caudally. They join on top of the nasal septum to form the central portion of the nasal bridge. Joseph was the first to define this anatomic relationship. The quadrangular plate and the upper lateral cartilage are not independent, as is often assumed, but a single unit.

This continuity of the upper lateral and septal cartilages exists in the cranial two thirds (as described by Straatsma and Straatsma [1951] and confirmed by Natvig et al. [1971] and McKinney et al. [1982]). Straatsma and Straatsma (1951) also demonstrated in 1951 that the nasal bones overlap the upper lateral cartilage by 2–11 mm. These findings were also confirmed in 1971 by Natvig et al. Only in rare cases is the space missing.

The terminal portions of the upper lateral cartilages are not attached to the septum but angle 10–15 degrees from the septum and move with the respiration towards and away from the septum, forming what is known as the nasal valve. Being thinner in this region they are also more flexible. The space between them and the septum is filled with connective tissue. In 1903 Mink first used the term valve when he referred to the limen nasi as a whole rather than to its medial fibrous attachment to the septum. Its tendency to curl away from the septum prevents the cartilage in this area from collapsing completely on inspiration.

Normal racial characteristics may show differences in the length and shape of the connection between the caudal end of the upper lateral cartilage and the caudal end of the septum. The cartilage in the Caucasian nose is rectangular or trapezoid and only extends 5–8 mm from the caudal end of the septum. In the negroid nose the upper lateral cartilage is triangular and comes down to the anterocaudal end of the septum.

The lower lateral cartilages are curved, shaping the nostrils and contributing to the form of the nasal tip and valve. The lower cartilages are suspended and maintained in position by fibrous tissue, which fixes them together at the dome level and also in the septum and to the upper lateral cartilages.

MUSCLES

The nasal muscles overlay the cartilaginous and, only partially, the bony framework. The procerus muscle and the pars transversa of the nasali muscles cover the upper and middle part of the nose. The procerus or pyramidalis (Fig. A) can be regarded as a continuation of the frontalis muscle. It acts to raise the dorsum and the lower lateral cartilages. The pars transversa of the nasalis muscle also called compressor naris arises from the lateral and cephalic section of the sub-pyriform crescent (Zide, 1985). The pars transversa joins with the procerus muscle in the middle as well as its opposite counterpart forming the nasalis-procerus aponeurosis, which covers the dorsum from the lower edge of the upper lateral cartilages in the radix, except for a muscle-free zone on each side. This muscle-free zone between the orbicularis oculi and the procerus is especially vulnerable to lateral trauma and also explains why a high osteotomy step is more easily palpable (Zide, 1985) (Fig. A) (see Osteotomies).

The aponeuroses of the procerus and the pars transversa of the nasalis muscle converge in the median lower part of the nose joining the domes of the lower lateral cartilages. This part of the aponeurotic sheet has erroneously been called ligament (Pitanguy, 1965). It is severed in

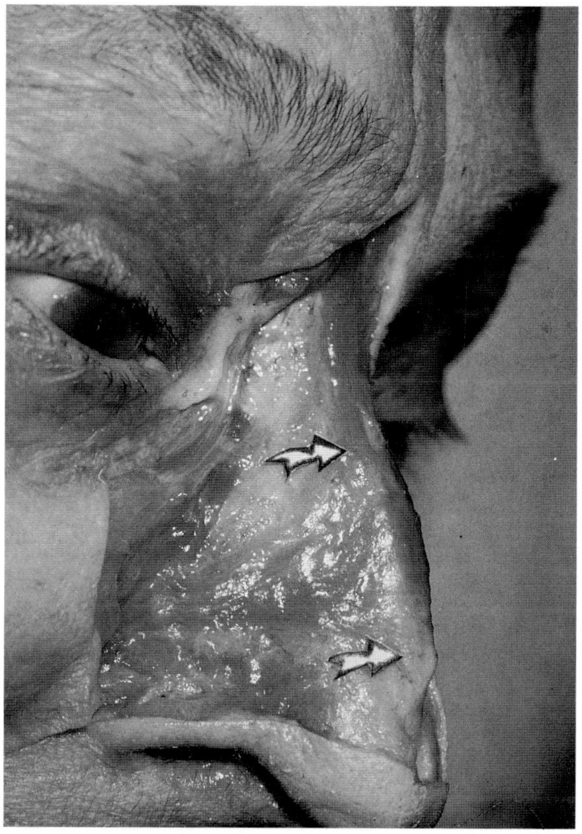

Fig. A. Muscles of the nose. Lower arrow points to aponeurosis of the dilator naris and the depressor alae nasi. Upper arrow demonstrates procerus muscle. Area without muscular covering superiorly is the site of nasal bone fractures with trauma. (With the permission of Dr. Zide)

most of the rhinoplasties for freeing the tip of the nose (see Chapter 12).

The pars transversa of the nasalis muscle effects the compression of the nose, lengthens the nose, contracts the nostrils, and narrows the vestibule. Its valve-like action on the nostrils and its physiologic role were especially studied by Mink (1920). When occasionally we want to counteract this valve-like action at the limen nasi in cases of collapsed valve, we resect the pars transversa musculi nasalis together with a section of the upper lateral cartilages from the septum. One must have also preserved the procerus muscles, which is the antagonist of the compressor.

At the lower part of the nose, the muscular covering is accomplished by three muscles that could be considered as three fascicles of the same muscle: the pars alaris of the nasal muscle, the depressor alae or myrtiformis, and the depressor septi. They arise from the cresentic origin of the maxilla. The pars alaris arises lateral to

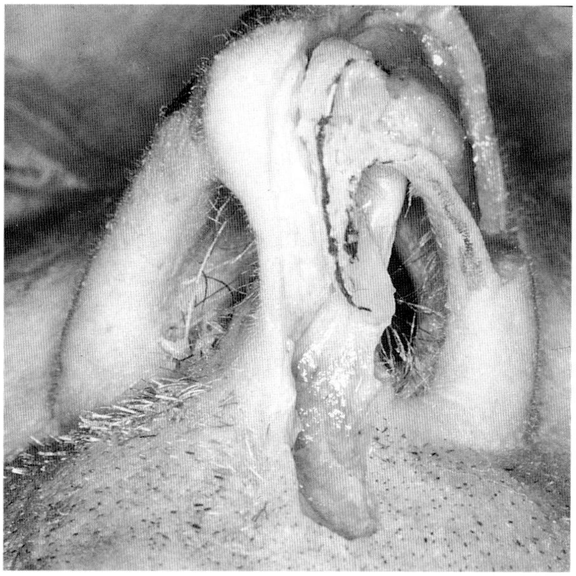

Fig. B. The Depressor septi muscle, which is thought to contribute to a drooping tip. (With the permission of Dr. Zide)

the bony origin of the depressor muscle (pars transversa) and a few millimeter inferior to the edge of the pyriform aperture (Zide, 1985). The alar part covers partially the lateral crus of the lower lateral cartilage at the lateral edge and assists in dilation of the naris. In the nonCaucasian nose it is more developed. The depressor alae or myrtiform muscle originates from the border of the pyriform crest and rises vertically like a fan up to the ala acting as a depressor and constrictor of the nostril.

The levator labii superioris alaeque nasi, which lies laterally in a vertical position, sends fibers to the cephalic part of the nostril, contributing to dilation and lifting of the naris. The lower medial part called depressor septi [Fig. B] arises from the periosteum above the central and lateral incisors as well as from the anterior spine. Some of the fibers may originate anterior to the superior fibers of the orbicularis oris muscle (Zide, 1985). The depressor muscle inserts into the membranous septum and the footplate of the medial crura. Vogt (1983) has shown that certain fibers pass between the medial crura and continue towards the tip. They pull down the nasal tip.

BLOOD SUPPLY

The arterial supply of the nose is achieved by the external and internal carotid system anastomosing both inside and outside the nose. The

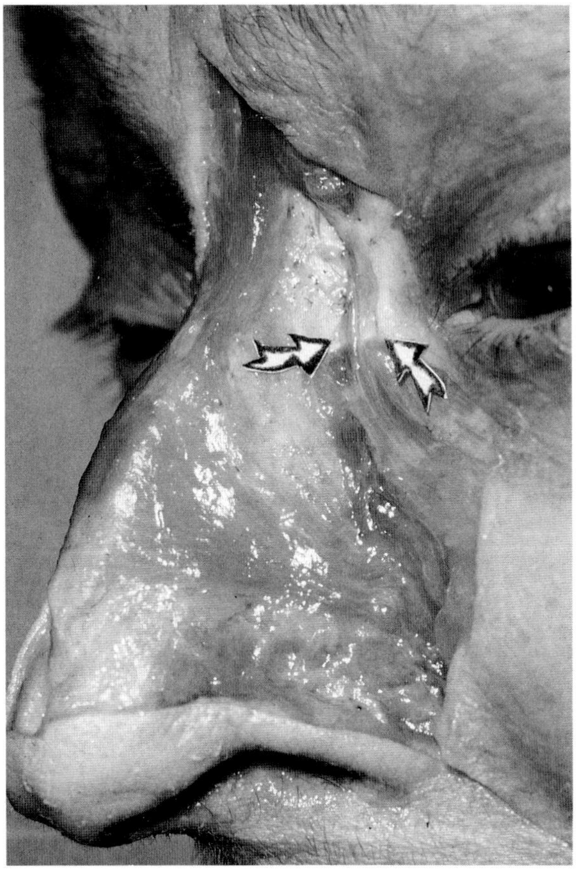

Fig. C. The angular artery, which is a branch of external carotid runs upward along the upper and lower borders of the alae and supplies the lateral wall and the dorsum communicating with branches of the infraorbital artery. (With the permission of Dr. Zide)

external carotid system contributes to the vascularization of the nose and the septum.

The angular artery [Fig. C] runs upward along the lateral wall of the nose, passing near the inner canthus of the lid, and becomes the dorsal artery, supplying the nasal dorsum. The angular artery itself arises from the facial artery. The dorsalis nasi artery arises from the ophthalmic artery which is a branch of the internal carotid artery. Also branching from the facial artery is the superior labial artery with the small columellar artery, which runs upward in the columella parallel to the contralateral one. It becomes visible and bleeds when we cut through the base or through the middle of the columella for an open access to the tip. The lateral nasal artery is also a branch of the facial artery. It runs along the lower and upper border of the ala.

The sphenopalatine artery contributes to the septal and turbinate blood supply. In addition there is an accessory supply contributed by both the palatine and the pterygo-palatine arteries. We find another anastomosis between the vascular area of the external and internal carotid artery between the upper alar artery and the terminal branch of the anterior ethmoidal artery.

The internal carotid system contributes to the vascularization of the superior portion of the septum by the anterior and posterior ethmoidal artery coming from the ophthalmic arteries in the orbital region. The posterior septal artery branches from the internal maxillary artery and anastomoses with the major palatine artery in the Canalis incisivus.

Venous drainage is achieved through the small external nasal veins that lead to the angular vein and from there into the superior and inferior ophthalmic vein as well as into the anterior facial vein. The anterior facial vein is connected with the pterygoid venous plexus by means of the deep facial vein. The latter is connected to the inferior ophthalmic vein by various anastomoses. Thus, in addition to the communication over the angular vein, a second connection exists here between the veins of the external nose and the cavernous sinus.

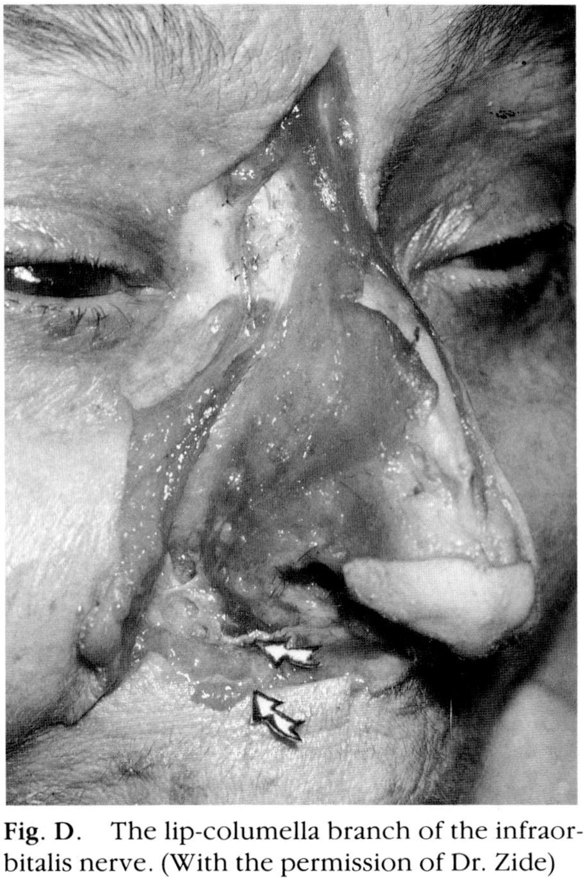

Fig. D. The lip-columella branch of the infraorbitalis nerve. (With the permission of Dr. Zide)

NERVE SUPPLY

The nerves of the external nose are divided into sensory and motor nerves. The sensory nerves branch off the trigeminal nerve and the motor nerves arise from the facial nerve. The nasal branch of the ethmoidal nerve runs behind the nasal bone, and sends out branches to the dorsum and tip of the nose.

The alae and lateral walls of the nose are supplied by the branching of the infraorbital nerve. A branch of this nerve extends across the lip to supply sensation to the columellar base (Zide, 1985) (Fig. D). Zide (1985) has pointed out that the terminal branch of the anterior ethmoidal nerve supplying tip sensation exits from under the caudal edge of the nasal bones (Fig. E) and is usually transected during the intercartilaginous incision, producing the hypesthesia commonly seen postoperatively. The innervation of the internal nose is supplied by both nasal nerve and the spheno-palatine nerve.

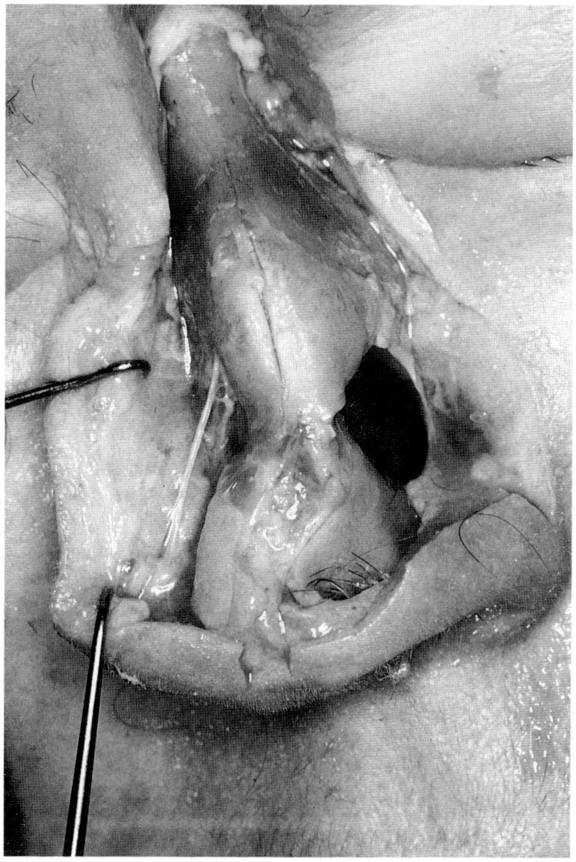

Fig. E. Terminal branch of anterior ethmoid nerve supplying tip sensation. This nerve is transected during the intercartilaginous incision producing tip hypesthesia commonly observed postoperatively. (With permission of Dr. Zide)

6

Physiology

The preservation and reestablishment of the nasal airways is an important problem in corrective nasal surgery. Still, today many rhinosurgeons consider nasal surgery mostly from the aesthetic standpoint, not paying enough attention to physiologic and functional, especially with regards to problems of the nose airway.

The nose has a multitude of functions. According to Cottle (1960) there could be more than 100 such functions, many of which are still not known. From the phylogenetic standpoint the sense of smell seems to be the oldest function of the nose. The nose has a great capacity to heat, moisten, and clean the inhaled air. This protects the lower respiratory airway with the delicate and easily damaged structures of the alveoli of the lungs. The proximity of the airway walls creates a slit-like nasal passage containing numerous serous and seromucous glands that promote, together with the vibrissae, the deposition of suspended particles and favor the exchange of heat and moisture. Air conditioning within the nasal cavity is effected by rapid changes in the arterial as well as the venous blood-flow through the turbinates which in itself depends on the humidity and temperature of the ambient air.

In order to prepare the air for the lower respiratory tract the nasal airflow has to be undisturbed in both sides. Most patients with nasal deformities also have breathing problems and will require a septorhinoplasty, incorporating its functional benefits with its aesthetic components. For this reason the surgeon should be concerned with nasal aerodynamics as related to the nasal structures.

From the physical standpoint the nares act like a funnel, guiding the airstream towards the valve area. This is the narrowest point of the nose. A slight stenosis in this area might cause severe disturbances of nasal ventilation because of the altered aerodynamics.

The nasal airway can be considered as a complex conduit having a varying roughness and different sectional diameters and a sinous course, comprised of expansions and valves.

Physically the nose acts like a tube with a pressure difference arising from variations in its diameter, with accompanying variations in airflow rates and pressures according to the Hagen-Poisseuille law. These structures affect the airflow in its pattern and its velocity.

The nose as the initial structure of the airway apparatus has the function of preparing the air in order to guide it to the olfactory area. To fulfill this task it needs a special shape and special equipment. In animals, we see many different types of noses meeting undoubtedly their special requirements. In humans we also note racial and ethnic variations in the nose, although for what different needs is less obvious. Yet on the whole it seems that the variety of noses found in the different species are the product of a specific evolution adapted to specific needs.

The nose can be similar to a radar station giving information to the organism, providing an alarm signal in the presence of toxic influences, or a warning of a hostile environment. The nose acts also as a reflex organ influencing or being influenced by other organs. In order to fulfill all required functions, the airflow has to pass through the nose under certain conditions. The airflow passage can be determined by measuring the nasal resistance or by inspecting the airway. By diminishing the cross-section of the tube by one-half, the pressure increases 16 times and vice versa. Experimental investigations have shown that the airflow in the nose is turbulent in almost all conditions. This means the airflow system becomes more sensitive to any changes in the cross-sectional area. It is obvious that the aerodynamic system of the nose is very sensitive in regulating the airspace in certain desired ways.

In the normal nose we find a rhythmic variation between congestion and decongestion of the cavernous tissues of the turbinates. This was first observed by Kayser in 1895, and the term *nasal cycle* was coined by Williams in 1972. One nasal airway is opening and its turbinates are shrinking and giving off secretions of serous fluid and mucus while the opposite nasal airway is closing. The total airway resistance remains relatively constant in spite of these continual changes. The cycle has been reported to occur over periods of 30 minutes to 4 hours (Williams, 1972). It seems now that every person has their specific cycle, which varies from between 2 and 8 hours and is related to the autonomous nervous system. After the investigations by Heetderks and Stockstead (1969) we now know about the nasal cycle, meaning the periodical shifting of the main flow from one side to the other. This phenomenon can be made visible by taking x-ray-tomograms in certain intervals over 24 hours.

This cycle also seems to function during the night. Movements of the body during sleep result from a properly established nasal cycle. Masing (1983) investigated sleeping children by monitoring their position. The difference between the sleeping behavior of freely breathing individuals as compared to those who experimentally had had one nostril blocked was significant. The human being needs a nose which allows the passage of sufficient air on both sides, thus one of the reasons to straighten a crooked septum and turbinate is to create equal aerodynamically stable conditions in both nasal airways.

During physical effort more oxygen is needed over a short time. An increased airflow is obtained through a widening of the airspace in the nose. Through stimulation of the little lower dilator muscles, the valve area opens and the turbinates shrink in correlation with an increased breathing frequency. When physical action stops, the nasal resistance returns to normal values. This is an important phenomenon which shows the great capacity of the nasal function to adapt. Holmes (1958) and Little (1963) have stated that the production of hypertrophied turbinates reflects a stimulation from either chemical, thermal, mechanical, or nervous trigger factors.

In cases where one side of the nose is completely or partially obstructed the patient is forced to breathe through the other side with a higher working index resulting. All nasal deformities of the cartilaginous vault will adversely influence nasal ventilation. For example, breathing difficulties are encountered in the drooping tip with its hanging configuration creating an acute nasolabial angle.

The air flow of the nose was first studied by Paulsen (1882). He found the passage to be curved using cigarette smoke in his experiments on a cadaver nose. Proetz (1949) repeated these experiments and discovered that the air current takes different paths on inspiration and expiration. According to him the airstream eddies twice during expiration. This intriguing statement incited Masing (1977) to undertake his own experimental studies using a nose model with a comparable steady waterflow. This system had the advantage of giving a more visible current. The waterflow was marked with a tiny blue ink stream, which permitted the investigator to determine its course under different conditions.

Masing found equal flow going through the whole nasal cavity and not only through the upper part of the nose as believed previously. Clinically speaking, this means that an intact functional nasal cavity is essential for good breathing. This also means that septal deviations and turbinate hyperplasia should be treated carefully even when these malformations are located in the lower part of the nose.

Small anatomic disturbances in the region of the nasal valve, which was first described by Mink (1903), can produce significant airway obstruction by narrowing the nasal valve angle. Normally, this angle between the caudal end of the upper lateral cartilage and the nasal septum is about 10–15 degrees. In all patients suffering nasal airway obstruction, a meticulous clinical evaluation of the nasal valve is required.

According to Cottle (1960), Bridger (1970), and Kern (1978), the nasal valve is usually considered to be the slit-like opening between the caudal end of the upper lateral or roof cartilage and the nasal septum. The valve actually forms a portion of the nasal valve area, and these two entities should not be confused—the nasal valve itself represents only a discrete and specific segment of the entire circumference of the nasal valve area. The nasal valve area is the narrowest portion of the nasal passage and has many synonyms: os internum, ostium internum, limen vestibuli, valve area, and valve region. The nasal valve also has several synonyms: the liminal valve, the flow-limiting segment, and the liminal chink Kern (1978).

The nasal valve area itself extends laterally from the region where the caudal end of the upper lateral cartilage meets the nasal septum to the bony point of the pyriform aperture and the soft fibrofatty tissue in this region. Bridger (1970) believed that the entire nasal valve area averaged approximately 55 mm^2, whereas Masing (1967) calculated the area 64 mm^2. The narrowest portion of the nasal airway is this opening in the nasal valve area, and the specific triangular slit-like portion between the caudal end of the upper lateral cartilage in its relationship to the nasal septum is the nasal valve.

As stated in Chapter 5, there are both constrictor muscles and dilator muscles. The constrictor muscles facilitate collapse or closing of the valve, whereas the dilator muscles increase the rigidity of the nasal valves and prevent collapse.

Bridger (1970) compared the internal part of the nose to a rigid tube, which has a short collapsible segment or flow-limiting segment. The transluminal pressure is the difference between the pressure outside the tube (or atmospheric pressure) and the intraluminal (or intranasal) pressure. The flexible external part of the nose tends to resist collapse primarily because of the way the cartilages are sprung open. Thus, a critical transmural pressure where the collapsible segment closes can be reached. This occurs when the inside or intraluminal intranasal pressure becomes negative from the effect of inspiration. Bridger (1970) demonstrated that a maximal inspiratory effort increases the flow-pressure curve to a point where the nasal airflow will no longer be increased by further increases in negative pressure.

In the Negroid nose with platyrhinia, the narrowest part of the nasal airway (the flow-limiting segment) is the area between the nasal septum and the anterior portion of the inferior turbinate. The angle of the valve is larger than in the Caucasians. Thus, in the Black person, the inferior turbinates probably constitute the most important inflow regulator, that is, the turbinal valve, whereas in the leptorrhine nose of the Caucasian, the nasal valve is probably the most important inflow regulator, accounting for most of the inspiratory resistance to airflow (van Dishoeck, 1942, 1965; De Wit et al, 1965; Hinderer, 1971).

Bridger (1970) noted that the most common site of deformity was the caudal end of the septum. We know that any abnormality in this nasal valve area could cause early collapse of the nasal valve and thereby produce nasal airway symptoms.

A valuable test that corresponds to the more sophisticated evaluations found with Rhinoscopy or Rhinomanometry is the Cottle test. While the patient breathes quietly, the cheek is drawn laterally away from the midline, opening the nasal valve, and the patient is asked if this maneuver improves airflow through the tested side. If this relieves the nasal obstruction, the Cottle sign is considered positive and indicates that the abnormality of the nasal valve is probably a significant factor in the genesis of symptomatic nasal airway obstruction.

Nasal valve abnormalities are multiple. The "all inclusive list" is found in a pathologic classification. The basis of the clinical classification is that nasal valve abnormalities are primarily caused by narrowing of the nasal valve angle. According to Kern (1978), this narrowing can arise from the soft covering mucocutaneous tissues, from skeletal supporting tissues, or from both. Symptoms may arise due to an already increased collapsibility of the nasal valve. Therefore, surgical intervention is directed toward reestablishment of normal anatomic relationships, usually by widening the nasal valve angle and preventing either extreme of rigidity or collapsibility, achieved by changing the position of the upper lateral cartilages and the lateral crura of the lower lateral cartilages.

The ciliary epithelium of the nasal cavity concerns itself with the cleaning function of the airway. The ciliary movements, however, are only possible if the mucosa is sufficiently moistened. Restricted secretion or absence of moisture may destroy the cilia, which then need to be regenerated.

Ginsel and Illum (1980) studied nasal mucociliary clearance by means of the saccharin-sky-blue technique in patients with septal deformities of the nose before and after plastic operation. Prior to an operation, the nasal clearance was statistically significantly slower than in healthy persons. The study showed that nasal mucociliary transport returns to normal after sufficient removal of anatomic obstacles such as spines and crests and with the reestablishment of normal air passage.

Filtration in the nose takes place in two ways: (1) the vibrissae in the vestibule filter out the big foreign bodies; and (2) entrapment adhesion of small particles is obtained along the moist mucosa as the air current is being projected against the mucous film. These small dust particles are swept from the anterior third of the membrane to pass on the lateral wall through the middle and inferior meatus.

The undulations carry the particles downward and backward into the nasopharynx where they are swallowed or expectorated. As already mentioned, the nose protects the lung by preparing the inspired air. The alveoli require relatively constant conditions for proper gas exchange. The delicate tissues must be protected from temperature extremes, insufficient humidity, and foreign bodies.

The mucosa holds moisture during inspiration and is humidified again to some extent by the warm expired air that condensates on the surface of the cool nasal structures. A little experiment may illustrate this: by inspiring through one nostril and exhaling through the other one, one feels quite uncomfortable after a short time as one side of the nose becomes dry and cool causing discomfort and headache.

The amount of nasal secretion depends on the location and region of the nasal mucosa. According to Eichner et al (1983), the average amount is between 125 and 75 ml. The protein concentration shows a very wide variation, with the normal secretion holding between 200 and 3500 mg. The average concentration in the upper nasal meatus is 950 mg, in the lower nasal meatus 1100 mg. Selective glycoprotein staining shows that the main constituents of nasal secretion proteins are glycoproteins. The electrolyte concentration for sodium is 90–148 mval, potassium 6–28 mval, and calcium 2–3.5 mval.

During inspiration the nose is able to moisten the air up to 80 percent relative humidity. For a short time the mouth and pharynx are also able to moisten the air to a similar degree. But, as we know, a mouth-breather has a dry throat in the morning and coughs to clean the pharynx. A dry nose is a severe handicap for a patient as the self-cleansing system is destroyed. A dry nose is the source of most infections of the upper respiratory tract.

Due to the turbinate system the nose is able to heat the air from 0 to 36 degrees quickly. This indicates a remarkable heating capacity, practically independent of the surrounding atmospheric temperature. As exhaled air warms the nasal cavity to maintain this performance, a regular alternation of nasal inspiration and expiration is mandatory to preserve this function as it is in maintaining humidification.

The nose has a reflex system which connects almost every organ of the body to the nose. Drettner (1970) observed the airspace of the nose while cooling the feet or the back. Remarkable differences in the airspace could be seen, i.e. a decongestion of the turbinates. Among all these reflexes we would like to mention the naso-pulmonal reflex, regulating the movements of the thorax. Ogura (1968) and coworkers investigated this relationship, finding significant differences between subjects with normal as opposed to disturbed breathing. This is one of the reasons why unimpaired breathing is important.

Cottle described the midcycle rest, which means a stop between inspiration and expiration. After septal surgery this phenomenon disappeared. This is a reason to operate on patients older than 60 years, because these patients particularly benefit from an easy working breathing system.

The exact clinical diagnosis of the degree of the impaired function created by obstruction must be the result of a critical analysis, thorough inspection, and precise rhinomanometry. Rhinomanometry takes permanent measures based on the physical laws of airflow by applying a standardized functional measuring gauge. This procedure, permitting the simultaneous measurement of nasal air pressure and flow during respiration, is not new. Donders in 1859 was the first to study nasopharyngeal pressure during respiration using a mercury manometer. Airflow was first measured in 1889 by Zwaardemaker with a hygrometer. Since then, many methods have been suggested. Rhinomanometry has today become a valuable aid in judging pre and postoperative function.

Anterior rhinomanometry (Franke, 1894) and posterior rhinomanometry (Kayser, 1895) already had their respective advocates in those early days. In 1939, Tonndorf emphasized that the removal of an obstacle in the nose such as a turbinate does not always result in improved nasal function. With respect to this, he was the first to stress the importance of Reynold's number.

The actual rhinomanometric techniques started to be developed in the 1960s. The airflow is measured by a pneumotachometer, which quantifies the difference in pressure across a known resistance. Pressure is measured by a transducer, which converts a pressure change into an electric current. Rhinomanometric methods actually used are:

1. Active anterior rhinomanometry using two nozzles, one in each nostril, one for nasopharyngeal pressure measurement and the other for flow measurement, or using a face mask, one nostril being sealed off with adhesive tape and a hard plastic tube passing through this tape for measurement of the nasopharyngeal pressure.
2. Active posterior rhinomanometry using a tube in the mouth for measurement of the nasopharyngeal pressure, while the patient breathes through both nostrils in a mask.

These techniques with different equipment attached have their advantages. In addition to rhinomanometry, other methods exist such as spirometry, intrathoracic pressure measurement, and body plesthysmography. These are used less frequently.

For Jessen and Malm (1984), rhinomanometry is necessary in the selection of patients for septal surgery.

In a comparative study of pre and postoperative rhinomanometry with standardized analysis of the patient's clinical state by Schmid and Markmiller (1983) it was found that in 3/4 of the 84 operated patients there was correlation of the three kinds of investigation. Courtiss and Goldwyn (1983) studied the effects of nasal surgery on airflow by means of anterior rhinomanometry to ascertain whether a rhinoplasty indeed affects the passage of air through the nose. They found that a rhinoplasty does not adversely affect the nasal airflow, and those patients who had procedures to improve their nasal airflow did indeed show this improvement. The data from their airflow studies frequently failed to correlate with the patient's assessment of their own nasal function as well as with the evaluations obtained by rhinoscopy. Furthermore, rhinomanometric findings varied considerably even when conducted by the same investigators. Courtiss and Goldwyn (1983) can not recommend rhinomanometry with enthusiasm because of its questionable reliability and validity.

Investigations by Fiebach (1983) gave similar results using anterior rhinomanometry in patients who underwent simple septoplasty. Pre and postoperative rhinomanometric investigations have also been reported by Mertz, McCaffrey, and Kern (1984), showing significant effect of septoplasty on airflow resistance. Thus, the effectiveness of a functional rhinoseptoplastic treatment and the possible need to modify a therapeutic program can be objectively assessed as it was proved by MacCaffrey and Kern (1979 and 1986) and confirmed by Friedrich at the ENT University Clinic of Lausanne with which we collaborate under the direction of M. Savary.

7

Preoperative Evaluation

While in other surgery, the complications are often determined by the character of the disease, the patients undergoing corrective rhinoplasty are almost always in good health.

The thorough observation and recording of the characteristics of not only the nose but of the person with the operated nose can only lead to improvements in results obtained with revision rhinoplasty as such maneuvers establish the basis for precise action in surgery. When seeing patients for the first time, we seek to know the purpose of their consultation, about the shape of the nose prior to undergoing surgery, details of a previous operation or operations, specifics regarding the patient's desire to change the shape of the nose, improving the air passage, and the likely psychological benefits of a planned intervention on the patient vis-à-vis his environment. We examine the nose externally, considering also the other facial structures, such as the forehead, eyes, cheeks, lips, and chin, with which the nose has to be in harmony. Furthermore, we examine the nose internally, the quality of the skin and of the mucosa, we check if there is an obstruction, and if necessary we undertake a functional examination of the breathing cycle.

Since it is generally assumed that there is a relationship between nasal obstruction and deformities of the nasal septum and diseases of the para-nasal sinuses, one has to examine patients for septal deviations and check their sinuses by radiography or endoscopy. In the management of postrhinoplastic deformities, a good doctor-patient relationship is very important. The plastic surgeon performing secondary rhinoplasties must usually spend additional sessions with an overanxious patient in order to define the suitable procedure, taking into account the desire of the patient and the technical possibilities for correction. Sometimes a compromise has to be accepted. In cases of an emotional crisis, a corrective procedure should be postponed or avoided. The surgeon should show the patient what he or she intends to change in the appearance of the nose by drawings and sketches.

We draw the nose in a frontal, profile, and axial view and in a chin forehead axis view. The whole profile should be drawn. This should be done in front of the patient. Then the same design should be repeated using a different color to outline the new contour expected.

We do, or request, preoperative black and white or color photographs, which include the two profiles, the frontal view, and the axial view. The profile of the dorsum and the tip of the nose should especially be discussed with the help of preoperative photographs and superimposed drawings. Not infrequently, photographic analyses reveal little facial abnormalities unrecognized during the consulting room examination. The drawings and photographs are always taken into the operating room, where the surgeon can refer to them during the intervention.

Palpation is of crucial importance to determine what structures may have been inadequately or excessively removed and to assess the quality of the skin and soft tissue with regard to firmness, mobility, resilience, and smoothness. These findings should be recorded and made known to the patient to help in understanding the limitations of the revision. Any adverse scar formation, pigmentation, grossly visible pores, or vascular changes must be called to the patient's attention and the chance of aggravating of these conditions with further surgery should be emphasized. Any potential embarrassments are to be taken into special consideration by preoperative inspection and palpation, such as by observing the nose during quiet and forced breathing, which generally shows if upper and/or lateral cartilage collapse is present.

The septum should be checked for deviations or anterior subluxation and the upper lateral cartilages inspected for protrusion into the nasal vestibule or cavity, which can be an important factor in the impairment of breathing after rhinoplasty. The collapse of a bony lateral wall into the nasal passage-way as well as web stenoses or cylindrical narrowing have to be excluded. When cartilage or bone grafting of the tip, dorsum, or alae is required one has to find out if some of this material is still available in the nose, especially in the septum.

One has to explain to the patient the possibilities of the procedure, and try to assimilate the wishes of the patient to the planned surgery. Sometimes one has to find a compromise. One should never say that the revision will be easy. One can promise that the result will be better but possibly not in one stage and that further surgery may be necessary.

We inform the patient of the results obtained intraoperatively and likely to occur in the postoperative phase. We speak about possible further pitfalls and complications. In revision operations, the patient has to know that the result may eventually be less satisfactory than that following an uncomplicated primary procedure.

In spite of the improved technical skill of the operators, the rhinoplastic interventions have not become shorter in duration, because today we have added important refining steps to the basic maneuvers. In secondary procedures these refining details are most important and time consuming, which makes a secondary operation often last longer than a primary rhinoplasty. If the secondary deformity is severe and particularly if internal and external scarring of the soft tissues exists, there may be little or nothing that can be accomplished by revision rhinoplasty. The severely "butchered nose" is extremely difficult to improve and presents a complex problem from both the technical and psychological point of view. The corrective rhinoplasty occasionally has to be converted into reconstructive surgery for those crucified noses.

We determine with the patient if the intervention should be carried out under general anesthesia with hospitalization, or under local anesthesia, as an outpatient procedure.

Many revisions are minor adjustments such as straightening of a still not straight dorsum or columella or eliminating a slight supratip prominence. These can be accomplished under local anesthesia without hospitalization.

8

Timing

If the surgeon decides to perform the revision, there arises the question of timing. For minor corrections at the border of the ala or the columella, we wait 5 months or more until the edema has practically resolved. For important revision we wait 12–15 months. During this time it is not always easy to convince the patient that this delay is absolutely necessary to ensure the stability of the tissue involved.

The timing is wrong when a revision is carried out too soon after the primary operation. Patients who are unhappy about the immediate result of the primary rhinoplasty quite often request a revision before the tissues have settled properly. The minimum time for complete wound resolution is about one year. Scar tissue may form beneath the skin over the lower half of the dorsum. It grows for up to 3–6 months and then slowly softens and thins. One should not operate until 9 or preferably 12 months have elapsed because the complete healing of the injured tissues and the setting of all scars must be allowed to occur. This can be psychologically a most stressful time for both patient and surgeon.

Should the operation be limited to correcting the unsatisfactory part of the primary result or should the whole nose be mobilized? To do too much leads to worse conditions. Since it is uncertain what has been left and what has been destroyed, complete dissection of all three layers (skin, cartilaginous and bony support, and lining) has to be carried out leaving enough attachment to maintain blood supply before any resection is carried out.

9

Anesthesia

In Switzerland most patients prefer to be asleep for aesthetic surgery of the face, especially for a rhinoplasty. In a study of patients undergoing rhinoplasty and face lift operations under local anesthesia, McNabb and Goldwyn (1976) found that 6 of 20 patients reported their experience in the operating room as being unpleasant.

McNabb and Goldwyn (1976) also carried out blood gas analyses on 20 cases. The mean arterial oxygen tension was 74.2 mm Hg, and the mean CO_2 tension was 53 mm Hg. These patients had significant respiratory depression attributed to the sedation associated with the local anesthesia. This is in comparison to a similar study on 20 patients under general anesthesia carried out by Coman and Reilly (1981).

In about 80 percent of the cases of primary rhinoplasty, we use general anesthesia administered by an expert anesthesiologist. It gives more comfort to the patient and to the operator, and is generally requested by the patient. In nearly all revision cases where an entire rhinoplasty has to be performed we prefer general anesthesia because of the important emotional and physical factors and because of the longer duration of the intervention. Good local anesthesia is more difficult to obtain in cicatricial nasal tissue than in a primary case. The inconvenience of greater bleeding seen with general anesthesia can be reduced by controlled hypotension.

The ambulatory office use of local anesthesia during rhinoplasty with osteotomy, especially for secondary procedures and hare lip nose surgery, can be particularly uncomfortable even when performed with a good supplemental intravenous sedation. On the other hand, a simple supratip revision or secondary refinement without osteotomies can be performed easily under local anesthesia as an outpatient procedure.

For such cases, outpatient surgery with local anesthesia requires utilization of an anesthetic agent that, in addition to providing good sedation and analgesia, also permits a relatively rapid recovery, with minimal incidence of intraoperative problems and postoperative side effects such as bleeding, vomiting, nausea, and hypotension. Of course, respiratory insufficiency is often associated with the sedative drugs that accompany the use of local anesthesia. The sedative drugs depress the respiratory center so that there is a decrease in the frequency and depth of respiration. We realize, however, that if the patient is relaxed and quiet and if the entire nose is well anesthetized, an easy secondary rhinoplasty with local anesthesia can be pleasant and problem free.

Some surgeons, such as Kabaker (1977) use ketamine 25 mg IV, diazepam 5 mg, and sublimase 1 mg IV, which is sufficient for the average 70 kg patient, prior to injecting the local anesthetic. The unpleasant dreams and hallucinations seen when ketamine is used alone are bracketed by the diazepam. Caution must be exercised in the patient with cardiovascular compromise, because of the potential tachycardia and hypertensive side effects seen with ketamine. Kabaker (1981) further uses pentothal when placing osteotomies. This is given by the nurse anesthetist or anesthesiologist, with all the available equipment for airway management and narcotic reversal at his disposal. Twenty-five years ago we operated on all our rhinoplasties under local anesthesia after administering a lytic cocktail, composed of chlorpromazin, phenothiazine, and derivatives of morphine.

Actually, the utilization of the controlled hypotensive anesthetic technique gives the best operating field for rhinoplasty. There are many ways in which controlled hypotension can be achieved. We induce hypotensive anesthesia with a premedication of atropine 0.5 mg and a morphinomimetic drug (1 mg/kg of weight), thiopentalum natrium (5 mg/kg of weight), fentanyl, 0.1 mg, and dehydro-benzo-peridol, 5 mg IV, and succinylcholine 50–100 mg IV prior to intubation. Hypotensive anesthesia is maintained with a NO_2/O_2 mixture plus halothane. Occasionally the addition of a betablocker is necessary. Immediately after intubation we locally infiltrate the nose with a solution containing POR (vasopressin) and, following the theory of Planas (1977), we wait about 30 minutes before beginning the surgery to reduce bleeding to a minimum.

Planas (1977) has carried out a clinical study on the physiologic effects of local anesthesia on serial blood pressure measurements before and during the operation. He believes that 20 minutes after the injection, when the blood pressure returns to normal, is the proper time to start surgery. He also observed that intraoperative bleeding increased as the duration of the operation extended into a more hypertensive period, approximately one hour after starting the intervention. When a local anesthetic is injected, some of the adrenaline-like substance escapes from the nasal tissue into the circulatory system, provoking hypertension. Metabolization of the drugs takes about 20 minutes. During this period increased bleeding would occur. Following this, during the second period local vasoconstriction is not countered by any hypertension and this appears to be the most opportune time to perform the operation. The third, or hypotensive, period seems to be stimulated by the apparent need for oxygen by tissue cells. Tissues exposed to a prolonged period of anoxia call for oxygen through the so-called "receptors" of tissue anoxia.

There are reflex mechanisms established via the spinal çord afferents as well as by means of chemical sensors (chemoreceptors) that provoke a vasodilation of the ischemic area and thus tend to increase bleeding. After the infiltration is completed, we delay the start of the operation by some 20–30 minutes, until the blood pressure has returned to normal and the nose of the patient has become pale. By varying the halothane dosage, the systolic blood presure is maintained at about 80 mm Hg and the relaxation is maintained with curare. The decurarization is accomplished by the use of prostigmine 2.5 mg and atropine 1 mg.

When the patient wants a local anesthetic, we first sedate the patient with diazepam (Valium) similar to the former lytic cocktail explained in the book by Denecke and Meyer (1964/1967). After a premedication of atropine and benzodiazepine we begin by inserting intranasal packs soaked in a topical anesthetic solution.

Some of our colleagues inject the following premedication prior to rhinoplasty: 1 hour before surgery between 20 and 40 mg of chlorazepam and 1/2 hour before surgery 50–100 mg of a morphinomimetic drug. As the patient becomes somnolent, we carry out the injection of about 10 ml xylocaine 1 percent with epinephrine or POR (vasopressin) beneath the skin of the external nose and beneath the septal mucosa, through the vestibular walls at the incision sites, and through the gingivo-labial fold. Injection at the base of the columella blocks the anterior ethmoidal branches and a branch of the infraorbital nerve. At the lateral wall, the needle is introduced just over the site of the incision for the lateral osteotomy and goes cephalad along the nasal and maxillary bones toward the glabella. At the end, the needle is advanced in the area of the dome for securing further hemostasis.

In secondary or posttraumatic rhinoplasty with scarred subcutaneous tissue, the dorsum of the nose is best injected percutaneously. Thc infraorbital nerve is blocked by field infiltration in the area of the exit of the nerve at the periosteal level. During the intervention, arterial blood pressure, pulse rate, EGG, and body temperature are monitored. The patient receives 500 ml of glucose-NaCl infusion with 10 mg of valium (benzodiazepine) to which occasionally rohypnol (fluorobenzodiazepine) is added. During the entire operation the patient is controlled by the anesthesiologist.

To operate with good visualization of the intranasal structures provided by a bloodless field is of prime importance in revision surgery, probably more so than in primary rhinoplasty. The type of anesthesia employed influences the vascularity of the operative field. Local anesthesia using a solution of xylocaine with POR (vasopressin or epinephrine) added after an effective premedication is, we believe, the procedure of choice for minor revision surgery, such as supratip correction.

10

Complications

BLEEDING

The general surgical risk due to cardiovascular disease, bleeding tendencies, diabetes, etc., which are present in many surgical operations, have practically no importance in aesthetic plastic surgery of the face. If such a basic disease is present, which can influence the operation unfavorably, surgery is rarely done. In spite of this, complications sometimes occur and can not be avoided even with the greatest caution.

One of the most common complications is hematoma and suffusion formation during and after rhinoplasty.

Epistaxis as well as postoperative bleeding in the region of Locus Kiesselbachii where the transfixion incision has been made is very rare and is generally considered as a harmless limited occurrence.

We have treated cases of Osler's disease with recurrent bleeding by excising an area of the septal mucosa about 2 cm × 2 cm wide and grafting it with buccal mucosa obtaining good results. This of course is not necessary for typical postoperative bleeding. Only once have we had to resort to arterial ligation, in a case with a nasal tumor. In a few cases after septorhinoplasty and fractures of the nose we succeeded in stopping troublesome bleeding by cauterization and secondary fixation of the dissected mucoperichondrium using transseptal mattress sutures. When the bleeding site is on the lateral nasal wall one can improve the visualization of the site by lateral displacement of the septum and fracture of the turbinates. This method of exposure has recently been confirmed by Anderson et al (1984).

In cases of severe intractable epistaxis there are various options for arterial ligation of vessels supplying the nasal cavity. These include the internal carotid system with its branches, the anterior and posterior ethmoidal arteries or the external carotid artery system with its branches, the sphenopalatine, labial, and major palatine arteries. The watershed area between the two systems is the middle turbinate. There are extensive anastomoses between the two external carotid arteries as well as between the external and the internal carotid artery systems through branches of the ophthalmic artery. For this reason procedures involving the unilateral ligation of the external carotid artery fail. So, actually, if a vessel ligation is considered necessary the best choice is the transmaxillary ligation of the internal maxillary artery belonging to the external carotid artery system. The transmaxillary access for this ligation has been advocated by Seiffert (1955). A surgical alternative to internal maxillary artery ligation for posterior epistaxis has been proposed by Maceri and Makielski (1984) who use an intraoral incision and identify the maxillary artery after removing buccal fat. Thus, a space is created between the mandibular ramus and the medial plerygoid muscle.

For the prevention of hematoma and seroma in difficult secondary rhinosurgical operations involving huge skin and mucosa dissections, we have been using fibrin tissue glue ever since 1979, as we do in all rhytidectomies, in all nerve anastomoses, and in many reconstructive cases using skin-flaps (Meyer and Kesselring, 1987, and Rheims, Meyer, and Daverio, 1987). The best way to prevent postoperative bleeding is to close by using the glue on all small vessels that do not bleed during an operation, due to the vasoconstrictive effect of the local anesthetic. One must somehow initiate local blood coagulation as the first step to wound healing. Combining a solution of fibrinogen with one of thrombin forms an almost instantaneous viscous biologic adhesive substance. Cronkite et al (1944), were the first to use this for the fixation of skin grafts but they did not achieve the desired success because the fibrinogen concentration that they used was too low.

Matras et al (1972) took up the idea of a biologic adhesive system. They anastomosed nerves in experimental animals with a highly concentrated cryoprecipitated fibrinogen, thrombin, and clotting factor XIII combination, and later used these substances for the same purpose in humans. Spaengler (1976) reported numerous experimental investigations and clinical experiences using these substances. He found that complete local hemostasis was always obtained, and that fibrin, a biologic material that is completely absorbable, has high adhesive properties, elasticity, and good tissue compatibility.

This is especially important in the glabellar region when the procerus muscle has been partially or totally removed and the skin has to be pressed against the underlying bone to prevent dead space formation. Another important area for gluing the skin against the remodeled structures is in the lateral osteotomy line up to the canthal level, where we fear hematoma formation. Finally, we introduced this preventive addition in the complex septal surgery for closure of small and middle size perforations (see Chapter 14), where after wide extramucosal dissection and suture of the fenestrations in the mucosa, the repositioned mucoperichondral and mucoperiostal leaves are brought together with or without interposition of cartilage, bone, or fascia. By gluing the walls together mattress sutures can be avoided.

The fibrin tissue glue is composed of two components: (1) a solution of fibrinogen and calcium; and (2) a solution of thrombin and topostasin. These two solutions can be injected in two separate syringes or simultaneously in a single or a double barreled syringe into submucous or subcutaneous pockets, immediately creating a clear fibrin glue (Fig. 6A) (see also Fig. 109C). After gluing, the mucosal or cutaneous layer is adapted to the underlying structure by slight manual pressure applied for over 3 minutes. In our experience there have been no significant allergic reactions or any other complications. Postrhinoplastic suffusion and edema are significantly reduced with this procedure.

Schoenfeld (1985) reported on about 30 rhinoplasties using fibrin tissue glue with no postoperative hematoma, while previously he had observed a 30 percent rate of effusions and hematomas. Hayward and MacKay (1987) avoid nasal packing by using fibrin glue in septal surgery. Wolf and Stammberger (1985) developed an autogenous fibrin tissue glue prepared from the patient's own plasma and used it in all fields of otorhinolaryngology including rhinoplasty and nose repairs with skin grafts. Hematoma of the lid region can occur in postoperative hours and days due to injury of the angular vessels during lateral osteotomy. Ice application is the only treatment possible. This complication only delays the healing time of the surrounding tissues but is not significant for the result of the operation (Fig. 1).

EDEMA

Another common complication is overly slow absorption of postoperative edema. In general, swelling of the nose gradually decreases during the second week after surgery, i.e., after removal of the dressing. After 2 weeks the swelling is only slightly visible. Usually there is still slight swelling of the lower lids while suffusion at this point has ceased. The nose then has a certain stiffness. At this time it cannot yet be wrinkled, as the mimic musculature of the nose

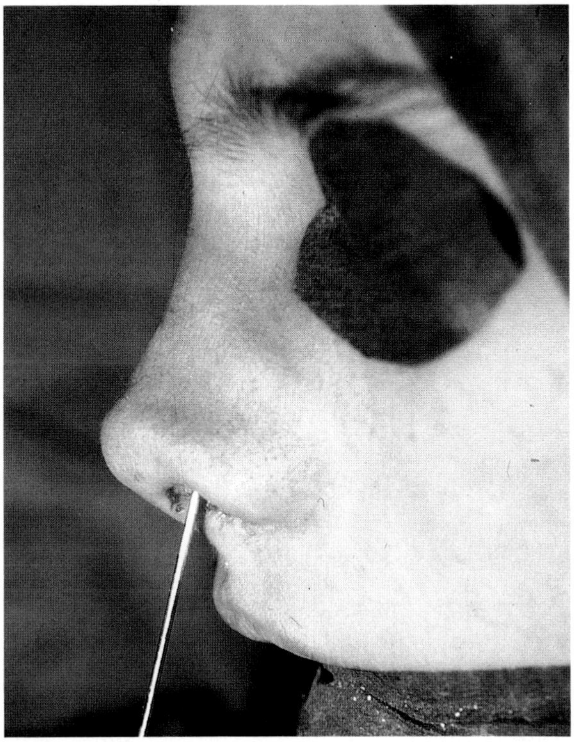

A

Fig. 1.(A) Injection of fibrin adhesive glue into the nasal dorsum.

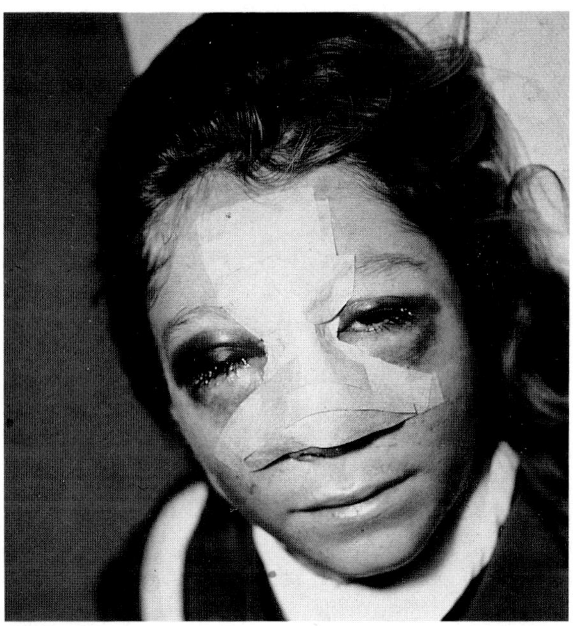

B

(B) Suffusion of the lids 4 days after primary rhinoplasty.

and its immediate vicinity is still inactive. If there has been greater than normal bleeding during the operation or if there is bleeding afterward, in spite of a well-fitting dressing, as a result of injury to a large blood vessel, then the swelling decreases slowly. Absorption of edema is also retarded by small infected hematomas and pustules on the nasal tip and on the dorsum, small necroses of bone splinters, and foreign body reactions to grafts. If sinus infections are present, no corrective surgery should be undertaken, unless there is indication because of obstructed nasal breathing. Surgery should then be done with antibiotic protection using doses higher than normal. Still we have observed stronger swelling and slower reduction of swelling in such cases postoperatively.

INFECTION

With the usual adequate preoperative cleaning of the nasal surgical field and maintenance of good sterile technique during rhinoplasty there should be minimal incidence of postoperative infection. Recent investigations on this subject by Slavin, Rees, Guy, and Goldwyn (1983) demonstrated that detectable bacteremia subsequent to the performance of osteotomies could not be found and that there were no instances of postoperative infections in healthy patients. Routine perioperative antibiotic prophylaxis is of questionable value in normal patients undergoing usual primary rhinoplasty, however, quite important in secondary procedures involving grafts or implants. Once the infection has developed, treatment should be aggressive in view of grave complications reported in the literature such as subdural empyema (Kubik and Adams, 1943), meningitis and right-sided cerebral abscess (Lacy and Conway, 1965), endocarditis (Coursey, 1974), central nervous system histoplasmosis (Gilden et al, 1974), septic cavernous sinus thrombosis (Causaborn et al, 1977), localized cerebritis (Lewin et al, 1979), and toxic shock syndrome (Thomas et al, 1960). Usually the organism implicated is pseudomonas (Kamer and Binder, 1980; Rudolph, 1982; Slavin and Rees, 1982), staphylococcus aureous (Cabouli et al, 1986), and streptococcus pyogenes (Huizing, 1986).

The incision and drainage of an acute septal abscess is not sufficient. It cannot prevent possible functional and cosmetic complications from developing. If, due to the dissolution or removal

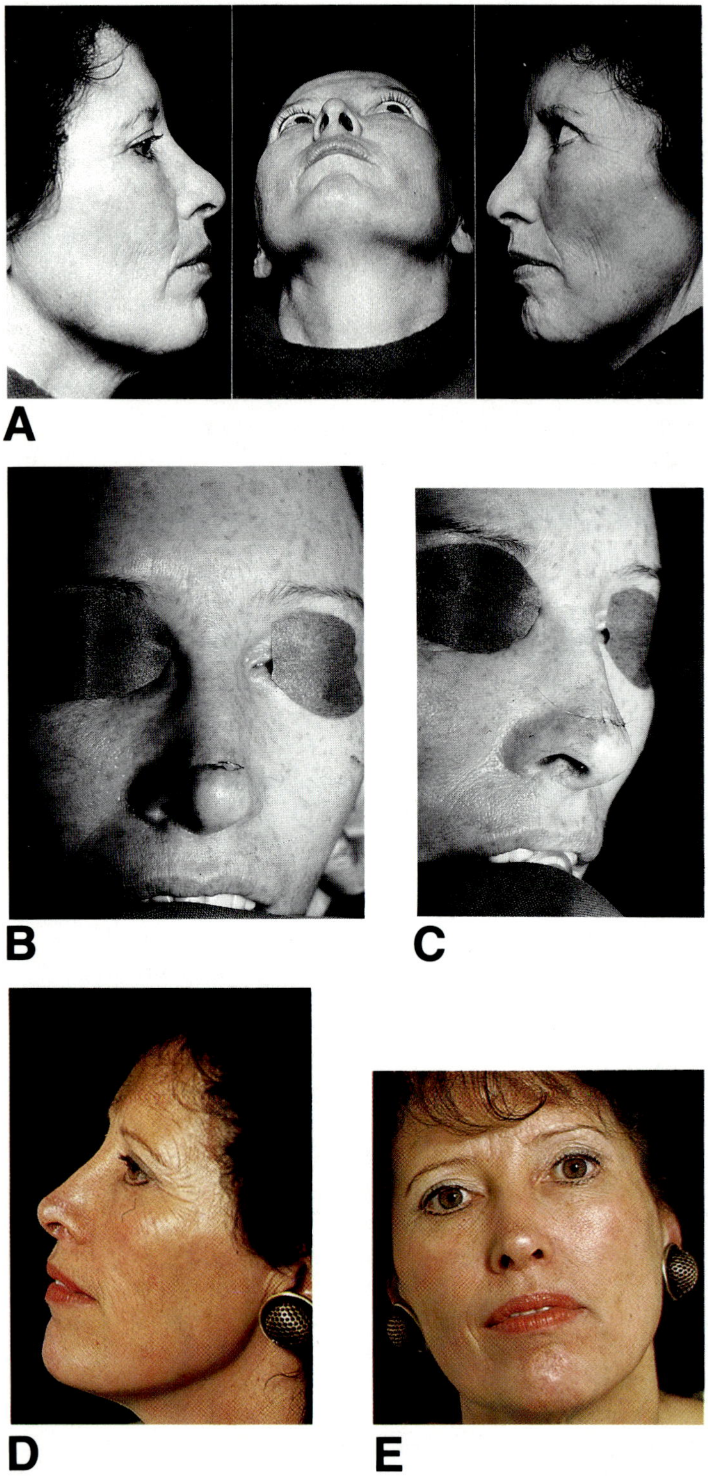

Fig. 2. After correction of a polly beak hypertrophy an infection of corticosteroid was made into the supratip area. This produced a little ulceration which had to be removed with a horizontal fusiform excision. (A) Polly beak before correction; (B) Outline of horizontal excision of the skin depression; (C) Suture of the wound; (D and E) Result after external suture.

of infected septal cartilage, a defect results that endangers the supporting function of the septum, this support must be replaced.

A septal abscess may occur after a nasal trauma. This should be evacuated as soon as possible and a cartilage graft should be immediately introduced into the cleaned pocket for prevention of shrinkage of surrounding tissues and late saddle formation or columella retraction with impairment of nasal function. Care must be taken in the management of cartilage grafts. Where adequate autogenous cartilage or bone from the posterior part of the septum is not available, grafting can be done with ear or rib cartilage, as we advocated in 1964 (Denecke and Meyer). Hellmich (1970) proposed homogenous bank cartilage for this purpose.

Postoperative infections occur most often in the columella, particularly in the puncture channels of the mattress sutures along the transfixion incision. Actual furuncles on the columella may form from these. If sutures were not removed and checked accurately, such suppuration could be observed at the base of the columella. This would be caused by infection of remaining bits of suture material.

COMPLICATIONS OF THE SKIN

Minor skin complications can occur as allergic tape reactions in highly sensitive patients. Sometimes they need a local treatment with corticosteroid creams.

Patients submitted to repeated rhinoplastic intervention may develop teleangiectasias, particularly in the tip, alar, and paranasal region. Their treatment is an electrocoagulation with a very fine needle passed under magnification into the lumen of the small spider shaped vessel complex.

Skin necrosis over the supratip area and the dorsum can result from too excessive pressure from the tape or splint in connection with circulatory problems. If this results in a scar it can be revised after a few months. Following the injections of cortisone, small areas of skin necrosis have been observed in the supratip area in a few cases with thick porous skin by us (Fig. 2) as well as Mahé et al (1975) (see Chapter 22).

Necrosis of the nasal tip can be caused by an excessive excision of cellulo-adipose tissue from the undersurface of the skin through the intercartilaginous or marginal incision in order to narrow the tip, or for better definition of the tip in thick-skinned noses, combined with too tight an application of an unpadded nasal splint providing a strong pinching pressure. Two cases which represented real surgical odysseys involved noses that presented with a total necrosis of the nasal tip and columella occurring after corrective rhinoplasty. Several reconstructive procedures had already been attempted unsuccessfully. We finally had to rebuild the lost parts of the nose by using a frontotemporal flap.

There are exceptional cases of butchered noses with catastrophic results in which a simple corrective rhinoplasty is transformed into a major reconstructive work because of loss of tissue at the tip, ala, and columella. If at the end of the operation we press structures into a new shape and retain them with a very tight packing, there is a danger of pressure necrosis caused by any of the following: tape dressing and plaster, metal or plastic stent on the nasal tip or ala. Such ulcers are extremely rare and almost always disappear after a few weeks without leaving visible scars. Nevertheless, too much pressure from the dressing should be avoided.

Particular attention must be given to the consistency of the nasal skin, especially in secondary correction. Occasionally we have to insert a layer of dermis or fascia between the skin and the underlying visible cartilaginous and bony structures. This will be illustrated in Chapter 13. Sometimes the skin is very thin and has little subcutaneous fat, especially in the region of the nasal tip. In such cases very careful handling of the underlying structures, particularly the upper and lower lateral cartilages, is indicated.

Postoperatively the skin is likely to become even thinner and reveals every irregularity and asymmetry of the underlying structures. If the skin over a healed graft or implant is under too much tension it also thins with risks of perforation. In such cases the graft or implant should be removed or eventually reduced in thickness before atrophy of the skin with later scar formation occurs.

INJURY OF THE LACRIMAL APPARATUS

Very little is published about this complication. An important study to determine the nature and the site of such injury was undertaken by Flowers and Anderson (1968). They demonstrated in cadavers that the lacrimal apparatus was especially vulnerable with relationship to the lateral osteotomy of a rhinoplasty. Significant disruption of the lacrimal sac after an osteotomy could be demonstrated by injection studies in the cadavers. This finding supported previous evidence that damage produced by the osteotomy is usually limited to the lacrimal sac, which is not protected by the medial canthal ligament or by the maxillary rim. The lacrimal canaliculi and the common canaliculus are protected from injury as they lie deep at the medial canthus and enter the lacrimal sac posteriorly. Postoperative obstruction of the lacrimal apparatus was observed by the two authors to be of short duration, resolving without sequelae.

The injured lacrimal sac generally heals rapidly without stenosis but with epiphora lasting two or three days being the only symptom. We can remember one case with persistent ephiphora where a lesion of the lacrimal sac probably occurred. We did not proceed to determine the patency of the lacrimal duct with fluorescein, as suggested by Flowers and Anderson (1968) in this case because of recovery after 5 days. There is no report in the literature regarding permanent damage to the lacrimal apparatus.

INTRACRANIAL INJURIES

Reports of intracranial lesions during rhinoplasty are extremely rare. They are found more in the neurosurgical literature (Lafuente, 1987). Cerebrospinal fluid rhinorrhea following rhinoplasty has been reported by Hallock and Trier (1983). The source of leakage was localized in the cribiform plate area. It was treated by temporal fascia grafting.

PERFORATIONS OF THE SEPTUM

The main causes of this complication are improperly executed submucous resections and unrecognized traumatic septal hematomas. They are less common today than they were a few decades ago because septoplasties are done more carefully and with less radical resections. The treatment of this complication will be discussed further in a later chapter.

ANOSMIA AND ALTERED SENSE OF SMELL

This complication should be a very unusual one since the olfactory area is located high in the nasal cavities far from the operative field of a rhinoplasty. We have observed anosmia or hyposmia only in cases of ozena and in one case where an overgenerous septal resection left only an anterior membranous pillar and a part of the vomer in the choanae. After the closure of this huge septal perforation (see Fig. 140), the anosmia remained and is now permanent.

Champion (1966) reported about 10 cases of temporary anosmia lasting from 6 to 18 months among 200 patients questioned after rhinoplasty. One patient had permanent anosmia. Goldwyn and Shore (1968) investigated by olfactory testing patients who underwent rhinoplasty or septoplasty and found that 80 percent had a normal sense of smell 2 weeks postoperatively and no patient had anosmia 2 months after surgery. So we are in agreement with them when they concluded that submucous septal resection and rhinoplasty very rarely produce a permanent alteration of smell.

CYSTS

Mucous Cysts

Postoperative mucous cysts of the nose are rare complications of rhinoplasty and have been reported only three times in the past by McGregor et al (1958), Mouly (1970), and Shulman and Westreich (1983). The first two authors attributed the cyst formation to herniation of the nasal mucosa into the infracture site. The third authors believe that the cysts are evidence of encystation of mucosal epithelium that is not cleared from the marginal field, a sort of mucosal graft in an ectopic position. Since it is probably not possible to ascertain the true etiology, we support both causes as being plausible.

Polyposis

A case of polyposis in a secondary rhinoplasty was reported by Pitanguy and Ceravolo (1982). Nasal polyps are not real neoplasm, but they are one of the common causes of a mass seen in the nasal cavity. Possible etiologies include infection, allergy, thermal causes, and/or trauma. In Pitanguy and Ceravolo (1922), Woakes described simple multiple polyposis associated with deforming pansinusitis in children. It is also possible that surgical trauma with a lesion of the mucoperiosteum and mucoperichondrium of the septum can act as a determining factor in inciting already predisposed tissue.

11

Residual Bony Deformities

Up to this point we have discussed immediate and early pitfalls. Residual deformities arising after primary rhinoplasty not stemming from those complications already discussed are due to errors in the conception of the surgery, errors in planning the different steps of the intervention, technical faults, and from unpredictable and uncontrollable pitfalls and vagaries in the postoperative healing process. We will analyze and discuss these faults and pitfall and the unfavorable results that follow as well as the techniques with which they eventually can be avoided and with which they can be secondarily corrected. To do this, we first would like to explain the different steps of both primary and secondary operations.

ORDER OF OPERATIVE STEPS

Usually for secondary rhinoplasties we proceed in the same order of operative steps as in primary procedures. These are as follows:

1. Separation of the mobile part of the nose, that means dorsal skin, the tip, and the columella from the stable part, i.e., bones, the upper lateral cartilages, and the septum
2. Removal of the hump (if present)
3. Correction of the septum (if necessary)
4. Modeling of the tip on the columella
5. Osteotomies
6. External resections and ancillary refining procedures

Other operators follow a different order of steps:

1. Septoplasty, hump removal, modeling of the tip, osteotomies
2. Modeling of the tip, hump removal, osteotomies, septoplasty
3. Hump removal, modeling of the tip, osteotomies, septoplasty
4. Hump removal, osteotomies, modeling of the tip, septoplasty
5. Hump removal, osteotomies, septoplasty, modeling of the tip

It is now obvious that the correction of the septum has to be carried together with external rhinoplasty. It can be incorporated at the beginning, in the middle, or at the end of the operation.

For the approach to rhinoplasty, we have 15 internal and external incisions, which are shown in Figures 3, 4, and 5. These are:

1. Erich incision (translobular)
2. Rethi incision (transcolumellar)
3. Rethi-Meyer incision
4. Transfixion incision
5. Basal incision (Cronin)
6. Mid columellar incision (Sheehan)
7. Intercartilaginous incision
8. Intracartilaginous incision
9. Marginal incision
10. Infracartilaginous incision
11. Gillies-Potter incision
12. Marginal columellar incision
13. Buffalo-horn-shaped incision
14. Horizontal glabellar (Fritz, Peterson) incision
15. Canthal (Straatsma) incision

Since we begin a rhinoplasty with hump removal we shall discuss the complications and secondary deformities after this maneuver first followed by postoperative deformities of the bony framework and their corrections.

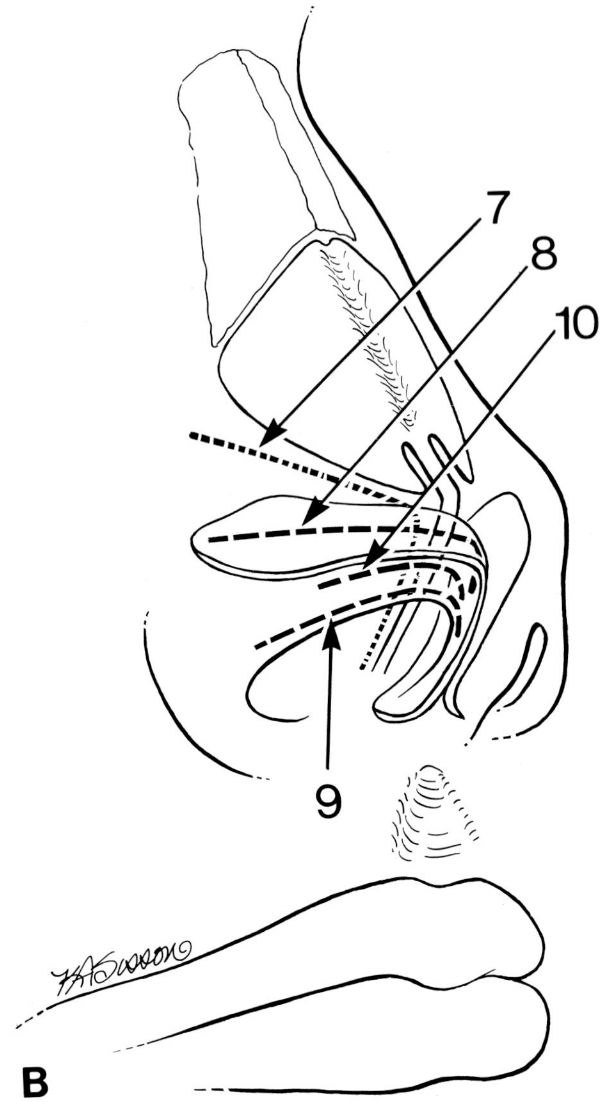

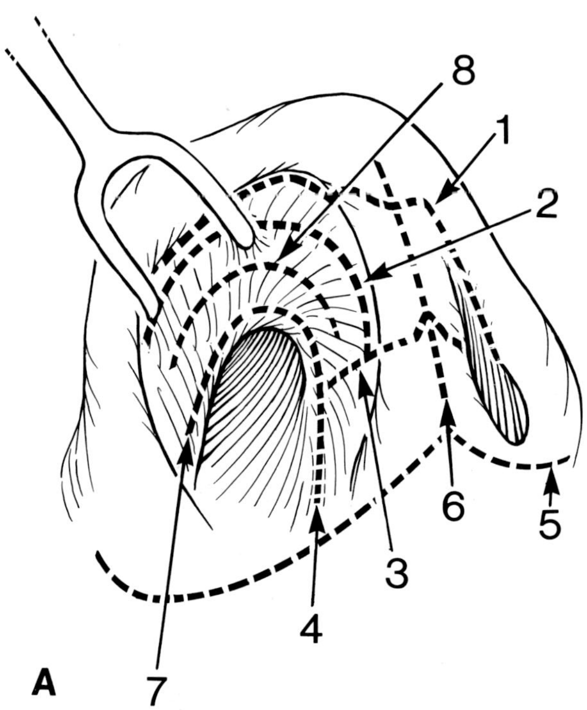

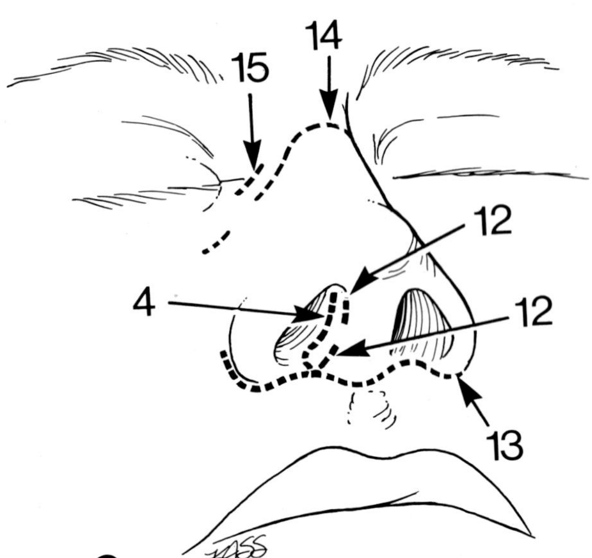

Fig. 3. A, B, and C: External incisons. The numbers in the figures correspond with the numbers in the above list.

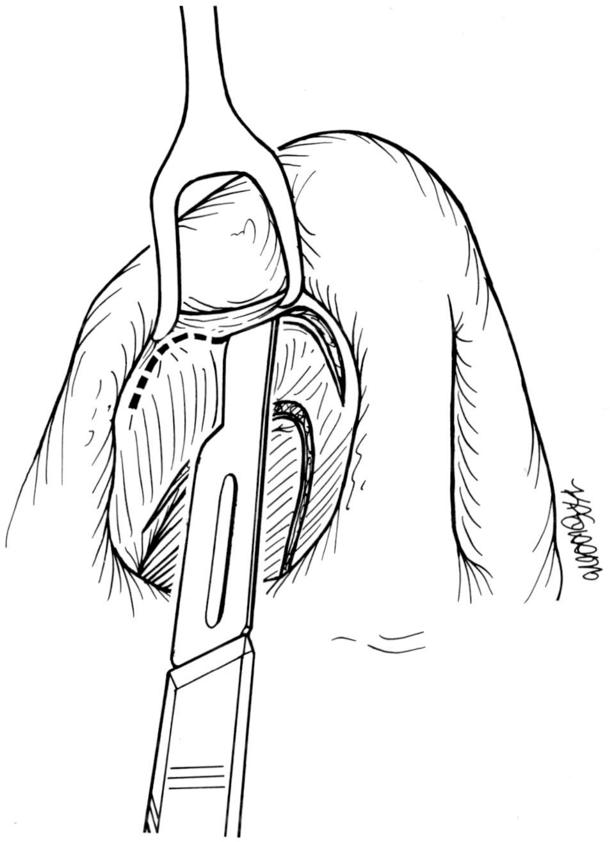

Fig. 4. Intercartilaginous incision already done. Infracartilaginous incision now performed.

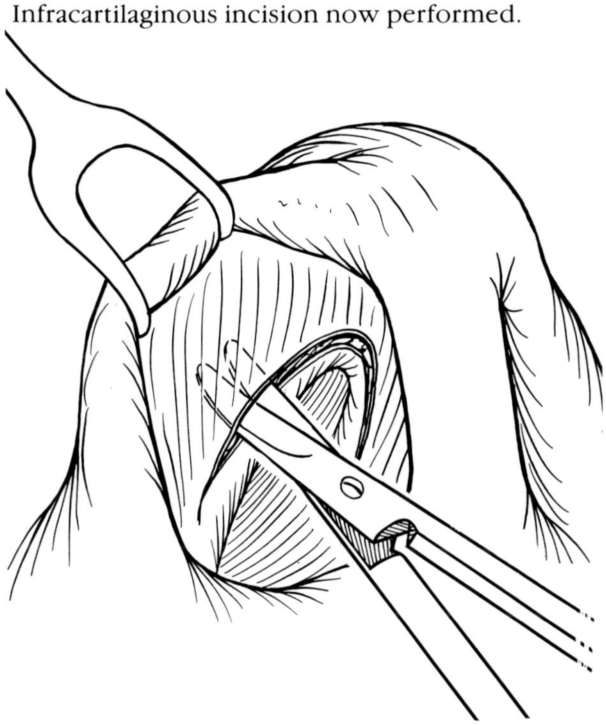

Fig. 5. Skin undermining in evertion technique.

Residual Bony Deformities after Rhinoplasty

There is little in the literature concerning pitfalls and dangers in correction of the bony part of the nose than there is about tip surgery because they are less frequent and easier to correct secondarily. Problems can involve the dorsum, the lateral walls, the base of the bony pyramid, and the glabella.

Postoperative Bony Deformities

The most common causes of postrhinoplasty deformities of the bony framework are:

1. Insufficient or excessive removal of the hump
2. Inadequate osteotomies causing bony irregularities
3. Insufficient correction of bony and septal deviation at the nasal root
4. Postoperative callus formation at the osteotomy site

REMOVAL OF THE HUMP

Insufficient Removal of the Hump

The decision concerning the extent of hump removal should be determined preoperatively with the patient. The surgeon should get a very clear idea of the patient's preferences by using preoperative photographs in which the profile view, placed under transparent paper, can be altered with a pencil in the presence of the patient. Thus, the reduction can be adjusted accordingly to fit the face.

The amount of the cartilaginous dorsum to be removed as evaluated by the preoperative assessment and the drawings can be outlined on the dorsal skin. Before reaching the bony skeleton of the nose, we proceed with the first maneuver, the separation of the mobile part of the nose from the stable portion using the intercartilaginous and transfixion incisions. The first one is carried out at the limen nasi between the vestibular skin and mucosa of the cavities and between the upper lateral and the lower lateral cartilages. The communication of these bilateral incisions at the border of the membranous septum is provided by the transfixion incision. Thus

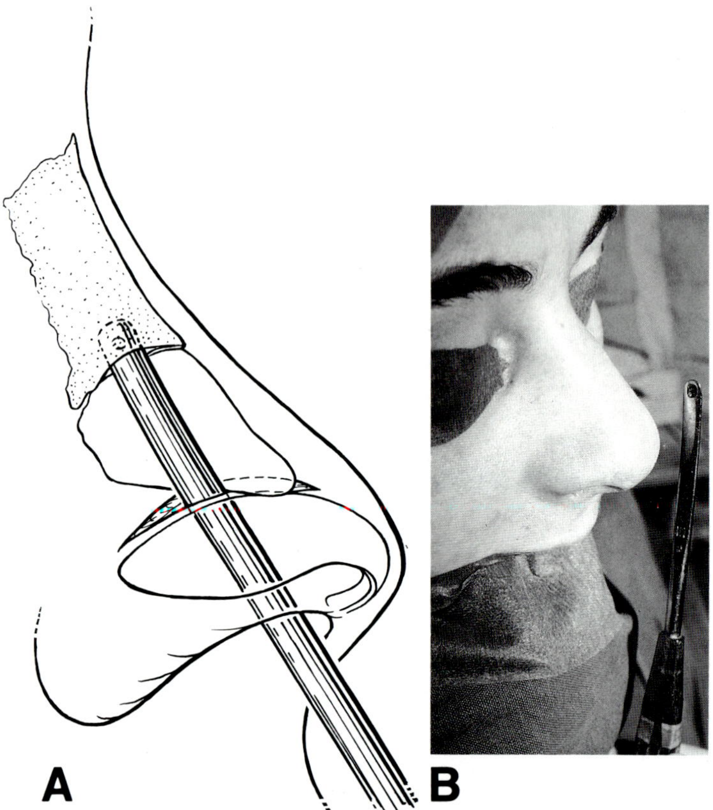

Fig. 6. (A) Subperiosteal dissection with Meyer's suction elevator. (B) Meyer's suction elevator.

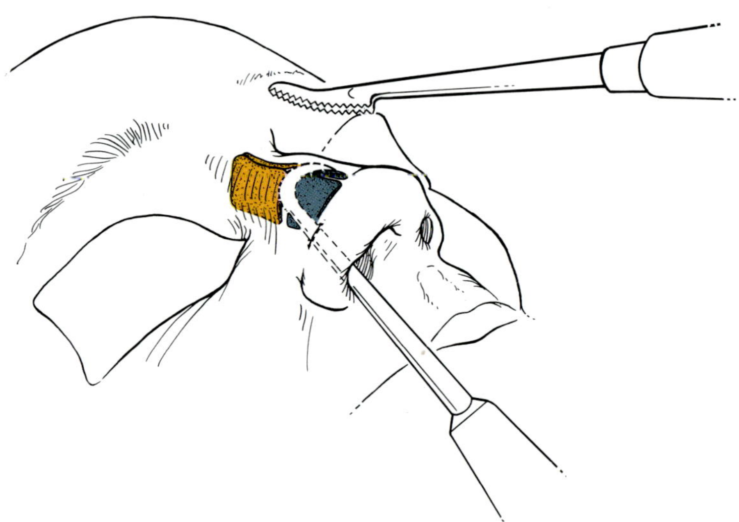

Fig. 7. Rasp for removing a small hump and for bony refinement. Trélat elevator for dorsal skin dissection.

we have separated the tip, columella, and the alar cartilages from the stable part of the nose, which is the bony framework, the upper lateral cartilages, and the septum.

The intercartilaginous incision is now spread and the skin undermined above the upper lateral cartilage. If there is a significant hump to remove in a primary rhinoplasty we provide an extensive skin dissection over the whole bony pryamid, to obtain an adequate apposition of the skin layer to the new shape of the dorsum and lateral walls at the end of the procedure.

While for a primary small hump the access for its resection can be gained with minimal undermining, we prefer to undermine widely in all secondary procedures in order to avoid irregular retraction of the skin. It can then be draped more effectively over the bony and cartilaginous framework if completely undermined, defatted, and freed from scar tissue. Distribution of any redundant nasal skin laterally into the cheek and into the glabellar area is facilitated by wide undermining, as stressed by Stucchi (1955) and Millard (1965). We perform a complete subperiosteal dissection with a fan-like maneuver using our specially designed straight suction elevator (Fig. 6) and finish the retrograde dorsal dissection with the curved elevator of Trelat (Fig. 7), in the same way as Mir y Mir (1956) uses an infant rib elevator.

For removal of a small hump the use of a rasp is sufficient (Fig. 7). Otherwise we apply the rasp only for bony refinement after hump resection. Fischer (1982) designed a special "hump shaver" with interchangeable blades for shaving off fine slices of bone, septum, and upper lateral cartilage.

Hump Removal Using the Extramucosal Technique

For removal of huge humps, as for the management of the stable part of the nose, the septum, the bony frame without a hump and the upper lateral cartilage, we choose to use the extramucosal method, which has become a routine technique in most rhinoplasties. We believe that for a secondary rhinoplasty this technique is particularly helpful.

Eitner (1932) (Fig. 8) and Fomon (1948) (Fig. 9) advocated the extensive dissection of mucoperichondrium from the septum and the upper lateral cartilages, providing an open approach to these structures. We have used this approach, in especially difficult cases such as deviated and harelip noses, since 1960, as mentioned by Denecke and Meyer (Fig. 10), and particularly by Anderson (1966), its importance for use in the routine rhinoplasty was emphasized by Anderson in 1966, and particularly by Robin, in 1970, Pollet, in 1970, and Jost, in 1972. Since 1970, we have used this technique routinely for most primary and secondary rhinoplasties.

We begin the blunt dissection of the septal mucoperichondrium through the transfixion incision on both sides up to the vault of the upper lateral cartilages. In order to facilitate the undermining along the septal cartilage, which is particularly difficult in the secondary procedures due to the fibrous adhesions, we blow up the soft tissues at the septal side of the transfixion incision, infiltrating and separating it from the cartilage with saline solution containing epinephrine or POR (vasopressin), resulting in a type of hydraulic dissection. We do this for both primary and secondary rhinoplasties.

We dissect bilaterally the mucoperichondrium from off the caudal cartilaginous end going up toward the insertion of the upper lateral cartilages into the septum. These cartilages are severed from their insertion and pushed into the nasal lumen together with their attached peri-

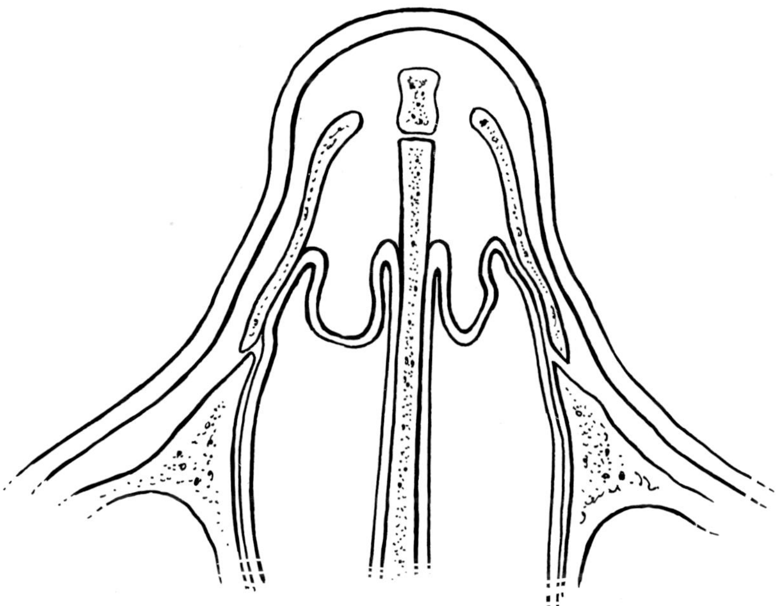

Fig. 8. Eitner's method of mucoperichondral dissection as designed in his publication.

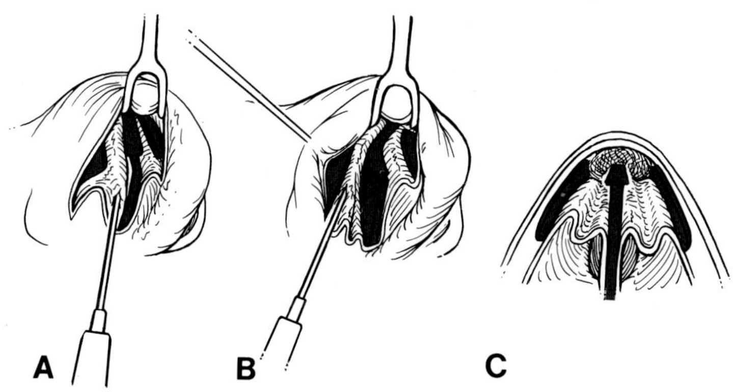

Fig. 9. Fomon's technique of dissection as presented in his book.

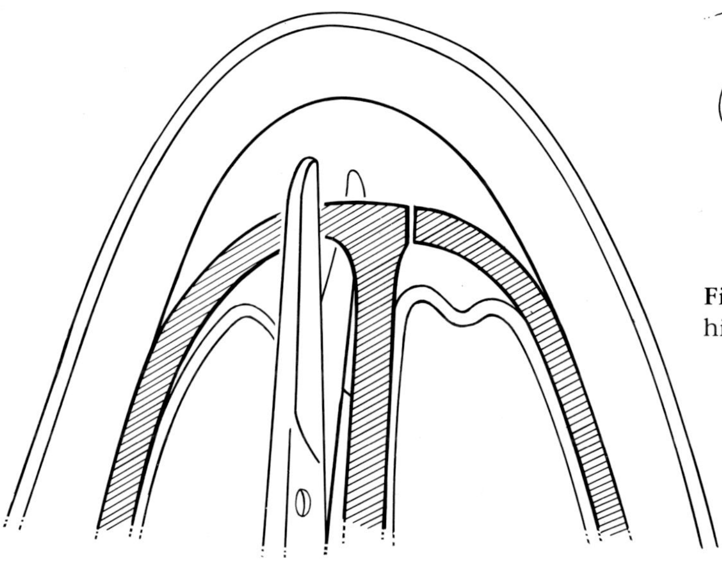

Fig. 10. Mucoperichondral dissection as shown in the book Denecke-Meyer.

chondreal vault. The dissection is extended as far as necessary. In the case of combination of rhinoplasty with septoplasty the perichondral elevation decollement is carried down along both sides over the entire septum. After pushing the mucoperichondrial vault laterally together with the freed upper lateral cartilages, we dissect the mucoperiosteal vault from off the bony septum and nasal bones, further cephalad and posterior.

Thus we have freed the dorsal edge of the septal cartilage and the bony dorsum so that we can proceed to the removal of the hump without cutting through the mucoperichondrial and mucoperiosteal vault as occurs in other techniques (Figs. 11 and 12).

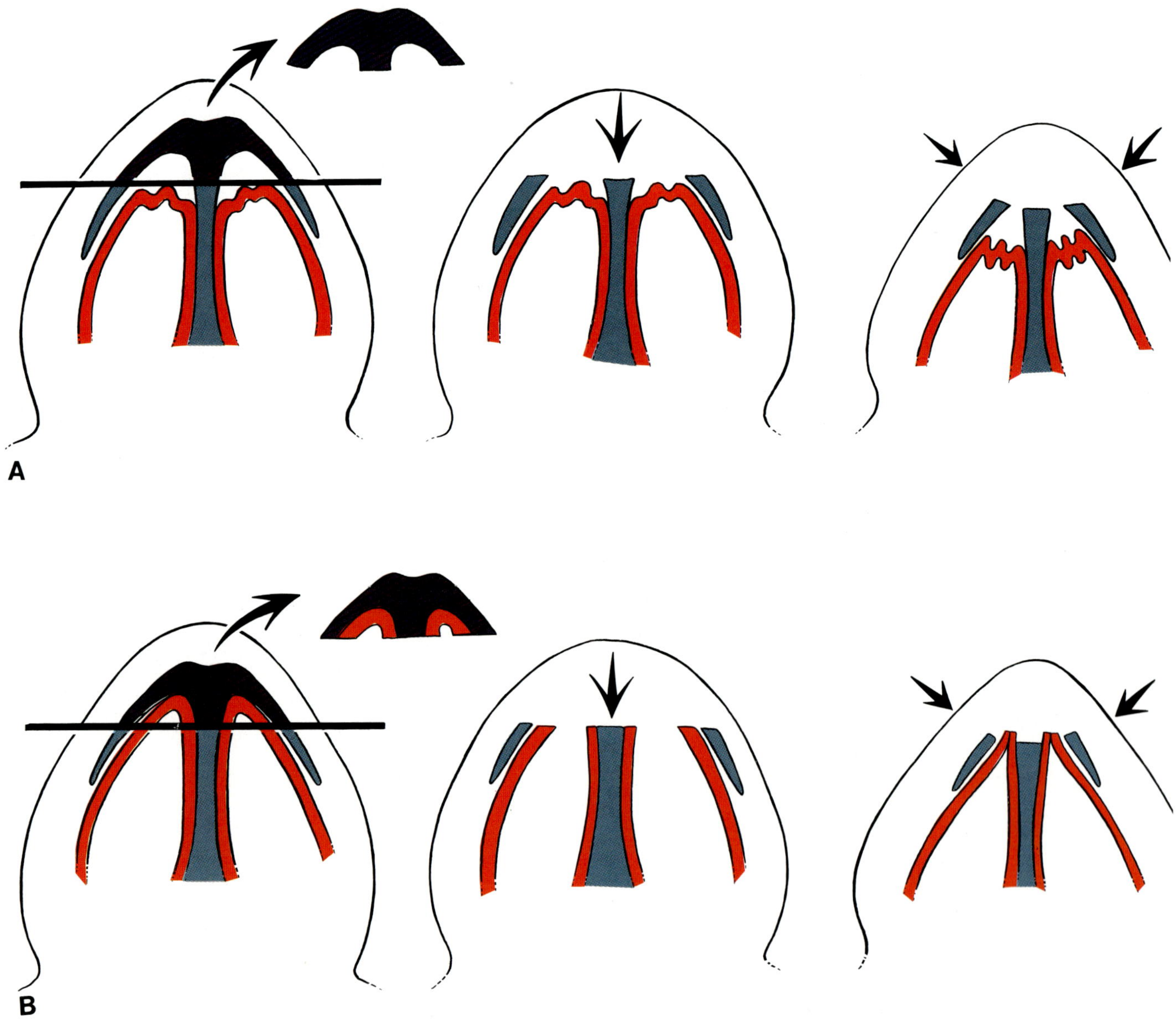

Fig. 11. (A) Resection of the cartilaginous hump with *extramucosal technique.* Mucoperichondral vault is dissected and pushed into the lumen while the trimmed upper lateral cartilages move toward the new dorsum thus reducing and narrowing the medial dorsal region. (B) Resection of the cartilaginous hump together with mucoperichondral vault.

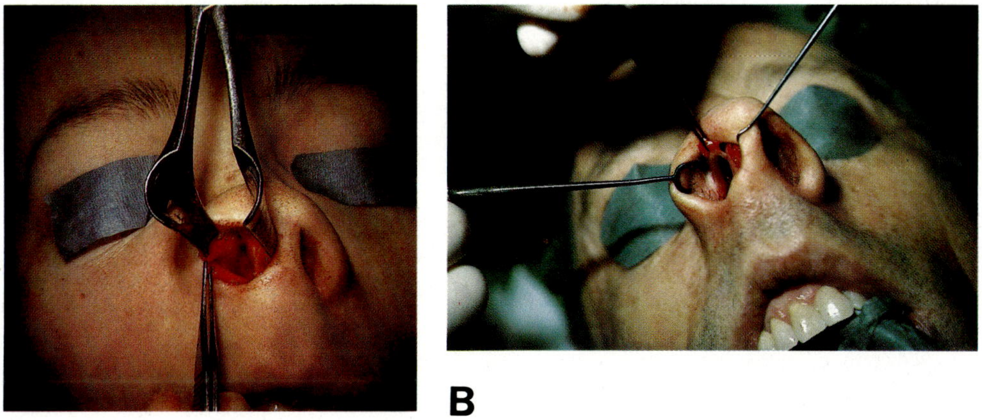

B

A

Fig. 12. Extramucosal technique. (A) Dissection of mucoperichondrium and of the median strip of the upper lateral cartilage to be resected. (B) Dissection of the mucoperichondrium from the septal cartilage on the right side and section of the upper lateral cartilage at its median junction.

First we resect the cartilaginous part of the hump using slightly curved scissors (Fig. 13A). We can then palpate the bayonet shaped dorsum and reassess the amount of bone to be resected (Fig. 13B). For the removal of small and medium sized bony humps we use a modified Rowland forceps, with slightly curved blades (Fig. 13C). When the gibbus is very prominent, we begin the resection with an osteotome inserted at the caudal end of the bony dorsum with only a few taps. Following this initial cut line we achieve the definitive resection using the forceps, cutting through the whole bony segment. We then resect a paramedian strip of the upper lateral cartilages.

Hump removal can be performed with the osteotome as well. For this purpose a sharp chisel is placed horizontally against the caudal edge of the bony hump at the level of the planned neo-dorsum. While the operator controls the course of the instrument, the assistant uses a hammer to drive the chisel.

To better guide the osteotome or forceps in the removal of the bony hump and to better appreciate the angulation needed, Aiach and Gomulinski (1982) locate the nasion with a needle that transfixes horizontally the soft tissues of the nasal root.

In most cases the bony resection of the hump should be extended into the glabellar region. A specially designed curved osteotome is most useful for this part of the procedure.

Other surgeons prefer osteotomes, saws, rasps, or the electrical bur for hump removal in primary as well as in secondary rhinoplasties.

In secondary procedures the cartilaginous septum often requires further trimming in order to plane it down to the level of the bony resection. This may also be true for the upper lateral cartilages. Slight overcorrection at both sites is desirable to prevent bulging above the nasal tip. Sparing the mucous membrane, fine adjustments are made with straight scissors. If the hump removal has been too deep, we reimplant part of the resected material of the septum and upper lateral cartilages as an osteo-cartilaginous or cartilaginous graft as advocated by Skoog (1966, 1974).

Postrhinoplasty deformities at the dorsum due to insufficient removal of the hump can be localized along the length of the dorsum or only at one of the three thirds. When an insufficient amount of tissue, cartilaginous or bony, has been removed in the dorsum and the glabella regions in a primary rhinoplasty, the secondary correction consists of additional removal of this carti-

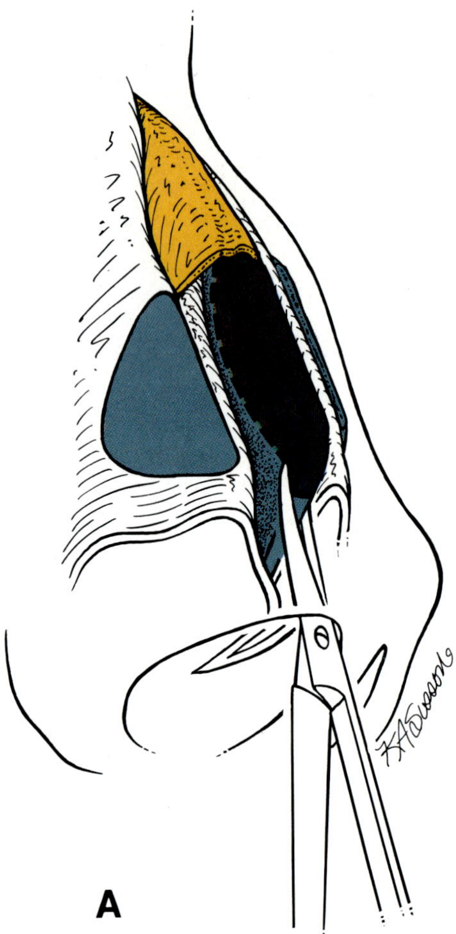

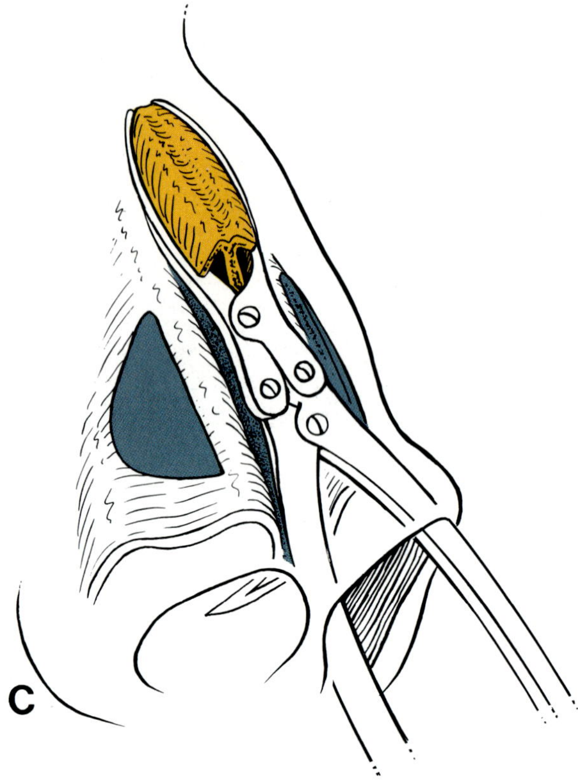

Fig. 13. Hump removal in two maneuvers with extramucosal access. (A) Resection of cartilaginous portion with slightly curved scissors. (B) End of the first step. (C) Resection of the bony hump with slightly curved Rowland forceps.

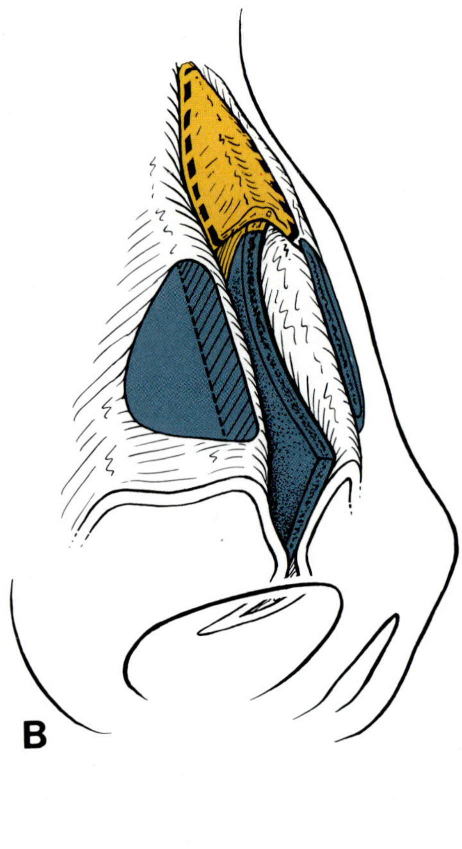

laginous and/or bony tissue (Fig. 14).

Cases with a residual excess of bone in the upper third of the dorsum are less frequent (Fig. 15). Thickening of the remaining periosteum or bone fragment left in place following hump ablation is commonly the cause. Patients who have a residual mid-third hump following surgery often represent a group in whom the surgeon failed to adequately manage the dorsal-most part of the cartilaginous septum that normally lies between the nasal bones. This can sometimes be difficult to remove, especially when one employs a rasp for hump removal. Cartilaginous tissues do not readily lend themselves to being rasped, and in many such cases, that cephalic portion of the dorsal septum has to be managed by excision, a technique that can be difficult because bone lies on either side of this cartilaginous segment.

Another failure that can lead to residual hump occurs when the medial most part of the upper lateral cartilages is not reevaluated following narrowing of the nose (Fig. 16). Thus, residual hump may be a false hump caused by failure to trim the dorsal borders of the thick upper lateral cartilages. Rogers (1972) describes these hump noses with overdevelopment of the upper lateral cartilage and an exaggerated overlap of their inferior borders as characteristic of Levantine people. Cephalically these cartilages are attached to the under surface of the nasal bone and, in some cases, when one fractures and mobilizes these bones the attached upper lateral cartilages are pushed forward along with the bones. In such cases trimming the dorsal protrusion of these cartilages eliminates the problem.

When the nasal hump has been inadequately removed in the mid-third of the dorsum, correction is best accomplished by wide dissection of the dorsum with extramucosal access to the upper lateral cartilages. These have to be trimmed medially where they still are in continuity and inserted to the septal cartilage. A paramedian strip of the cartilage is resected with scissors or knife. If there is also an excess of the quadrangular plate at its dorsal edge, this is removed with scissors or a Rowland forceps. Irregularities of the lower border of the bony bridge are eliminated by use of rasps.

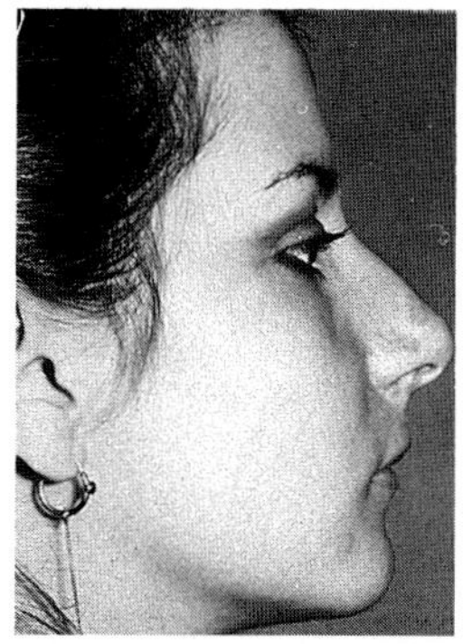

A

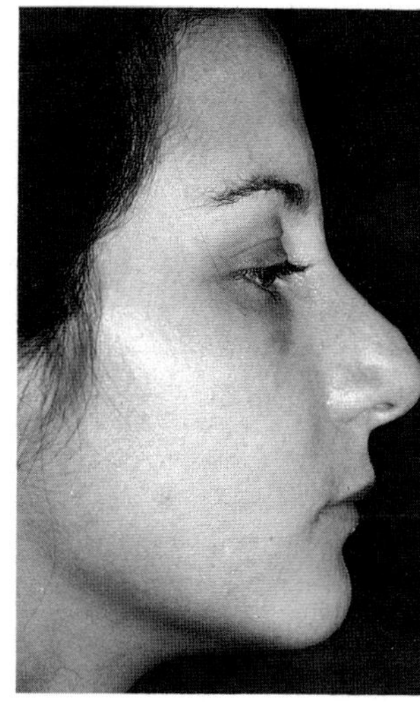

B

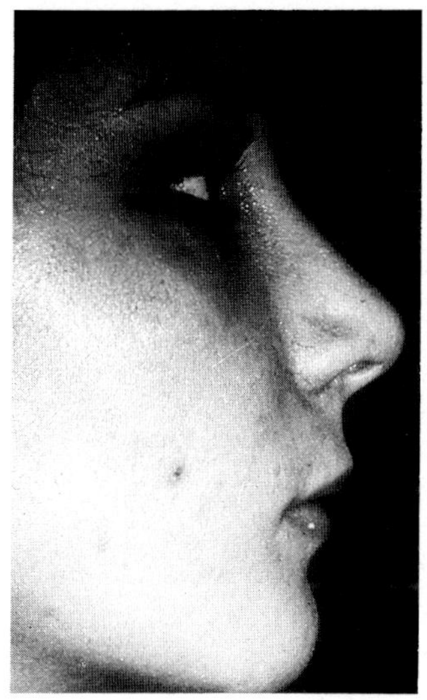

C

Fig. 14. This young female underwent a primary reduction rhinoplasty with hump removal by an assistant. (A) Preoperative view. (B) the patient developed a polly beak that was corrected secondarily one year later. (C) Result 8 months after revision.

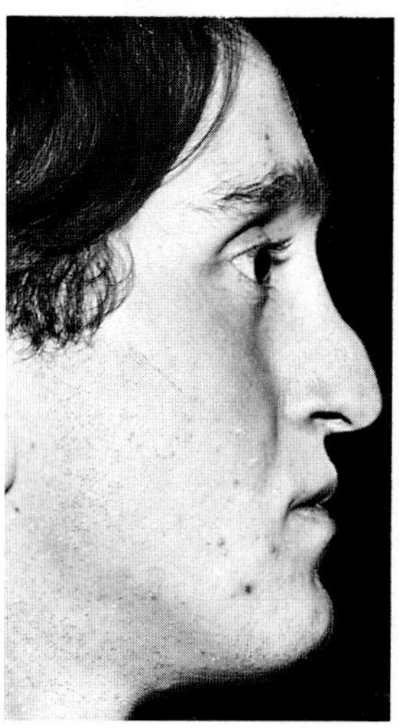

A

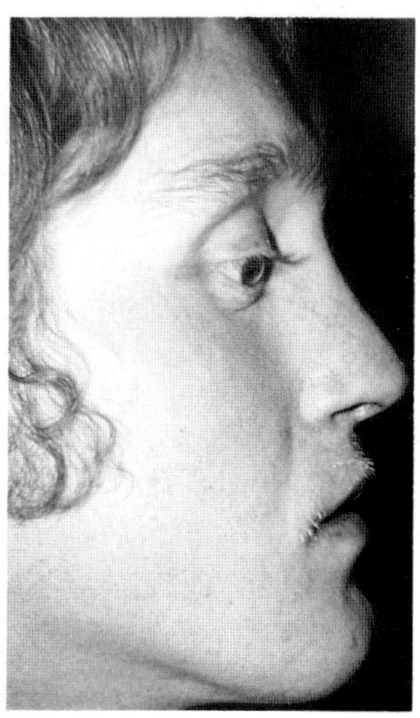

B

Fig. 16. (A) High polly beak with too much cartilaginous tissue left in the primary operation. (B) Patient after revision (Removal of fibrous tissue in the upper part of the supratip area and septal cartilage and upper lateral cartilage reduction).

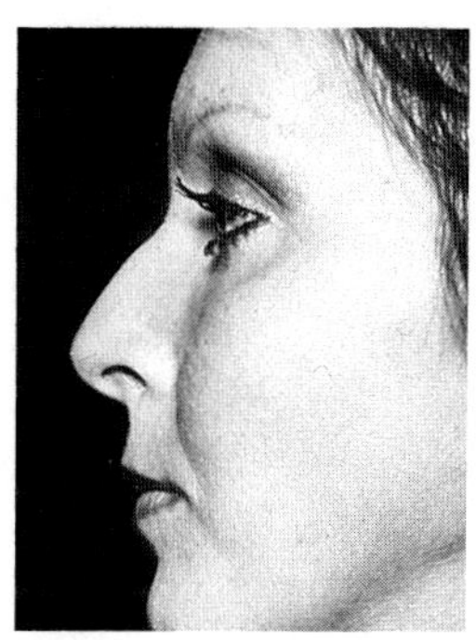

A

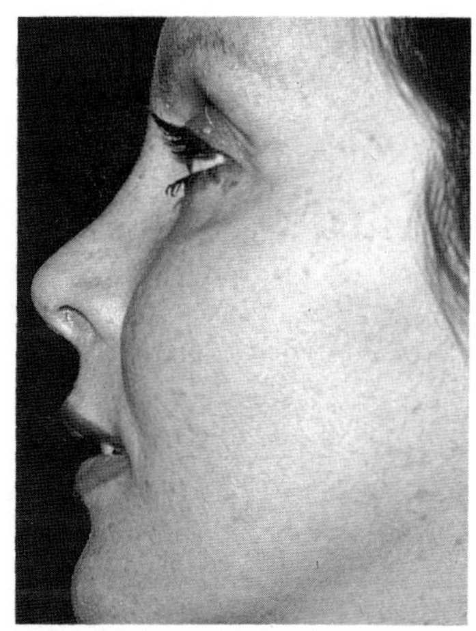

B

Fig. 15. Young female with a polly beak in the upper portion of the supratip area. (A) Before and (B) after secondary correction (Removal of fibrous tissue and lowering of the dorsal line of the septal cartilage that was left too high in the primary surgery).

Persistent hump in the lower one third of the nose, due to failure in deepening the antero-superior border of the septal cartilage, is part of the deformity known as "parrots's beak" or "polly beak" (Figs. 17 and 18). This most difficult secondary correction after requiring bony, cartilaginous, and fibrous tissue removal will be considered separately later on.

Depression of the septal and lower lateral cartilage in the lower portion of the nose may give the illusion of a persistent hump in the bony region. If the surgeon removes this false hump, the profile will be lowered even more, thereby replacing one deformity with another. In such a

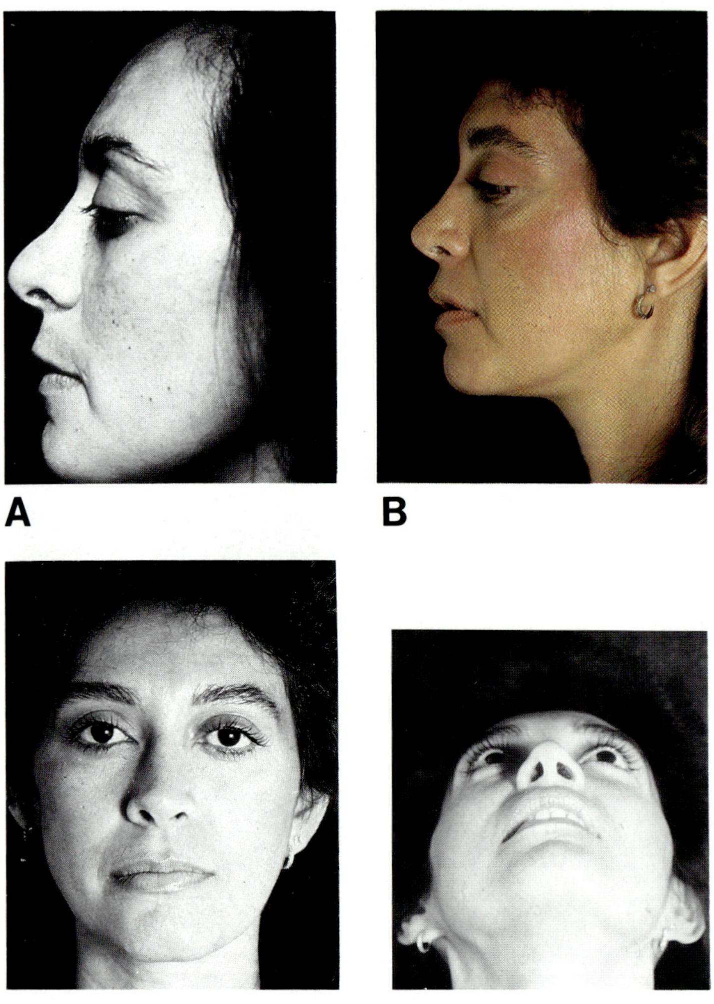

Fig. 17. Polly beak with retracted ala in a young female. (A) Before and (B, C, and D) after correction. Removal of fibrous tissue in the supratip area and cartilage grafting into the alar rim (see chapter on Lowering of the alar rim.)

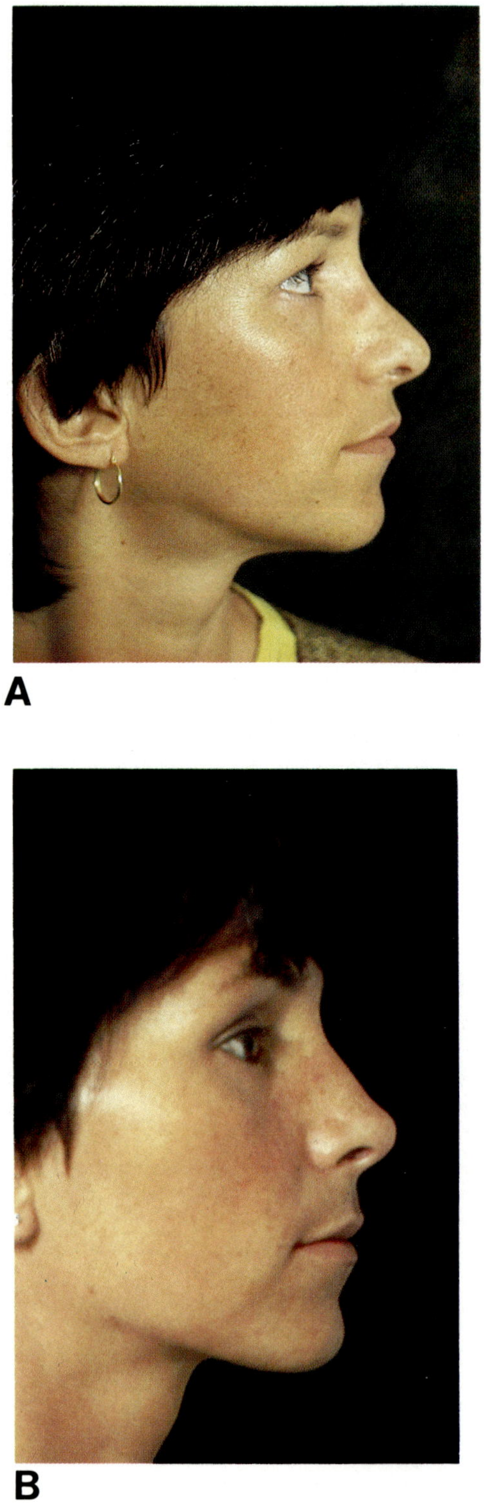

Fig. 18. Slight supratip thickening corrected with fibrous tissue removal and tip projection with cartilage graft. (A) Preoperative and (B) Postoperative view.

case the fault was excessive rather than insufficient removal of the hump. Because of this delicate relationship some surgeons feel that once the tip has been appropriately positioned with proper projection, it is easier to evaluate the corresponding level of the dorsum, which then must be adapted to the tip. Thus, for Rees (1973) and other surgeons, it is often desirable to correct the cartilaginous part of the nose before removing the hump, particularly when the hump is small. We prefer to manage the easier part of the reduction rhinoplasty first and then adapt the tip to the new dorsum, which has been reduced.

Excessive Removal of the Hump

In general, for any part of the nose, the more significant complications occur when too much tissue has been removed as opposed to insufficient removal. Excessive removal of the dorsum and in the lining of the vestibule is often associated with pinching, scarring, and restriction of nasal breathing. Thus, some of the most deforming and least correctable "errors of excess" are seen when too much dorsum has been removed, usually at the nasal bones and the perpendicular plate of the ethmoid. The deformities created vary from relatively slight to extreme, but all tend to disturb the facial appearance, creating a "flat" middle third of the face. Typically, the dorsum has been amputated, widening the frontal appearance of the nose, giving the typical boxers look. In addition to being self-conscious about their appearance, the patients often complain of sensitivity and tenderness of the nasal dorsum, a symptom that is probably due to the unprotected nasal mucous membrane lying adjacent to the external nasal skin.

There is a lesser version of this same problem that is caused by a failure to narrow the nasal bridge with osteotomies following dorsal hump removal. This is called an "open roof" or "open vault" (Cottle, 1954) deformity and is not necessarily associated with excessive bone removal, but rather a failure to close the dorsum after it has been flattened by hump removal.

After the osteotomies of both nasal bones and the frontal process of the maxilla, the infracturing has to be performed in such a way that the bones cannot separate again afterwards. Thus, the roof of the bony vault will not remain open. The syndrome described by Cottle (1954) is characterized by headaches, attacks of dizziness, and cold sensitivity in the nose. Sometimes the overlying soft tissues sink into the two bony gaps, which gives an additional ugly look to the nose.

In the case of "open roof" deformity the remedy is simple. One usually has to narrow the nose with lateral osteotomies and infracturing. Furthermore, when excessive dorsum has been removed, one must resort to the placement of a graft or implants. Generally, correction of an excessive removal of upper and lower lateral cartilages is best managed by replacement of cartilage, harvested either from the patient's septum or auricle. Restoration of a natural contour after excessive removal of these cartilages is difficult to accomplish. In some extreme cases in which both cartilage and mucosa are deficient, one is best advised to use composite grafts.

Furthermore, in cases where the lower part of the dorsum is too prominent, giving an inferior hump in the cartilaginous part of the nose while the bony part is too depressed, the correction would be an upward shifting of the cartilaginous hump towards the bony pyramid (Fig. 16). Such displacement of dorsal material is sometimes useful in secondary procedures as well.

As mentioned previously, Skoog (1974) advocates the partial replacement of large osteocartilaginous humps (Fig. 19) as a routine procedure so that many of the objectionable features of hump removal, such as irregular edges and especially the "open roof syndrome" of Cottle, can be avoided. Occasionally it is required to leave a small remnant of the preexisting hump, which gives a minimal waved line (Fig. 20). In these cases, the method of Skoog (1974) with partial reimplantation of the hump can be applied.

Deformities resulting from too radical a resection of the bony and/or cartilaginous hump, leading to saddling of the dorsum with a wide nasal bridge and nasal bones too short for proper infracturing, can be corrected with a cartilage or bone graft, as we will discuss later in the description of the management of the saddle nose. The same secondary deformity can result from an overdone "push-down" procedure (Fig. 21). This technique, advocated by Cottle and used by some ENT surgeons, can be appropriate if applied in the correction of minimal hump nose (Fig. 21A). Today it has been practically abandoned. We use the septal push-down only for the management of certain septal perforations (see Chapter 14).

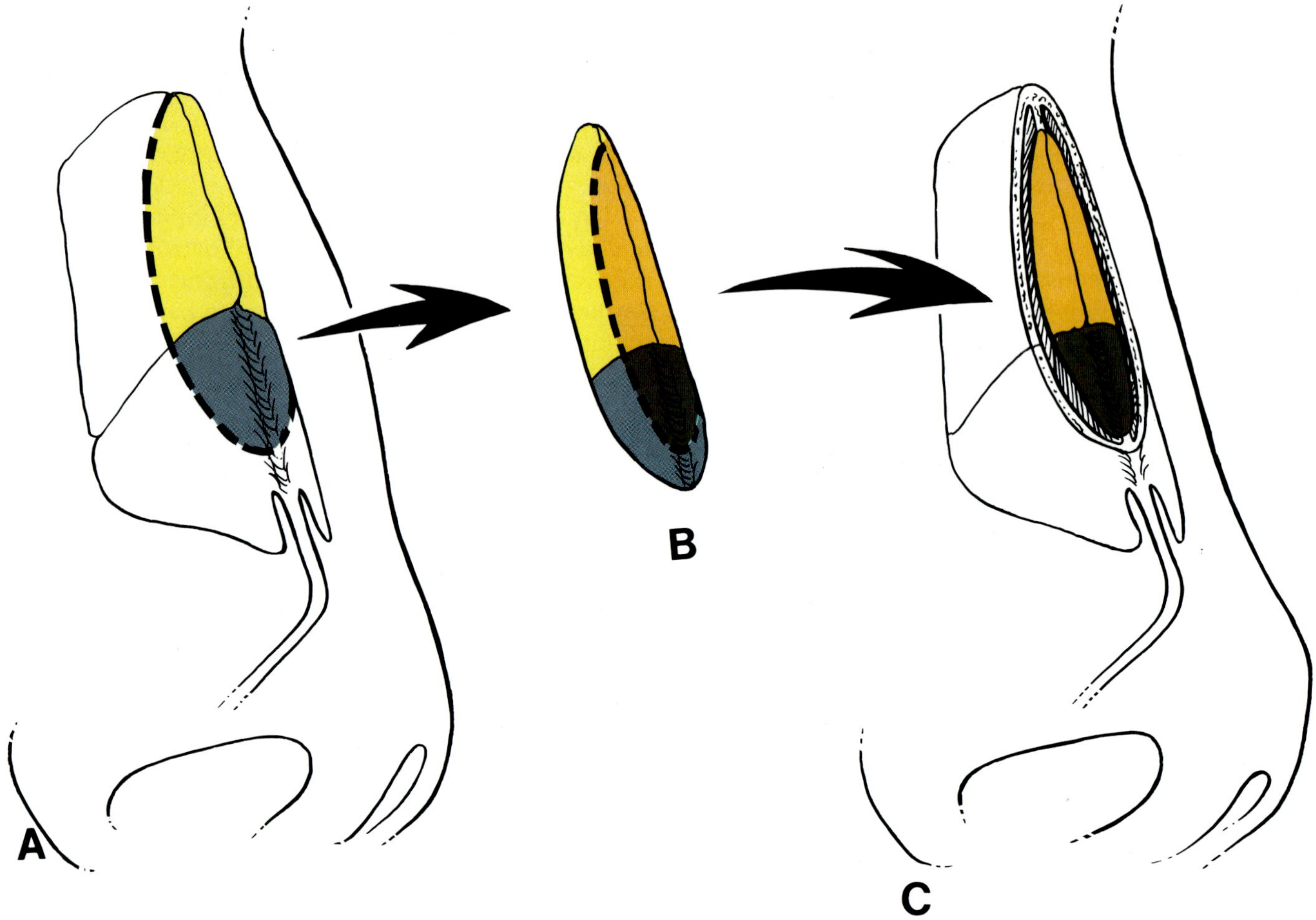

Fig. 19. (A,B,C) Skoog's technique reducing and reintroducing the removed and reduced hump.

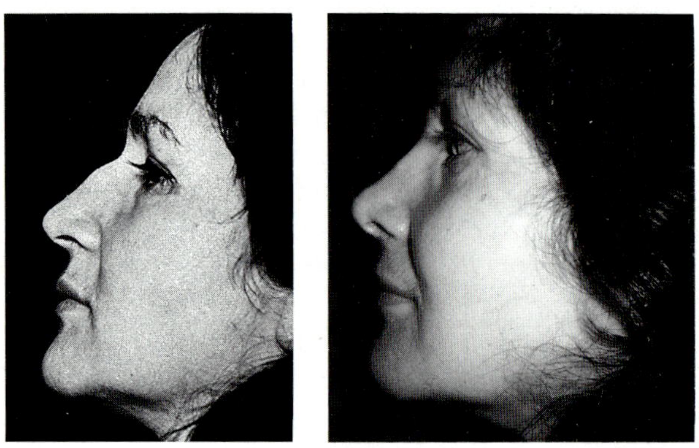

Fig. 20. (A and B) Hump removal and reinsertion of the reduced hump according to the method of Skoog in a 30-year-old patient.

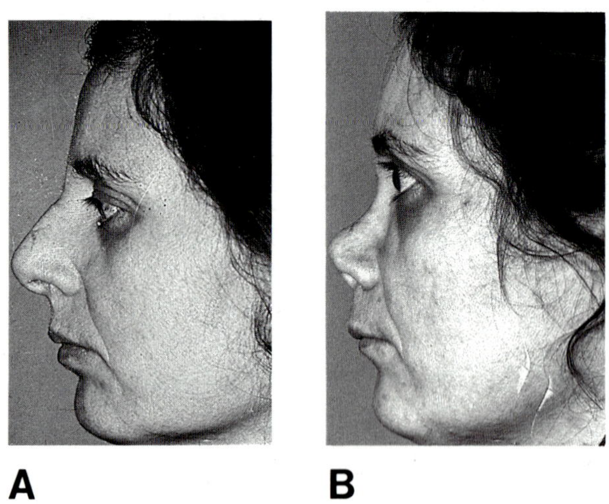

Fig. 21. Excessive reduction of a hump nose by an overdone "push down" procedure of Cottle in a 45-year-old female operated by an overzealous assistant. (A) Patient before primary reductive operation. (B) Result of the primary surgery. Secondary correction (see Fig. 98). (*Fig. 21 continues*)

Excessive removal of tissue can make a secondary rhinoplasty very difficult because of the inelasticity of the tissues, particularly of the vestibular lining. When correcting a bird's beak deformity with a cartilage graft, the extramucosal approach has proved in our hands to be very helpful. It permits an elongation and amplification of the lining in the nasal cavities as well as in the vestibules.

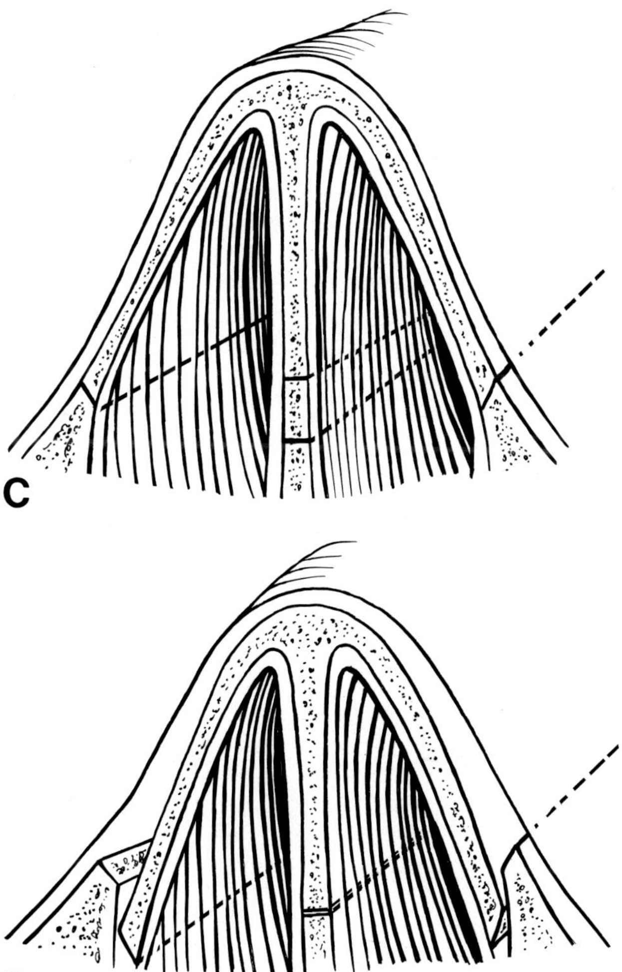

C

D

Fig. 21. (*continued*) (C and D) "Push down" technique of Cottle. Lateral osteotomy on both sides and resection of a strip of cartilage and bone from the septum after elevation of the mucosa from the septum and from nasal bones. The bony and cartilaginous nasal dorsum can be pushed to a deeper level with an intact medial vault. If necessary a strip of bone can also be removed bilaterally at the lateral osteotomy line.

As already mentioned, we usually proceed to the osteotomies as one of the last steps of a rhinoplasty after septal correction (if necessary), hump removal (if necessary), and modeling of the tip and columella. But we will analyze this maneuver and the difficulties encountered as well as revisions possible in the context of bony deformities.

OSTEOTOMIES

Many secondary deformities result from inadequate or irregular osteotomies and particularly from insufficient mobilization of the nasal bones and approximation of their median borders, i.e., the cut edge after hump removal. Any hump removal calls for an exact and symmetric narrowing of the nasal bones in the same way that a large flat nose needs narrowing without hump removal in order to reconstruct the nasal arch and build a triangular pyramid in cross section. For this purpose the bones must be mobilized and detached from their footing by precise osteotomies.

In secondary surgery the manipulation of the nasal bones has to be limited to the particular requirements, determined as needing correction as the nasal bones heal more by fibrous union and less by callus formation as in primary rhinoplasty. The excessive fibrous tissue encountered at the osteotomy lines has to be reduced by excision and the mobilization of the bones must be complete and clean.

Prior to the osteotomies the operative field has to be inspected and meticulously cleaned of all cartilaginous or bony particles. It is also advantageous to smoothen any irregularities of the dorsum at this moment with a chisel, a small Kazanjian forceps, or a rasp because after the osteotomies the bones will be too mobile for this maneuver. On both sides we perform three osteotomies: the paramedian (called median by many authors), the lateral, and the transverse osteotomy. It is not important whether the paramedian or lateral osteotomy is performed first. In primary cases we begin with the lateral osteotomy, in secondary cases sometimes with the paramedian.

Paramedian Osteotomy

The paramedian osteotomy is carried out on both sides along the dorsal bridge of the septum. After hump removal one only has to complete the osteotomy from the interosseous gap to the nasion in order to separate the nasal bones from the perpendicular plate of the ethmoid.

When the hump removal goes right to the nasion the paramedian osteotomy become superfluous. Obviously, paramedian osteotomies are also necessary in flat noses with broad bony bridges and in crooked noses in which hump removal has not been required.

We insert the straight osteotome vertically into the upper corner of the interosseous gap and cut the bone in a vertical paramedian line. In cases of correction of the osseous nasal pyramid by osteotomies without hump removal, the osteotome is driven from the caudal border of the nasal bones right up to the root of the nose in a paramedian plane parallel to the septum.

To allow the medial transposition of the nasal bones without incongruity, at the osteotomy line a bone wedge should be removed on either side of the perpendicular plate of the ethmoid at the root of the nose. This maneuver, if necessary, is executed very meticulously with an osteotome or a cutting forceps. We consider this detail a necessary completion of the osteotomy only in cases of thick bones and in very broad bony pyramids, and find it unnecessary when the osseous skeleton is delicate. The opportunity still exists to eliminate bony irregularities at the moment of approximation of the bones with a small Kazanjian forceps.

Lateral Osteotomy

Lateral osteotomy, to narrow the base of the nasal pyramid, is performed in a routine rhinoplasty through an internal or external incision. Either an osteotome or a saw can be used, placed subperiosteally or supraperiosteally with or without tunneling of the overlying subcutaneous tissue. In performing a lateral osteotomy we make a stab incision low in the wall of the vestibule through the skin and periosteum over the margin of the piriform aperture. We introduce an unguarded straight osteotome and advance it to the inferior margin of the nasomaxillary process at the piriform aperture. From there the nasal process of the maxilla is split at the base, sloping in a slightly outward bent osteotomy line, passing at some 5 mm distance from the inner canthus but remaining far enough away from the lacrimal system (Fig. 22A). Thus, like Webster (1977), we avoid a step-like prominence at the lateral osteotomy by an angulated or curved osteotomy, which also prevents an excessive undesirable narrowing of the nasal cavity.

The osteotomy can also be performed through a small external incision in the alar-lip crease (Jordan, 1958) or through existing incisions after an alotomy. The excisions at the alar base, as described by Weir (1892), Seltzer (1949), Aufricht (1943), and Sheehan (1936) (see Chapter 16), are an ideal site for introducing the osteotome. So if an alar base resection is needed, we take the opportunity of this external incision to carry out the lateral osteotomy, thus avoiding a special incision in the vestibule (Fig. 22B).

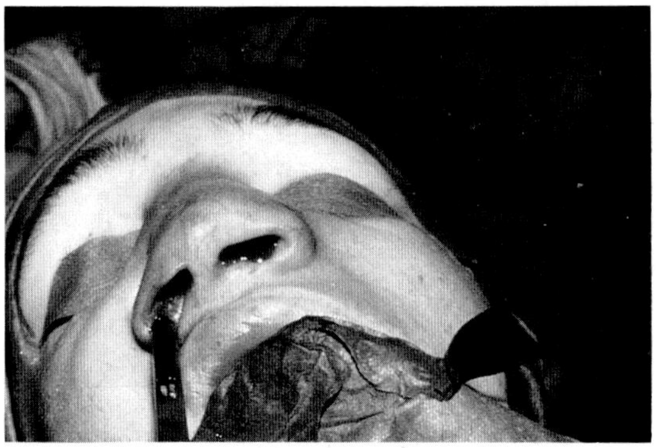

A

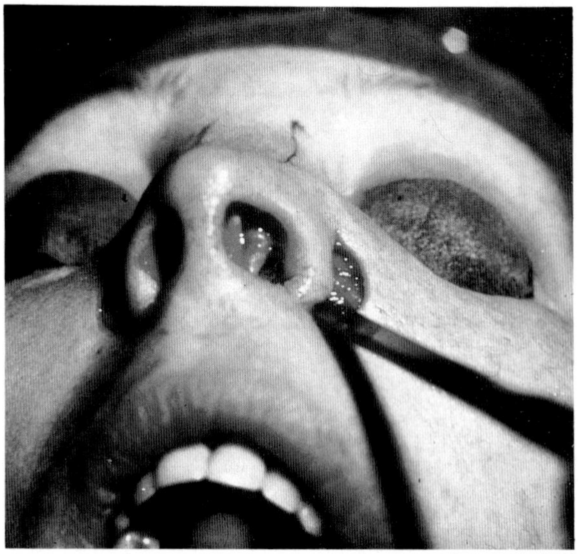

B

Fig. 22. (A) Lateral osteotomy as we perform through a stab incision in the lateral wall of the vestibule. (B) Lateral osteotomy through alotomy.

Some surgeons, as Schmid (1983), use a sublabial approach, making an incision through the gingivolabial mucosa. Straatsma (1951) and Silver (1952) inserted a 2 mm osteotome through the skin at the midpoint of a line extending from the middle of the lower eyelid to the external border of the ala. Actually, Mir y Mir (1983), Ortiz-Monasterio and Olmedo (1977), and others routinely use a small oblique incision below the canthus for lateral and transverse osteotomies. We do so occasionally when the bony structures are very fine. The frontal process of the maxilla is then cut in an oblique line (Figs. 23A and 24).

In some cases of female noses with exceptionally fine bones we chose to use a 1.5 mm chisel for lateral and paramedian osteotomies. Tardy (1973, 1977) utilizes such a very narrow osteotome for all osteotomies. Many surgeons, especially the Commonwealth plastic surgeons and ENT surgeons, prefer to use the saw. We began by utilizing the saw for hump removal and lateral osteotomies in our first rhinoplasties and prefer over the last 15 years to use the chisel. For many years we also used an electric burr for lateral and transverse osteotomies with the help of the Aufricht speculum or of a special tissue-protecting metallic shield, as described in 1964 (Denecke and Meyer). We have since abandoned this previously quite valuable technique and now prefer the chisel, which is much easier to handle. Recently Goodman (1981) readvocated the use of the burr, which provides many advantages.

After the lateral osteotomies are performed we check to ensure that the osteotomies have been made at the appropriate level. If the testing finger already finds a step at the lateral edge of the lateral osteotomy, the cut has not been placed laterally enough. A parallel osteotomy must be added immediately, leaving the resulting bone strip in place (Figs. 25, 26, and 27). This can be done with a 2 mm osteotome.

Many secondary deformities such as an ugly flat appearance of the bony bridge and a visible step at the base of the nasal pyramid result from carrying the lateral osteotomy too far medially. If it has not been performed at the appropriate location, a new osteotomy should be carried out further laterally.

Transverse Osteotomy

A precise transverse osteotomy at the nasofrontal suture is in our view extremely important

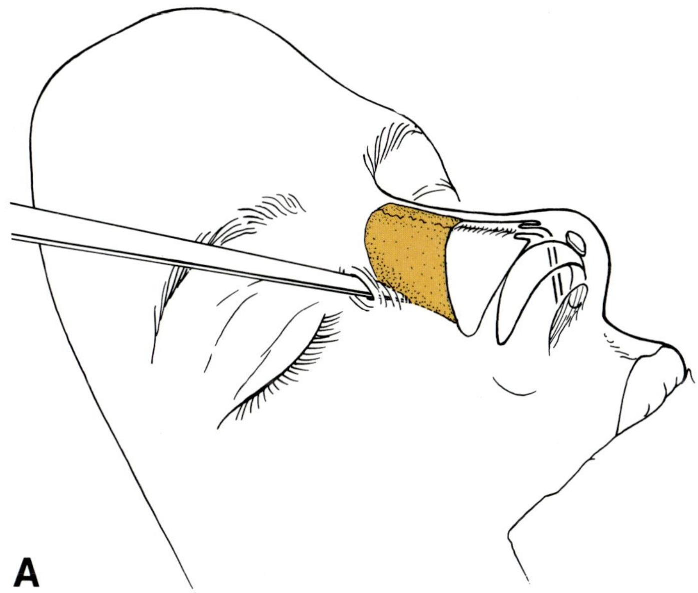

A

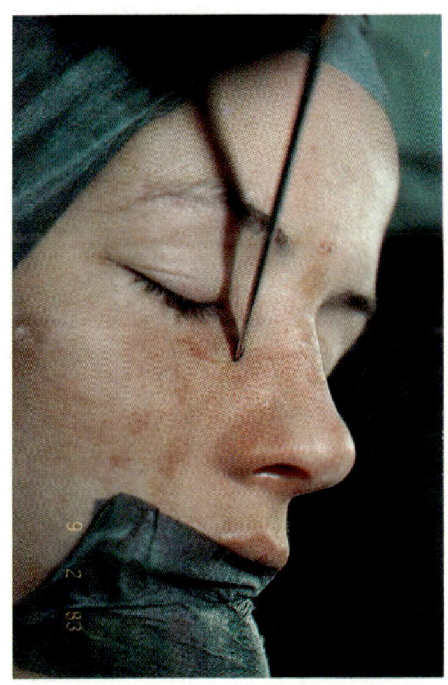

B

Fig. 23. (A and B) Lateral osteotomy through cutaneous stab incision.

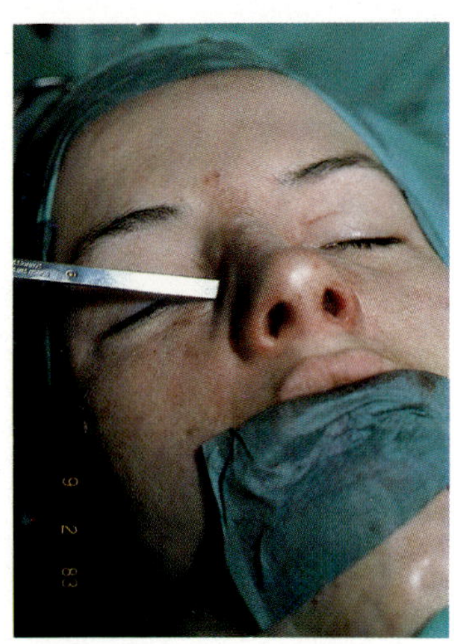

Fig. 24. Transverse osteotomy through the same lateral incision.

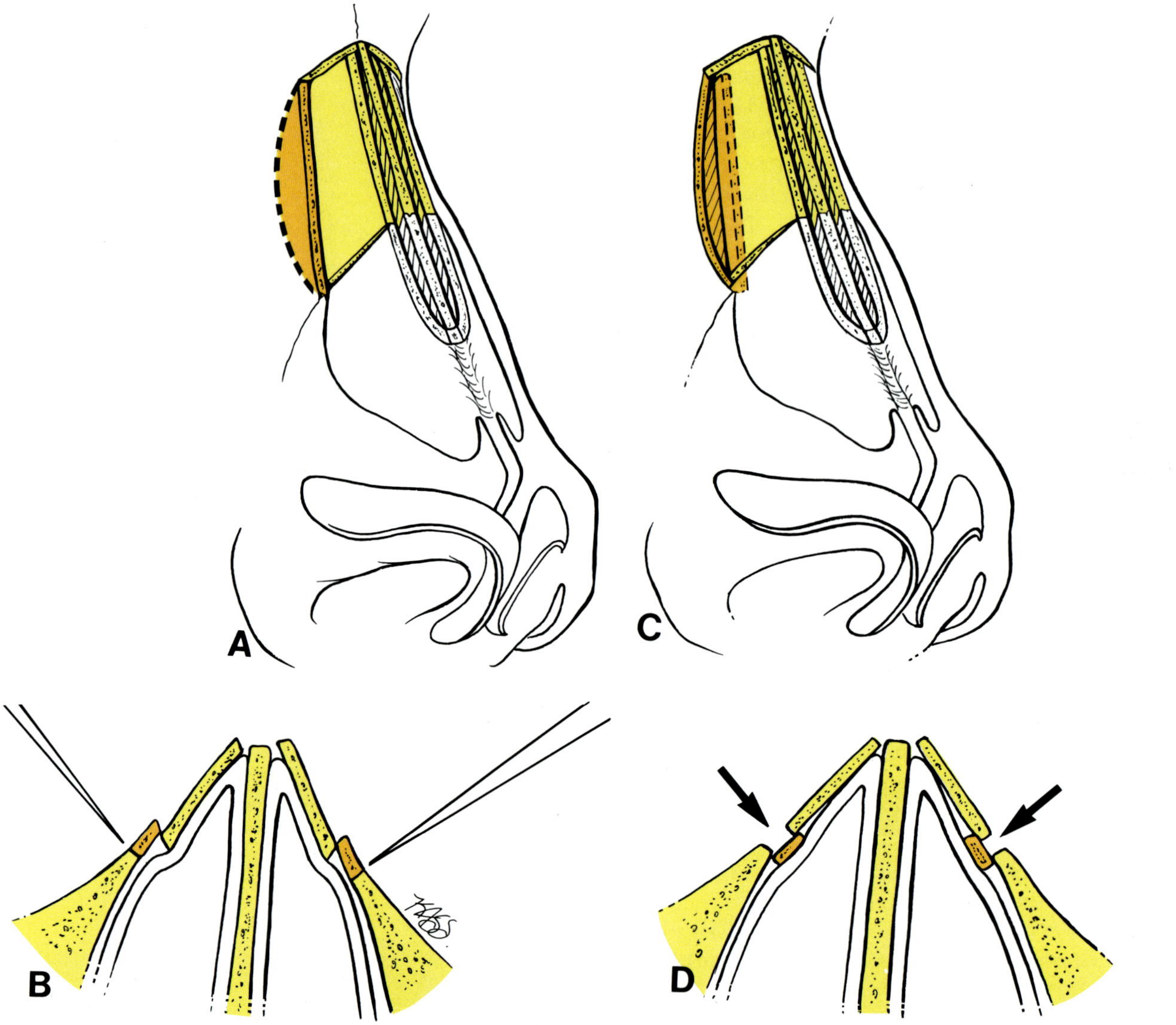

Fig. 25. If a stairstep at the lateral osteotomy line can be palpated, we have to reduce the osteotomy a few millimeters more laterally. (A) Outline of the new osteotomy. (B) New osteotomy shown in section view. (C and D) The obtained strip of bone is pushed towards the lumen.

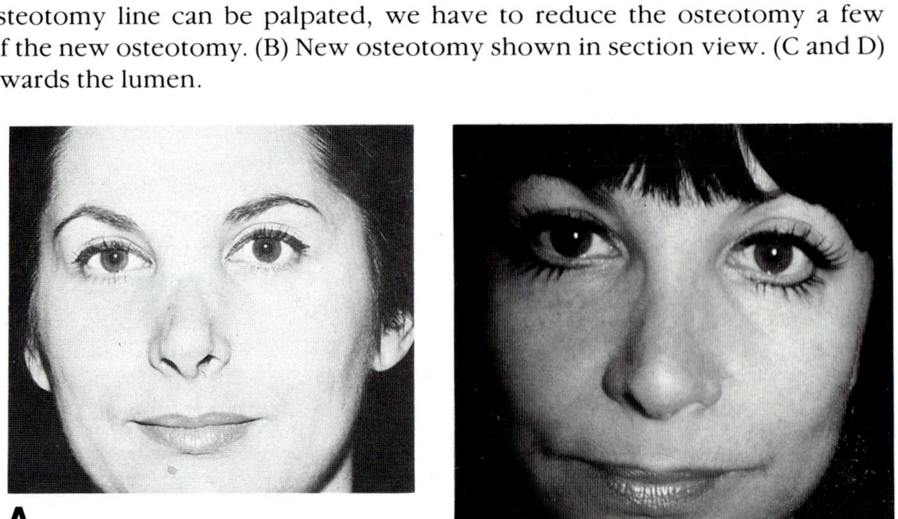

Fig. 26. Inadequate lateral osteotomy led to visible step formation at the osteotomy line. (A) The osteotomy had to be redone in a more lateral line. (B) Result of the secondary procedure.

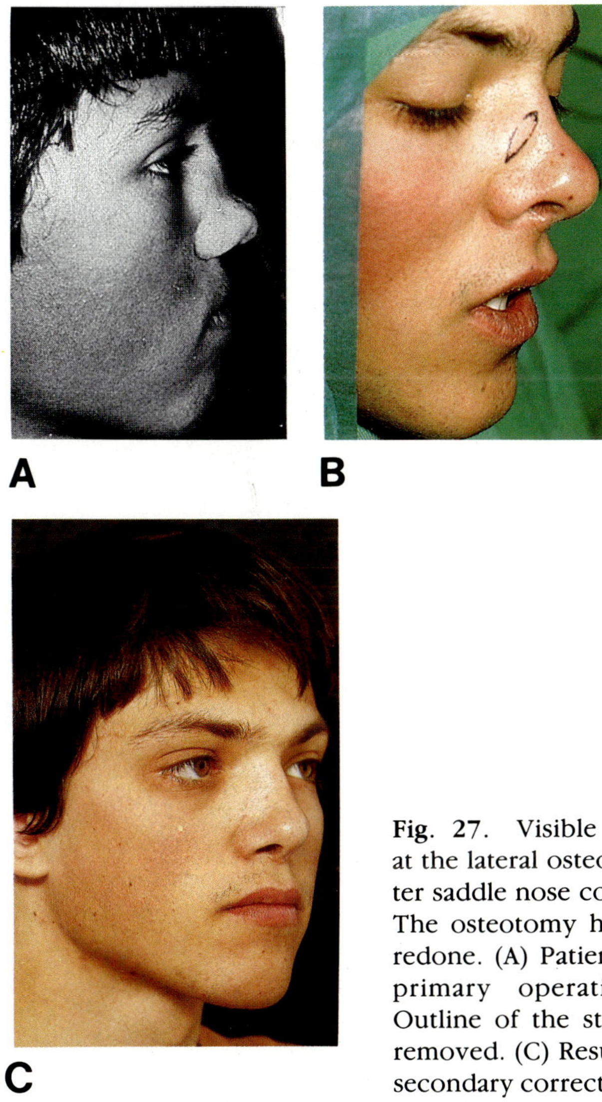

Fig. 27. Visible stairstep at the lateral osteotomy after saddle nose correction. The osteotomy had to be redone. (A) Patient before primary operation. (B) Outline of the step to be removed. (C) Result of the secondary correction.

for the symmetrical mobilization of the bones. It has to be approximately horizontal forming the small branch of an inverted L, the other branch being the lateral osteotomy.

The transverse osteotomy can be avoided by driving the lateral osteotomy medially toward the nasion at the Sulcus prelacrimalis of the frontal process of the maxilla. Such a curved line is difficult to achieve with only one incision. Another way to avoid the transverse osteotomy is to carry the lateral osteotomy in an oblique line joining one another in the nasion. This method, still used by some surgeons, can lead to unsightly bony deformities in the cranial part of the nose. For this reason we do not recommend it.

Instead of cutting the bone horizontally with an osteotome, many surgeons prefer to achieve this fracture by using only thumb pressure. For this to be possible, the upper ends of the paramedian and lateral osteotomies have to be quite close to one another, leaving only a short bony bridge for easy manual fracture. We consider that by doing so, one obtains too short a horizontal branch of the "L," not corresponding to our desired osteotomy line.

To obtain a clean and approximately horizontal osteotomy in the area of the naso-frontal suture may cause great difficulties. We use a curved chisel to carry out the osteotomy starting at the ascending lateral osteotomy line and extending to the midline toward the glabella on both sides. This osteotome is introduced through the intercartilaginous incision (Fig. 28). Other surgeons prefer a transcutaneous access as already mentioned (Fig. 24).

For performing a precisely controlled infracture of the lateral walls, Schrudde (1970) devised a special pushing and biting forceps, which he called a Rhinotome, which he introduced into the nose like a Walsham forceps). A similar instrument, a chisel forceps, was devised in 1981 by Straith. His goal was to create a proper L-shaped fracture without avulsing and tearing the periosteum and muscle attachment in the area of the nasion. Another similar forceps was described by Neves-Pinto (1983) for the same purpose of achieving a more precise and easier transverse osteotomy.

Rubin designed in 1969 a special nasofrontal osteotome to permit the surgeon to produce a transverse osteotomy and to impact parts of the superior nasal pyramid into the radix area while leaving the mucosa intact. Another similar instrument, a lateral osteotome, used to make the longitudinal cut of the lateral osteotomy, is introduced superiorly by the same author below the medial canthus and directed inferiorly without need of mucosal incision.

Incomplete lateral and transverse osteotomies and incomplete infracturing are among the more common postrhinoplasty problems. Refracture with eventual comminution of the bone complex helps to correct these problems.

After the precise approximation of the dorsal edges of the nasal bones by in or out fracture, it becomes obvious whether the transverse osteotomy is truly horizontal, or oblique, or whether a wrong fracture line with medial spur formation has occurred, which may happen especially with thick bones. Maliniac (1947), Barsky (1950), and Koechlin (1951) first pointed out the possibility of this mistake. Such a spur must be resected with the curved chisel and removed subsequently with the Luer or Levignac biting forceps (Figs. 29 and 30). The lateral fracture line can be too short, leaving the upper part of the nose too wide. It can be lengthened in the revisional procedure in the same way, continuing the primary osteotomy upward guided by its groove until it reaches the requested level. To ensure proper secondary reosteotomy when the primary lateral osteotomy in the upper part and the transverse osteotomy have failed, Bruck (1981) introduced a narrow chisel through a stab incision in the glabellar region.

Mobilization of the Bones

After separation of the bones on all sides we can proceed to the mobilization and medial realignment of the two bony plates. If they appear too large, one should resect a straight strip from the median edge with small Kazanjian forceps, Luer forceps, or the bone biting bayonet forceps of Levignac. It is always important to check the smoothness of the superior edge of the converging nasal bones and septum to avoid overprojection of the septum. The septal edge must be covered by the nasal bones and any distortion must be removed with the rasp.

The dorsal edge of the cartilaginous septum may be trimmed if necessary. Should the upper lateral cartilage still be connected, it must be divided and the medial edge trimmed with scissors using an extramucosal technique.

The median realignment of the mobilized nasal bones with part of the frontal processes of the maxilla is accomplished either by thumb pressure or, when more resistance is encountered, with forceps. We usually try to bring the anterior or medial border of the nasal bones into the midline with gentle thumb pressure. The bone are also pushed medially at the lateral osteotomy sites. One must be sure that the mobilized lateral borders of the osteotomies are locked there and do not drop. This wedging occurring at the medial portion of the frontal processes must be achieved in the appropriate site of the lateral osteotomy, i.e., deep in the nasomaxillary groove in the region of the thick portion of the nasofrontal process. Should a step deformity arise, it can sometimes be corrected secondarily by comminuting the frontal process with an osteotome or by rasping away the bony ridge.

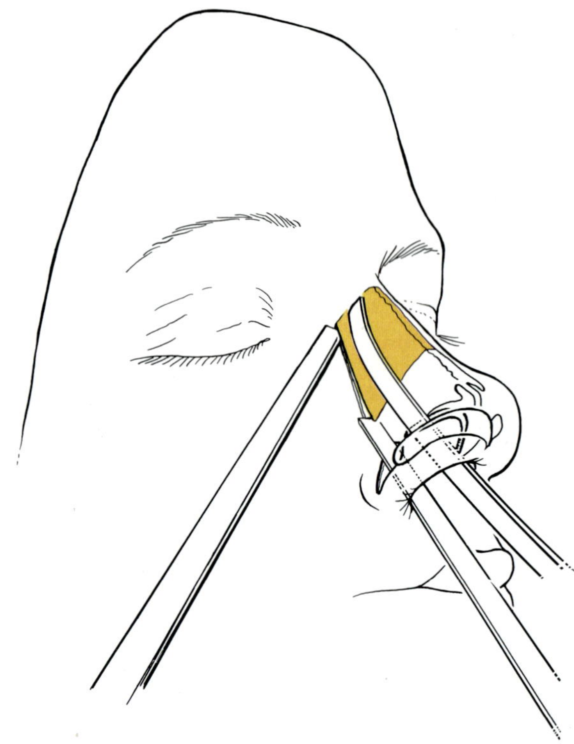

Fig. 28. Curved osteotome for transverse osteotomy through the intercartilaginous incision. Straight osteotomes for transvestibular or transcutaneous lateral osteotomy.

There is the danger in many primary cases of mobilizing the lateral walls too much, thus excessively narrowing the nasal cavity, especially when the nasal bones are very convex. According to Wright (1963), the narrowing of the bony pyramid without stenosis can be achieved by producing vertical fractures of the nasal bones so that their caudal portion can be packed away from the septum while the upper and middle portions are kept narrow. Where narrowing of the airway has already been produced in a previous nasal plastic procedure, the caudal half of the bony pyramid can be outfractured separately.

The nasal cavity may also be further narrowed postoperatively when the lateral walls are pulled down into the nasal cavity by progressive scar contracture, as Straith (1981) has pointed out. In these cases the depressed lateral walls have to be repositioned. There are situations in secondary rhinoplasty where we have to correct a bony pyramid by performing longitudinal osteotomies parallel to the lateral osteotomy.

A saddle nose can result from too much infracturing of the nasal bones so that they drop

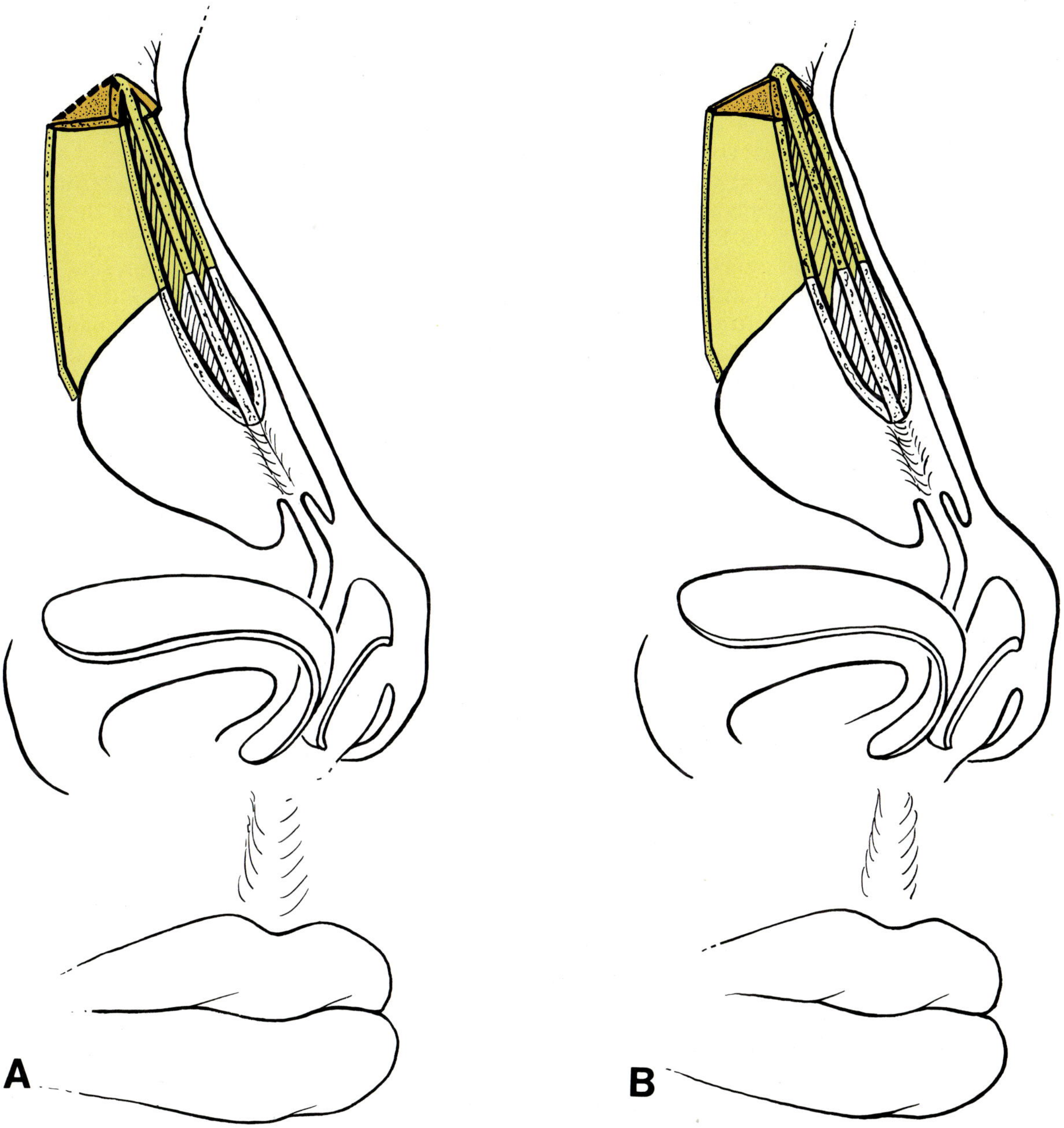

Fig. 29. Inadequate transverse osteotomy with incorrect fracture line and medial spur formation. This can occur essentially in thick bones. The osteotomy has to be redone. The spur must be mobilized and realigned or removed subsequently with the Luer of Levignac grasping forceps. (A) Spur formation with visible step. (B) Realignment of the mobilized bony spur.

Fig. 30. A 29-year-old man with sequelae of an incorrect lateral and transverse osteotomy and bony spur formation. (A) Preoperative front view. (B) Front view after revision and realignment of the bones in a secondary procedure.

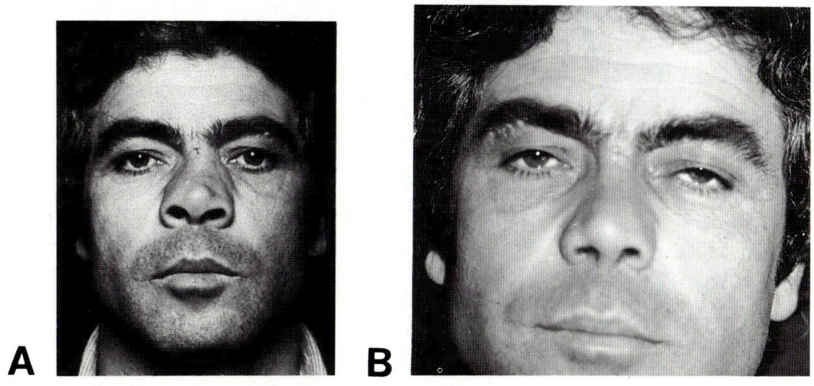

into the piriform aperture. That is why some surgeons (Rees [1973] and others) try to preserve the periosteum so that the soft tissue attachment can support the mobilized bones.

If the realignment of the bones cannot be achieved with thumb pressure, one has to use a Walsham, Ash, or Martin forceps (Fig. 31). The inner blade is placed against the mucosa at the nasal atrium (agger nasi) and the upper nasal cavity. The other blade is introduced into the subperiosteal pocket above the bone. One can feel the bone solidly between the two blades. The forceps is closed tightly and pushed carefully toward the midline. The lateral edge is tilted inward and then back again. This maneuver, called *infracturing,* can also be performed in the opposite sense, termed *outfracturing.* Most important is the careful inward setting and locking of the lateral edge of the mobilized bones as a final step.

In revision procedures, the mobilization and displacement of the nasal bones is not as easy as in primary cases. In order to bring the dorsal edges into contact with the septum we often have to use the Walsham or Ash forceps to mobilize the bones inwards or outwards.

One of the most common residual bony deformities is the protruding perpendicular plate of the ethmoid. Often this is not obvious until after 6 months following surgery. If it is accompanied by an "open roof" (see next column) in which a space or gap exists between the septum and the lateral walls, this hallmark of the operated nose may represent a real problem during revision. Simple rasping or nipping away of the protruding ethmoidal bone leaves an even broader flat bridge. Performing new osteotomies and correcting the open roof with adequate splinting are likely to make the protruding septum relatively more prominent, because the medial edges of the lateral walls move somewhat posteriorly and laterally when the desired medial movement takes place.

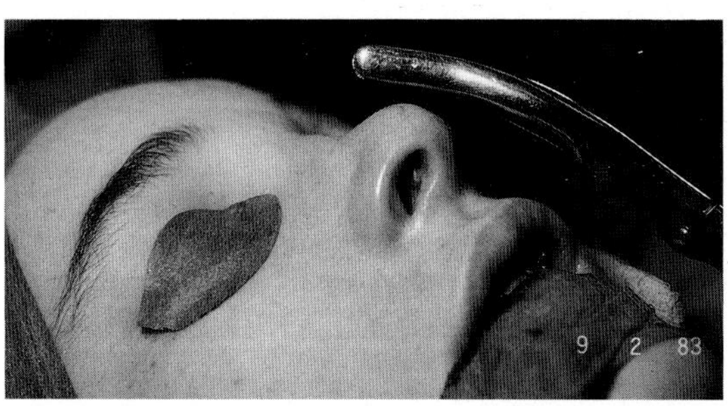

Fig. 31. Walsham forceps for repositioning of the mobilized bones in case of fracture and in difficult secondary realignment.

If the position of the nasofrontal angle and tip are such that the profile of the bridge can be projected forward with a cartilage or bone graft, a pleasing appearance may result, often providing the best result in many of these cases. If clinical and aesthetic judgment dictates that the profile of the bridge be retropositioned, the protruding ethmoidal bone may be shaved or rasped down. Any projecting upper lateral or septal cartilage can be trimmed and the septal bones rasped precisely.

The same rhinoplastic osteotomies and bone mobilization maneuvers are also appropriated for the correction of many posttraumatic bony defects in which the same anatomic components are involved by fracture. The ideal management of a recent traumatism consists of immediately reducing the fracture, immobilizing the fragments with packing, taping, and plaster, and splinting the eventually associated septal fracture. Occasionally, an excessive edema or hematoma may make immediate reduction undesirable. In such an instance reduction might still be attempted after some delay, during which time soft tissue is apt to subside.

Correction of Wide Flat Dorsum (Open Roof)

This deformity can be inherited or caused by trauma or by a poorly performed rhinoplasty. Traumatic or iatrogenic flat and wide noses usually have a heavy frontal process of the maxilla and the lateral nasal walls are placed too far apart from one another. They are joined in the midline by a wide flat bony plate, composed of bony callus formation and fibrous tissue.

Paramedian, lateral, and transverse osteotomies have to be carried out to permit the bilateral medial approximation of the bony walls. Fibrous tissue has to be removed. Instead of locking the free lateral edge of the mobilized bony walls below the maxillary edge of the lateral osteotomy, we place the medially displaced bone in a somewhat more vertical position in order to obtain a slight rise in the midline. This is especially desired in a low degree saddle nose deformity. This additional elevation should not be exaggerated at the cost of undesirable shaping of the nasal walls. One has to keep in mind that the bones at the osteotomy line will be drawn laterally by scar tissue formation in the postoperative period. A widening can thereby occur once again. For this reason the narrowed nose should be held in place for at least 10 days in a slightly exaggerated position by transnasal nylon mattress sutures or by a transnasal suture of tantalum wire, as described by Fomon (1954) and Nervert (1955). They placed the suture through the skin, the nasal cavities, and the septum, then subcutaneously to the midline of the dorsum where it again emerged from the skin.

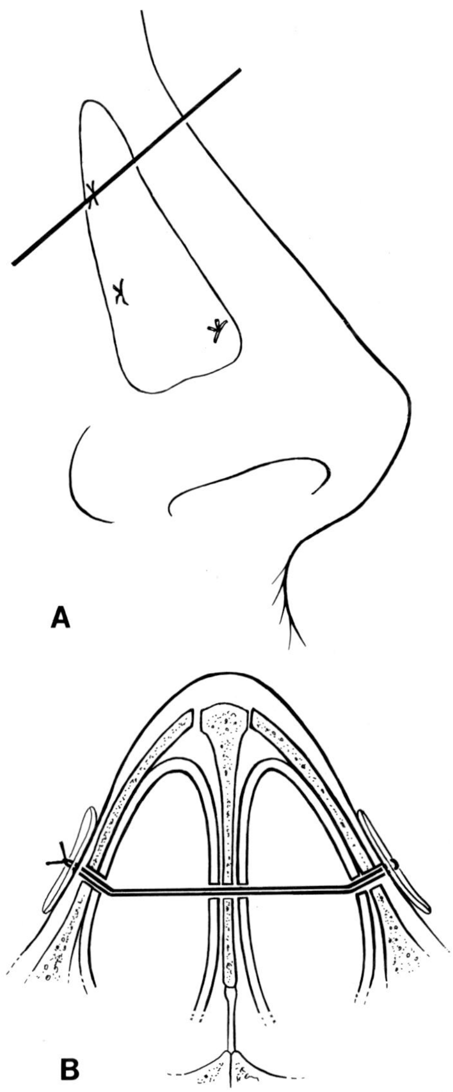

Fig. 32. Transnasal mattress suture for fixation of the narrowed bony pyramid. The thread is passing through the lateral osteotomy and through the septum. (A) Lateral view and (B) sagittal view.

We use mattress sutures in a similar way and tie them over a sheet of plastic material. For this purpose we use the plastic packaging of a suture turned on itself to provide a double layer. We place the sheets on the nasal slope and guide a straight needle of a 4-0 nonabsorbable suture (Prolene or Dermalone) through the sheets, the skin, and the dehiscence found at the lateral osteotomy line into the nasal cavity. From there we pierce the septum, and pass the thread through the opposite nasal cavity, bone gap, skin, and sheet. The needle is then introduced at a point 3–4 mm away to follow the above described route towards the other side. The two ends of the suture are then tied there over the sheet. The two bony plates are fixed in a slightly overcorrected position (Figs. 32, 33, and 34). We usually place two mattress sutures, one in the cephalic part and the other in the caudal part of the lateral osteotomy line or one at the level of the lower lateral cartilages. It is important to cut the excess plastic sheeting around the knot in a smooth fashion to prevent pressure marks on the surrounding skin.

This method of narrowing noses can be combined with the insertion of bone or cartilage grafts, or of implants in cases of saddle nose deformity. The treatment of these defects will be discussed later.

Bony Deviation

In cases of deviation of the bony pyramid, we proceed by performing all the usual osteotomies and by resecting a strip of bone from the dorsal edge of the overly large side. Many authors, such as Feuerstein (1985), correct such deviations by resecting bone at the lateral osteotomy site on the flatter side, which permits one to pivot the whole nasal pyramid toward that side. We prefer to manage the mobilization and displacement of the bony and cartilaginous elements of the pyramid by detaching them from each other and placing them in a new straight and equilibrated position (Fig. 35). As already mentioned, we perform paramedian osteotomies in all cases of bony deformities if a hump does not have to be removed. In addition to the deviation of the bony pyramid in crooked noses, one has to adapt the septum to the straightened position of the bones and upper lateral cartilages by scoring, cross-hatching, or resecting strips of it.

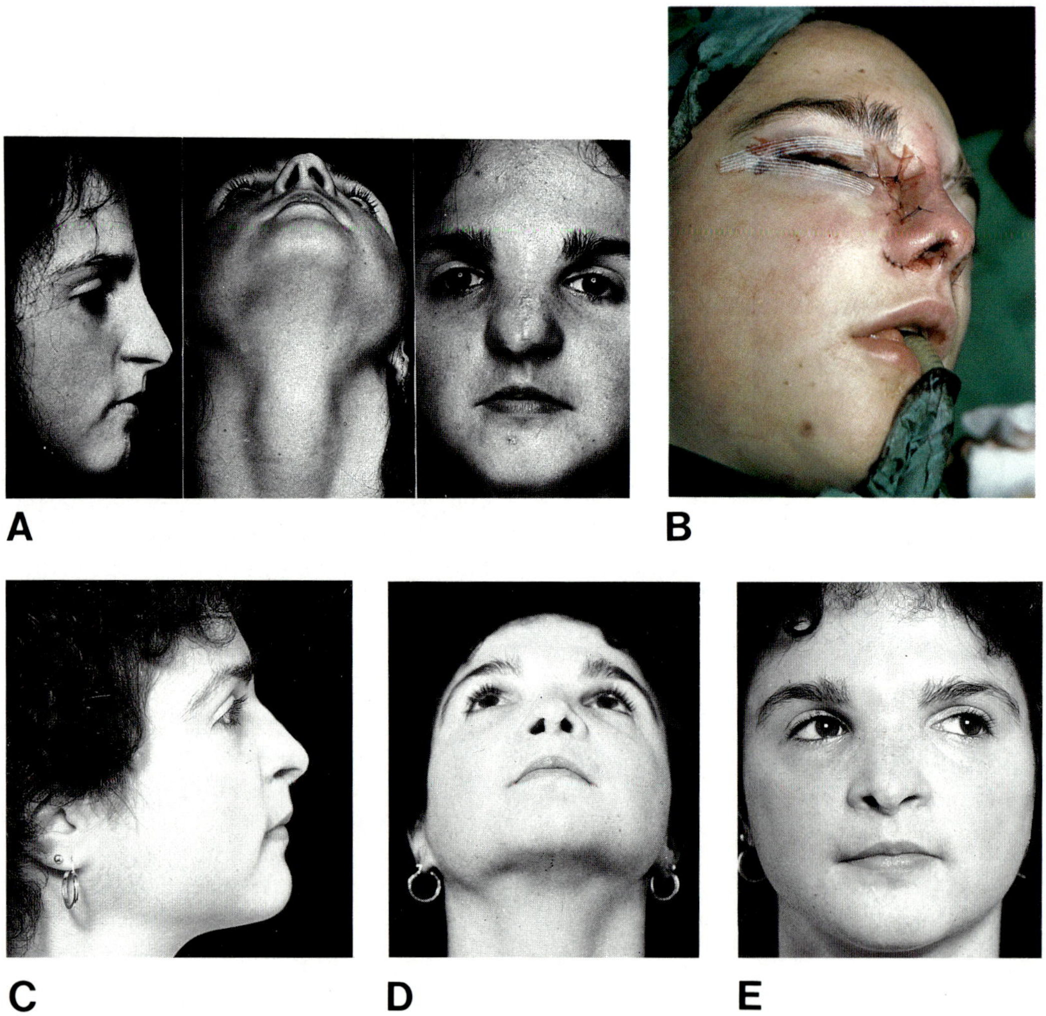

Fig. 33. Platirhyny and slight hyperthelorism corrected in two stages, the first for skin and median bone resection, the second for mobilization of the bone narrowing of the nasal pyramid, fixation of the bones with transnasal mattress sutures, as well as marginal alar resection and wedge resection at the alar base. (A) Preoperative view of the 18-year-old girl. (B) End of the second intervention. (C, D, and E) Late result after 1 year.

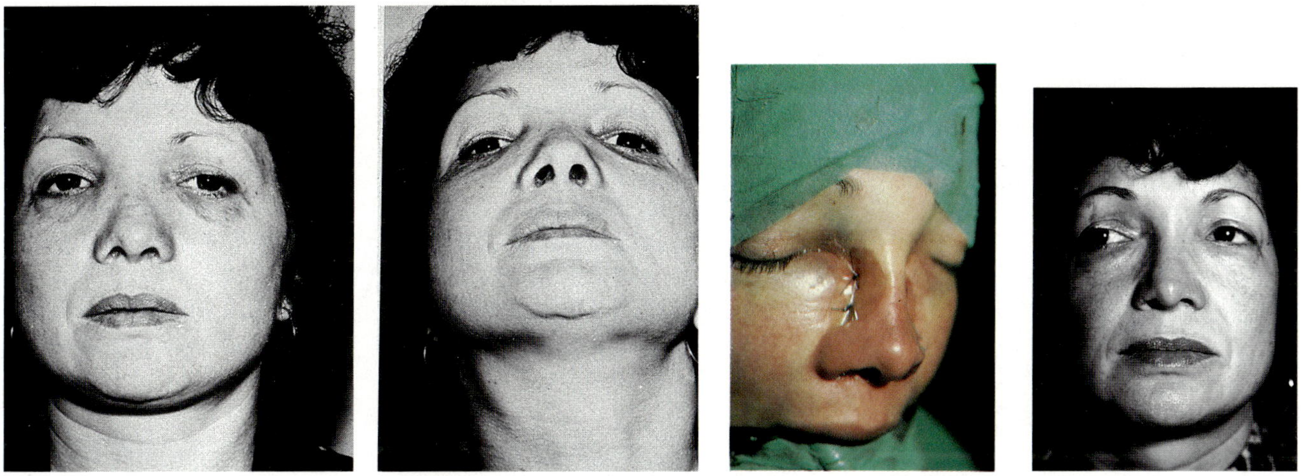

A B C

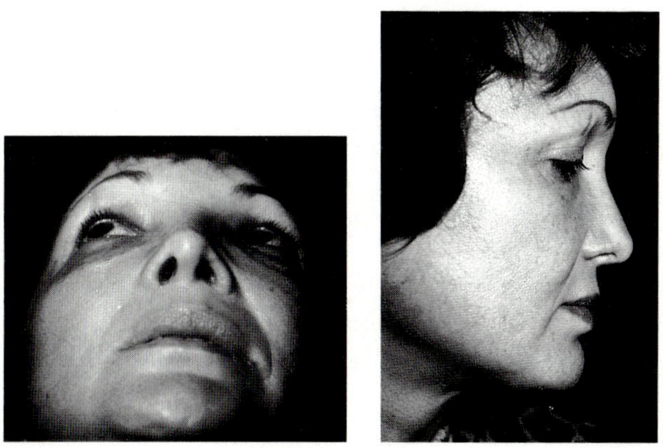

D E

Fig. 34. Secondary correction of wide flat dorsum by simple osteotomies, push-up of the nasal bones, transnasal mattress sutures passing through the lateral osteotomy dehiscences and the septum and plaster of Paris. The mattress sutures are removed after 7–10 days. The plaster is then renewed and left for another week. (A) A 35-year-old female after insufficient primary correction. (B) End of the revisional surgery with transnasal mattress suture tied over plastic sheets. (C) Postoperative front view. (D) Postoperative axial view. (E) Postoperative profile showing an acceptable prominence of the dorsum and tip projection.

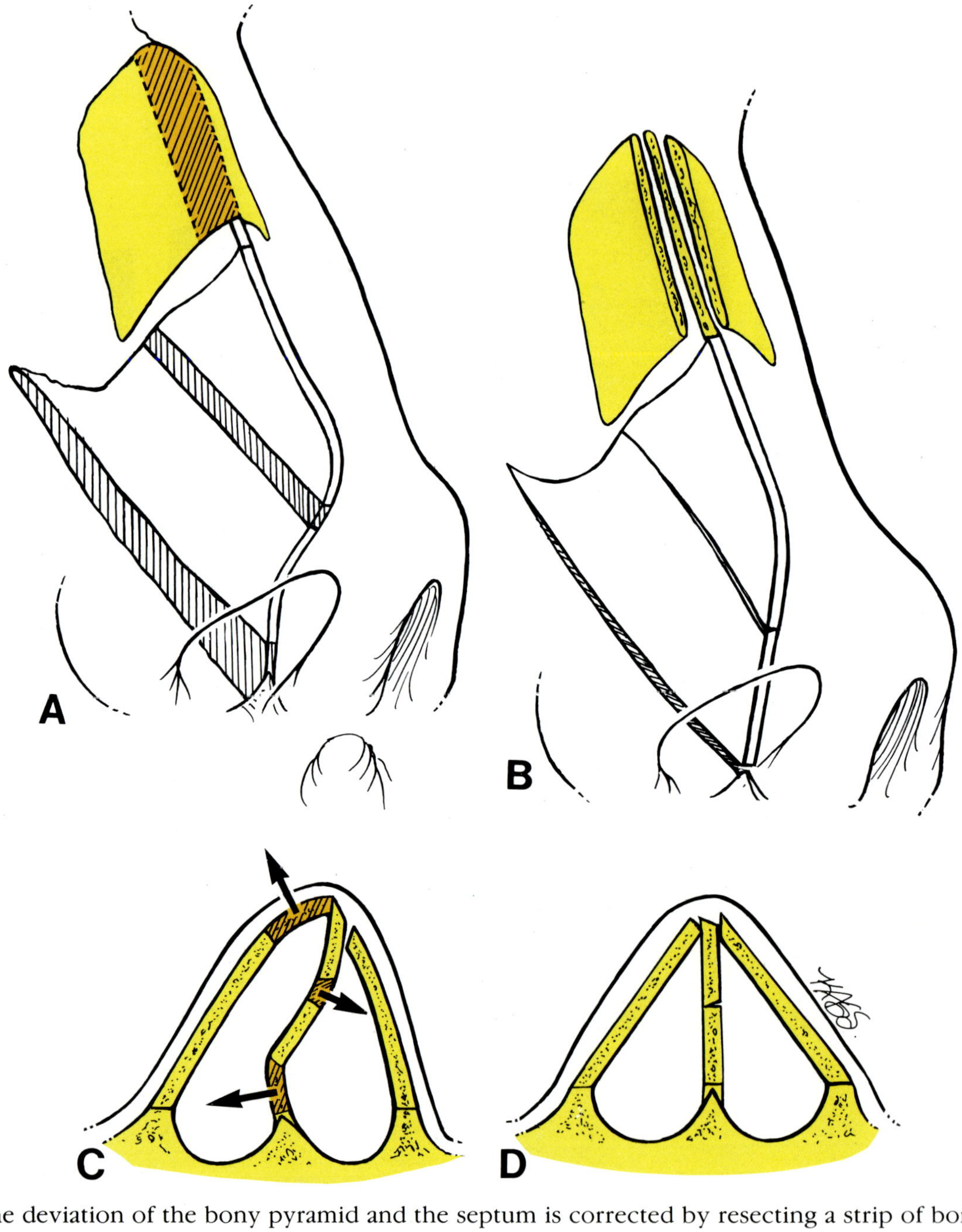

Fig. 35. The deviation of the bony pyramid and the septum is corrected by resecting a strip of bone of the too large side of the pyramid at the dorsal edge and not at the lateral base corresponding to the lateral osteotomy. One or two strips of septal cartilage are also removed for the adapted balance of the septal plate. (A and C) Strips of bone and cartilage to be resected. (B and D) Resulting straight position of the bony pyramid and septal plate.

The twisted nose presents either a C-shaped or S-shaped external deformity. In the first case, there is a lateral deviation of the nasal bones with a similar displacement of the nasal mid-third and a nasal tip that roughly ends up in the midline. The S-shaped deformity is similar in its bony upper-third, but then in the mid-third abruptly deviates to the opposite side of the midline and again the nasal tip ends up roughly in the midline.

In all cases, but especially in S-shaped dorsal deviation, it is important to section the upper lateral cartilages at their insertion into the septum using the extramucosal technique. These cartilages must be trimmed paramedially and placed into a symmetric position, as we shall explain later in Chapter 14. Sometimes we encounter patients with crooked dorsums combined with rare congenital, pronounced asymmetry of the face consisting of a displaced lower half. The face presents two parallel vertical midlines, one corresponding to the intercanthal midline and the other corresponding to the philtral and labial midline. After corrective rhinoplasty, the asymmetry of the face still remains and the nasal dorsum must follow a slightly oblique line in front view (Figs. 36 and 37).

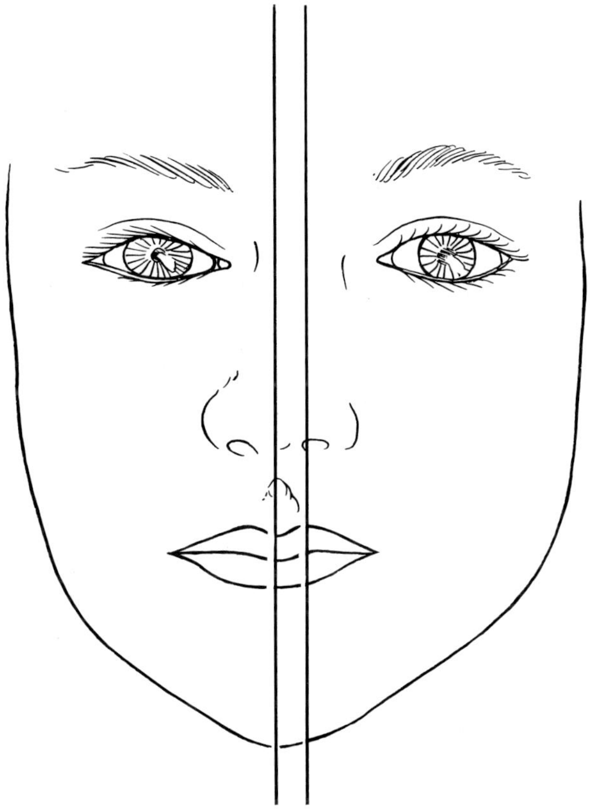

Fig. 36. Face with two parallel vertical axes one corresponding to the intercanthal midline and the other corresponding to the philtral and labial midline. This deformity can be congenital or acquired.

Nasofrontal Angle

The nasofrontal angle is obtained from a line drawn along the nasal dorsum and another line that intersects the glabella and the gnathion. Several craniometers have been devised to measure this angle. Many cephalometric studies have been carried out. In some cases, the nasal root presents an osseous hypertrophy that must be taken into consideration. Teleradiography or xeroradiography may be helpful in the study of these structures and in the evaluation of the amount of bone to be removed or added. No allowance is made for the slope of the forehead. The angle is not measured in the not too uncommon cases of macro or micrognathia.

An aesthetically desirable nasofrontal angle lies in the range of 30–35 degrees. It is frequently positioned improperly after rhinoplasty. Its shape and position should be related to the entire profile and especially to that of the forehead and brow profiles. Within limits it can change with the addition or substraction of bone or soft tissue or with implants.

The profile resulting from cephalometric measurement may not always correspond to the ideal, which complements the whole face and physiognomy. As Fontana and Muti (1983) have stated, there is no absolute and constant validity of geometrical measurements in rhinoplasty, although they are of fundamental importance in maxillofacial surgery. The profile as a whole must be harmonized by balancing the volumes and lines of the face as we do in profiloplasty. We have to correct not only the nasal profile and the nasofrontal angle but also the forehead and chin, with the necessary artistic sense and proper technical execution. Nasofrontal deformities mainly concern angles that are too shallow or aesthetically overly deepened.

A shallow ill-defined nasofrontal angle is by far the most common postoperative problem. Modifications are usually provided in conjunction with profile alignment and measures used to gain tip projection. The patient with a sloping forehead shows little improvement after a rhinoplasty unless the nasal root or nasofrontal angle is deepened. This surgical maneuver is very difficult despite the availability of numerous published techniques. The difficulty is primarily due to the thickness of the bone at the nasal root.

Marked thickness of the bone may prevent adequate narrowing at the radix; selective resection of a medial angle of the nasal bone with chisel or bone-biting forceps may be necessary to allow enough room for medial displacement of the bones during the infracturing. We don't use the lateral transcutaneous approach for deepening the angle as used by other surgeons. Excision of the procerus muscle and soft tissue in the region of the root of the nose may be sufficient to improve the too shallow or insufficiently deepened angle, but often bony removal is needed.

Since the skin is thicker at the nasion it has to be defatted. At the same time we may remove the subcutaneous tissue where the fibers of the pyramidal muscle end. We perform a more or less extended "procerectomy" in about 20 percent of our cases.

After total or subtotal removal of the procerus muscle, which may be helpful to further deepen the glabella, we use fibrin tissue glue at the end of the operation, applying the skin to stick to the underlying bone without dead space formation. By this perfect adherence of tissue we prevent effusions of blood and serum in an area where the pressure of the dressing and the plaster cannot always be efficient enough. The glue is inserted into the subcutaneous pocket by means of two syringes containing the two components (fibinogen plus calcium and thrombin [topostasin]) or with a double syringe, as explained in the chapter on complications (hematoma).

The Etruscan or Greek nose in which the nasal root continues uninterruptedly into the forehead is corrected by deepening the glabella-nasion area with a slightly curved osteotome as used to make the transverse osteotomy. Biting forceps may then remove the irregularities resulting from this difficult bone resection.

If the nasofrontal angle has to be corrected and the frontal prominence accentuated, a bone graft obtained, if possible, from the removed hump, can be placed at the desired height. In very narrow nasal pyramids the nasal bones may be pushed laterally after the osteotomies in order

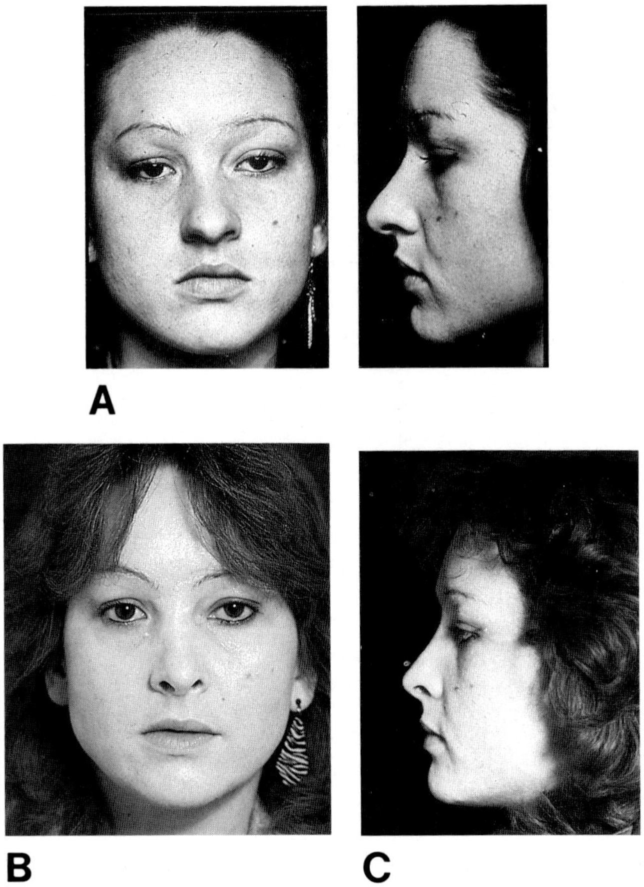

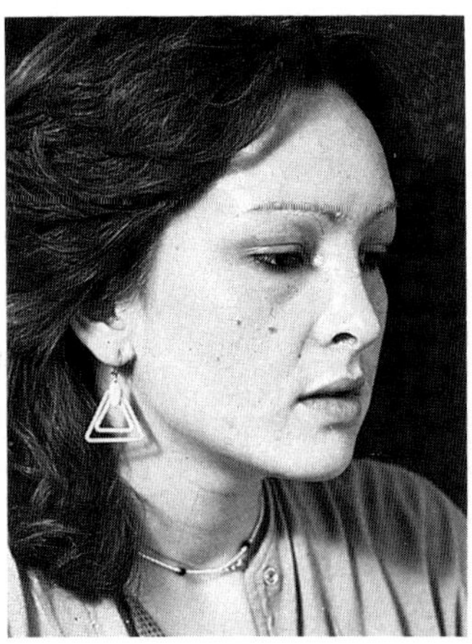

D

Fig. 37. Face of young female as example for a lateral displacement of the lower part, in this case traumatic in etiology. The intercanthal midline does not cover the vertical axis corresponding to the labial and philtral midline. The two axes are parallel with a delay of about 1 cm. The aesthetic correction cannot be perfect. The dorsum of the nose must have again an oblique position since the midline of the upper bony part has to remain exactly between the canthi, and the midline of the tip has to stay in the same vertical line as the philtrum and the middle point of the cupids bow. (A) Preoperative front and profile view. (B) Front view after septorhinoplasty with osteotomies and tip reshaping. (C) Postoperative profile. (D) Postoperative half-profile.

to diverge and cause them to overlap the maxillary bones.

An illusion of depth can often best be obtained by augmenting the glabellar region or by creating a forehead bossing with iliac bone "onlay" grafts or with silicone or proplast implants. It is important to maintain firm pressure at this site for at least a week in order to prevent hematomas and the later formation of fibrous tissue in the new bony crease.

The overly deepened nasofrontal angle may be a congenital condition or the result of excess bony hump resection, particularly when the forehead is too prominent. In order to reduce the glabella-forehead prominence the bone is incised using a straight osteotome after which a curved one, such as the one used for the transverse osteotomy, achieves the resection in a curved profile line (Fig. 38).

For decreasing the overly deepened angle, auricular or septal cartilage is an excellent source for autogenous cartilage and makes an ideal graft for this area.

Attempts to reduce the overly accentuated angle can lead to excessive lowering of the bony-cartilaginous pyramid combined with overcorrected hump removal leading to a bird's beak profile.

The concept of altering the nasofrontal area by decreasing the nasofrontal angle using a sliding nasal bone graft has been demonstrated by T. Smith (1981). This technique involves the

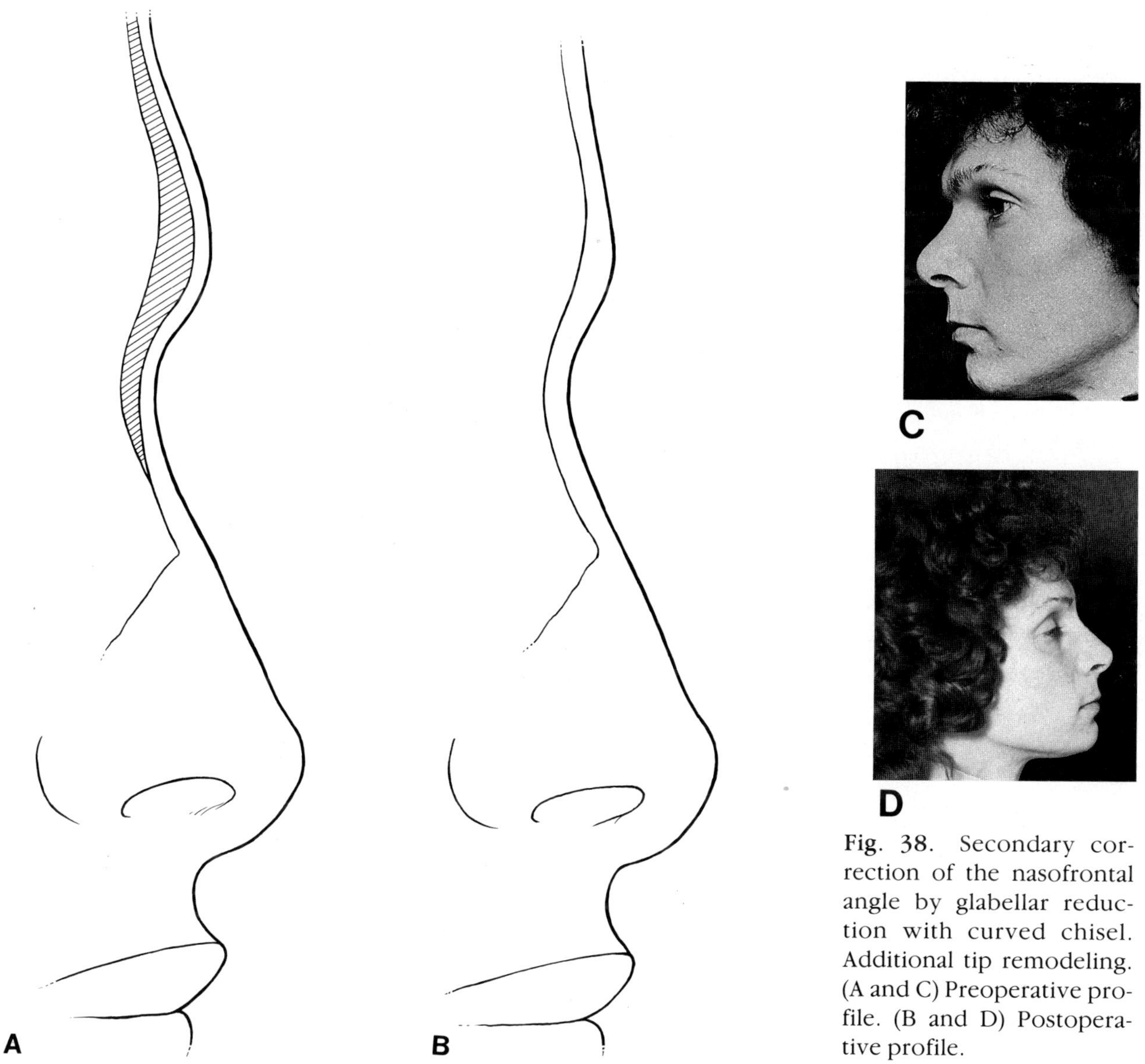

Fig. 38. Secondary correction of the nasofrontal angle by glabellar reduction with curved chisel. Additional tip remodeling. (A and C) Preoperative profile. (B and D) Postoperative profile.

usual dorsal skin dissection followed by progressive osteotome detachment of the nasal hump to its upper limit, leaving the periosteum on the bony hump and the procerus muscle intact. This muscle is not separated from its frontal attachment. The nasal hump with periosteum and pedicle of procerus muscle is then mobilized superiorly into the nasal spine area. We believe that the hump, when too large, must be reduced under the skin, leaving the upper attachment intact before being slid upward. This would then classify as a reduction and reimplantation in the way proposed by Skoog (1974), but only localized to the uppermost part of the nasal profile.

Lowering of the nasofrontal angle may produce shortening of the nose by an illusion effect. The poorly developed nasofrontal angle can be accentuated as well as lowered. Alteration to the nasofrontal angle can be accomplished with a chisel, a special nasofrontal gouge, a rasp, and the rotating burr, as we have advocated in the book by Denecke and Meyer published in 1965/1967.

We currently use the burr only in exceptional cases to smooth out irregularities at the upper transverse osteotomy and to deepen the nasofrontal angle. Goodman (1981) also found that the rotating burr greatly facilitates the modeling of the nasion area. The Aufricht retractor improves the visualization and the ease of this maneuver especially when combined with an open rhinoplasty using the decortication technique of Rethi. Once again we would like to state that excessive lowering of the nasofrontal angle and excessive hump removal lead to a "bird's beak" profile. This deformity has to be corrected by the use of a bone graft as we will see in Chapter 13.

12

Residual Deformities of the Cartilaginous Framework

INTRODUCTION AND GENERALITIES

Deformities of the cartilage are often more difficult to correct than those of the bone. External deviation of the nose in the lower part after rhinoplasty may be due to deviations of the dorsal border of the septal cartilage, forming a C- or S-shaped curve. We classify deflected noses as: (1) deformities restricted to the external nasal skeleton, (2) deformities of the inner skeleton, and (3) deformities affecting both. All three categories can be encountered in postrhinoplastic deformities. In the first and third categories it is necessary to bring the displaced nasal bone into normal position by means of the usual osteotomies and by paramedian wedge resection on the side where the nose is too wide. The deflected nose can have a residual hump. This hump then has to be removed in the usual way, assuring the same asymmetrical resection of a strip of bone on the flatter side of the bony pyramid, as for the simple crooked nose (see Chapter 14).

Along with the work on the external bone, it is also important to adequately mobilize the cartilaginous and bony septum. This should be done with the extramucosal technique that we use for all primary and secondary septal deviations and nasal deformities. We believe that particularly in secondary procedures and for correction of the crooked nose with septal deviation the *extramucosal method* is extraordinarily helpful.

We proceed as follows: After having separated the mobile from the stable part of the nose by undermining the skin over the upper lateral cartilages and bony framework we extend the cartilaginous incisions into the transfixion incision between the membranous and cartilaginous septum down to the anterior nasal spine. We then separate the septal mucoperichondrium from the cartilage beginning at the transfixion incision by using hydraulic dissection as already explained. In secondary rhinoplasty, the dissection of the skin from the upper lateral cartilages with fine blunt scissors and the subperiosteal elevation of the skin over the dorsum is usually much more laborious than in primary cases. For dorsal dissection we utilize our suction elevator, as mentioned before. At the level of the weak triangle of Converse in the supratip area we join the intercartilaginous incision with the transfixion incision. Any scar tissue of an operated tip can make this maneuver difficult with an ordinary knife or a Joseph's button-ended-knife.

If an approach to the anterior nasal spine is necessary, we enlarge the transfixion incision with scissors placed at the base of the columella, at the spine level, sectioning the fan-shaped depressor septi nasi muscle. This maneuver separates the mobile part of the nose, which consists of the tip, the columella, and the alar cartilages from the stable part, which is the bony frame, the upper lateral cartilages, and the septum, as mentioned.

In about 80 percent of primary and secondary rhinoplasties, the rhinoplasty is combined with a septoplasty. In these cases of septorhinoplasty we dissect over the basal crest of the maxilla and vomer along the floor of the nose and backward over the whole area of the bony septum. This is done on both sides to provide good vision and to facilitate the correction of the deflected cartilaginous and bony septum. The deformed septal cartilage is cut vertically and brought into a midline position while the bony deviation is corrected by fracture and replacement. If some of the cartilage has to be removed in the anterior and upper part of the septum, the resection should not be carried too far dorsally, otherwise the remaining cartilaginous bridge might be too thin, leading to a duck beak deformity. The removed cartilage or some bony strips from the posterior aspect of the septum can be reimplanted in a straight position between the perichondrial sheets. If the deviation is in the antero-inferior part of the septum, we incise the cartilage parallel to the edge of the vomer some 3 mm away from it and remove the freed cartilage strip along the vomerine groove. Multiple incisions in the deviated portion of the cartilage lead to a straightening of the septum in this region.

In cases of subluxation of the septum at its basal edge, we obtain the swinging-door effect of Metzenbaum (1929) and Seltzer (1944). Several parallel perpendicular incisions mobilize the septal cartilage, which is necessary for straightening. Cartilage should only be removed if necessary to improve the airway.

Too radical a submucous resection of the ethmoid plate and vomer as well as of the septal cartilage is ill-advised during septorhinoplasty, because of the hazard of collapse of the nasal pyramid into the pyriform aperture. Instead of removing parts of the septum, the crooked nose once mobilized should be corrected by repositioning the cartilaginous fragments or by fracturing the perpendicular plate. If bony fragments are completely mobilized, they are reimplanted and kept in situ by gluing with Fibrin sealant and by packing while reimplanted cartilaginous strips are held in place by gluing or transseptal mattress sutures. For this purpose we use a nonabsorbable suture on a straight or curved needle to stabilize the reconstructed septum in a sagittal position reinforcing it with bilateral packing.

In some cases of secondary septorhinoplasty we find a defect in the cartilaginous and/or bony support of the septum. The extramucosal approach is then particularly useful to facilitate the difficult separation of the mucoperichondrium and mucoperiosteum from their lateral counterparts and the interstitial fibrous tissue present at the site of loss of cartilage or bone.

The extramucosal technique is indicated for the crooked nose with severe septal deviation and asymmetric position of the upper lateral cartilages, which we occasionally encounter in this difficult secondary procedure. We advise surgeons to use the extramucosal technique, even if it does not belong to their routine regimen. As we shall discuss later, the extramucosal technique is indispensable for surgical correction of septal perforations of up to a diameter of 3 cm.

In the anterior part of the septum, both mucoperichondrial leaves are approximated with mattress sutures. They are tied in the nasal cavity by the knot sliding maneuver.

At the end of the secondary correction we have to make sure that all osteotomies that had to be repeated after incomplete or inadequate primary fracturing are this time complete and adequate on both sides and not "green stick" fractures with persistent fibrous adhesions. We have to ascertain that the septum no longer exerts unilateral pressure to the bony vault of the nose. The paramedian osteotomy and the section of the upper lateral cartilages from the septum has to be especially complete, because failure to correct the dorsal cartilaginous and bony arch would again be a cause for late recurring deviation and crookening of the dorsum months after the revision procedure, even if the nose was symmetrical at the conclusion of the operation. For the same reason, the bony as well as the cartilaginous medial transposition should be overcorrected, i.e., at the end of the operation the nasal dorsum has to deviate slightly to the opposite side. This dogma is more important in revision cases than in primary rhinoplasty. The overcorrected nose must be kept in the new position by the dressing and splinting. The dressing and plaster should be left for at least 10 days or, even better, 2–3 weeks. Due to the swelling of the skin, the plaster might have to be changed after a week to 10 days. The second splinting should then tend to overcorrect less.

DEFORMITIES OF THE CAUDAL EDGE OF THE SEPTAL CARTILAGE

After hump removal, we proceed to further corrections of the stable part of the nose, the quadrangular cartilage, in order to vertically shift the nasal tip by the visor flap mechanism of the lower lateral cartilages (Fomon, 1960).

At the limen nasi not too much cartilage and especially limited vestibular skin should be trimmed to avoid an ugly retraction of the ala. An overlapping of cartilage and vestibular skin or mucosa can still be resected at the end of the procedure. We must always keep in mind that no gap should occur in the inner vestibular lining.

Now one can perform the border resection at the septal cartilage (Figs. 39 and 40) to the extent necessary and in the shape desired for shortening and reducing the nose. The amount of excision of septal cartilage requires a certain amount of experience. An overcorrection would lead to a hidden columella. The level of the columella should always be 2 or 3 mm beyond the alar border.

The length of the nose is determined primarily by the length of the septum and secondarily by the soft part of the nasal tip. The reduction of the caudal border of the septal cartilage, which forms a ridge, defines the new dorsal contour. The line of resection should be an extension of the line formed by the bony dorsum.

The extent of the border resection at the caudal edge of the septum is determined by the planned retrusion of the columella for shortening the nose. One must overcorrect to a certain degree. This is done because the soft parts of the nasal tip and the columella tend to undergo a slight ptosis even months after the operation. If the nasolabial angle is satisfactory before the operation, (i.e., at least 90 degrees) then a rectangular strip of cartilage can be resected along the caudal edge (Fig. 39). The line of the excision should run parallel to the former border. If the angle is too acute, which is usually the case with long noses, a wedge-shaped piece with its point toward the maxillary spine is excised along the edge (Fig. 39 D). In an opposite manner, a wedge of cartilage with its flat end toward the spine must be removed from the edge of the cartilage if the nasolabial angle is too obtuse and the upper lip too short (Fig. 39 E). In these cases, we find the anterior nasal spine enlarged and quite prominent. This requires its removal at least in part with chisel or with the Luer or Levignac bone forceps.

The nasolabial angle must harmonize with the rest of the profile. With a slightly prognathic jaw, for example, or with strongly receding chin the angle should not exceed 90 degrees. In general it may be larger in women than in men, especially in women with very delicate features (Fig. 39). An exaggeration of the obtusity of the angle leads to a retroussé nose, which fits with the rest of the facial contour only in very rare cases (Fig. 41). An increase in the nasolabial angle can be achieved when refining the tip-columella region at the end of the operation, but it can also be prepared initially by cutting the septal border according to the lower border of the medial crus after the lower lateral cartilage is reduced as required. The new line of the caudal border of the septal cartilage should have an angle in the anterior third (Fig. 39 F).

To avoid pronounced postoperative drooping of the nasal tip, we cut a small depression in the dorsal border of the septal cartilage (Lipsett, 1959), just above the nasal tip (Fig. 39 A). This should take up any excess subcutaneous tissue. In relation to the dorsal line, the tip must be very slightly prominent in order to give the nose an attractive shape. The depression in the cartilage in the supratip region reduces the danger of postoperative formation of a so-called polly beak with a small hump above the tip.

To prevent postoperative sagging of the base of the columella and upper lip, we utilize the lip-freeing technique of Fred (1955) (see Fig.

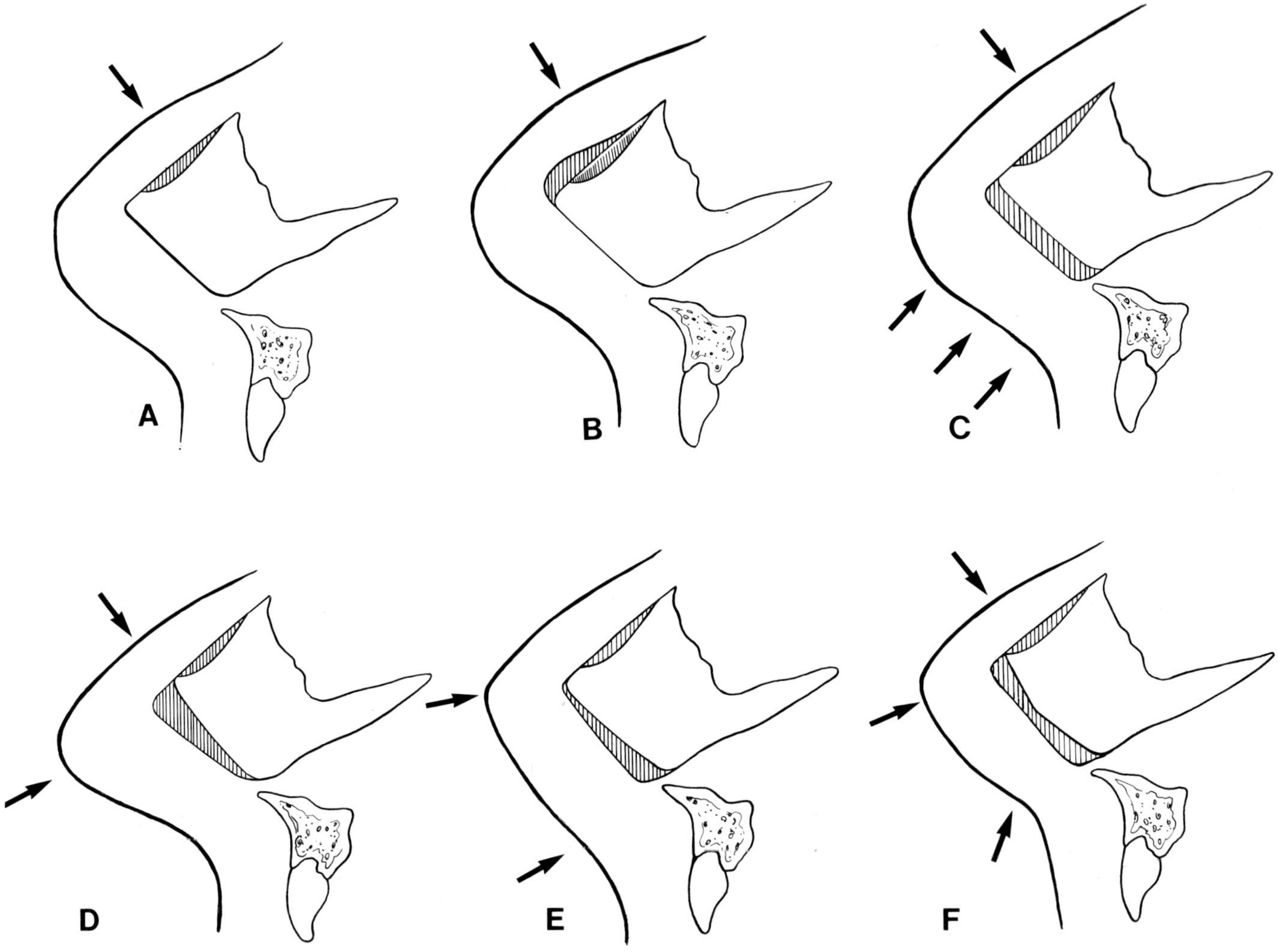

Fig. 39. Trimming of the septal cartilage. (A) Lipsett depression in the supratip area. This has to be emphasized in secondary polly beak correction. (B) Tip-supratip trimmed to be performed in cases of too prominent tip and supratip swelling. (C) Lipsett depression and inferior border resection for correction of supratip swelling and sagging of the columella. (D) Lipsett depression and anteroinferior resection of the septal border for cases of drooping of the tip and supratip swelling. (E) Lipsett depression and basal resection of the inferior septal border for correction of too obtuse nasolabial angle. (F) Lipsett depression and appropriate trimming of the inferior septal border for producing a double angle and for correction of supratip swelling.

113). The upper lip and the base of the columella is occasionally stretched too tightly against the anterior nasal spine, giving an open-mouth look to the lip. The typical anomaly of the tethered upper lip is usually associated with the hump nose deformity and a prominent nasal spine (see Chapter 15).

SUPRATIP DEFORMITIES

A common poor result after rhinoplasty is a supratip curvature in the region of the "weak triangle" of Converse. After complete reduction of the nose, a hard soft hump occurs just above the tip, the parrot's beak of Sarnoff (1950) and Lenz (1954) or *polly beak.* This can be the result of inadequate technique but also may occur unpredictably even to the most experienced surgeons. Thus, Rogers (1972) states that "there is probably not a plastic surgeon alive, no matter how competent and experienced, who has not suffered the disappointment of having more than several patients present themselves following primary rhinoplasty with a parrot's beak." Millard (1969) puts it: "Even when special precautions are taken, it surreptitiously creeps into being. Instead of the bridge running gracefully straight until it takes a slight kick-up at the end of the tip the bridge rises in a slow well-rounding off into a hook at the tip."

Generally speaking, we distinguish two kinds of such a supratip elevation: the polly beak of the novice and the polly beak of the experienced surgeon. For us, even after over a quarter of a century in aesthetic surgery, rhinoplasty being one of our major interests, always paying attention to surgical detail, with routine long-term follow-up, participating in courses on advanced rhinoplasty, and debating in detail with other experienced surgeons, the supratip still remains a dilemma dependent upon an individual's characteristics and upon the unpredictable nature of the postoperative healing process. There remains some uncertainty as to whether the cause of the supratip deformity arises from too much tissue being removed in the supratip area, leaving a dead space with resulting overproduction of subcutaneous fibrous tissue, or from too much subcutaneous tissue or cartilage being left behind producing a supratip prominence.

There are many causes of failure in managing this delicate area. For this reason, before proceeding to a secondary correction, a precise di-

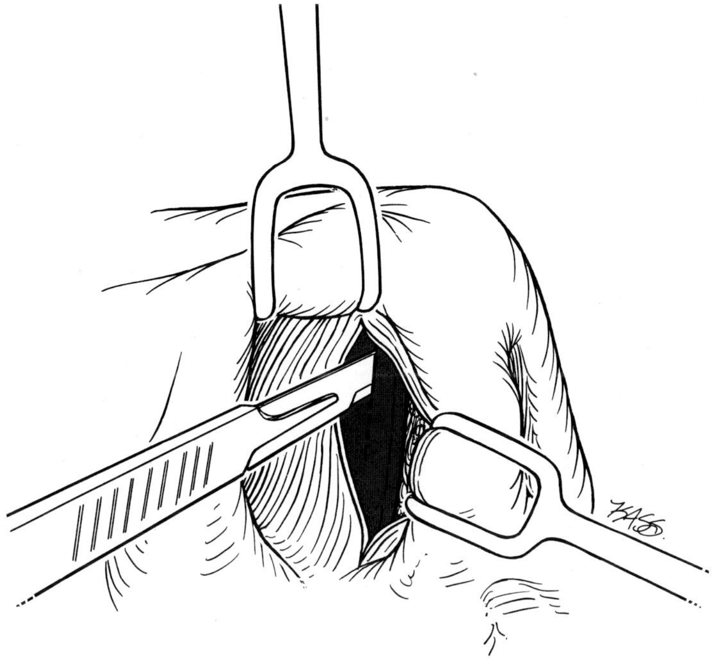

Fig. 40. Strip resection at the inferior septal border.

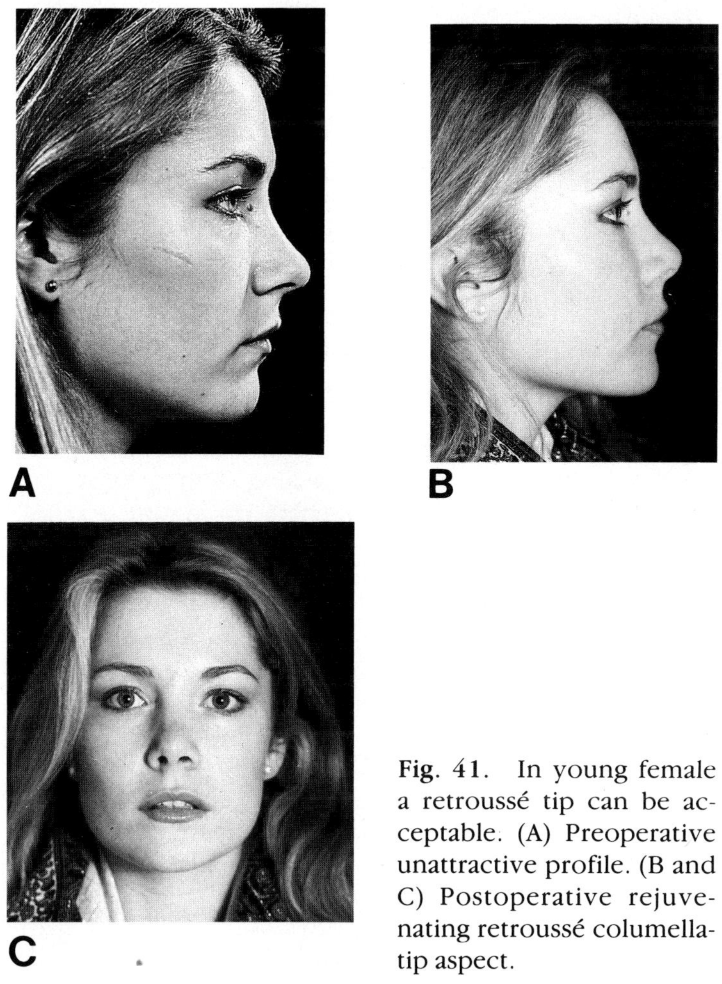

Fig. 41. In young female a retroussé tip can be acceptable. (A) Preoperative unattractive profile. (B and C) Postoperative rejuvenating retroussé columella-tip aspect.

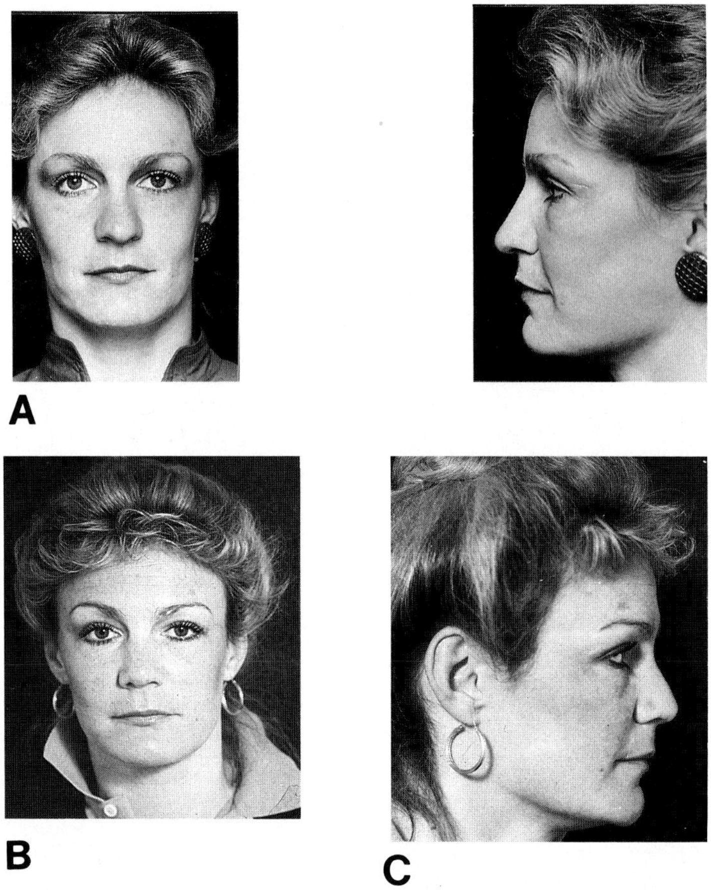

Fig. 42. (A) This woman shows a hooked drooping tip with a straight columellar-lobule profile. (B and C) It is corrected in a secondary procedure with tip and columellar onlay grafts from the septum obtaining a double beak in the new profile.

agnosis must be made, and this is only possible when time for final healing of the primary surgery has elapsed, which means about 1 year.

Among the principal elements present at the weak triangle in the dorsal or supratip region are the septal cartilages, upper lateral and lower lateral cartilages, and the procerus, transverse, and lower lateral portions of the nasal muscle, which support the tip. All these structures may be involved in the supratip deformity. The most usual of the causes are: (1) insufficient lowering or trimming of the dorsal border of the septum; (2) insufficient trimming of the dorsal borders of the upper lateral cartilages; (3) insufficient trimming of the septal mucosa; (4) excessive resection of intranasal lining; (5) excessive resection of the lower lateral cartilage domes; (6) short columella; (7) misplaced or misshaped grafts or implants; and (8) inherent thickness of the skin and subcutaneous tissue.

Insufficient Lowering of the Septum

If the septal dorsum is not sufficiently lowered, a postoperative convexity of the supratip area results. To prevent this after removal of a nasal hump one also removes a strip from the septal cartilage just above the caudal anterior angle. The surplus subcutaneous tissue can then sink into this recess. Lipsett (1959) even recommends cutting a small notch in the cartilage at this point. The Aufricht scoop undertaken in the dorsum to obtain space for telescoped skin is precisely the same maneuver as the Lipsett depression.

At the end of a primary rhinoplasty there must exist a slight depression just above the nasal tip and in secondary procedures this depression must be even deeper. This area is determined by segments of the lower lateral cartilages and can subsequently fill with connective tissue. If at the end of the operation one leaves a straight dorsum just above the tip, then a hump is unavoidably formed by fibrous tissue filling in the supratip region due to the lateral compression of the dressing. The hump is then very difficult to eliminate after removal of the dressing. It is even necessary to emphasize the slight depression just above the tip by means of tight horizontally placed strips of adhesive tape. Careful application of the adhesive tape dressing is very important. One must avoid forming too large a dead space in the "weak triangle," i.e., in the depression of Lipsett. This is especially true if thick skin, which adapts poorly to the underlying tissues, is present.

This overcorrection of the septal profile line has to be exaggerated in patients with a preoperative hooked tip, as Millard (1969) recommends, assuming that they have a greater chance to develop a postrhinoplasty parrot's beak. The primary hooked tip is encountered in patients with a short columella, while in the secondary nose the cause is a failure in tip protrusion and columella lengthening (Fig. 42). Lowering the projection of the cartilaginous portion of the septal dorsum interferes with tip definition, like the shortening of the cartilaginous septum at the anterior-caudal angles and leads to a polly-beak.

Insufficient Trimming of the Dorsal Borders of the Upper Laterals

The insufficient trimming of the dorsal border of the upper lateral cartilage has already been discussed as one of the possible deformities after removal of the nasal hump.

Insufficient Trimming of Septal Mucosa

If in a primary rhinoplasty the hump is resected without using the extramucosal technique, the septal mucoperichondrium must be trimmed lower than the dorsal border of the septum, otherwise it may grow over the dorsum to unite with the opposite mucoperichondrium and become interposed between the skin and the septal cartilage. This is one of the reasons why the extramucosal technique is advantageous, since there is no cutting of the mucoperichondrial vault under the cartilaginous arch of the upper lateral cartilages, at least not in the caudal part of that vault. It is, however, obvious that when using the extramucosal method one has to be careful when pushing the preserved mucoperichondrial vault toward the lumen in order to avoid interposing it in the roof. This danger is minimized by leaving the vault intact. On the other hand, in the posterior or cephalic part of the nasal cavity, resection of the mucoperiosteal vault is of no importance because in that region one must only pay attention not to produce an open roof by perfectly aligning the bones.

At the level of the supratip groove of Lipsett, Bruck (1981) stabilizes the weak upper lateral cartilages by through and through catgut suture going from one side, across the septum to the other side. By choosing this technique, we would be afraid to add to the scar formation in this dangerous area. Through one nostril, Jost (1973) sutures the two mucoperichondrial walls together in the midline, covering the anterior-superior edge of the septal cartilage. In doing so he tries to avoid parrot's beak formation.

Excessive Resection of Intranasal Lining

This fault of the primary surgeon leads to scar retractions in the vestibules and compensatory scar hypertrophy in the soft tissue found between the upper and the lower lateral cartilages. The correction involves careful removal of the scar tissue and in extreme cases the vestibular lining may need restoring with skin grafts or small composite grafts taken from the inner aspect of the crus helicis of the ear.

Excessive Resection of the Lower Lateral Cartilage

There are cases in which the dorsal profile cannot be lowered as much as desired because of underdevelopment of the nasal tip. One then has to rebuild the tip, sculpturing the lower lateral cartilages, which in cases of parrot beak deformity have been altered by too aggressive reduction. One finds a lack of lower lateral cartilage that has been insufficiently proportioned in relation to the profile.

To prevent this failure some authors (Rees [1973], Wright [1972], and others) recommend shaping the nasal tip before reducing the dorsum in patients with thick skin. The lack of tip projection due to excessive resection of the lower cartilages at the dome has to be compensated with struts as a support, with additional modeling provided by mattress sutures in the remaining stumps of the lower lateral cartilages. The concomitant advancement of the columella after rearrangement of the lower lateral cartilages is provided by inserting a batton of cartilage, as we will explain later on.

Short Columella

The failure to elongate the columella and advance the tip of the nose produces a supratip elevation with a hooked tip. In secondary surgery these corrections must be done utilizing all technical possibilities available in the same way as is used to correct excessive resection of lower lateral cartilage.

Misplaced or Misshaped Grafts or Implants

This complication can occur in the supratip area as well as in any other region of the nose where bone or cartilage grafts have been applied. We shall discuss this as it relates to the problems seen in augmentation rhinoplasty (see Chapter 13).

Inherent Thickness of the Skin and Subcutaneous Tissue

In these cases the supratip swelling is accentuated by fibrous tissue formation in the dead space between the dorsal skin and the septal border. The thicker the skin of the tip and the dorsum the more obvious the deformity will be.

This deformity can be considered as being unpredictable to a certain degree. It is this soft tissue that can cause a polly beak deformity even after a rhinoplasty carried out by the best of specialists. Sometimes one has to correct nothing else but this type of parrot's beak some 6 months to 1 year after the primary surgery by removing fibrous tissue from the weak triangle of Converse through bilateral intercartilaginous incisions.

In such cases we inform the patient that a third intervention may possibly be necessary in spite of all the efforts to eliminate the source of the distressing uncontrollable tissue growth. Such a secondary operation limited to the supratip area can be done in certain cases on an out-patient basis.

We reduce the excessive fibrosis and thickening of the supratip skin using the eversion or retrograde access technique through an intercartilaginous incision. Beginning on the right side this incision is enlarged, with the knife cutting obliquely through the fibrous tissue in a bevelled way toward the border of the nostril, preserving meticulously the skin lining the lateral vestibular wall. The lower border of the intercartilaginous incision is grasped with a retractor and pulled downward until the cephalic border of the residual lower lateral cartilage is exposed. We dissect the external surface of the remaining cartilage from the thickened skin with small blunt scissors, extending the incision to reach fibrous tissue situated over the antero-caudal angle of the septal cartilage, and if necessary we remove some of the upper border of the alar cartilage. From there we carry the intercartilaginous incision through the fibrous tissue into the membranous septum, reaching the posterior edge of the medial crura of the lower lateral cartilage through this transfixion incision. We always use this transseptal incision and extend it below the flared end of the medial crura. We don't believe that it compromises support, as stated by Anderson (1976). Always preserving the vestibular skin at the domes, we continue the incision and dissection of the anterior dorsal border of the septal cartilage where we create a depression of that border according to the notch of Lipsett. At that point a strip of cartilage has usually to be resected together with the scar tissue. The sharp dissection is then continued over the upper lateral cartilages up to the point where the dorsal profile is adequate.

The extent of scar tissue removal in the membranous septum and columella is defined at the beginning of the intervention. Behind the lobule there is rarely fibrous tissue that has to be removed. This delicate and meticulous maneuver is repeated on the opposite side until the under surface of the skin is completely freed from the underlying skeleton of the stable part of the nose.

Now we proceed to the most dangerous and delicate part of the correction, the undermining of the skin in the tip and supratip area, which has to be kept in the right layer, not too far and not too close to the dermis. Again we use fine blunt scissors and begin just behind and cephalic to the very top of the tip, the region where in primary surgery we cut through the superficial fascia that supports the tip-columella complex (Fig. 43). This aponeurosis of the procerus and trans-

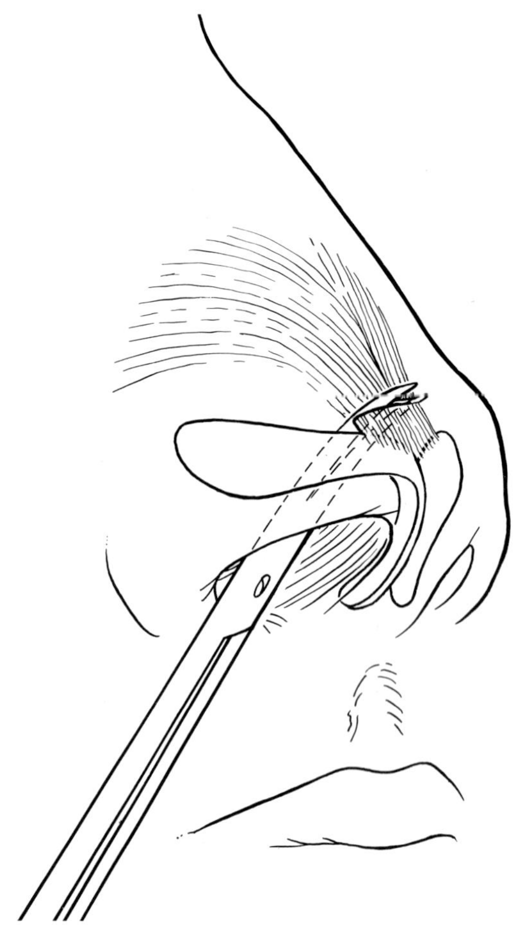

Fig. 43. For freeing the tip, we cut the dorsal aponeurosis in the supratip area.

verse nasal muscle which converge and join the medial end of the lateral crura was erroneously called a dermo-cartilaginous ligament (Pitanguy, 1965, 1982), as we mentioned in Chapter 5. The section of this aponeurosis in the weak triangle of Converse is a tip freeing maneuver that cannot cause tip drooping. It gives a certain degree of independence to the tip-columella complex. Its section is important in primary as well as in secondary procedures, because it allows the shifting up of cartilaginous and soft structures of the lobule. Once the skin of the whole supratip area is completely freed from the fibrous subcutaneous layer and its pliability reestablished, the scar tissue complex can be removed like a tumor together with the detached strip of cartilage from the Lipsett supratip notch of the septal cartilage. This small piece of cartilage will eventually be useful as graft for supporting the tip. Ashley (1976) advocated a double wing excision of scar, soft tissue, and septal dorsum for secondary supratip hump correction. We do not resect any tissue at the very tip and use our two-pocket procedure.

We proceed to restore projection of the tip after having emptied the supratip area. To this end we shape the strips of cartilage from the septum or lower lateral cartilage into a triangular or trapezoid graft and introduce it into a superficial pocket at the top of the nasal tip, which we create through a small marginal incision at the anterior border of the columella. The pocket in the tip and lobule should not communicate with the presently empty supratip dissection (Figs. 44 and 45). The anterior pocket with its cartilage graft shifts this area forward, accentuating the protrusion of the tip. At this point in the procedure the profile of the dorsum, tip, and columella is checked and eventually perfected by reimplanting small strips of cartilage longitudinally in the supratip area.

We stabilize the nose with Scanpor tape, which is somewhat more elastic than Micropore tape. In the supratip area we apply slight pressure on the skin in order to adapt it to the depression of Lipsett in the septal cartilage (Fig. 46). Long-term taping of 2 weeks is sometimes necessary. A small plaster of Paris splint helps to slightly exaggerate the new profile across the supratip depression.

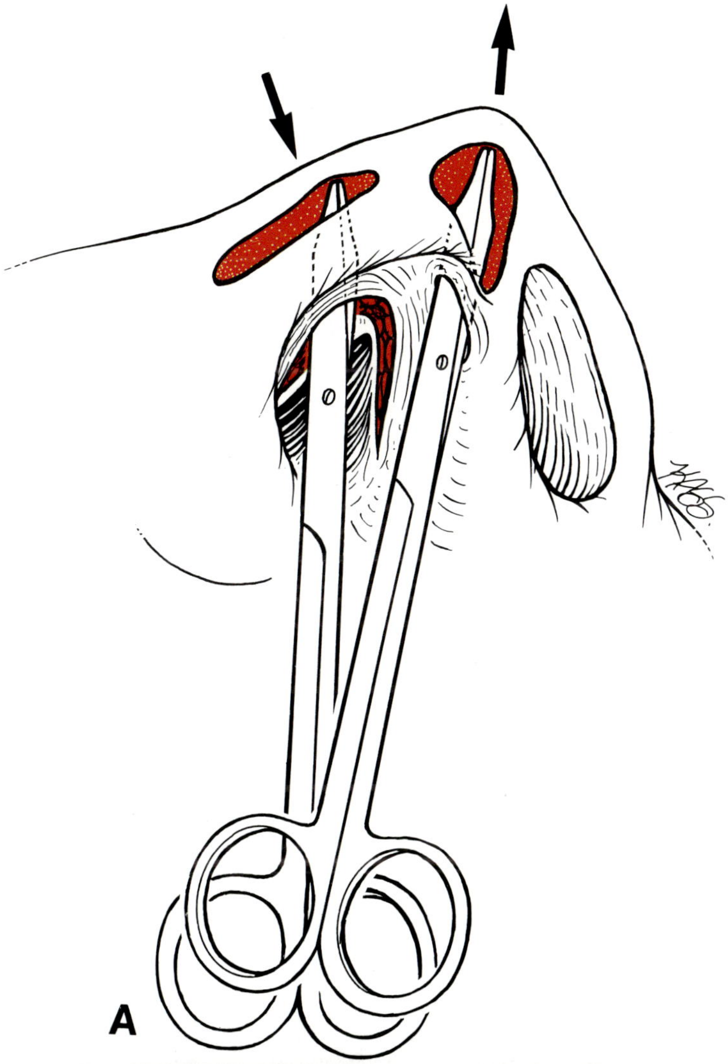

A

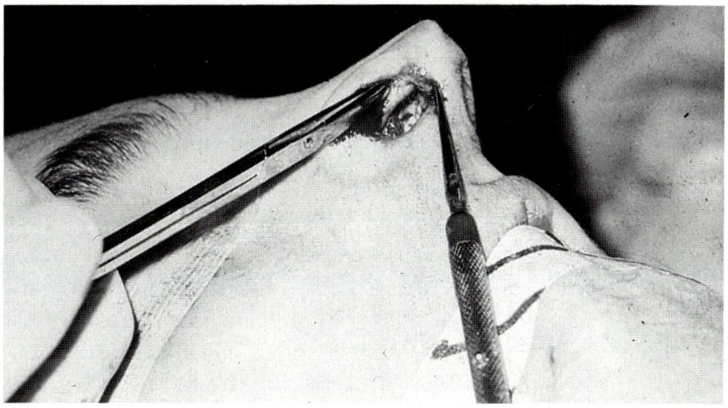

B

Fig. 44. (A and B) Formation of two subcutaneous pockets, one in the supratip area for removing the fibrous tissue producing the polly beak and the other in the tip-lobular area: The first one is achieved through the intercartilaginous incision, the second through an incision at the columellar border.

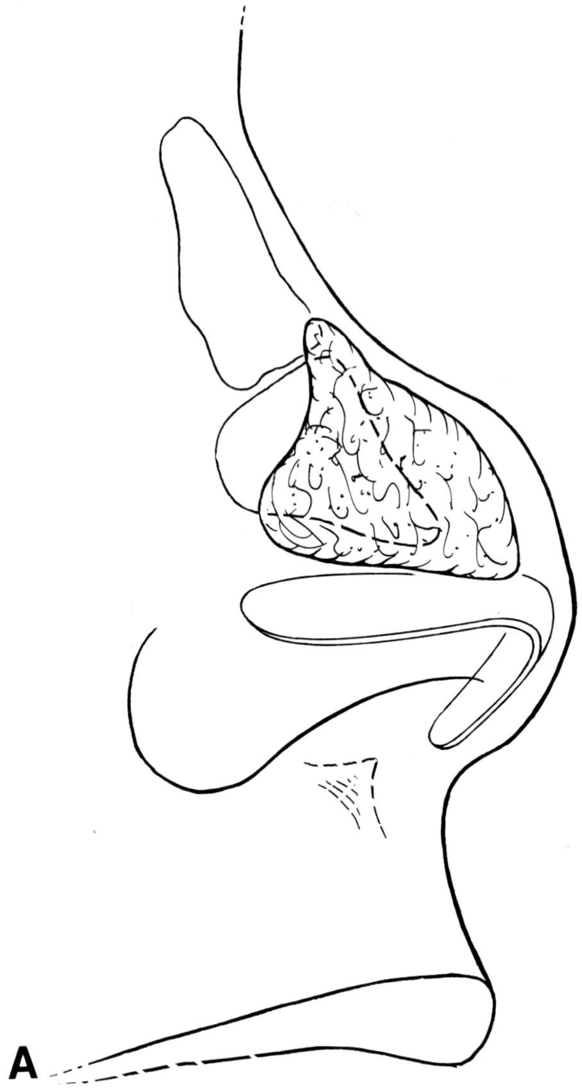

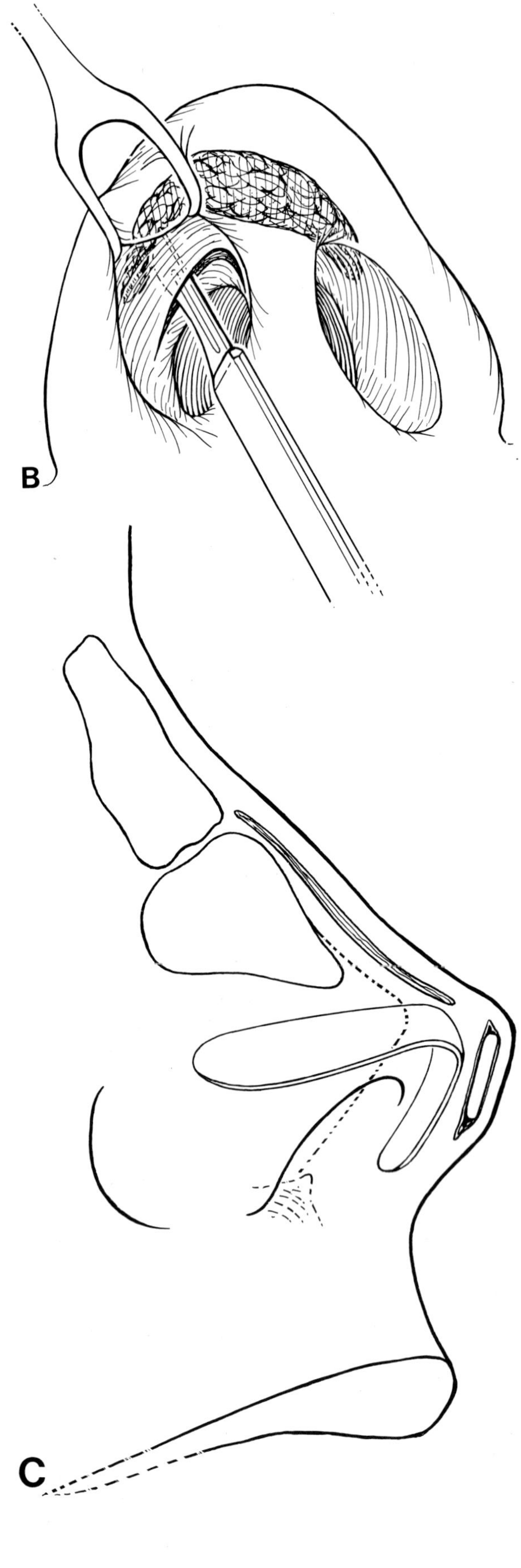

Fig. 45. Correction of polly beak. (A and B) Retrograde bevelled dissection from the intercartilaginous incision freeing the part of the remaining lower cephalic lateral cartilage with supratip fibrous tissue. This dissection is extended with blunt scissors toward the caudal border of the remaining upper lateral cartilage then further cranially between these cartilages and the skin freeing the whole mass of fibrous tissue that is grasped with a moskito clamp and removed through both intercartilaginous incisions. (C) Supratip pocket is emptied. A strut of cartilage is placed into a tip-lobular pocket to increase tip projection at the end of the revisional intervention.

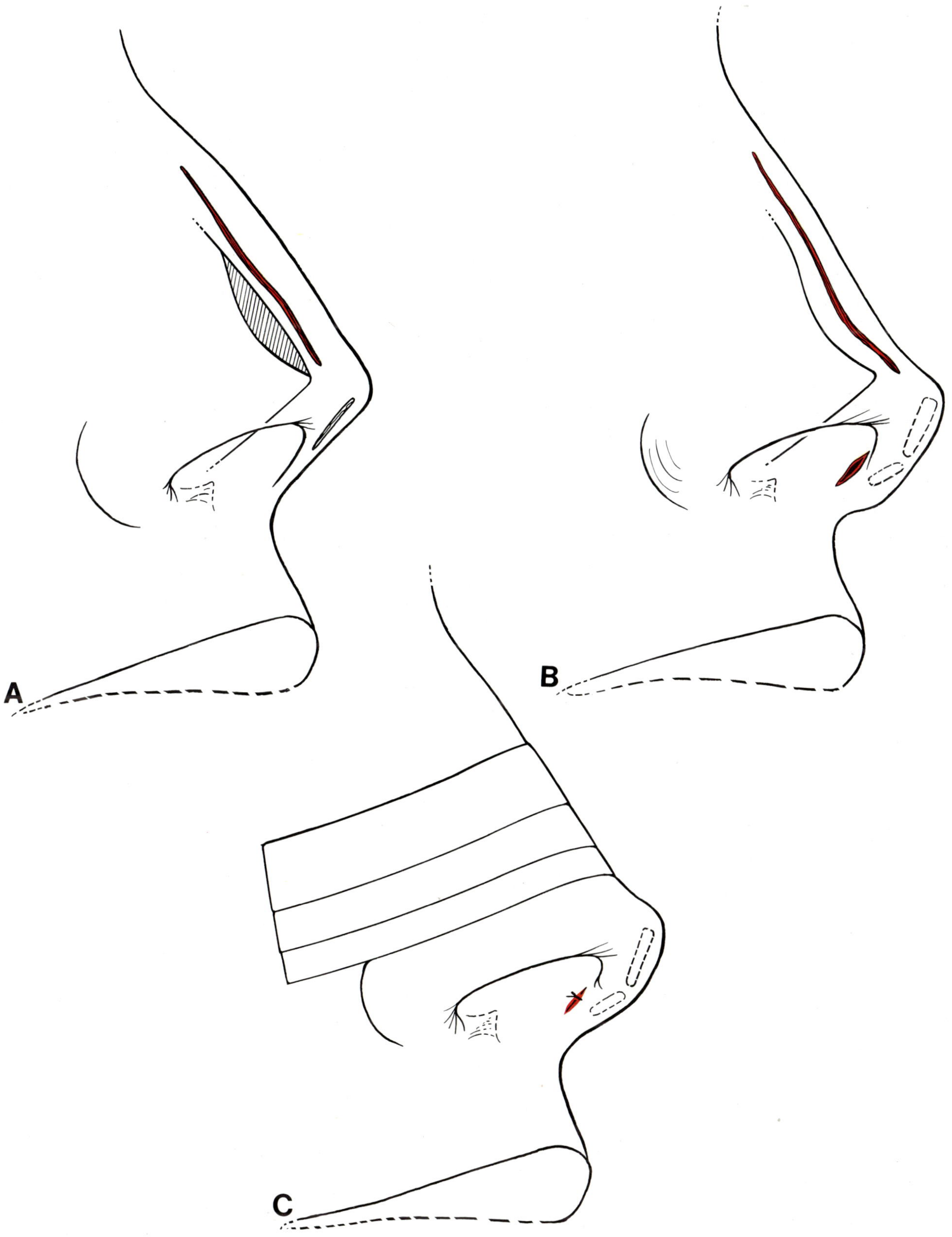

Fig. 46. (A) After removal of the supratip fibrous tissue we cut a slight depression in the antero superior border of the septal cartilage, which should take up the excess of subcutaneous tissue. (B) The supratip pocket is emptied and the tip-lobule pocket is filled with a tip onlay cartilage strut and another cartilage graft for accenting the double angle. (C) The supratip depression is emphasized with scampor tapes.

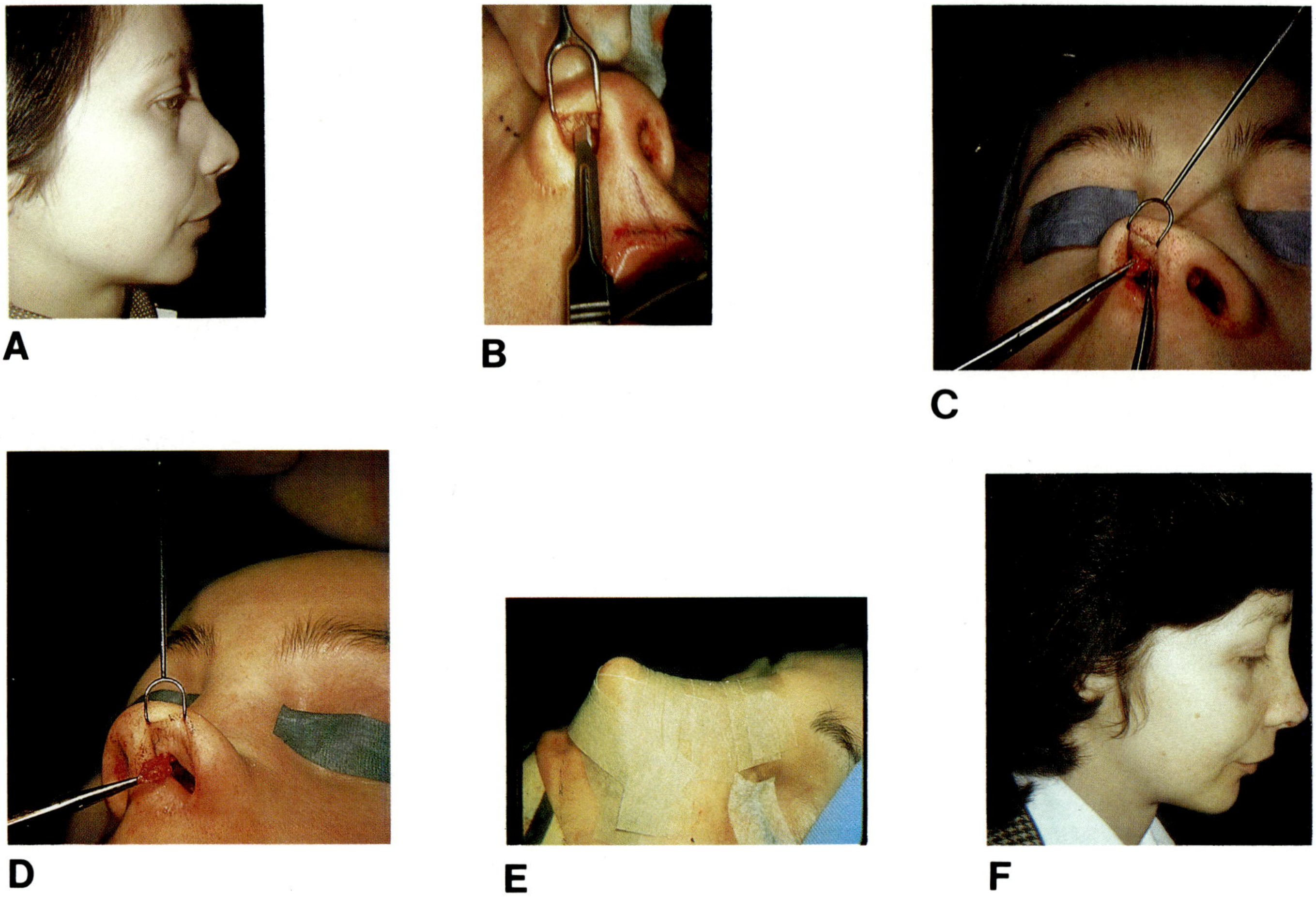

Fig. 47. Young woman with polly beak underwent a secondary septorhinoplasty with osteotomies, narrowing of the bony pyramid, modeling of the tip, and removal of the supratip fibrous tissue. (A) Preoperative profile view (B) Bevelled dissection with the knife as in Figure 44. (C) Resection of fibrous mass. (D) Insertion of cartilage graft into lobule. (E) Dressing with Scampor tape. (F) Postoperative result.

Postoperative care is important (Figs. 47-52). Palpable or visible irregularities of the supratip and tip skin have to be controlled by injections or dermo-jet applications of corticosteroids. Massage and resplinting for another few days or one week are sometimes advisable. Uneven trimming of the septal border or upper lateral cartilages can occasionally cause irregularities of the supratip and dorsal contour and may require tertiary intervention for smoothing of such subcutaneous imbalances. Dermabrasion, as advocated for cases of surface irregularities of the skin with furrows, is to be applied only in exceptional cases (see Chapter 22).

Rounded and Tipless Thick Tip

Secondary techniques must be performed to correct an ugly round lobule without sufficient projection of the very tip. Cartilage has to be harvested from the septum by submucous resection and inserted into the lobule and columella to define the nasal tip.

DEFORMITY OF THE TIP AND NOSTRIL DUE TO FALSE SHAPING OF THE ALAR CARTILAGES

Complications involving the tip and nostril may occur after (1) insufficient resection; (2) in-

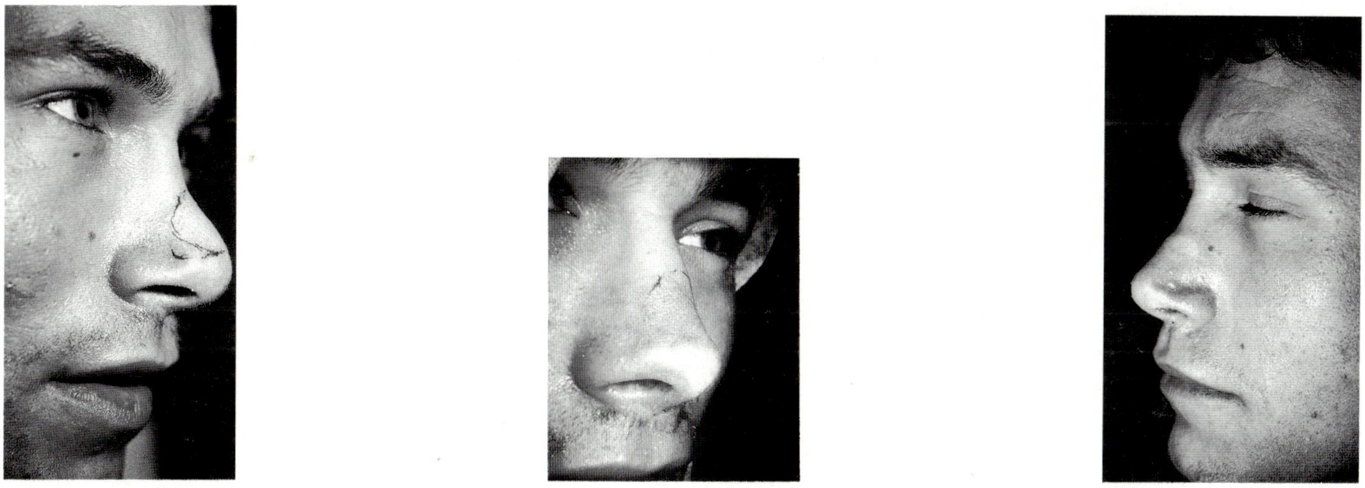

A B C

Fig. 48. Polly beak in a young man operated secondarily in an outpatient procedure. (A) Patient before revision. (B) Patient at the end of the intervention with an exaggerated deepening of the supratip area. (C) Late result: the overcorrection has disappeared and leaves an acceptable dorsal line.

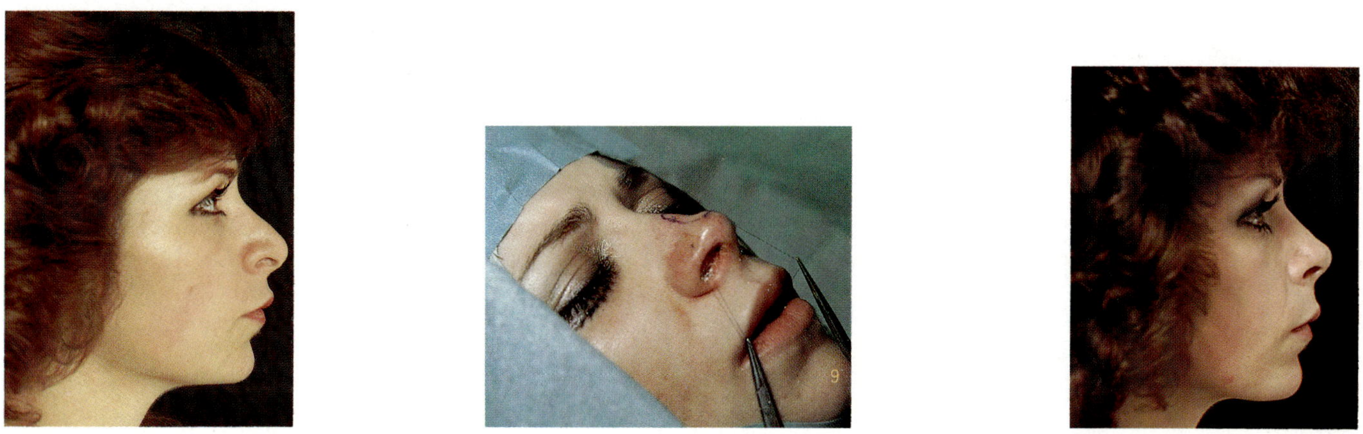

A B C

Fig. 49. Out-patient revision in a young woman with polly beak. (A) Preoperative view. (B) End of the operation. Notice the exaggerated deepening of the supratip area. In addition, the alar border has been slightly lowered. (C) Result.

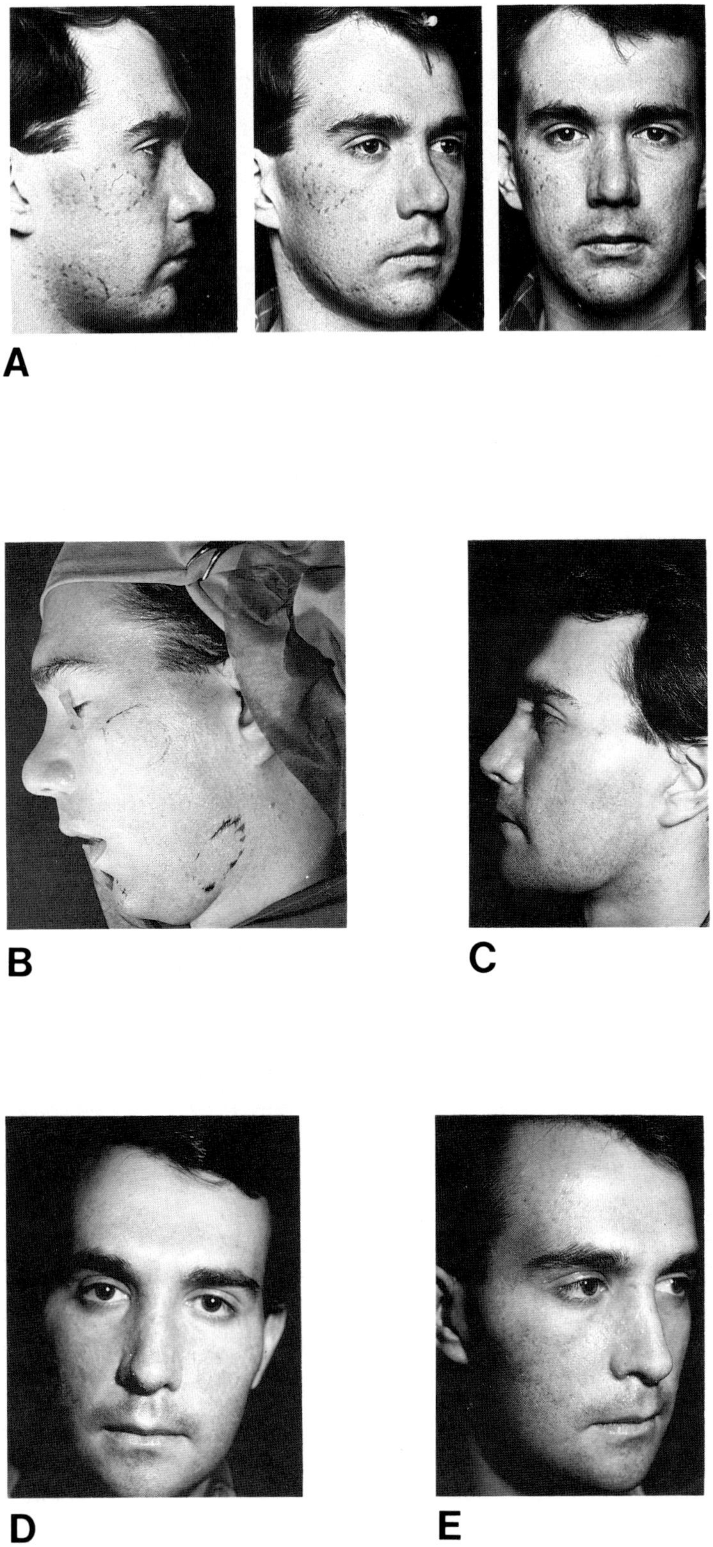

Fig. 50. Septorhinoplasty for secondary supratip deformity combined with malar mandibular and chin augmentation. (A) Young man before revision surgery. (B) Outline of adjunctive augmentation procedures. (C, D, and E) Early result after three weeks.

sufficient trimming of the septal cartilage; (3) insufficient trimming of the upper lateral cartilage (Parrot's beak); and (4) insufficient trimming of the lower lateral cartilage. For primary and secondary rhinoplasty, we have three main endonasal incisions to gain access to the structures of the tip and two external incisions: (1) the infracartilaginous incision for the luxation or delivery technique; (2) the intracartilaginous, transcartilaginous, or cartilage splitting incision; (3) the already mentioned intercartilaginous incision for eversion or retrograde technique; (4) the transcolumellar incision for the decortication method of Rethi (1929); and (5) the columella circumcising incision of Gillies (1920) and Potter (1954).

Technique of Access

The intercartilaginous incision is made through the mucosa at the limen nasi between the caudal border of the upper lateral cartilage and the cephalic border of the lateral crus of the lower lateral cartilage (Figs. 3A an B). The intracartilaginous incision is made through the vestibular skin and cartilage over the long axis of the lateral crus of the lower lateral cartilage. The infracartilaginous incision runs through the vestibular skin caudal to the caudal margin of the lateral crus of the lower lateral cartilage and is carried through the skin of the columella caudal to the caudal margin of the medial crus. The marginal incision, or "rim incision," is made through the vestibular skin close to the inner margin of the lower lateral rim and columella (see Figs. 3A and B).

Each of the above incisions is used separately or in combination in aesthetic rhinoplasty: the delivery technique with infracartilaginous incision presents the lower lateral cartilage in anatomic relationship. Visualization in this position facilitates alteration of contour.

As we have, Sheen (1978) also champions the use of infracartilaginous incisions, which he calls a "rim incision," in concert with intercartilaginous and transfixion incisions and delivers the lower lateral cartilage externally as a bipedicle flap. We always found this method highly satisfactory. The infracartilaginous incision alone may be used in selected cases for access to undermining and delivering of the alar cartilages. This incision gives adequate access for completion of the entire rhinoplasty. Elimination of the intercartilaginous incision at the limen nasi avoids intranasal scar in the valve area.

To better understand the modifications possible in the lower lateral and tip structures we will first describe the different accesses to the lower lateral cartilage that we use in primary surgery. We shall then discuss which techniques are applied in secondary procedures according to the situation encountered.

In the *luxation or delivery technique* (Fig. 53) we create through the two more or less parallel incisions in the vestibule a bipedicle flap of vestibular skin and cartilage. One of these incisions is the previously mentioned intercartilaginous incision. The second one is the infracartilaginous incision at the caudal margin of the lower lateral cartilage. This incision extends medially past the dome and courses vertically downward along the caudal edge of the medial crus. The infracartilaginous incision does not exactly correspond to the marginal incision (Dingman and Natwig, 1982). It remains 1 or 2 mm from the rim and may extend into the lateral third of the ala, where the cartilage diverges from the ala rim. The lateral end of the incision may also turn away from the rim of the vestibule, corresponding to this divergence, unlike the marginal incision, which runs parallel to the ala border. After undermining the soft tissue layer over the lateral crus, this cartilaginous arch with the attached vestibular skin can be luxated from the nostril as a bipedicle flap. The delivered flap is held on a broad flat elevator.

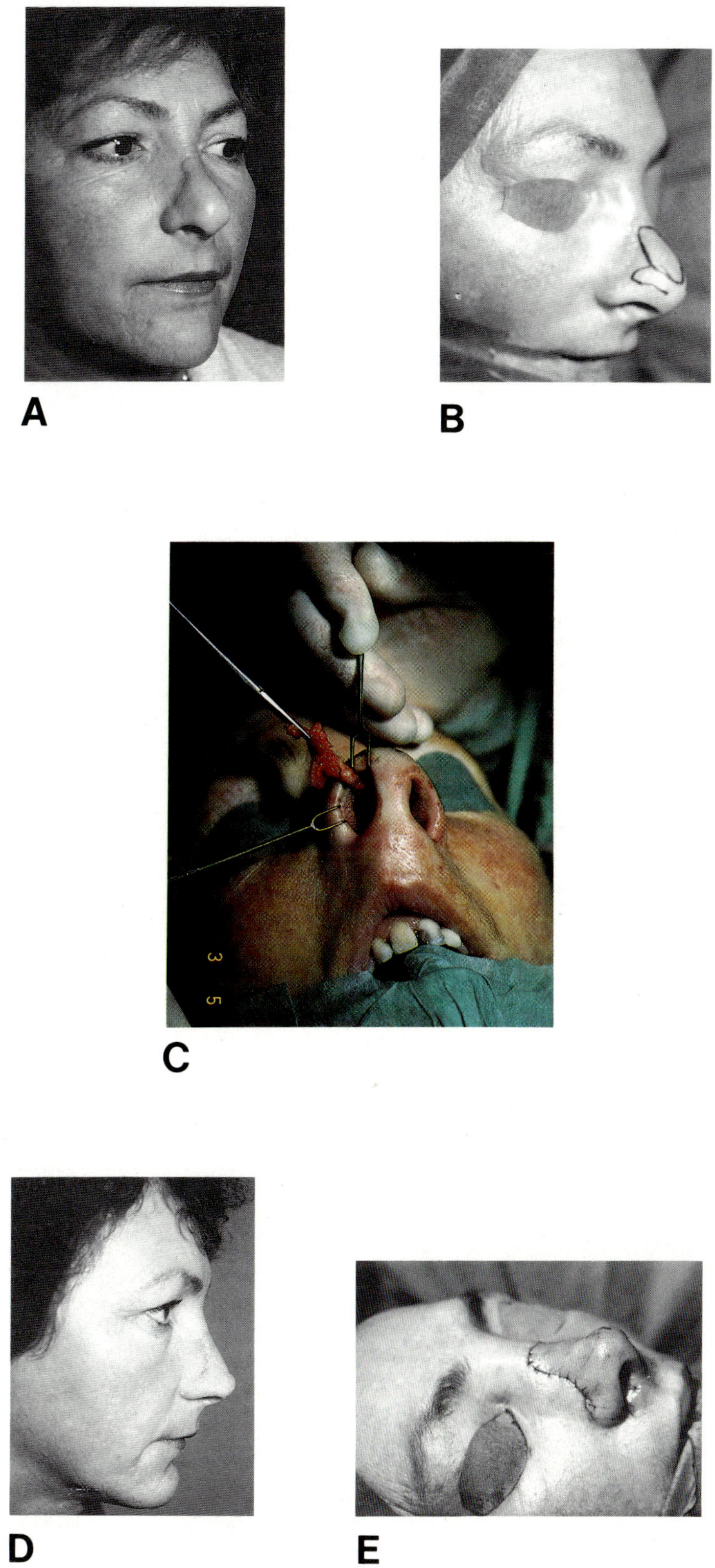

Fig. 51. Supratip thickening after posttraumatic correction. In the secondary procedure the polly beak is corrected contemporaneously with the scar revision on the right side of the nose. (A) Female patient, after first correction. (B) Outline of fibrous tissue resection area at the beginning of the revision surgery. (C) Removal of fibrous tissue. (D) End of the secondary correction with revision of the scar and supratip modeling. (E) End result.

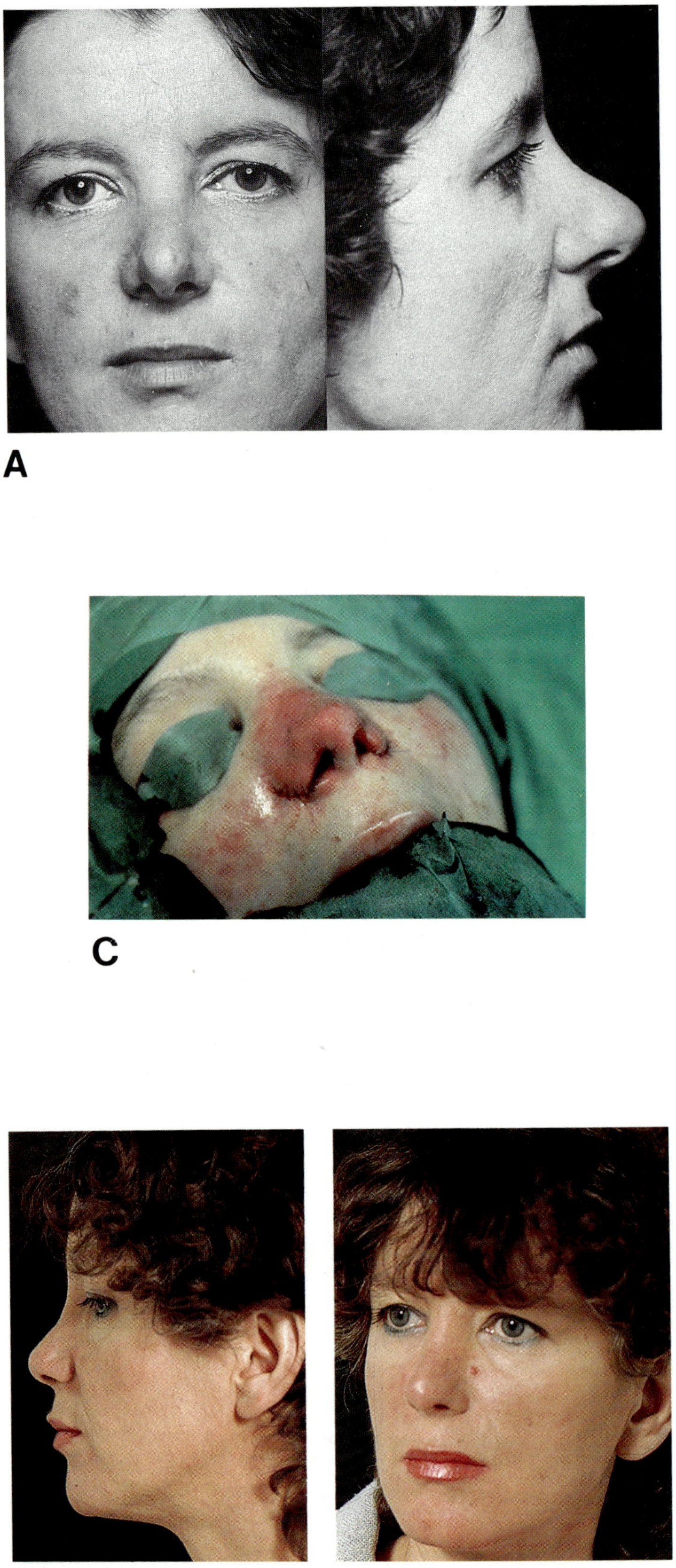

Fig. 52. Enormous hard fibrous tissue formation in tip, supratip, and alar region after several rhinoplasties. There were practically no residual cartilaginous elements at the domes of the lower lateral cartilages. (A) Preoperative view. (B) Outline of tip-supratip area to be reduced. (C) End of revision surgery with reduced dorsum tip and alar bases. The skin has to be adapted to the new shape of the underlying structures. The dressing must be kept for 2 weeks. (D, E, and F) Late result after revision of the alar border.

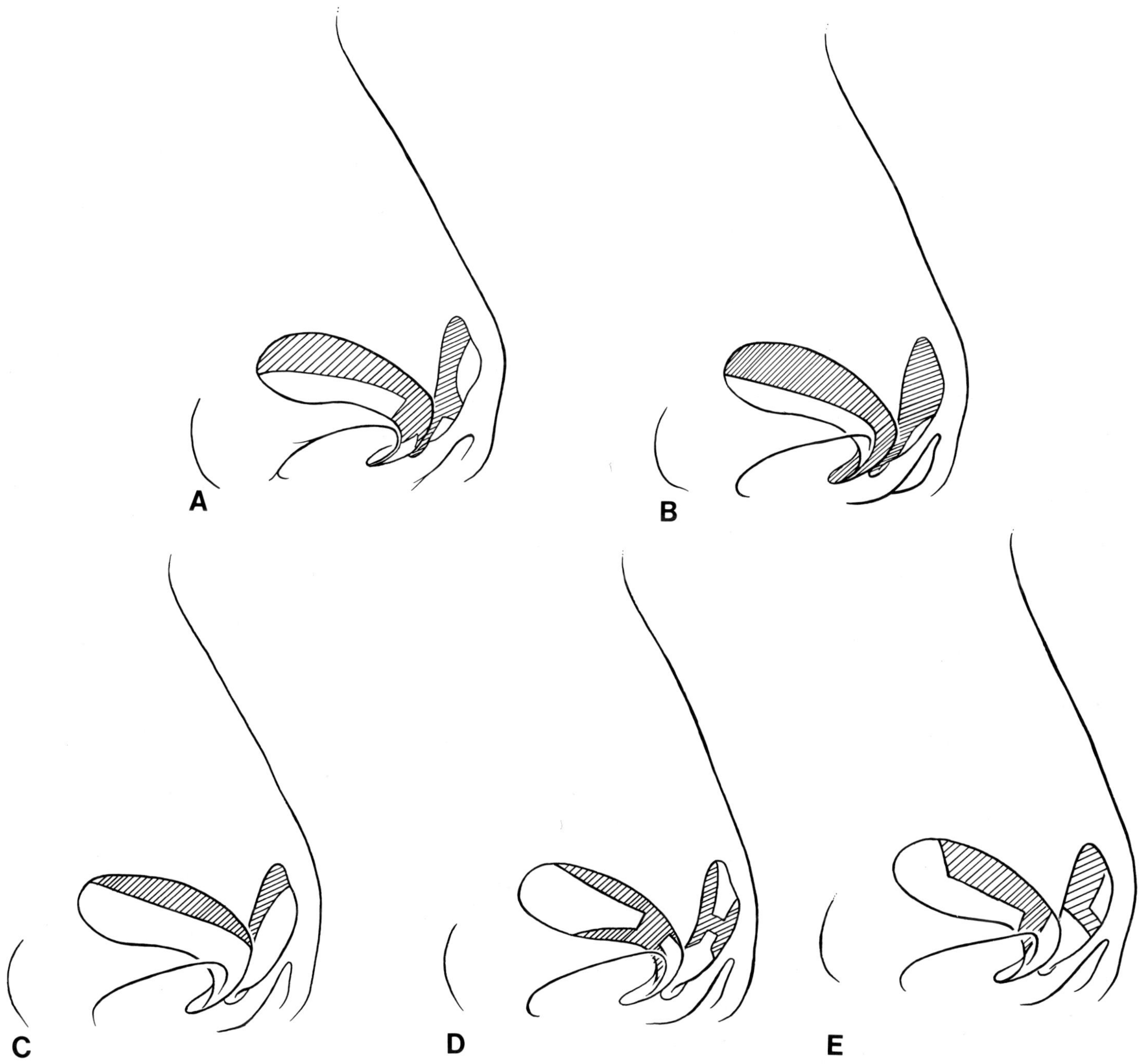

Fig. 53. Luxation technique. The bipedicle flap between the intercartilaginous and the infracartilaginous incision is delivered and rest on an elevator A. The amount of cartilage usually to be removed is cross-hatched in B.

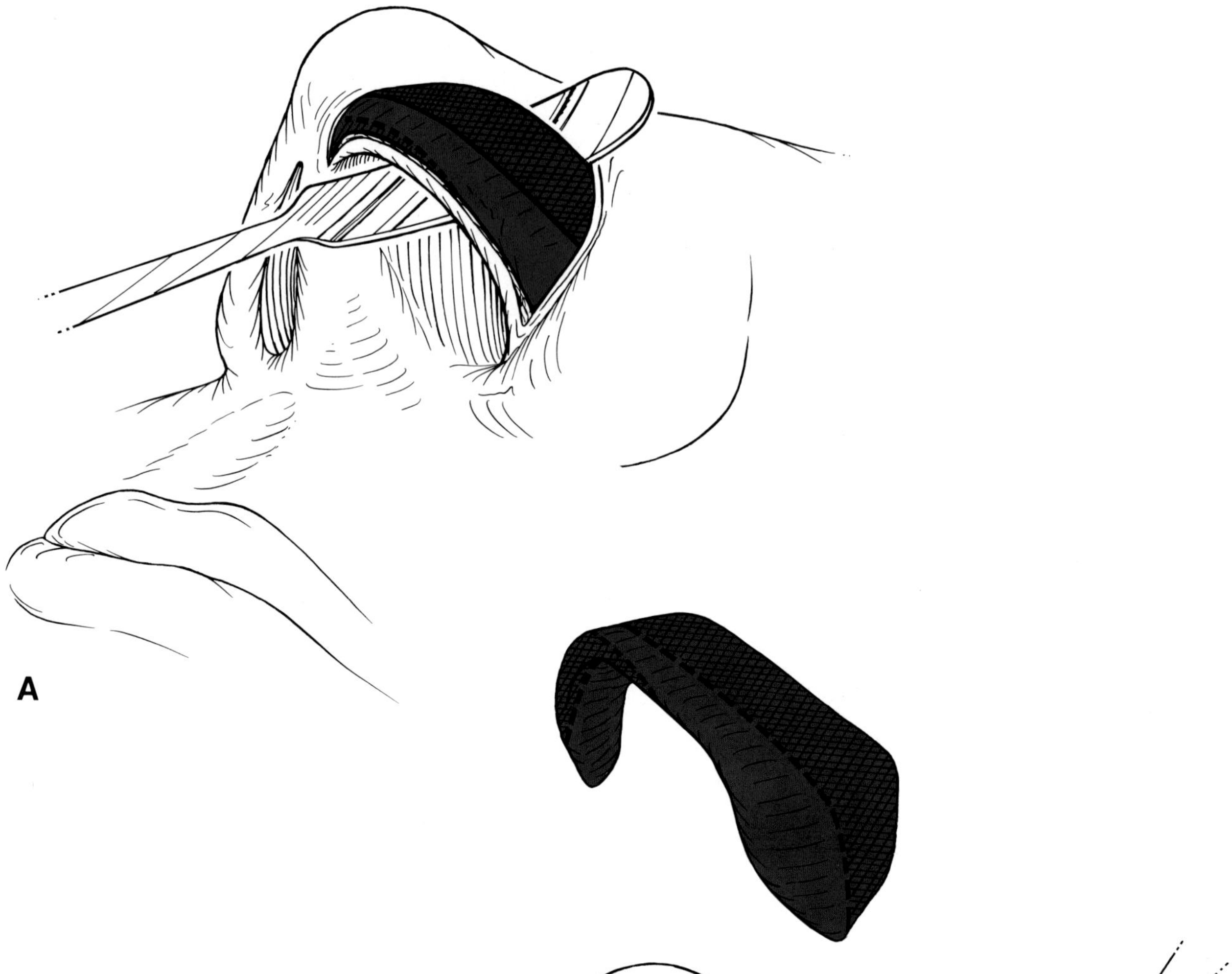

Fig. 54. Resections usually performed by American and European surgeons according to (A) Converse, (B) Seltzer, (C) Aufricht, (D) Becker, and (E) McDowell.

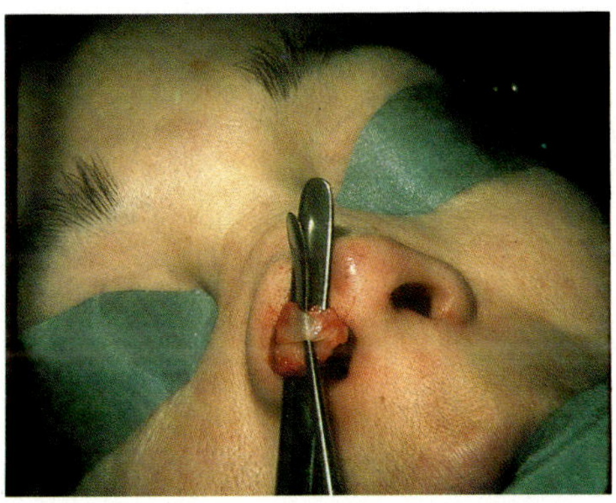

Fig. 55. Luxation technique. The cephalic 2/3 of the lateral crus are dissected from the vestibular skin and will be removed.

Hueston (1982) introduced a wishbone shaped metallic fork for holding both delivered domes at the same time. We recommend it for cases of minimal resection. Exposing the lower lateral cartilages in this way and joining the intercartilaginous with the infracartilaginous incision, provides a clear comprehension of the patient's anatomy and allows precise symmetrical remodeling. If necessary, a fibrofatty cushion is removed from the lateral crus.

Various geometric excisions can now be performed in the lower lateral cartilages (Fig. 54). We usually remodel the cartilage in the following way: we resect about two-thirds of the cephalic portion of the lateral crus by incising it along its whole length, beginning at the medial knee at the dome 1 to 2 mm from the caudal border and proceeding to the lateral end of the cartilage, diverging a bit from the caudal edge (Fig. 55). With a sharp elevator the upper portion of the lateral crus is dissected from the underlying perichondrium and vestibular skin and is removed. Using the knife, we score the remaining cartilaginous arch with multiple parallel cuts. These incisions, which are about 1 mm apart, start at the medial crus about 1–2 mm medial to the medial angle. The cuts are somewhat deeper between both angles, and more superficial at the lateral side. At the point where we want to place the lateral angle of the new domes in the corrected nasal tip, we transect the cartilage to the underlying perichondrium during the carving. This produces an emphasized curvature, especially at this point of the dome. In the relatively wide tip, we make this deep cut as far medially on the cartilage as possible; which is about the site of the medial knee. We do the contrary in cases where we want to make a pointed narrow tip by accentuating the angle farther laterally. If in a bulbous nose the carving correction is not sufficient one can always remove one, two, or more of the cartilage rectangles between the incisions. This is done when the circumference of the nostril is too wide (Fig. 56).

If a cartilage rectangle has to be removed from the arch for reducing the circumference, this excision should not be carried too laterally but extended only a little beyond the lateral knee. Thus we prevent the complication of the pinched nose.

In order to narrow and shorten the tip, we excise 2–5 mm of cartilage between the medial and lateral knee or we even extend the resection into the medial crus if we want to lower the dome considerably. By doing so, we may produce a little fold of vestibular skin at the dome where the bipedicle flap is deprived of its cartilage. By resecting this fold, we transform the bipedicle cutaneo-cartilaginous flap into a monopedicle, which results in a laterally based pedicle flap, as described by Lipsett (1959) under the name of "chondroplastic flap" (Fig. 57). This flap is similar to that of Safian (1935), only narrower and extending further medially.

An increased protrusion of the tip can be achieved by folding the cartilaginous arch of the dome medially under the skin of the tip on both sides, thus elongating the medial crura. In this case, the rectangular cartilage excision or the deep carving must be placed at the lateral knee but under no circumstances more laterally, otherwise there would be again the danger of producing a pinched nose.

The elongated medial crura can be held together by one or more mattress sutures going from one dome to the other. The two stumps can be sutured together with absorbable suture material. The mattress suture can also include the vestibular skin bilaterally. One then ties the suture in the nasal vestibule. If the suture is tied over the vestibular skin, nonabsorbable material can also be used. Using a straight needle a suture is passed from medial to lateral with a hollow tube pressed against the lateral aspect of the columella at a point corresponding to its medial insertion site (Fig. 58). After the penetration of the medial crura, the point of the straight needle emerges precisely at the point located symmetrically on the columellar-vestibular skin of the opposite side. It is important to keep the needle absolutely horizontal so that no distorsion of the tip and columella occurs.

In wide, flat, nasal tips that sometimes have a slight depression in the skin between the domes and may be considered a sign of dog nose, we make a double approximating suture suggested by Joseph (1928), grasping the cartilage farther laterally and thus effecting an elevation of the tip.

Many surgeons, like Bloom (1956), Walter (1966), Ponti (1969), Simons (1975) and Micheli-Pellegrini (1975), use the erection of the elongated medial crura in the tip of the nose according to Goldman (1953) as a routine procedure (see Figs. 65, 66, and 67). T. Smith (1978) abandoned this technique.

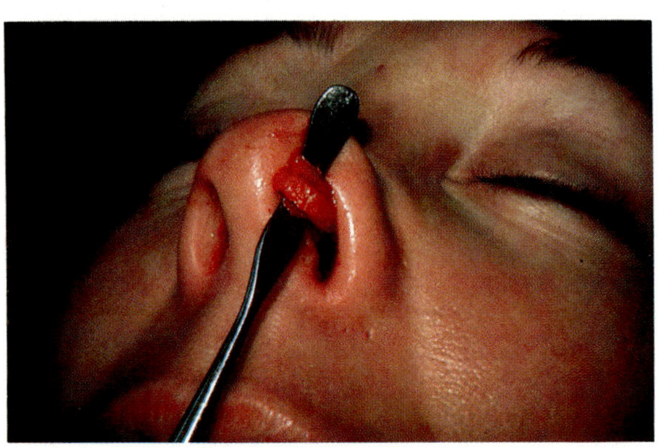

Fig. 56. A segment of the cartilaginous arch at the dome is removed.

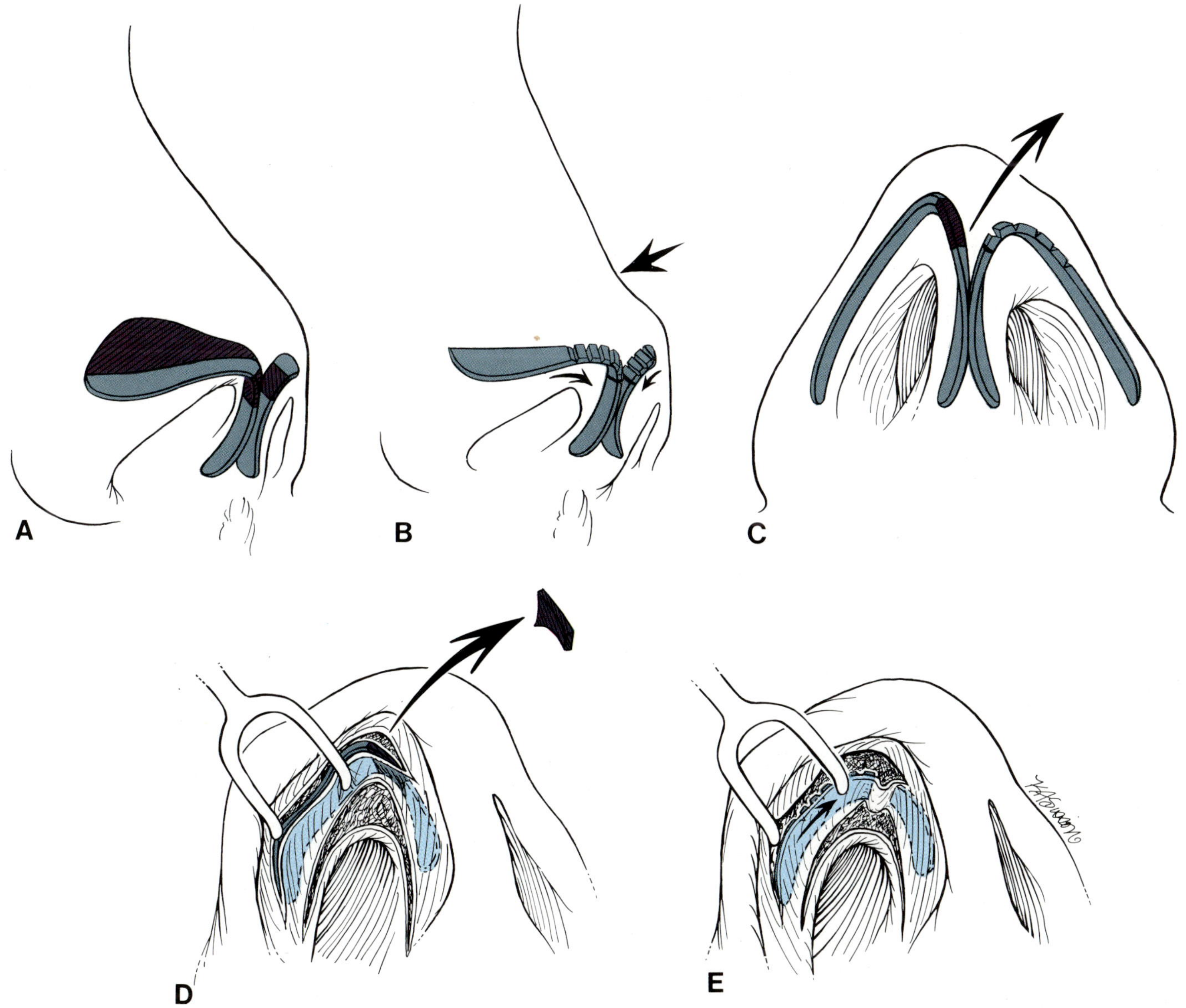

Fig. 57. Lipsett technique for reduction of the tip protrusion. (A) Outline of the resected area of the lower lateral cartilage: the upper two-thirds of the lateral crus and a strip from the anterior part of the medial crus on both sides. (B) Situation after partial resection. (C) Dome reduced on the right side. (D) Segment of the cartilaginous arch removed. (E) The lateral crus is pushed medially and joins the reduced medial crus. The vestibular skin fold can be left in place or removed.

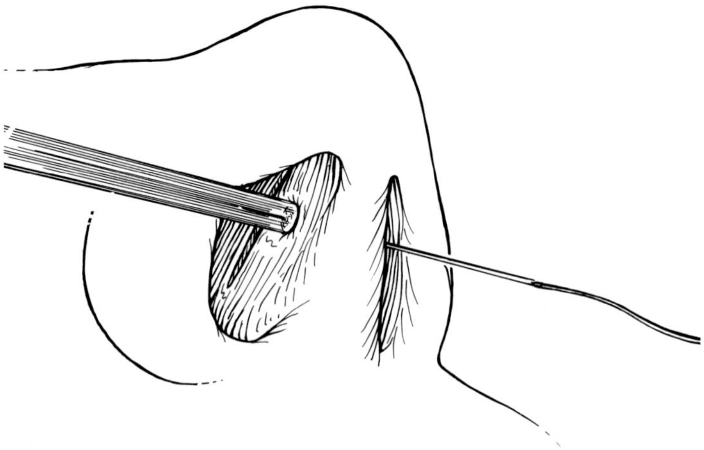

Fig. 58. Using a straight needle, a suture is passed from medial to lateral with a hollow tube pressed against the lateral aspect of the columella at a point corresponding to its medial insertion site.

Since the posterior edges of the erected cartilage stumps come higher than the anterior because they include parts of the broader lateral crura, the two pillars have to be trimmed obliquely to the level of the septal cartilage (Gallanti, 1954; Micheli-Pellegrini, 1975; Willemot, 1969). The disadvantage of this method is that the cartilaginous median pillars can bend backward if they are too weak. Furthermore, this technically very interesting trick is fraught with the danger of producing sharp cartilaginous edge stumps that can become visible after a few months. We believe that there is less danger for this complication the way we do the modeling of the domes by carving the cartilaginous arch. However, we also have to be very careful with

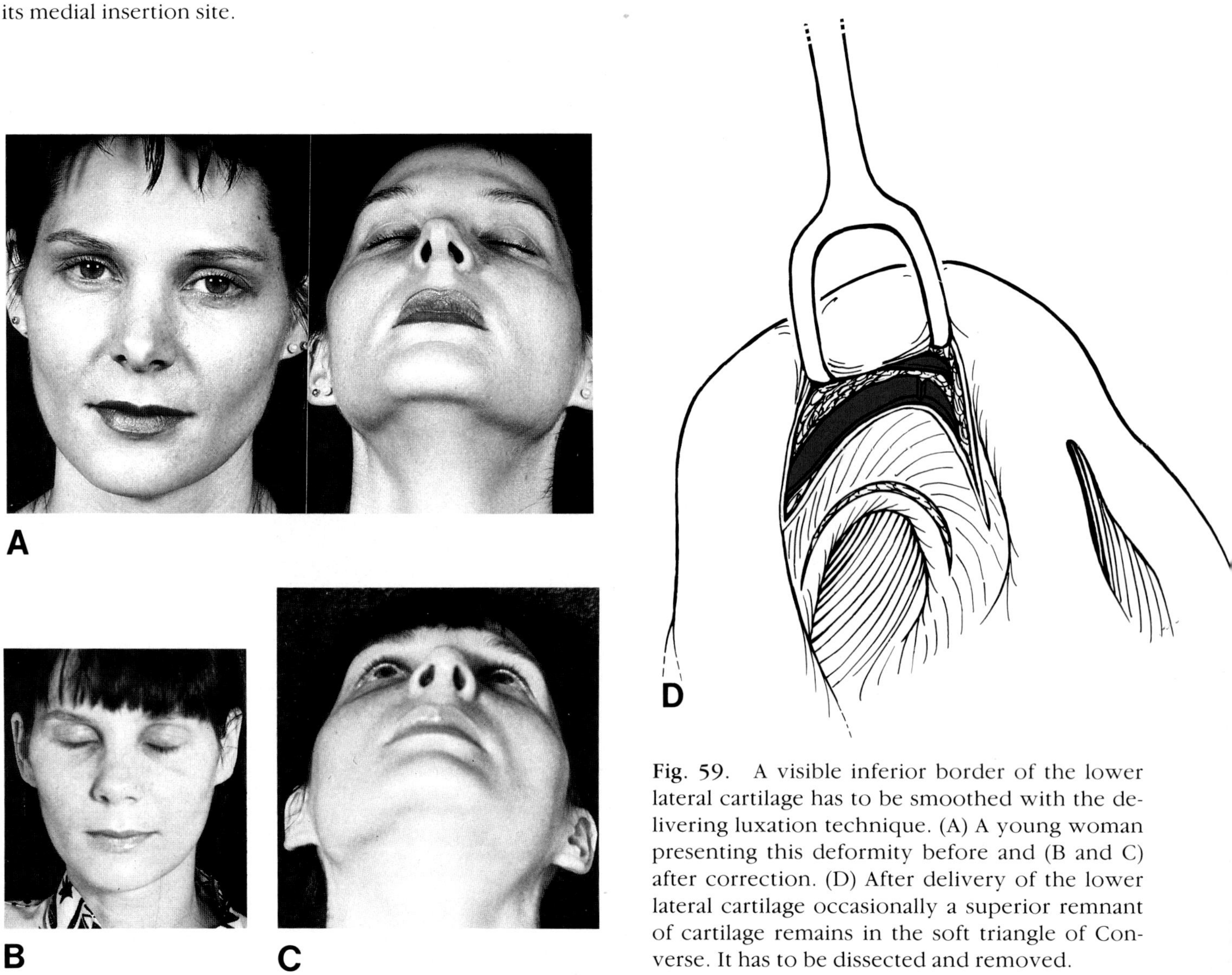

Fig. 59. A visible inferior border of the lower lateral cartilage has to be smoothed with the delivering luxation technique. (A) A young woman presenting this deformity before and (B and C) after correction. (D) After delivery of the lower lateral cartilage occasionally a superior remnant of cartilage remains in the soft triangle of Converse. It has to be dissected and removed.

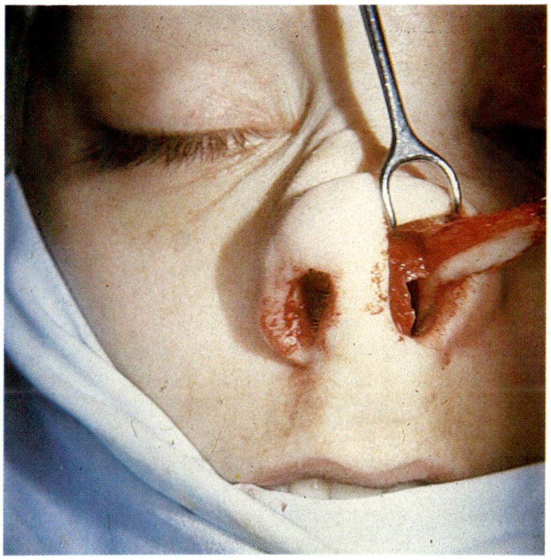

Fig. 60. Lateral crural flap of Webster.

our technique in cases with thin skin where we leave parts of the domes uncurved. In many thin skinned noses, the distal edge of the lower lateral cartilage is visible near the dome towards the weak triangle of Converse and even along the anterior part of the lower lateral rim (Fig. 59A, B, and C). This border must be resected and the residual strip of cartilage has to be carved very carefully in a crosshatching way. For this special correction, the luxation method is of great value because it allows a complete exposure of the lower lateral cartilages and symmetrical, precise reduction and sculpturing. It can happen that, using the delivery technique, the very caudal edge of the dome is not taken with the bipedicled flap. If such is the case this strip of cartilage will be palpable in the tip, distorting it. One has to remove it in a further maneuver (Fig. 59D).

Transcartilaginous, Intracartilaginous, or Cartilage Splitting Incision

Kazanjian and Converse (1959) introduced the partial exposure of the lower lateral cartilages using an intracartilaginous incision that splits the lateral crus. The incision is carried through the vestibular skin and the lower lateral cartilage at the level that is determined by the amount of cartilage to be resected. The strip of cartilage proximal to the incision is dissected free from the vestibular and external skin and in this way easily removed. We described this approach, which we use sometimes, in the book by Denecke and Meyer (1964/1967). Dingman (1956), Anderson (1966), and Mahé (1982) advocated this incision.

If a narrowing of the tip is necessary, a triangular piece from the marginal part of the lower lateral cartilage with the point toward the vestibular rim has to be resected. Nowadays this approach has become very common. It is particularly indicated when only a reduction of the cephalic portion of the lower lateral cartilage is required and the caudal border can be left intact.

Instead of removing the proximal portion of the lower lateral cartilage, it can be reduced and shaped together with the attached vestibular skin, as a laterally based composite flap. Such a flap, which is trimmed on the three free borders, has been advocated by Cinelly (1958), Webster (1975), and Rish (1955). Webster calls it the "lateral crural flap" (Fig. 60). In contrast to Safian's (1955) vestibular flap, which includes the whole lateral crus and to Lipsett's (1959) "chondroplastic flap," which consists of the caudal part the lateral crus, this very narrow but relatively long flap contains the cephalic part of the cartilage. We use this technique in primary surgery for modeling the tip when we want only a reduction of the convexity of the lower lateral cartilage in its upper aspect, leaving intact the lower margin of the cartilage and the circumference of the nostrils. We obtain a slight, natural looking depression at the level of the lateral crural flap, i.e., in the cephalic portion of the ala towards the tip as well as a cephalic rotation of the nostril and the tip.

Eversion Method (Retrograde Approach from the Intercartilaginous Incision)

This method, already mentioned in corrections of supratip thickening, has been introduced by McIndoe (1951, 1958) and is used mainly by English Commonwealth, and South American surgeons. Instead of being luxated and keeping its original position, the lower lateral cartilage is everted, i.e., turned outward and upside down. The lower border of the intercartilaginous incision is grasped with a retractor and pulled downward out of the nostril. Thus, the upper border of the alar cartilage is exposed and can be carefully separated from the overlying skin and from the vestibular skin, which is partially excised together with the upper part of the lateral crus in the retrograde way.

Additional exposure can be gained through a vertical incision in the vestibular skin at the

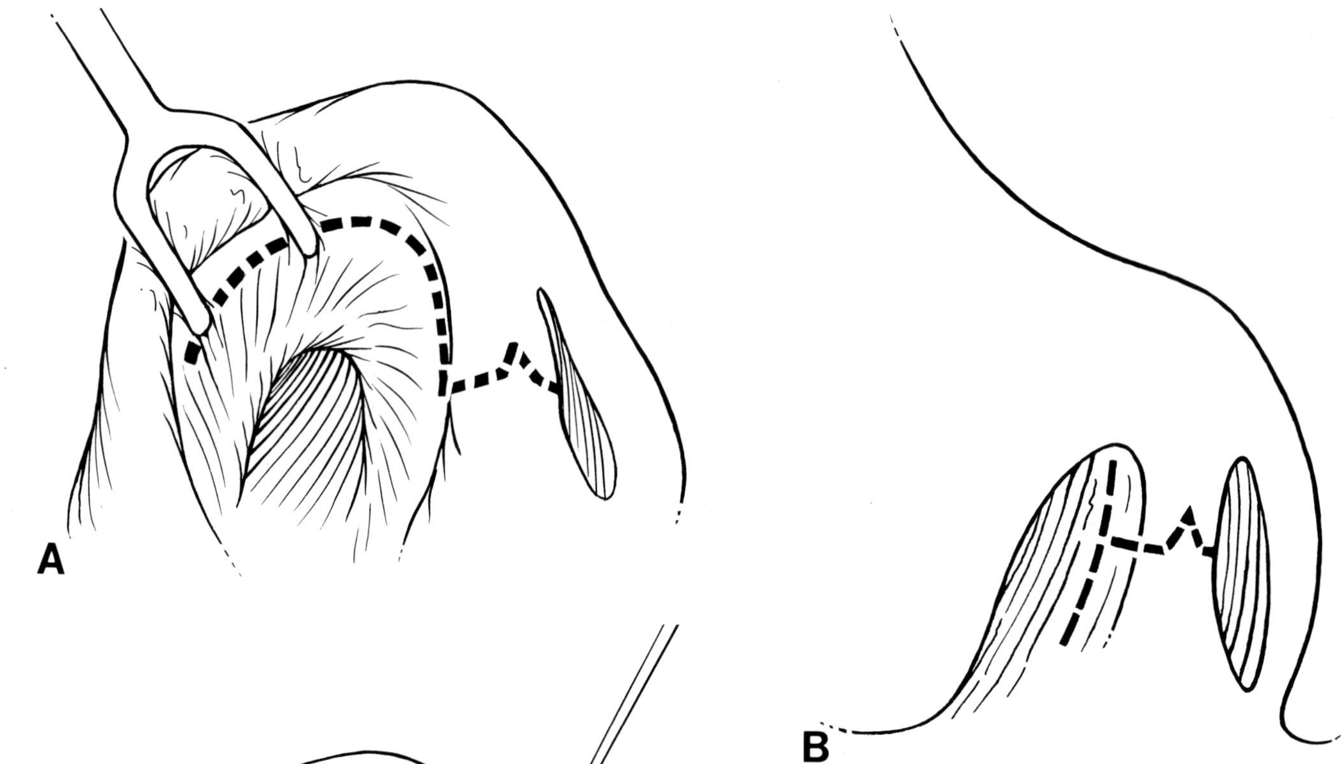

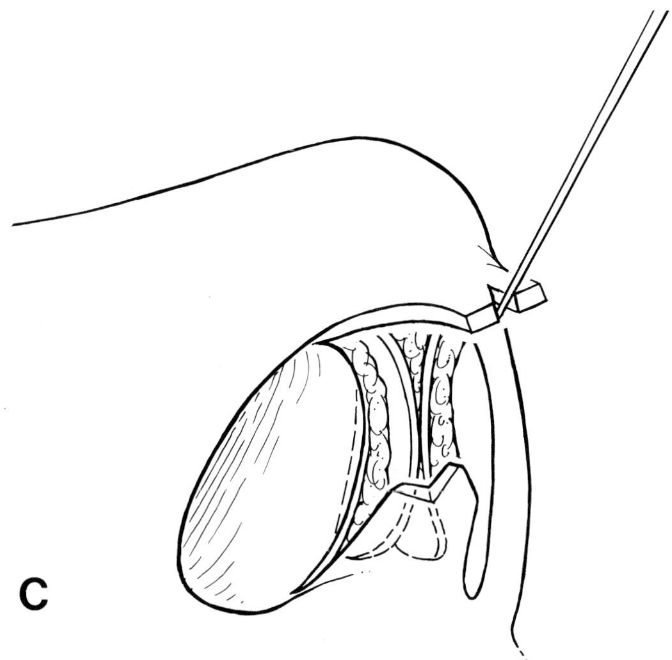

Fig. 61. (A) Incision of Rethi. (B and C) External incision with Goodmann's modification.

dome where, if necessary, a triangular excision of cartilage can be added. In primary rhinoplasty we use this technique only in rare cases in which very conservative sculpturing of the alar cartilage is demanded as well as in corrections of harelip noses and saddle nose deformities. However, we choose this incision in secondary surgery, as already mentioned, for selected polly beak correction not necessarily requiring a complete revision rhinoplasty.

Incision of Rethi and Similar Methods Using External Incisions

An open approach to rhinoplasty is not a new concept. Historically, one of the earliest descriptions of nasal surgery dates back to the Sushruta Samhita, which was described circa 600 B.C. The Indian method of rhinoplasty was essentially an external approach to the nasal dorsum.

When Joseph (1932), who is generally considered the father of modern rhinoplasty, executed his first rhinoplastic procedure (termed *rhinomyosis*), he performed some reduction rhinoplasties by an external approach, resecting the redundant overlying nasal skin along the subjacent cartilage and bone. Thus the evolution of the present technique of external rhinoplasty can be traced back to Rethi (1929) in Budapest. He described in 1921 an approach to the nasal tip using a high transverse columellar incision. The columellar skin is severed in the anterior third and swung upward like a flap (Fig. 61 A).

Bending around at right angles bilaterally, the incision joins the vestibular rim incision. Rethi incision comes from an older one that Gilles (1920) called *elephant trunk incision*. In the latter, a columellar flap that has to be put over the tip starts at the columellar base.

Sercer, in 1958, published a modification to uncover the entire infrastructure of the nose. He termed the procedure *decortication of the nose* and defined decortication as temporary separation of the skin from the nasal pyramid. In the same year, Hauberisser (1956) published a modification of the Rethi technique. He extended the vestibular rim incision further lateral to the alar-facial junction, and continued in the external skin all the way around this junction. By doing so he could fold back the skin of the nasal tip and dorsum, still further to a maximum. Coughlin (1925), May (1947, 1957), de Kleine (1950), Rehrmann (1959), and Hage (1960) have particularly advocated the advantage of the mediocolumellar incision, and added some minor modifications to this method. Thus, this technique was introduced in the United States for the first time in 1947 by May. Padovan (1966), who was an associate of Sercer in Zagreb, Yugoslavia, extended this approach further to expose and allow for corrective surgery on the nasal septal structures.

We have used this technique since 1960, proceeding in the following way. The incision is made along the line of the caudal border of the lower lateral cartilage, which lies in a variable distance cephalic to the alar rim. The dome area is freed by blunt dissection before making the transverse columellar incision at the medial columellar level. As we wrote in 1964 (Meyer in Denecke and Meyer), the incision is especially suitable for cases in which one wants to achieve a more pronounced raising of the nasal tip folding forward the domes, by straightening the curved cartilage bow and suturing them together according to the method of Straith (1936) and Goldman (1953, 1957). The cartilage is severed perpendicularly to the border in the region of the lateral crus, a few millimeters from the dome and is then dissected out as far as the medial crus.

We do not consider such an access to the nasal tip necessary in simple tip corrections since the luxation and eversion methods suffice. In our book (1965/1967) we pointed out "it can be advised for the correction of hare lip nose and other malformations as well as for correction of the saddle or deflected noses due to scarring." For the special cases of hare lip nose and saddle nose we modified the technique, passing with the horizontal incision bilaterally over the medial crura to join the transfixion incision (see Fig. 3A). In this way, the medial crura are also cut through at the level of the horizontal incision so that their anterior part and the dome as well as the upper part of the lower lateral cartilages are exposed from the rear. This exposure has special advantages in the harelip nose. We still use it beside the original Rethi incision in such surgery.

Padovan, Sercer's successor, wrote about the technique of his master in 1966 and considered that the indications for external approach were: (1) the long hump nose; (2) a hump nose combined with cartilaginous deformities; (3) any deformity of the nose associated with congenital anomalies of the lip, upper jaw, and palate; and (4) all marked deformities associated with trauma of the nasal pyramid. He presented his experience with the external approach in 1970 in New York and from that year on this technique has been used in North America by the members of the Academy of Facial Plastic Surgery, while plastic surgeons had not previously followed the technique introduced in their country by one of their own, May.

Goodman published in 1973 a little modification (see Fig. 61 B) of Rethi's incision, breaking the horizontal line at the midcolumellar level by notching the central portion with an inverted V. A similar notch has been advocated by Figi (1952) (see Chapter 20). Goodman was followed later by Wright (1981) and others. At that time Anderson (1974) disagreed with Goodman's statement that one cannot see what one is doing in the ordinary rhinoplasty. However, Anderson conceded that this is probably a good procedure in some cases in some hands. But he was concerned that this technique may be used in more cases than are really indicated. He did not think it should replace the endonasal approach. This is about the same consideration we always have expressed concerning this splendid technique, which has a series of good indications, without having to be adopted routinely in all rhinoplasties, easy cases included.

Goodman stated in 1978 that the following deformities should be considered for applying the open access of Rethi: (1) congenital deformities of the nose, (2) major nasal septal deformities, (3) large hump nose with cartilaginous deformities, (4) major augmentation procedures with cartilaginous deformities, (5) excision of dermoid cysts or other pathology, (6) correction of the bifid tip, (7) excision of subcutaneous scar tissue, and (8) reoperation with major deformities. Pech et al wrote in 1981 about their experience with this technique, considering that it should be limited to cases in which the normal procedure is not satisfactory, particularly in rhinoplasties after severe trauma and in secondary operations. In such cases predictable osteocartilaginous damage and scar adherence may render difficult the dissection in the right cleavage plane.

One year later, Anderson (1982) made a similar suggestion, including the following indications for this technique: (1) secondary rhinoplasty, (2) traumatic noses, (3) important septal deformities, (4) long noses, (5) flat nasofrontal angle, (6) negroid noses, and (7) columella asymmetry. This is to show how controversial such an important problem of access in rhinoplasty may be. Late follow-up will probably enlighten us regarding this uncertainty.

As we do, McCollough (1981) stresses the advantage of the open procedure in corrections of crooked noses where the openly visible dissected dorsal strip of the septum can be separated from the upper lateral cartilages and straightened by means of a morcelizer (see Fig. 119E). In 1983 Vogt reviewed her experience with the straight transverse columellar incision, pointing out that no long lasting swelling of the tip, no supratip deformities, no unsightly scarring, and no scar retraction at the incisions occurred. The author recommends the open approach to be used routinely in primary corrective rhinoplasty. Goodman, Wright, McCollough, Anderson, and others are actually using this technique routinely. Anderson and Ries (1986) wrote a book entitled *Rhinoplasty: Emphasizing the External Approach.*

The external access of Rethi is used by Peck (1981) for inserting an L-shaped bone graft from the iliac crest in correction of saddle noses. We now apply these approaches only in the correction of crooked noses (see Chapter 11), saddle nose (see Chapter 12), retracted columella (see Chapter 15), harelip nose (see Chapter 20), and special cases of revision.

Another similar incision used for the correction of harelip nose and advocated by Erich (1953, 1959) follows an undulating line along the nostril borders and through the columella, exposing the lower lateral cartilages in the same way as Rethi's incision (see Chapter 20). A more extended exposure of these cartilages in unilateral and bilateral harelip noses is provided by the method of Potter (1954), circumcising the columella, but leaving the lobular attachment, and carrying the incision along the alar rim and into the lateral vestibular wall. It is derived from an older method of Gillies (1920) in which the flap starts at the base of the columellar and is pulled up over the tip like an elephant trunk.

Same Incisions in Secondary Procedures

Many of the surgeons dealing with secondary procedures avoid incisions along or close to the nostril margin and prefer the eversion technique. We do not share this opinion.

If the whole cartilaginous arch, especially the dome, has to be remodeled, in about 80 percent of revisions, we choose the *luxation technique* using the infracartilaginous incision that, as mentioned, does not correspond to the marginal or rim incision. Obviously the best exposure of the alar cartilage, apart from the external approach, may it be intact or trimmed or otherwise manipulated or enveloped in scar tissue, is provided by the luxation technique. This exposure is the method of choice for all difficult primary rhinoplasties, as mentioned before, and for most secondary procedures. When we encounter a retracted alar border and fibrous thickening of the vestibular surface of the residual lateral crura, however, we apply the *cartilage splitting method* using the intracartilaginous incision. Through the transcartilaginous incision we are then able to lower the alar rim by cartilage grafting.

On the other hand, if the alar rim is low and has to be elevated to a harmonious level by marginal resection, as we shall explain later, it is advisable not to apply the luxation method with partial rim incision because the latter would probably interfere with the marginal resection line or leave a too narrow intermediate strip of skin at the border of the ala. The use of the *eversion technique* with retrograde approach of the alar cartilage through the intercartilaginous incision has already been mentioned in secondary corrections of the polly beak deformity.

While in primary rhinoplasties the occasional sacrifice of a small strip of vestibular skin together with the upper portion of the lower lateral cartilage is permitted we have to spare every millimeter of cutaneous vestibular lining in secondary correction of supratip subcutaneous thickening.

Pinocchio Nose

The overprojected tip of the Pinocchio nose is an example of unbalanced structures. When it is encountered in a secondary nose it emphasizes the undercorrection performed by the first surgeon, as a consequence of underestimating the magnitude of the initial nasal deformities. The overprojection of the tip can also result from an excessive hump removal without adequate sculpturing of the excessively wide alar cartilages.

In secondary revisions we approach the patient as we do for a primary Pinocchio tip. The main point of the procedure is to expose widely the alar cartilages from the anterior third of the medial crura to the anterior third of the lateral crura. This can be best achieved with the luxation technique.

The resection of the dome has to be exceptionally wide, in addition to the resection of the cephalad two-thirds, and of the lateral extremities of the lateral crura (Fig. 62), which in these cases particularly extend into the cellulo-adipose lateral flare of the nostril (Jost, 1972, 1975). Such an important dome resection leads to some difficulties with tip modeling, but it is absolutely necessary. In addition we have to resect the excessive vestibular skin in order to contour the lining. The Lipsett's flap is sometimes useful.

Wedge resections at the alar bases (Figs. 63 and 64) are usually necessary, to prevent excessive flaring of the ala, which results after tip reduction. If possible the Weir resection should be limited to the caudal part of alar-cheek junction. We occasionally have to adapt the columellar length to the reduced apico-alar structure by resecting the medial crura and/or removing a horizontal strip of skin at its base, as shown in the chapter on columellar correction (see Fig. 148).

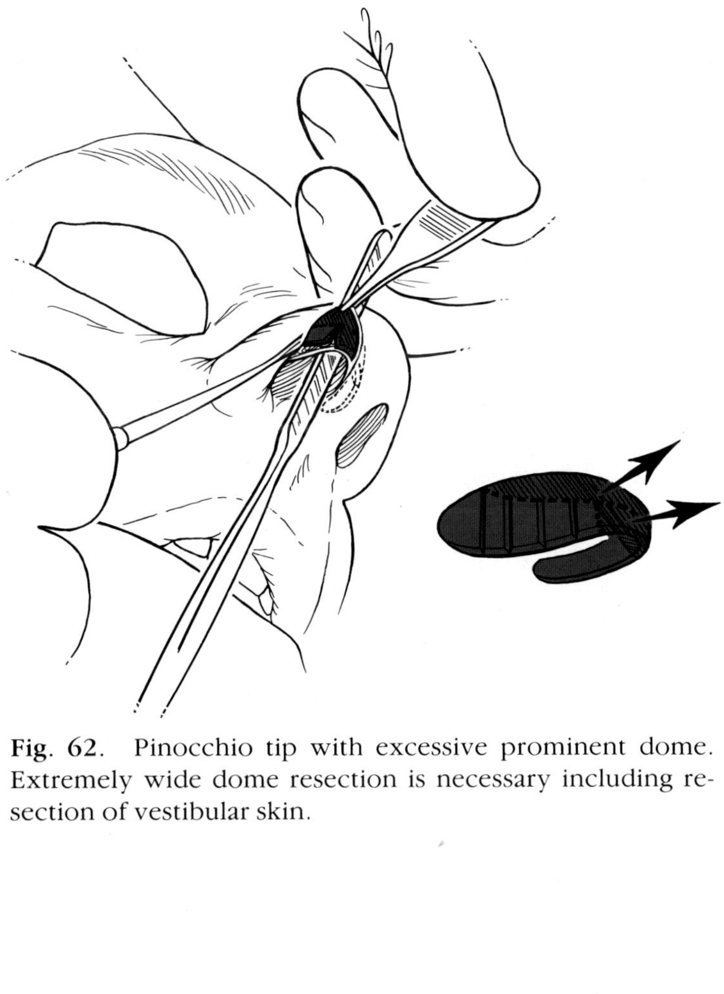

Fig. 62. Pinocchio tip with excessive prominent dome. Extremely wide dome resection is necessary including resection of vestibular skin.

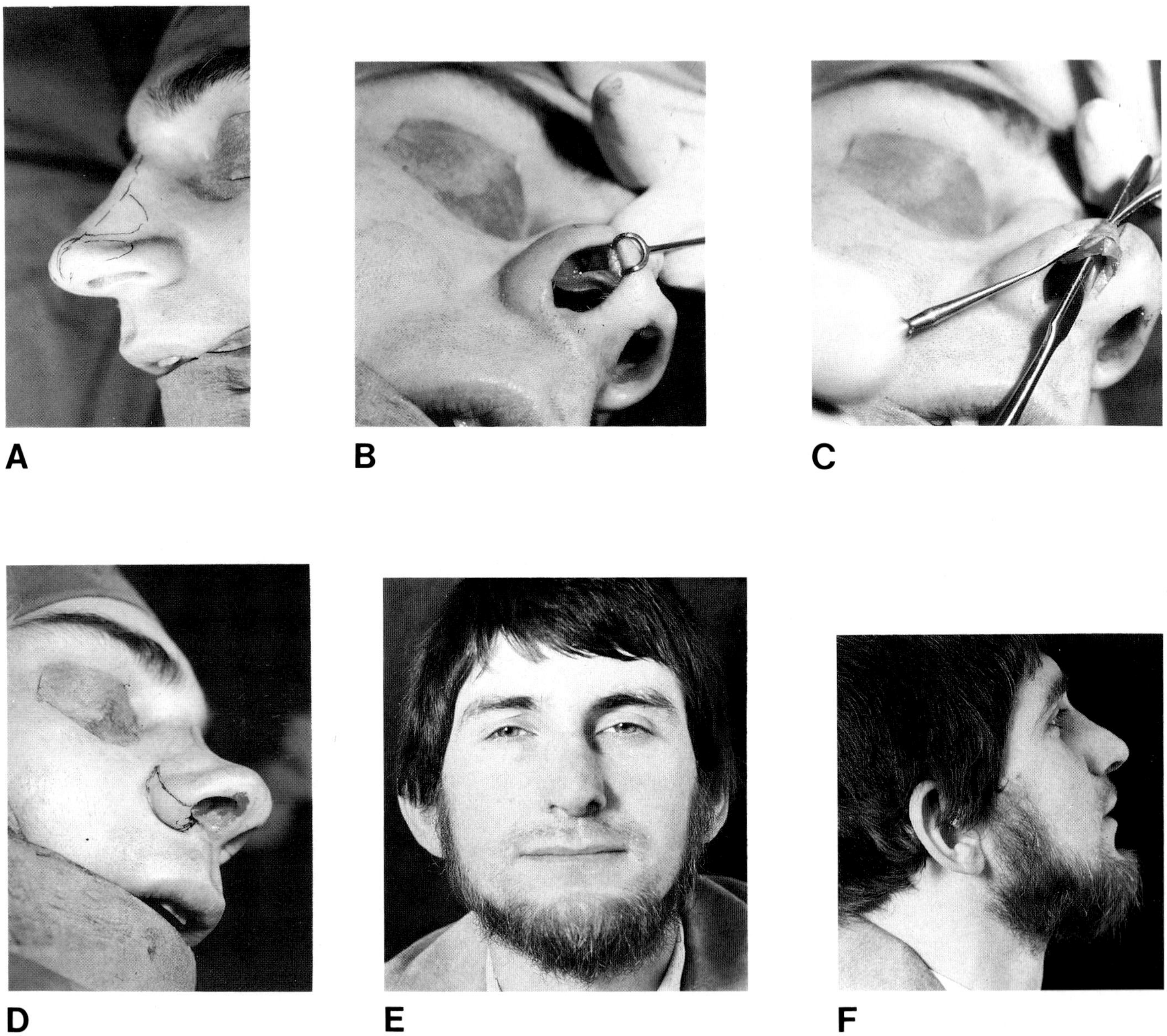

Fig. 63. Corresponding case to Fig. 62. (A) Pinocchio tip before correction. (B) Cartilaginous arch to be reduced. (C) Reduction of the dome. (D) Wedge resection at the alar base. (E and F) End result after shortening of the columella.

Too Broad Tip

Like the Pinocchio nose, the too broad, squared, and flattened tip also has an unaesthetic aspect. To thin and appropriately project the tip, the memory of the flattened alar cartilages is broken by scoring the lower lateral cartilages at their anterior and central thirds. The lateral aspects of the domes are sectioned (Fig. 65). The medial crura are subsequently exposed and approximated with mattress sutures, thus lengthening the columella and projecting the tip.

The "Butterfly" method of Ponti (1969) can also be used to refine a broad tip, when the columellar length and its support are already appropriate. We section the lateral crura at the dome and suture together the erected medial crura, leaving the medial knee of the dome intact (Figs. 66, and 67).

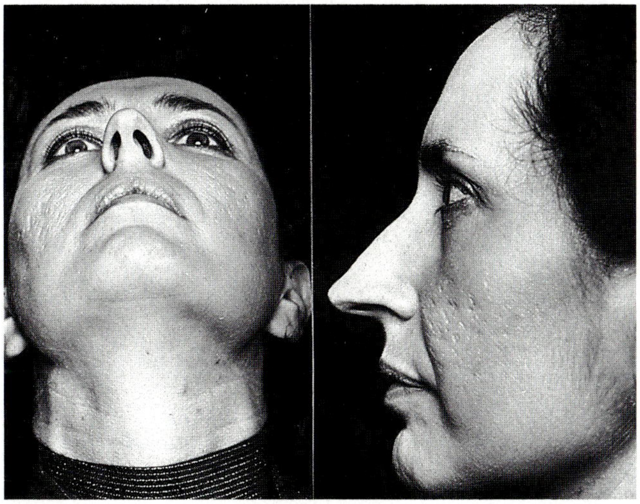

A

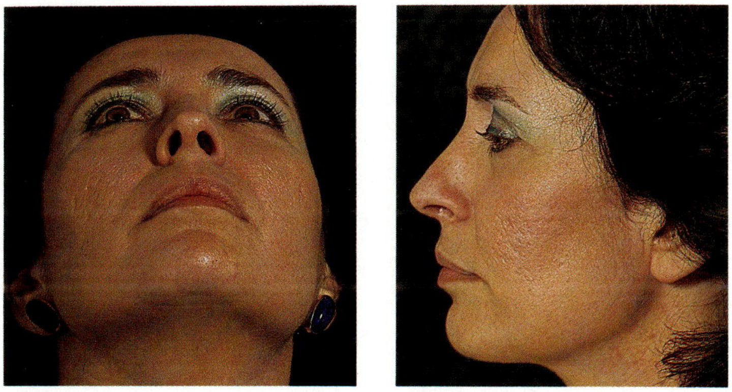

B C

Fig. 64. Similar Pinocchio nose in middle-aged female. Procedure performed as in Fig. 62. (A) Intraoperative axial and profile views. (B and C) Same postoperative views.

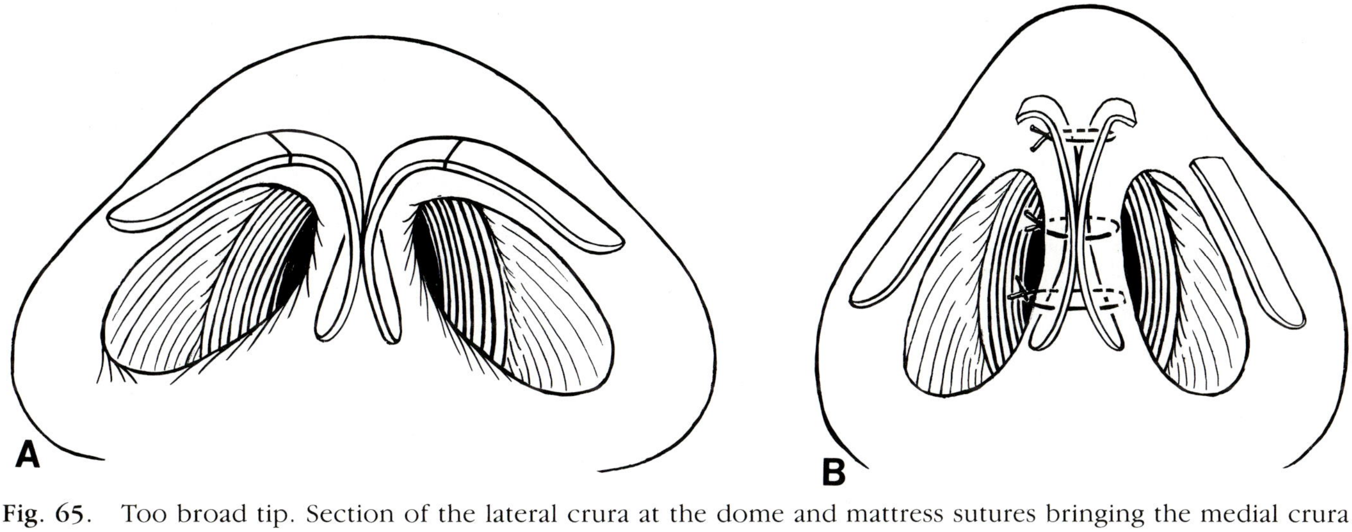

A B

Fig. 65. Too broad tip. Section of the lateral crura at the dome and mattress sutures bringing the medial crura together. This can be done with or without resection of a segment at the dome.

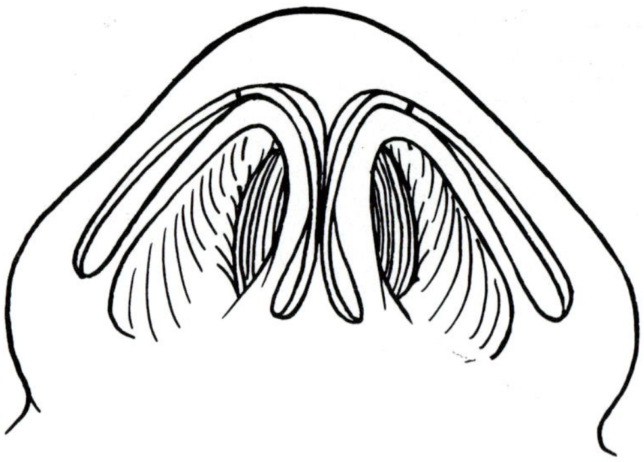

A

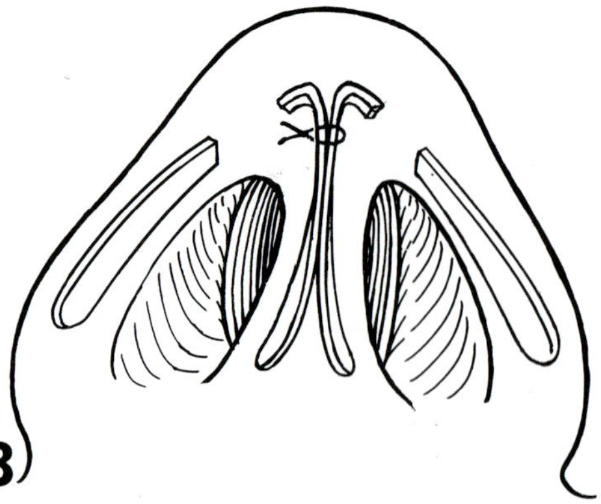

B

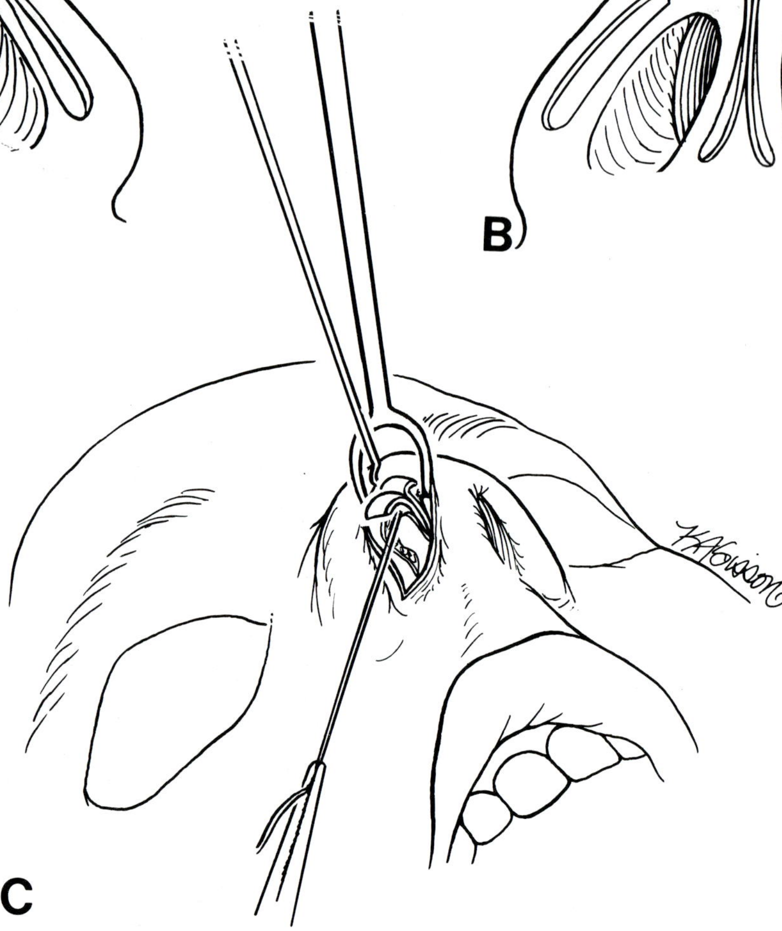

C

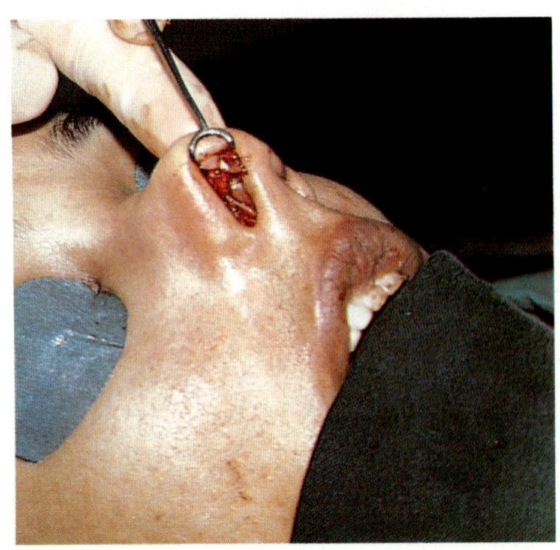

D

Fig. 66. "Butterfly" method of Ponti. (A) Section of the lateral crura at the dome. (B) Suturing together the erected and lengthened medial crura leaving the medial knee of the dome intact. (C) Exposure of the anterior portion of the medial crura for passing the mattress suture. (D) Exposure of the dome and suturing of the "butterfly" tip complex of Ponti. Cartilage fragments of the dome ready to be sutured together.

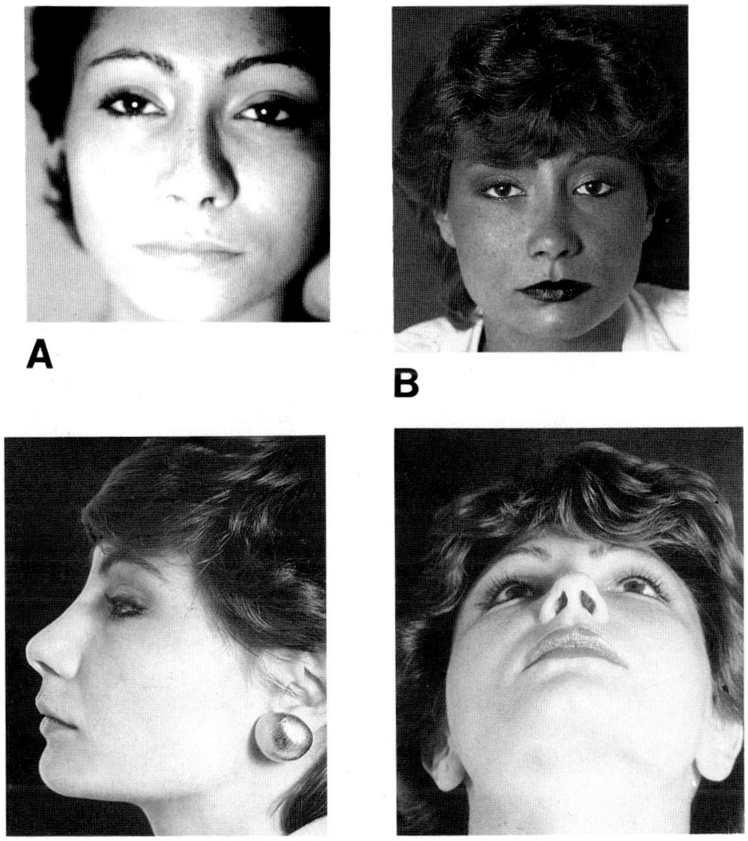

A B C D

Fig. 67. Secondary correction of a broad tip with Ponti's butterfly technique in a 25-year-old woman. (A) Preoperative view. (B, C, and D) Postoperative views.

Deformities of the tip, such as a bulbous tip with a broad lobule, can also be very unattractive following primary rhinoplasty and necessitate secondary revision. This revision must be done meticulously to refine and contour the tip by the excision of scar tissue in the tip and supratip area. Finally we place a cartilage onlay in a tip lobular pocket. This kind of tip onlay can be complimented by another columellar onlay, accentuating the double break at the lobule-columellar junction (Fig. 69 A and B). Lobular and tip grafts were described by Eitner (1935), Straatma (1951), Fomon (1948), and Meyer (1964–1967) in Denecke and Meyer (Fig. 69 C). They were presented by us in several international courses for cases of lost tip projection. In primary tip sculpturing we used and still use segments of removed lateral cartilages in two layers. Later this technique was popularized in the United States by Sheen (1975) and Peck (1977).

Ojeda (1985) recommends a spring cartilage graft to be placed into the tip as a supplementary lobular graft (Fig. 69 D). The tip graft usually has a rectangular, trapezoid, or triangular shape. We insert two trapezoid shaped pieces into the lobule area and two small pieces at the lobule-columella junction. All of these are introduced through a stab incision at the columellar border. Most of these are harvested from the cranial edge of the lower lateral cartilage. It can be double or triple layered. The pocket is made just long enough to accommodate and hold the cartilage graft in the desired position.

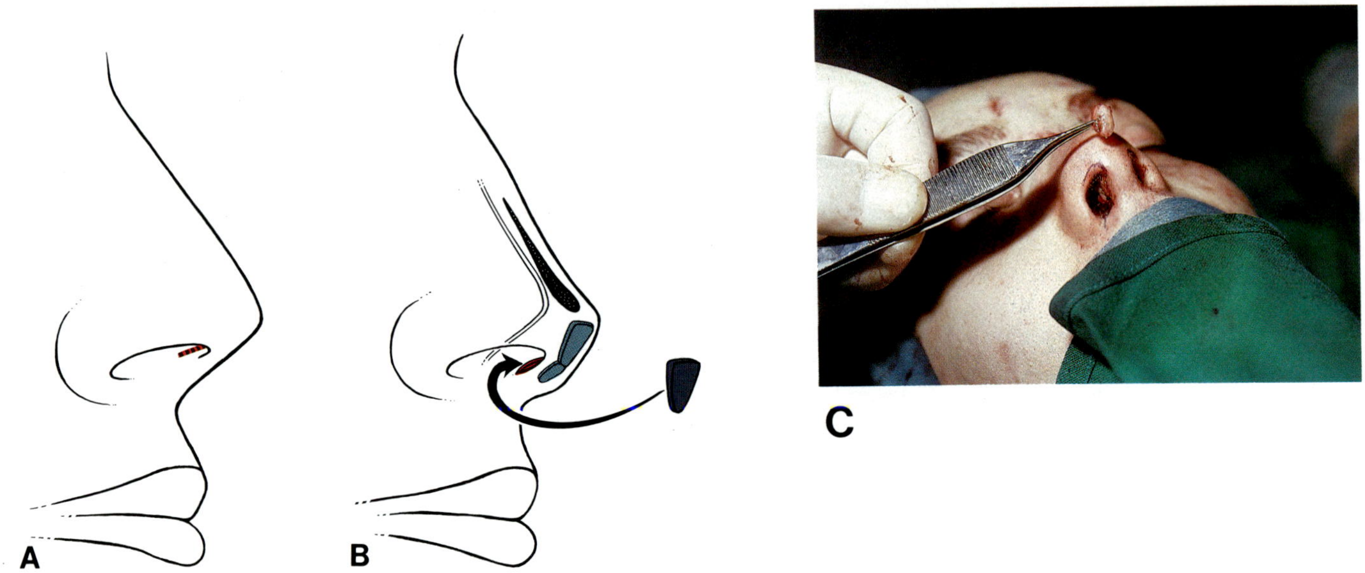

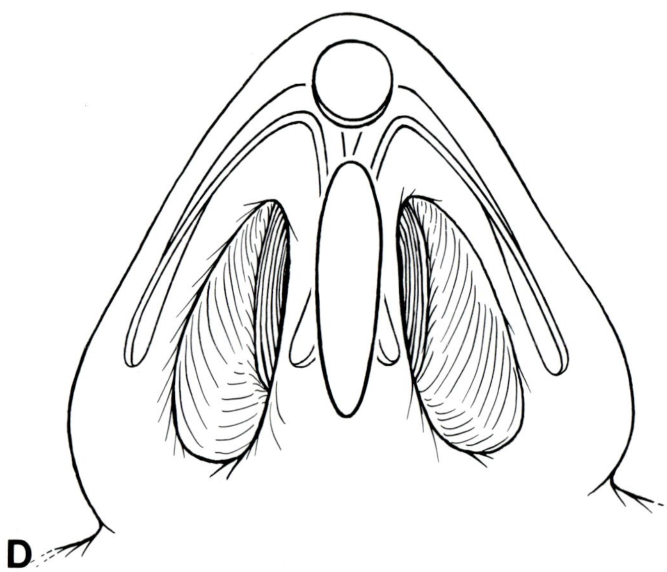

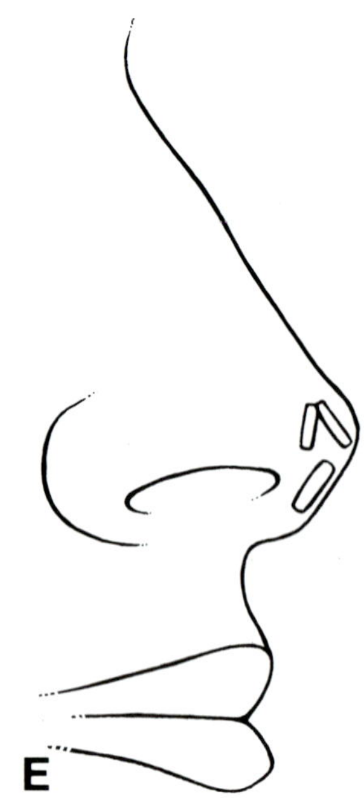

Fig. 68. (A–E) Lobular tip onlay advocated by Eitner and further described by Meyer and Sheen. It can be combined with a smaller cartilage graft in the middle of the columella for emphasizing the double angle (see Fig. 139). (A and B) Both onlays. (C) Lobular-tip onlay shown preoperatively. (D) Columellar batten and lobular onlay as presented in the book by Denecke and Meyer (1967). (E) For tip definition, Ojeda uses in addition to a lobular onlay graft, a spring-like folded cartilaginous graft.

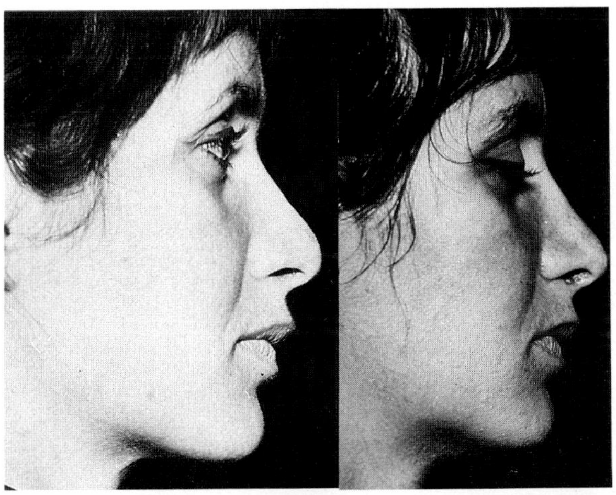

Fig. 69. (A) Retracted tip or tipless tip after overzealous resection of the septal border and the dome, is now requiring definition by means of a tip-columella support. Preoperative profile view and postoperative profile. *(Fig. 69. continues.)*

In cases of thick skin we prefer to transplant a triangular or trapezoid piece of stronger septal cartilage, like Ortiz-Monasterio (1977, 1981), rather than the soft alar cartilage. To represent the two domes of the lower lateral cartilages, trapezoid conchal cartilage grafts are recommended.

This technical detail for sculpturing the tip lobule complex, producing a harmonious double break in profile and a double light reflex (alar cartilage high lights) in the front and the axial views has been used by us for over 20 years. Only in a very rare case have we had to perform a little local revision of the lateral edge of the onlay which became secondarily visible. Resorption of the onlay graft is minimal.

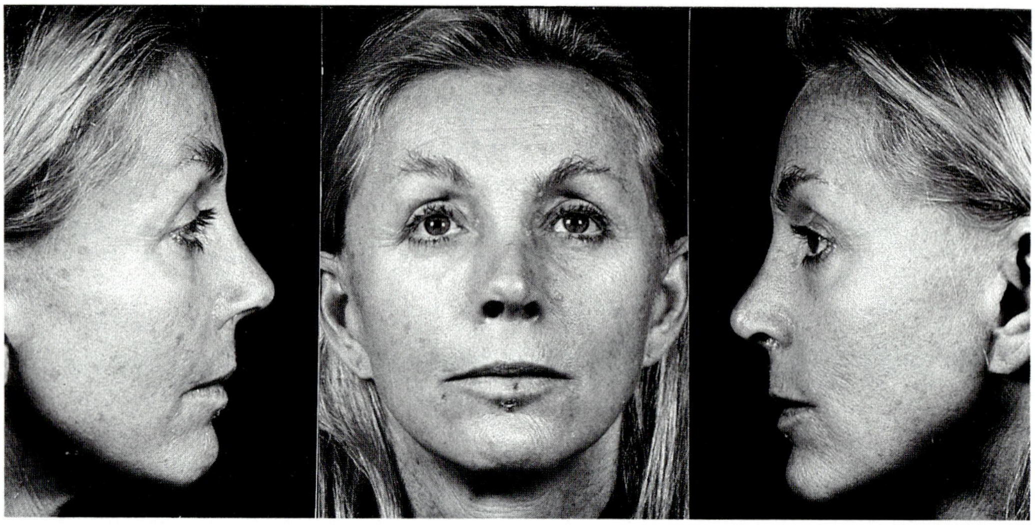

B

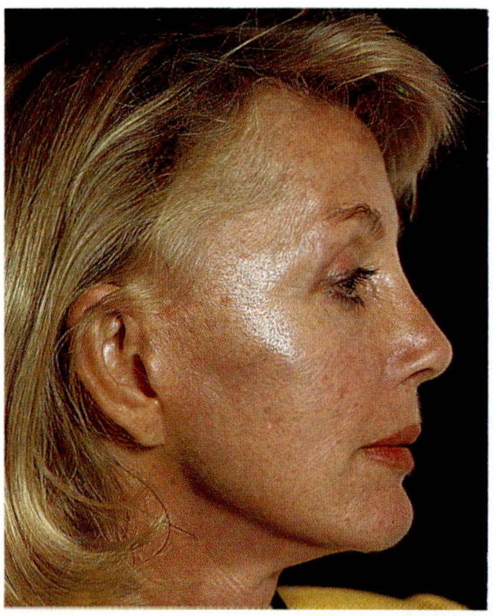

C

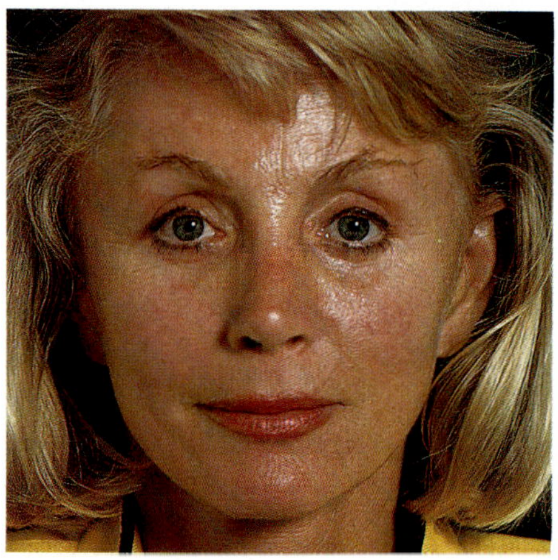

D

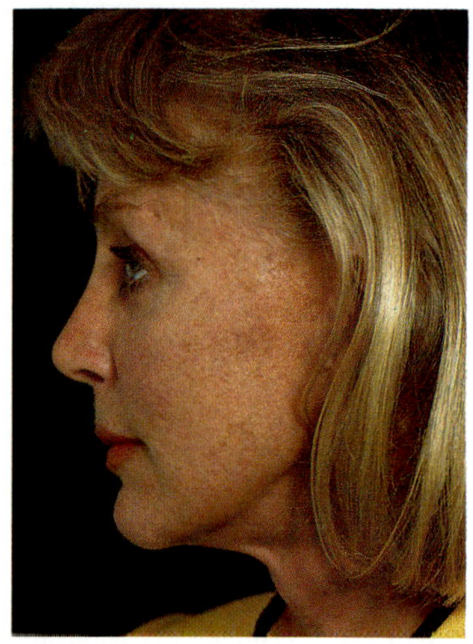

E

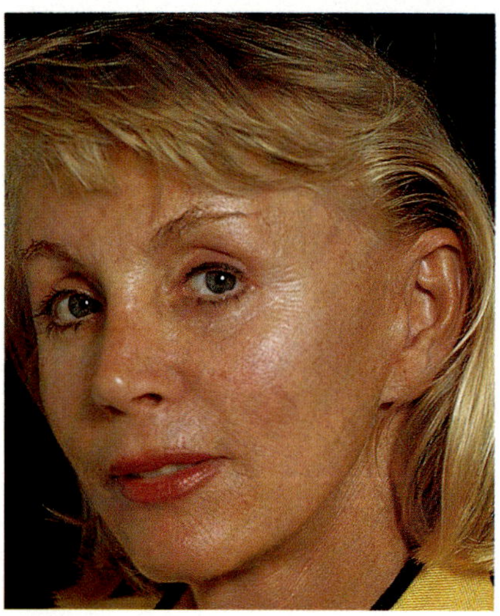

F

Fig. 69. (B–F) A too straight columellar profile line has to be broken to obtain a double break by augmentation at the lobule-columellar junction. (G) Young woman showing this secondary deformity before and (H, I, J, and K) after revision.

Collapse of the Middle Third of the Nose

Excessive narrowing and depression of the middle third of the nasal dorsum creates two problems. It produces an unattractive profile, but, above all, it disturbs the function of the nasal valve. This functional pathology results from over-resection of the upper lateral cartilages along with the hump removal.

When we encounter this overcorrection during a primary rhinoplasty we have to reinsert immediately a part of the hump, as advocated by Skoog (1966, 1974), in order to prevent the collapse (Fig. 70). Usually, however, this collapse of the nose appears progressively after a primary intervention. The spreader technique of Sheen (1984) is a good way for secondary correction of the collapse of the middle third of the nose (Fig. 71). This procedure consists of taking a basal strip from the septal cartilage and reinserting it over the trimmed lower lateral cartilages in order to spread these and correct their collapse (Fig. 72). Another method to augment and normalize the dorsal ridge is the "tile graft" of Planas (1987).

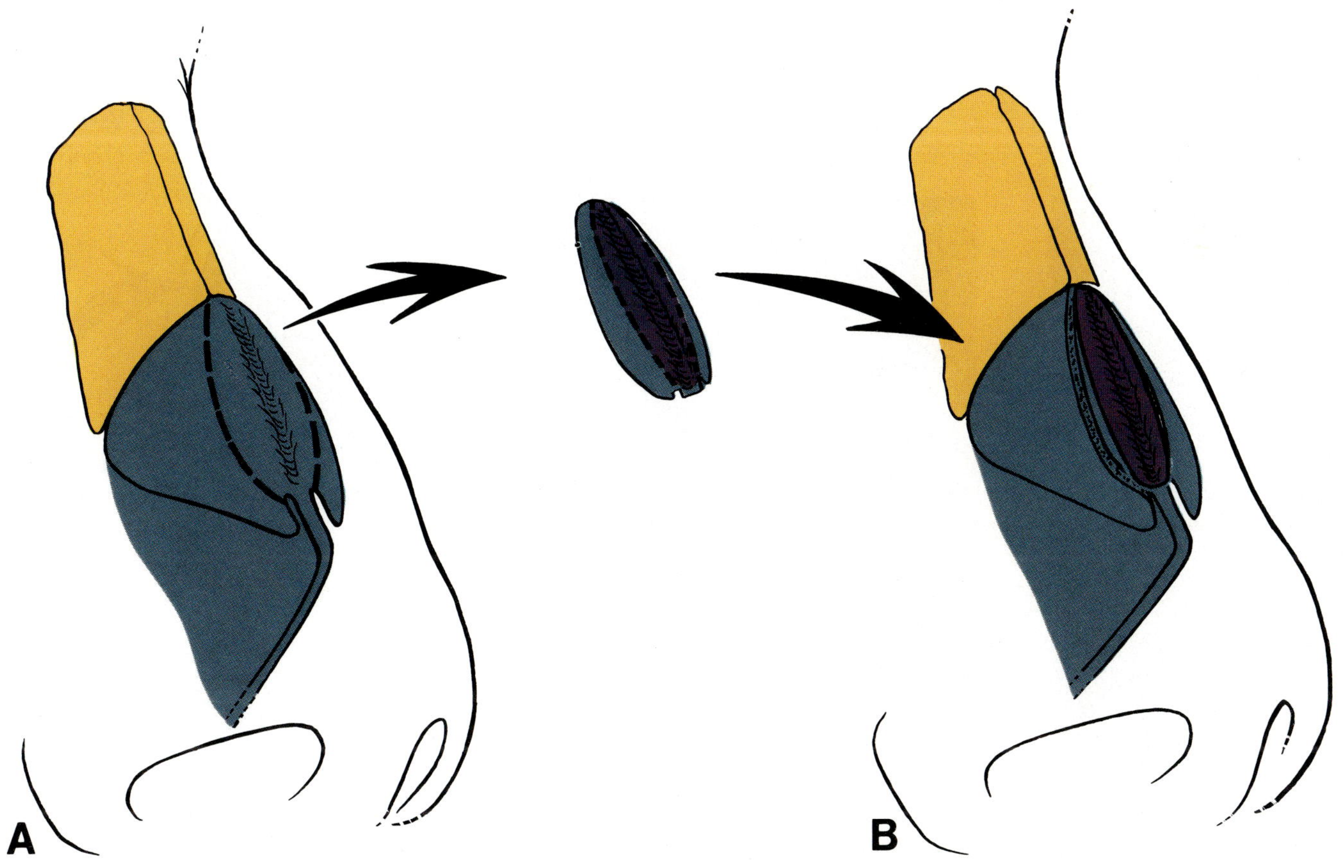

Fig. 70. If in a hump removal an excessive resection of the upper lateral cartilages with the corresponding portion of septal border has been made, the resected piece can be reduced and inserted in order to prevent a depression and narrowing of the ridge at that level. (A) Resection of cartilaginous hump. (B) Reinsertion of the reduced hump.

The depression of the middle third of the nose may also include the supratip area. In these cases we insert a septal cartilage graft in the cartilaginous part of the dorsum, reaching the supratip area to create a harmonious profile (Fig. 73). The dissection of the recipient pocket must be meticulous, to avoid trauma to the dermis. It may be dangerous to place a cartilage graft into the very supratip area, which could cause a polly beak deformity. It should be done only in secondary rhinoplasties after scar removal and the creation of a Lipsett depression at the septal ridge. Such a fine longitudinal graft (or two or three tiny strips of cartilage) in the supratip pocket must be combined with a cartilage onlay in the tip-lobule-pocket. We increase in this way the tip projection and minimize the risk of producing a polly beak.

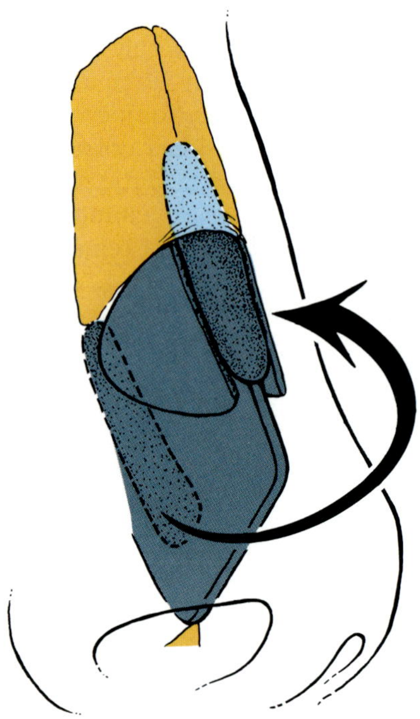

Fig. 71. Spreader technique of Sheen. A strip of cartilage is placed between the medially trimmed upper lateral cartilages in order to prevent or to correct a collapse of the middle third of the nose.

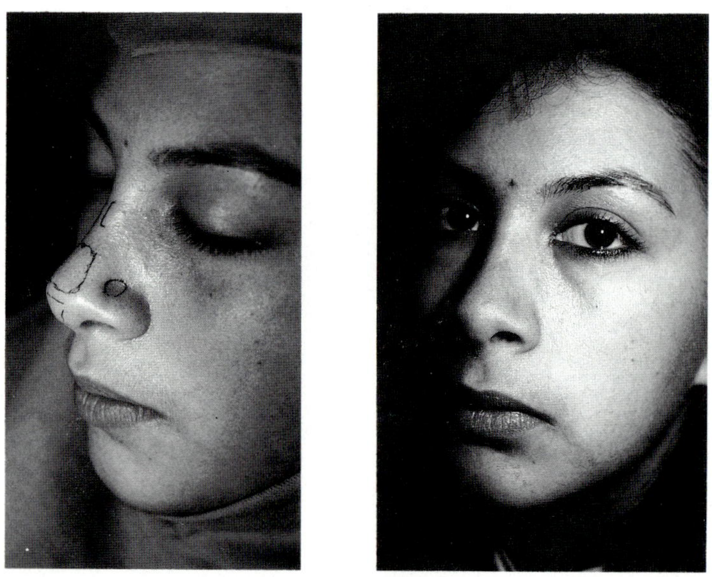

A **B**

Fig. 72. Collapse of the middle third of the nose corrected with a reduced piece of the cartilaginous dorsum (medial portion of the upper lateral cartilages and the corresponding dorsal marginal strip of septum) (A) Preoperative view of collapsing nose in a girl. (B) Half profile view after correction.

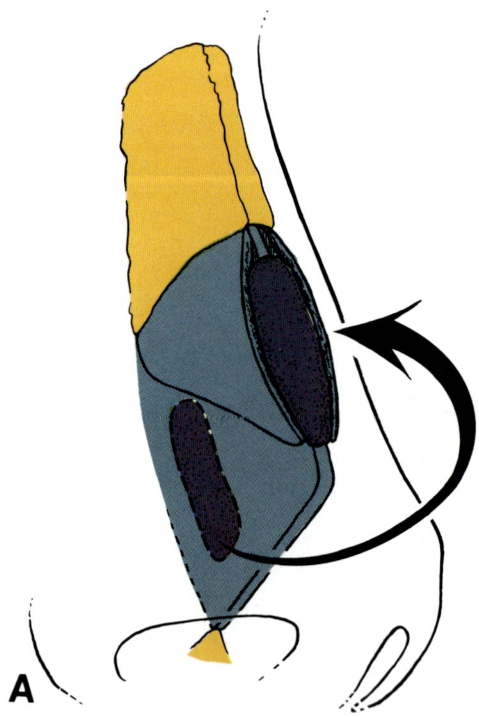

Fig. 73. After hump reduction and osteotomies in a young female, a spreader graft from the cartilaginous dorsum is reinserted and a strip of septal cartilage is placed medially into the supratip area in order to achieve a harmonious dorsal ridge and middle third of the pyramid. In addition a septal cartilage graft is inserted as onlay into the tip-lobule complex. (A, B, and C) Pieces of cartilage ready for being reinserted. (D and E) Corrected nose at the end of the operation.

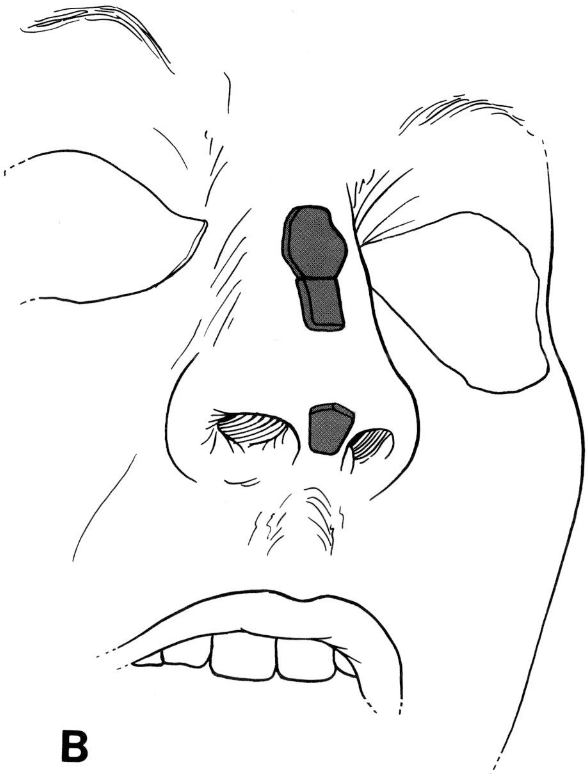

B

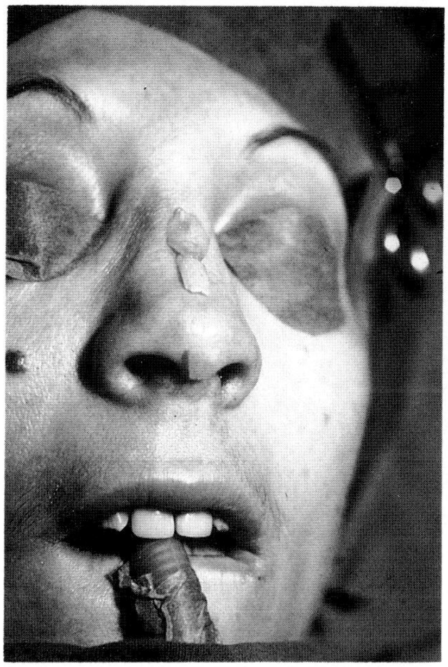

C

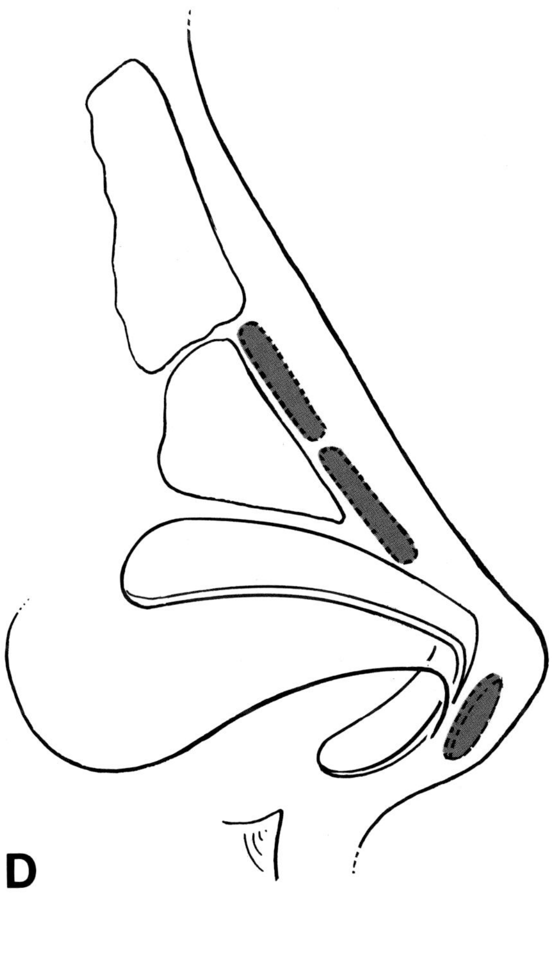

D

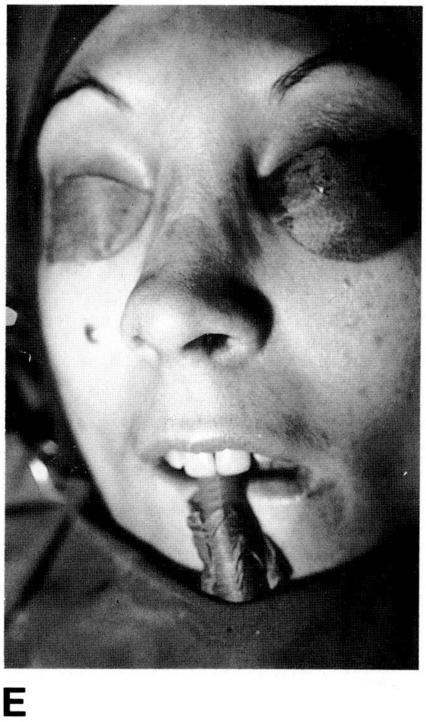

E

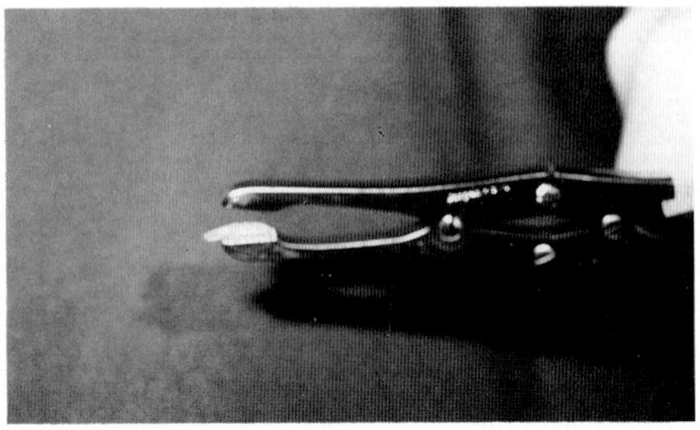

Fig. 74. Cartilage morcelized.

For these procedures using septal grafts for ridge revision, we usually soften the rigid cartilage graft with a morcelizer. By this maneuver the sharp angles and edges of the graft are softened and the spring forces in it eliminated. The morcelizer can be a forceps (Fig. 74) with scored inner surfaces, as we utilize, or a cartilage crusher as used by most of the ENT surgeons and by Sheen (1978). The reinsertion of the morcelized cartilage graft above the irregular nasal ridge is a valuable procedure in secondary rhinoplasty (Fig. 75). Sometimes it is necessary to achieve stability of the graft by a transfixion suture through the dorsal skin.

Collapsing Ala

Alar collapse is more a functional disturbance than a cosmetic one. To underline this, some authors used to speak of "aspiration phenomenon," instead of collapsed ala.

The cause of alar collapse during inspiration is the particular slackness of the alar and/or the upper lateral cartilage, so that the ala nasi is unable to resist the suction effect caused by the inspired air stream and its negative pressure. Establishing the tension of the triangulo-alar skeleton, according to the Cottle test (see Chapter 4), clinches the diagnosis. Collapsed ala can be a primary pathologic finding in cases with too narrow a nasal cavity, like in tension nose, occasionally accompanied by septal deviation.

The too thin nasal lumen increases the respiratory negative pressure, especially during physical exertion, and results in alar collapse. In elderly patients, this disturbance can even occur with normal breathing, because of frequently deformed alar cartilages along with the loss of muscle tone.

The secondary etiologies are usually due to the inappropriate resection of the cartilage framework and to the loss of muscular action consequent to a previous rhinoplasty. Special care must be taken when operating on a nose with a long thin tip, where the upper lateral cartilage forms an acute angle with the septum. This kind of nose, like those where the upper lateral cartilage overlays the lower lateral cartilage, increases the risk of postoperative collapse.

The surgical correction of collapsed ala, recommended in the literature, includes two principles: (1) the stiffening of the cartilage by additional grafts (Fomon, 1960; Meyer, 1964 (in Denecke and Meyer); Wedig, 1965; Podvinec and Maksinovic, 1966; Marino, 1968; Hage, 1969, and Mosing, 1977; (2) the displacement or alteration of cartilage already present by repositioning or fixing it to the upper lateral cartilage (Fomon, 1960; Meyer, 1964; Walter, 1976). Since, on the basis of long-term studies, the methods mentioned so far have not always functionally satisfied us, we have added in the last years, for particular cases, a modified rotation technique, as Farrior (1962) described for the correction of collapsed ala due to harelip nasal deformities. In such cases the alar base is moved laterally, by V-Y plasty, thereby widening the floor of the vestibule.

Hage (1969) diagramed a bilateral conchal "butterfly graft" for stiffening of the tip-alar complex. The standard tip correction, with luxation technique, resection of the upper two-thirds of the alar cartilage, scoring the remaining alar arch, and sectioning the upper lateral cartilage at its insertion into the septum using the extramucosal procedure, does, in our hands, correct most cases of collapsing alae. Usually, we fix the ala, and the upper alar groove, in a less concave position, with 5-0 mattress sutures tied over small silicone sheets at the level of the upper lateral cartilage, or of the lower lateral cartilage, or of both (Figs. 76 and 77 D). Additionally we resect the pars transversa musculi nasalis together with the resection of the upper lateral car-

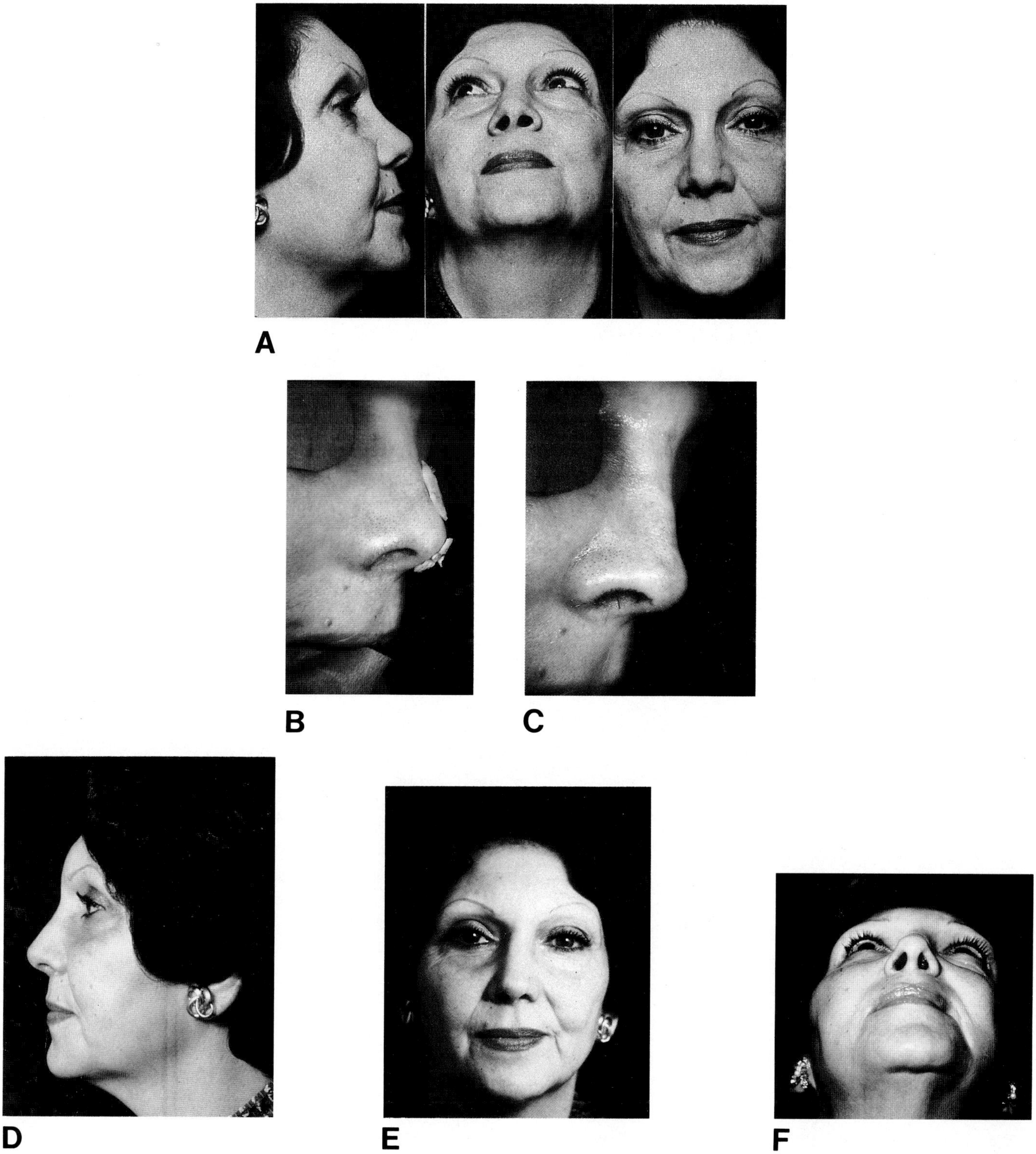

Fig. 75. Middle-aged female with secondary asymmetries of the dorsum tip, alae, and columella, requiring remodeling of these structures. Morcelized tip, columella, and dorsal cartilage struts were used in a revision procedure. Furthermore, a marginal alar resection on the right side and a narrowing of the left vestibular floor was performed. (A) Preoperative views. (B) Cartilage graft from the septum and cephalic alar portion are ready for being morcelized and reinserted. (C) End of the operation. All nasal structures are remodeled. The right alar border and the vestibular floor are sutured. (D, E, and F) Result.

tilage from the septum. One must also preserve the procerus muscle, the antagonist of the compressor. If the lateral crus shows a marked concave deformity, it can be resected, turned, and sutured in place in the opposite position, thus giving the ala a convex appearance.

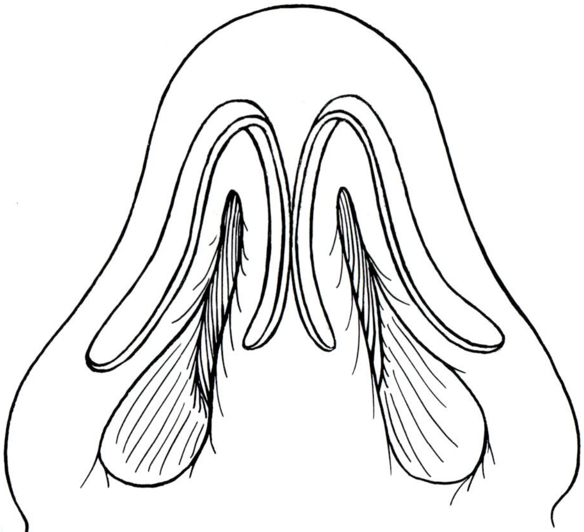

A

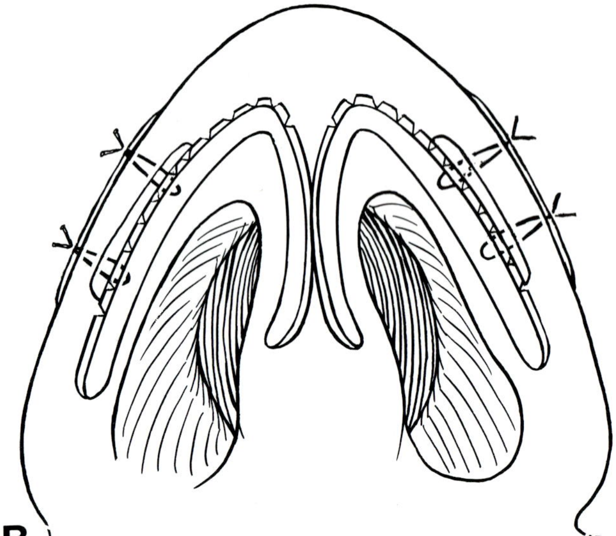

B

Fig. 76. For correction of collapsing ala, the lower lateral cartilages are also fixed in a new spread position after being reduced, scored, or cross-hatched, and if necessary cut vertically at the dome. (A) Preoperative position of the lateral crura. (B) New position with transalar mattress sutures.

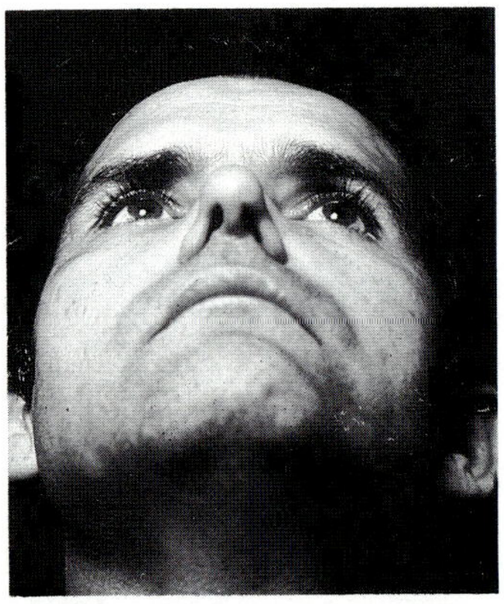

A

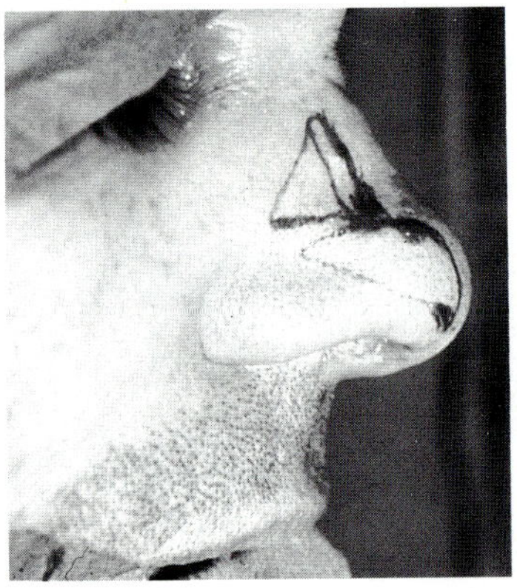

B

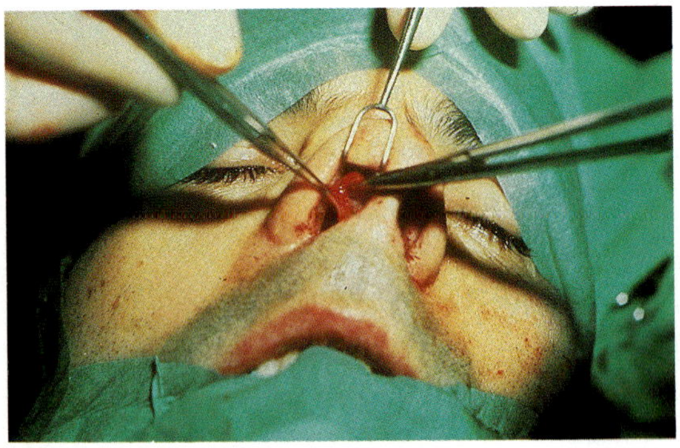

C

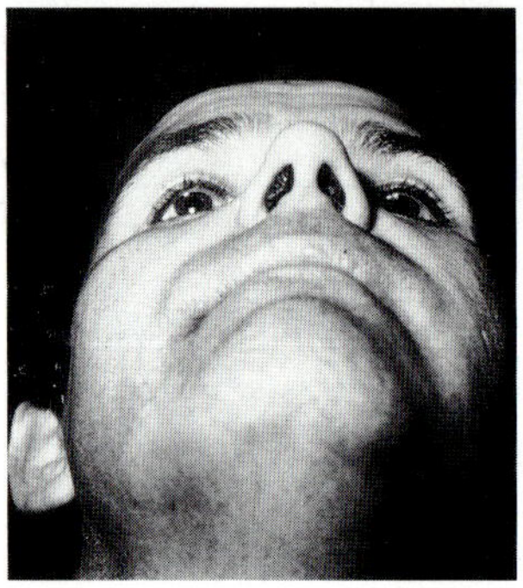

D

Fig. 77. Correction of collapsing ala. (A and B) Preoperative views. (C) Section of the upper lateral cartilage with the extramucosal technique. (D) Corrected alae in spread position.

In cases of collapsing ala due to a deficiency of the cartilage framework of congenital etiology, we reconstruct the valve skeleton by using a conchal graft or a septal slice graft or one cortical layer of the perpendicular ethmoid plate, which are all appropriate in replacing the missing cartilages. We introduce the graft through an intercartilaginous incision into the receptor pocket, prepared by a very meticulous and precise dissection, in order to minimize the operative trauma. A subtotal resection of the lateral crus of the lower lateral cartilage also gives appropriate material for the same lateral support. We can introduce the graft into a subperiosteal pocket formed in the external or internal aspect of the nasal bones, as Bridger (1981) and Lapidot (1985) have suggested. Bridger uses split rib graft and Lapidot uses septal cartilage. In all our cases, to help the healing of the graft in the right position and to diminish the formation of fibrous tissue around the graft, we apply trans-alar mattress sutures and fibrin sealant (Fig. 78).

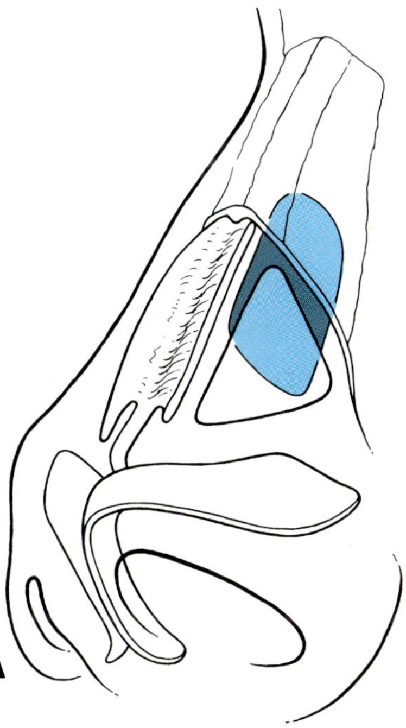

A

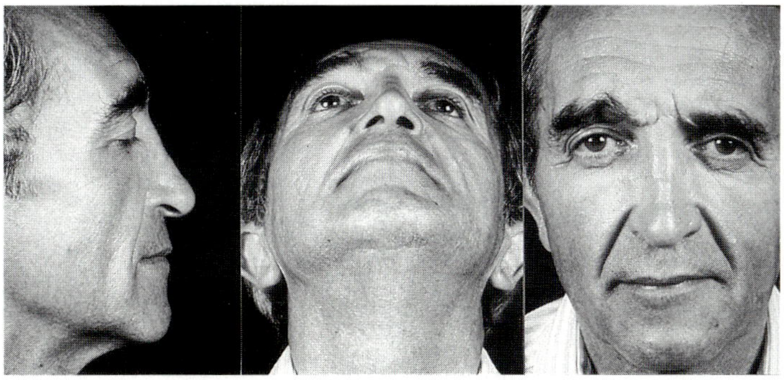

B

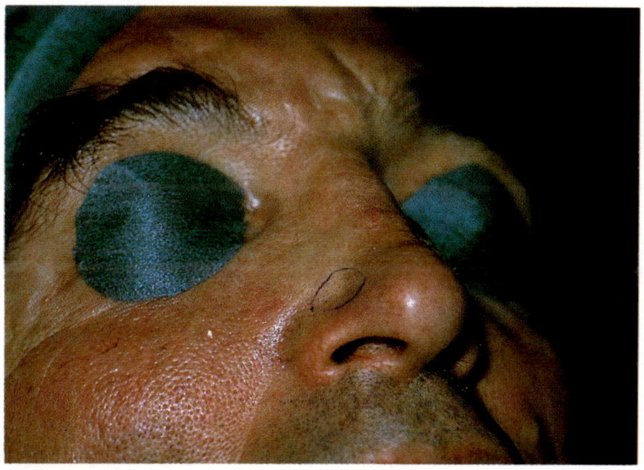

C

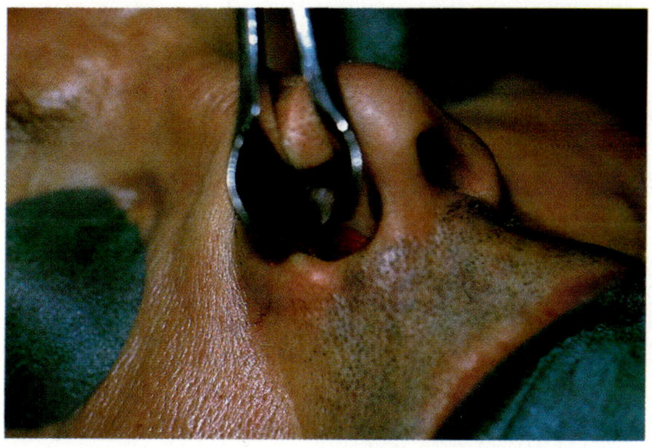

D

Fig. 78. (A) To correct collapse of the valve and middle third of the nose we introduce a septal slice graft into a subperiosteal pocket of the nasal bone through the intercartilaginous incision leaving the half of the graft underneath the upper lateral cartilage. (B-L) Correction of collapsing upper and lower lateral cartilage in an aging nose. (B) Preoperative views. (C) External depression of the nasal wall at the level of the valve. (D) Internal view of the collapsing valve.

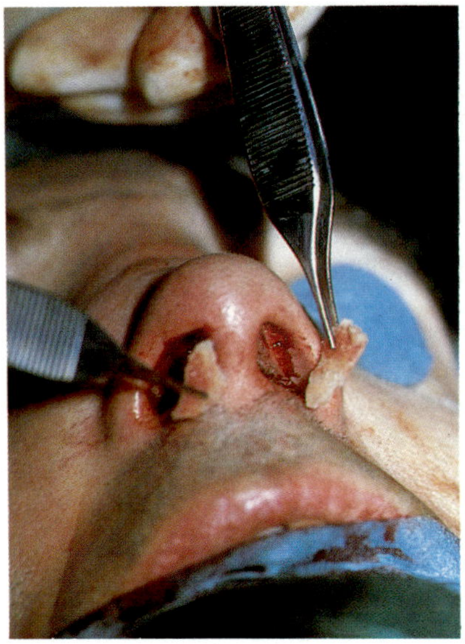

E

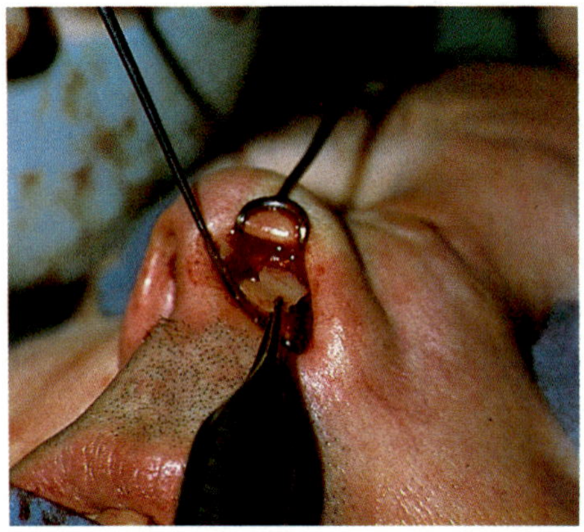

F

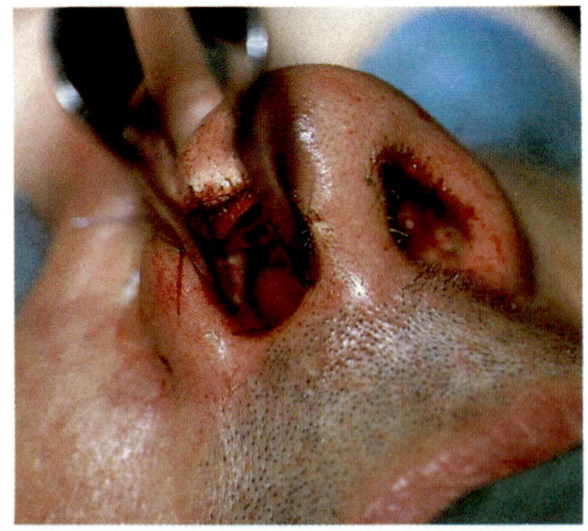

G

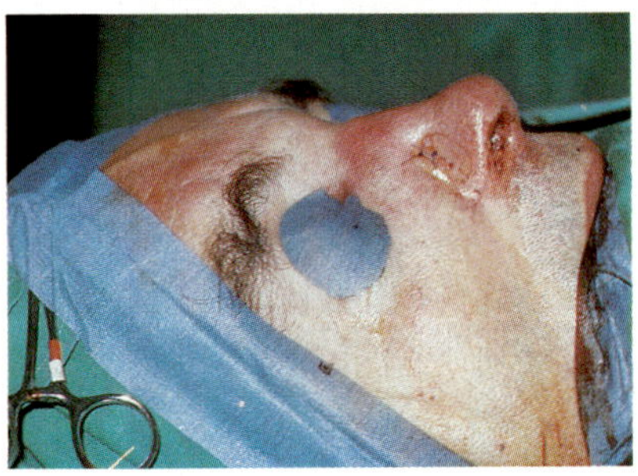

H

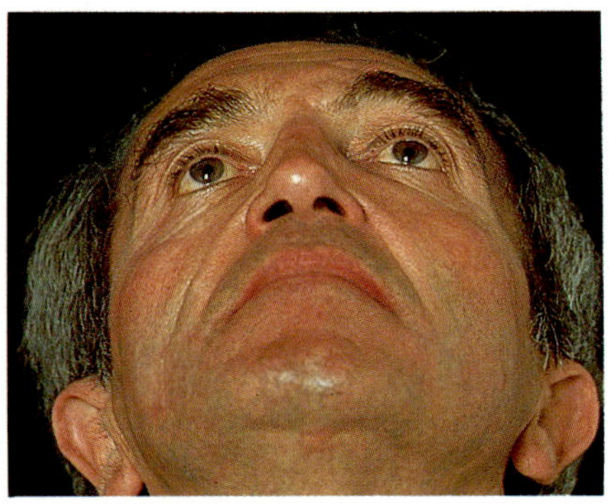

I

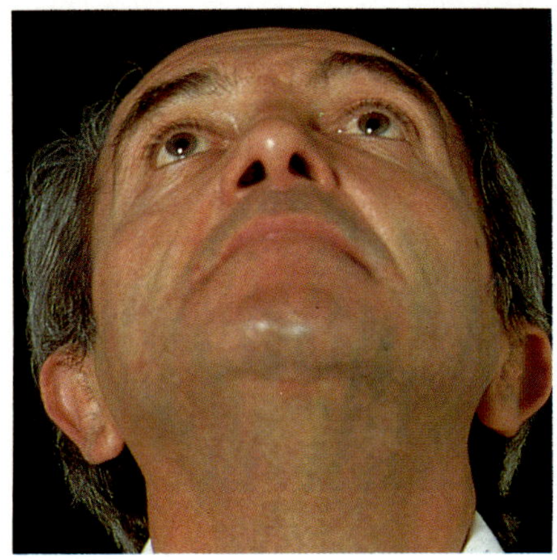

J

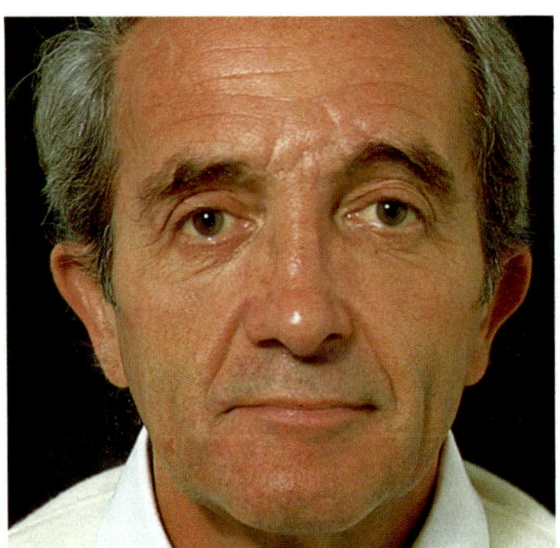

K

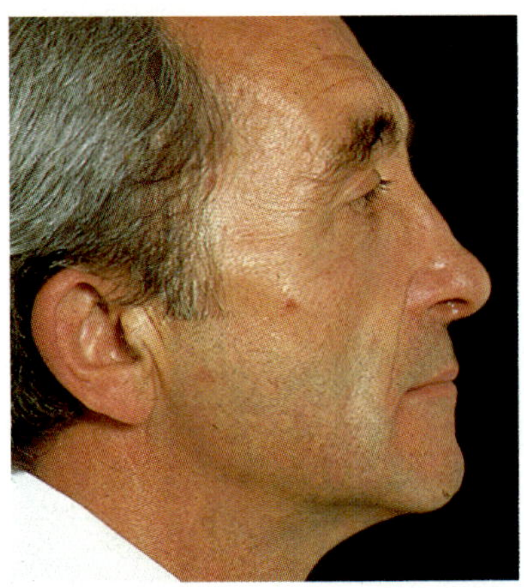

L

(E) Sheets of septal cartilage and ethmoidal bone ready to be introduced into a lateral subperiosteal pocket. (F) Insertion of the ethmoidal plate on the right side. (G) The same bone graft visible in the subperiosteal pocket at the nasal bone. (H) End of the operation. Fixation of the grafts with mattress sutures. (I and J) External result. (K and L) Preoperative and postoperative axial view.

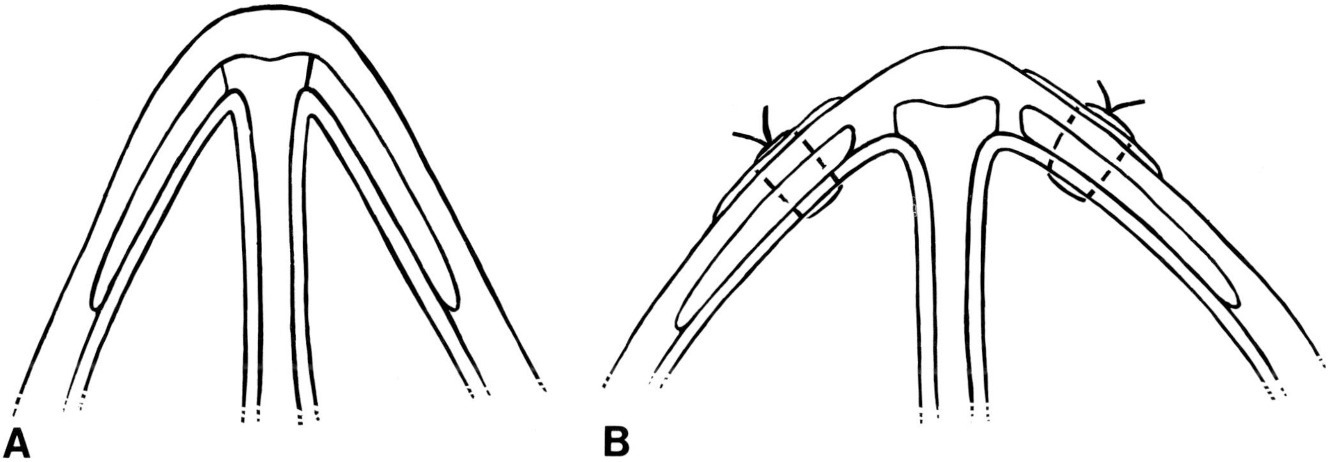

Fig. 79. For correction of collapsed ala we use the extramucosal technique with section of the upper lateral cartilages at their insertion to the septum and we fix them in a new more lateral position, with obtuse valve-angle by means of transcutaneous mattress sutures. The alar cartilages are handled as usual with vertical section at the dome. (A) Upper lateral cartilages in a narrow position with acute angle at the valve. (B) These cartilages kept the new position by mattress sutures with more obtuse angle at the valve.

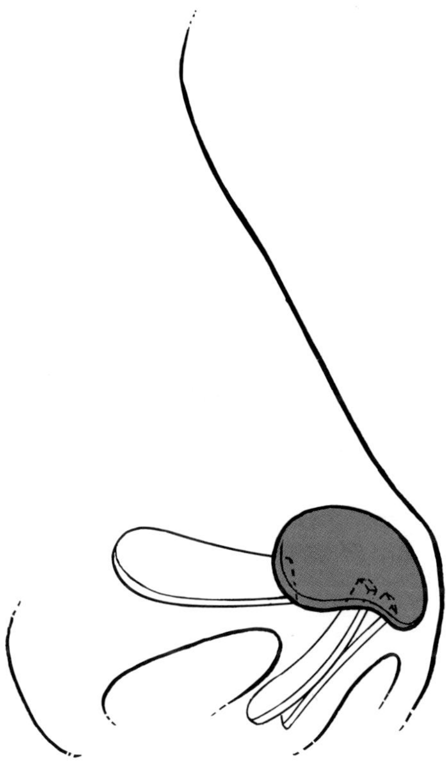

Fig. 80. Cartilage graft from the ear concha for correction of a pointed narrow tip.

Various interventions have been proposed by Fomon (1960) to cure this deformity, such as severing the insertion of the upper lateral cartilage at the septum and to fix it, after rotation, in a new curved position (Fig. 79). The same author also suggests using a suture with luxation effect at the lower edge of the upper lateral and at the upper edge of the alar cartilage.

While Masing (1971) utilized a posterior shifting of the lateral crus of the lower lateral cartilage, securing it to the upper lateral cartilage, Georgi (1982) devised a modified flap for the correction of the collapse of the ala. The inner valve is widened and stabilized using a cartilage transposition flap from the upper border of the lower lateral cartilage brought into a pocket in the membranous septum. This effect can be supported by filling the resulting cartilage defect at the intercartilaginous incision with septal or auricular cartilage.

We believe that the fixation of the inward rolled medial border of the upper lateral cartilage after its section at the junction with the septum, as advocated by Fomon, is not necessary if transalar mattress sutures are applied.

The Pointed Narrow Tip

The pointed narrow tip results from excising the entire dome of the lower lateral cartilages, including the vestibular lining, during the primary procedure. The treatment of this deformity often requires more than just a trapezoid or triangular strut. The acute angles formed by the residual stumps of the lower lateral cartilages have to be trimmed secondarily, and in most cases the nose should also be shortened. The medial segments of the lateral crura are spread and a carved piece of cartilage is interposed between them, producing a smooth, broader, and more rounded tip.

As is often the case, after a primary rhinoplasty, we don't find any excess of the lateral

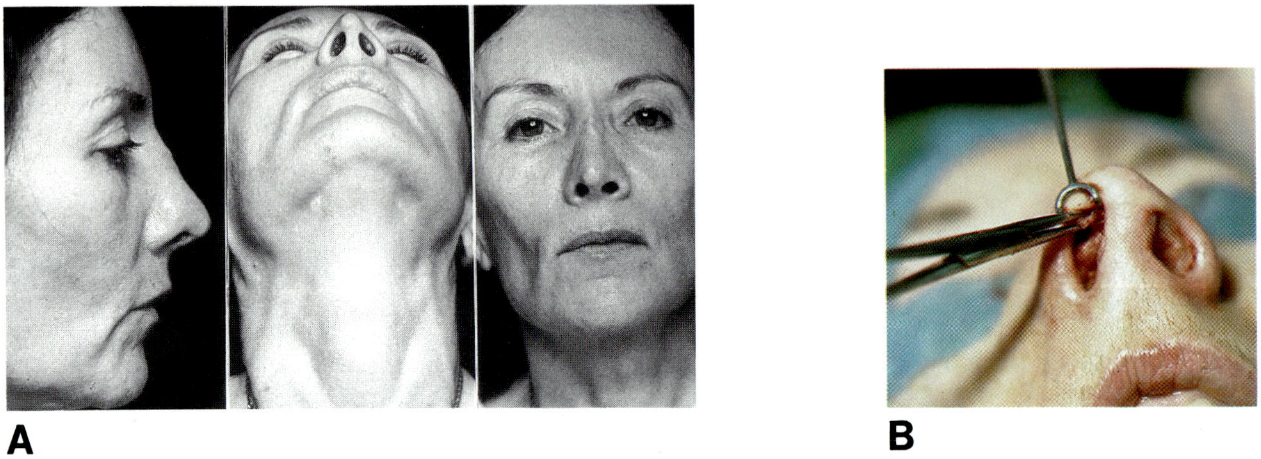

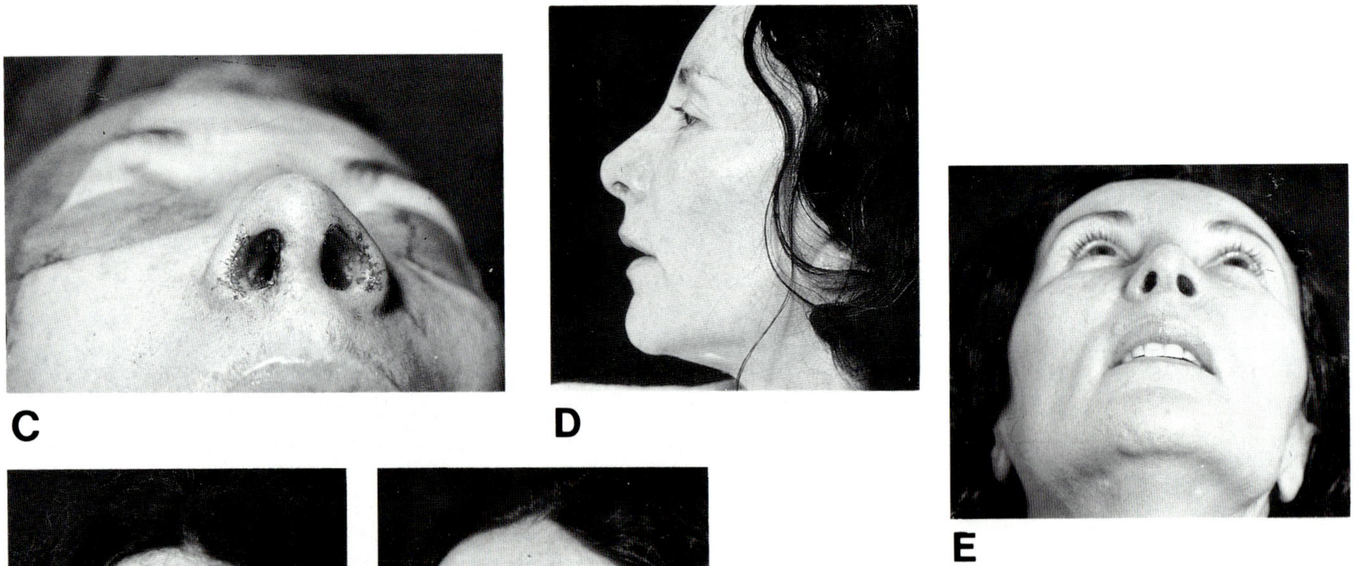

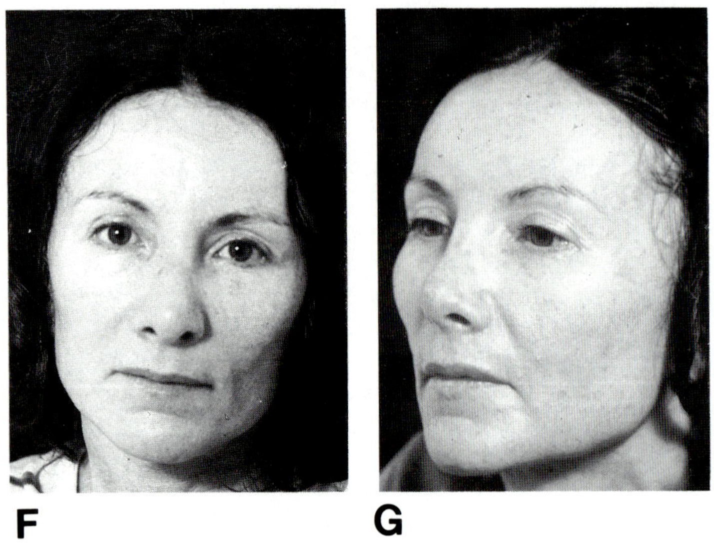

Fig. 81. Fifty-year-old lady with a too narrow tip and low posterior part of the alar rim. In a secondary procedure fibrous tissue has been removed from the tip and an ear concha umbrella-graft inserted at its place on the top of the still existent medial crura. Posterior marginal alar resection was also performed. (A) Postrhinoplasty sequelae with too pointed tip. (B) Placing umbrella-graft into the tip. (C) End of the operation with a more rounded tip by insertion of ear cartilage graft as designed in Figure 78. Over and over suture of alar rim wound. (D, E, F, and G) Result after secondary rhinoplasty.

crura which can be harvested for the tip and lobule augmentation. In this situation, we can apply an "umbrella" graft (Fig. 80). With this technique an ear conchal graft is inserted on the top of the still existant medial crura (Fig. 81). This kind of graft is best positioned through the infracartilaginous incision. The umbrella graft gives an excellent result with harmonious tip projection and softness. It may be further supported by a strut of cartilage from the septum in front of the remaining medial crura or between them if the tip projection is still too poor. Thus, the umbrella is supported and protruded into the vault of the tip skin, which has been meticulously freed from underlying scar tissue.

Bifid or Cleft Tip

A double light reflex at the nasal tip is a sign of beauty. However, if the double peak of the tip is exaggerated in height and width in primary cases it has to be corrected. If encountered in operated cases this deformity is due to fibrous tissue, which separates the medial crura or to insufficient modeling of the cartilaginous domes. To correct this exaggerated bifidity of the tip, we first have to dissect the two lower lateral cartilages and remove the fatty fibrous tissue between them. Then we must sculpture the alar cartilage in an appropriate way, reducing and scoring occasionally the domes by vertical resections, and suturing them together (Fig. 82). Occasionally, a cup shaped cartilage graft from the ear is necessary to fill the cleft (Fig. 83).

Pinched Nose

A pinched nose is a permanent sinking of the vestibular wall, obstructing the nostril and

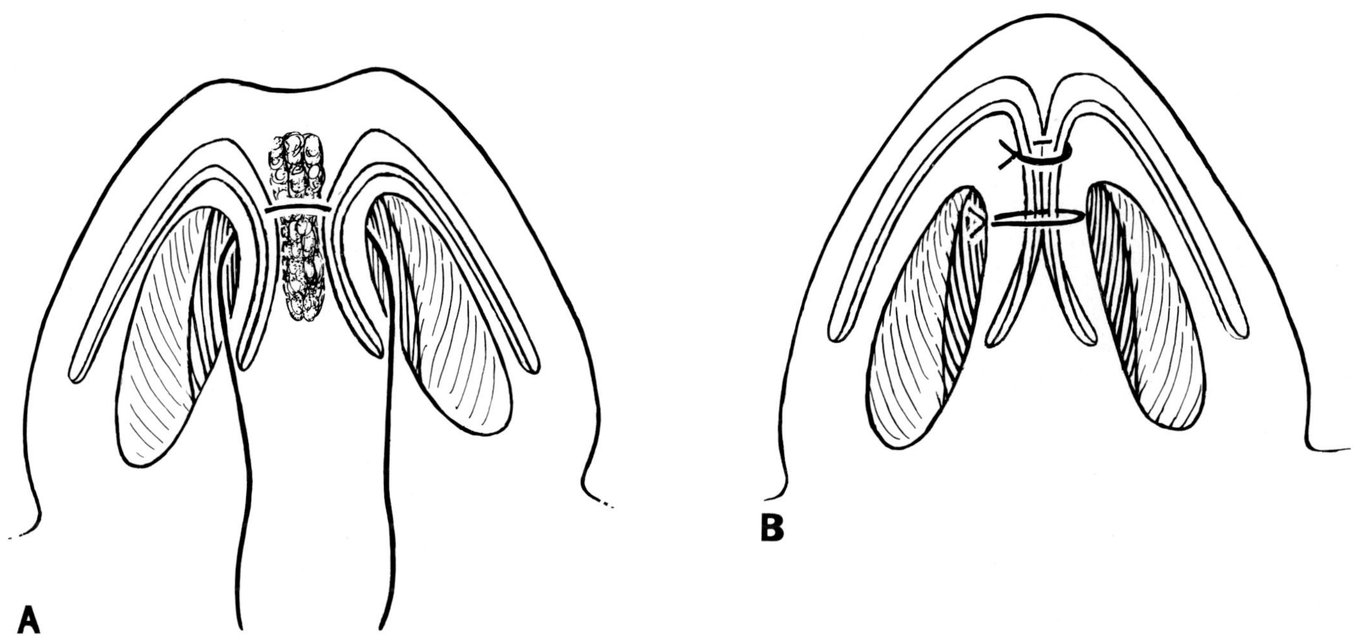

Fig. 82. Correction of bifid or cleft tip. (A) Fatty-fibrous tissue between the medial crura will be removed. (B) The lower lateral cartilages have been sectioned vertically at the dome and remodeled. The medial crura are sutured together. Eventually, a cup-shaped cartilage graft from the ear is necessary to fill the cleft and thus to correct the bifidity of the tip.

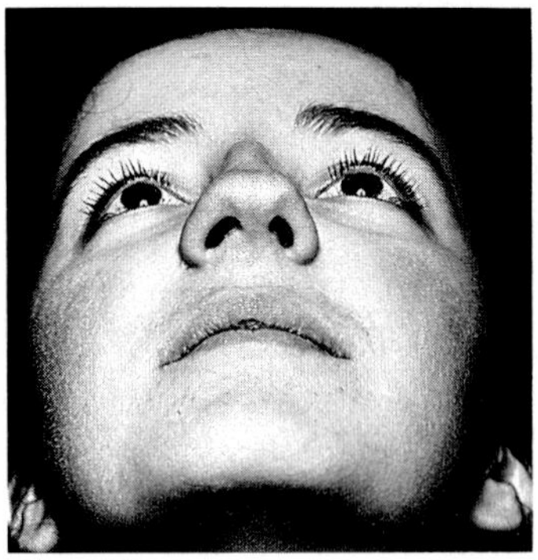

A

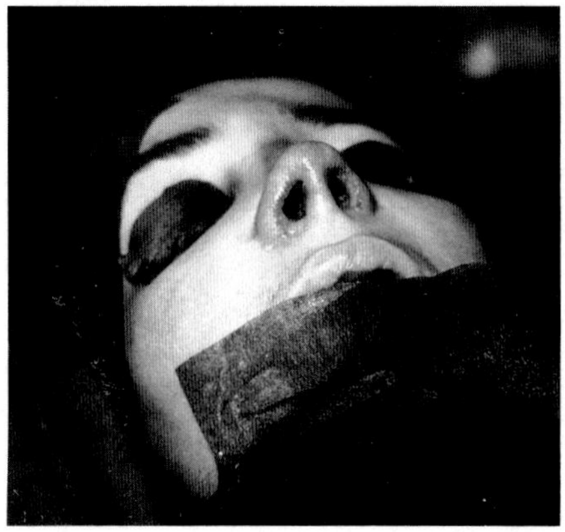

B

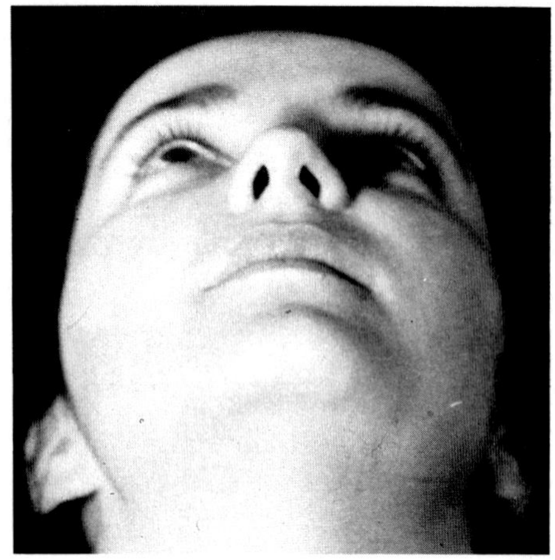

C

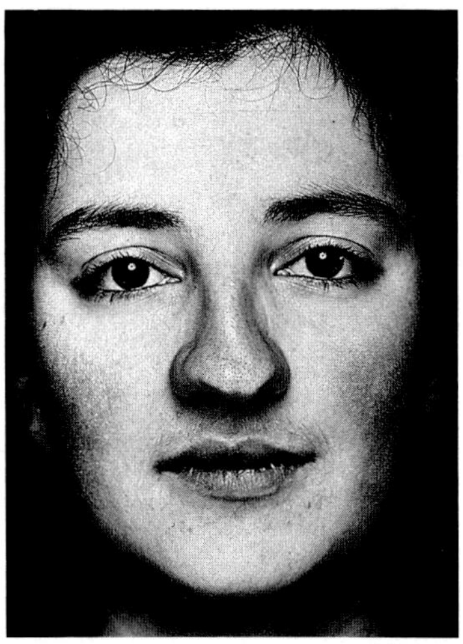

D

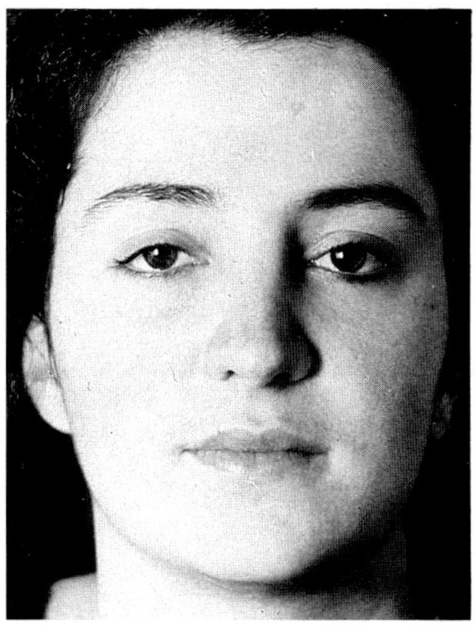

E

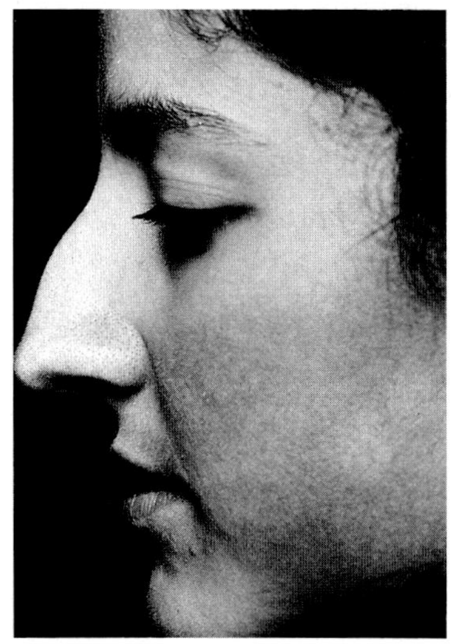

F

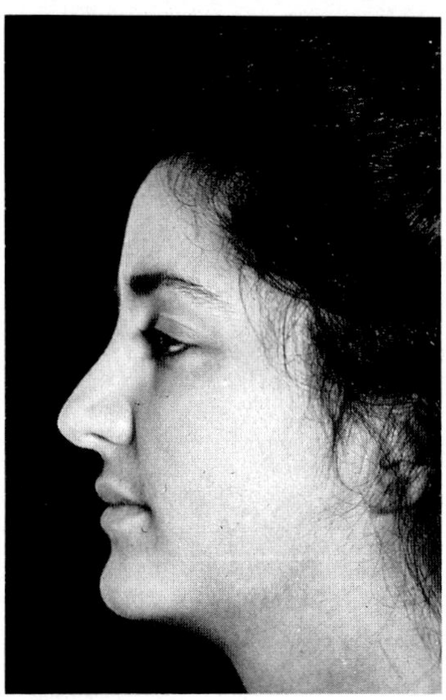

G

Fig. 83. This bifid nasal tip of a young girl was corrected with a cup-shaped cartilage graft from the ear inserted into the tip-lobule area and with a cartilaginous columellar strut from the septum. (A) Postoperative axial view. (B) End of the operation with two grafts in place and resection wounds at the alar rims sutured. (C) Postoperative axial view. (D and E) Frontal views. (F and G) Profile views.

creating an unaesthetic alar groove on one or both sides. This nasal deformity is always secondary to an excessive lower lateral cartilage resection, and must be differentiated from the collapsing ala, which is only seen on inspiration, due to its particular slackness. The pinched nostril results from the loss of a wide part of the lower lateral cartilage and often also from a concomitant vestibular scar retraction.

If for the reduction of the alar cartilage during a primary rhinoplasty a resection of a segment is necessary, this should not be performed in the lateral part of the lateral crus, but in a more median or paramedian section, otherwise the postoperative loss of continuity of the cartilaginous vault produces a pinched nose in the next few months. This precaution must be absolutely observed in any method of tip and ala sculpturing, but especially when using the procedure of Ponti (1969), where the "butterfly" structure of this technique should be cut as narrow as possible in the dome.

When the vestibular lining is intact, one just has to reconstruct the alar cartilage framework. For that, we insert meticulously a discoid cartilage graft from the septum. This graft is carved slightly convex and fixed, like a bridge, over the remaining parts of the lateral crus, with trans-alar mattress sutures (Figs. 84 and 85). For this purpose Nicolle (1986) inserts through an alar rim incision a bevelled elliptic septal cartilage graft of the whole length of a lateral crus and dome. In case of severely pinched nostrils with cicatricial retraction, a simple cartilage graft is not sufficient. For these patients we have to use a composite graft, which is best harvested from the inner side of the crus helicis, to rebuild at the same time the vestibular lining and the missing cartilaginous framework, after removal of scar tissue. This graft is sutured into the gap at the level of the intracartilaginous, intercartilaginous, or infracartilaginous incision and, if necessary, maintained in position with trans-alar mattress sutures, tied over a plastic sheet (Figs. 86 and 87).

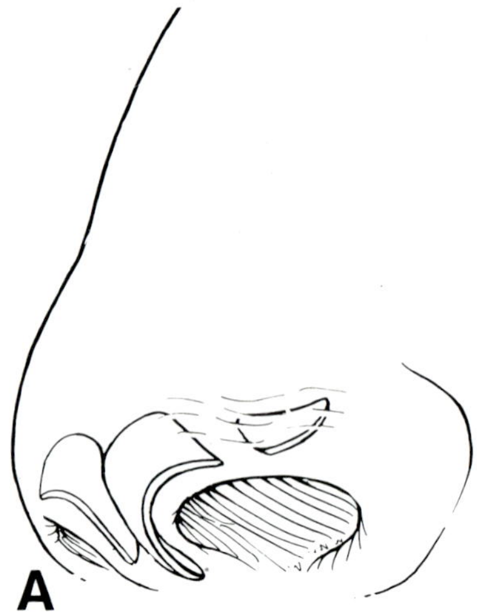

A

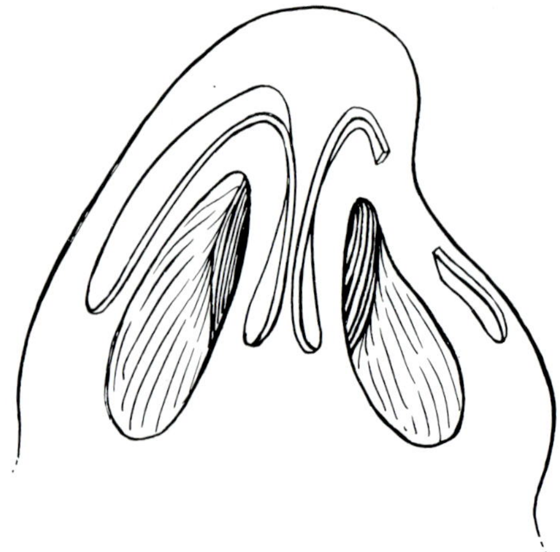

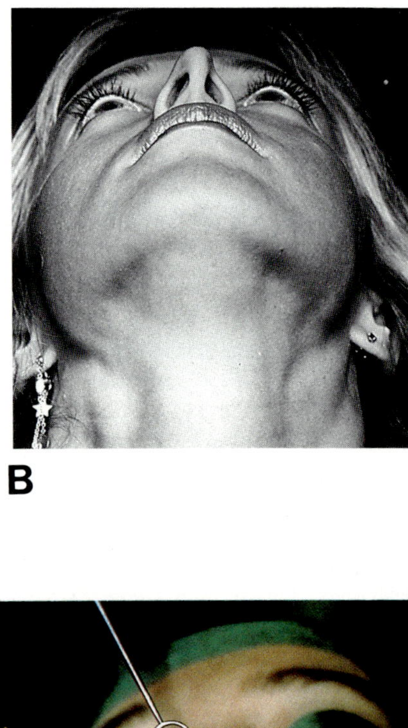

B

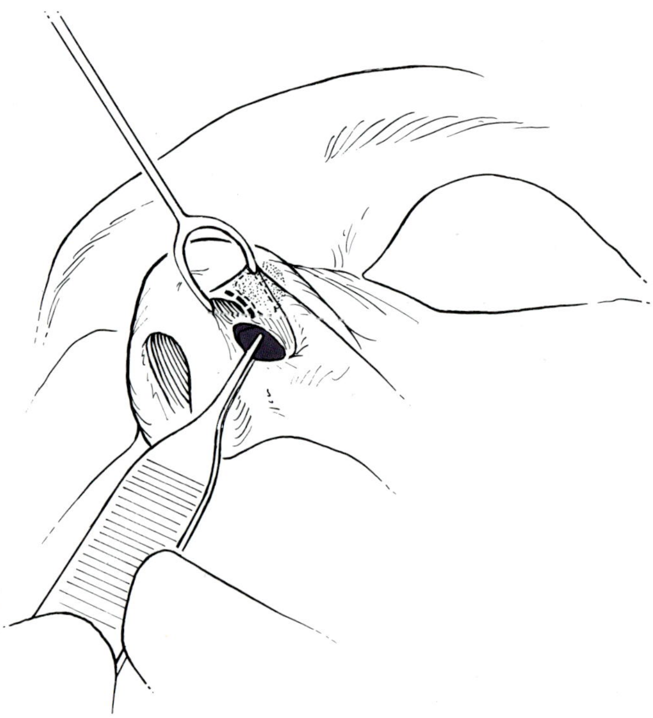

C

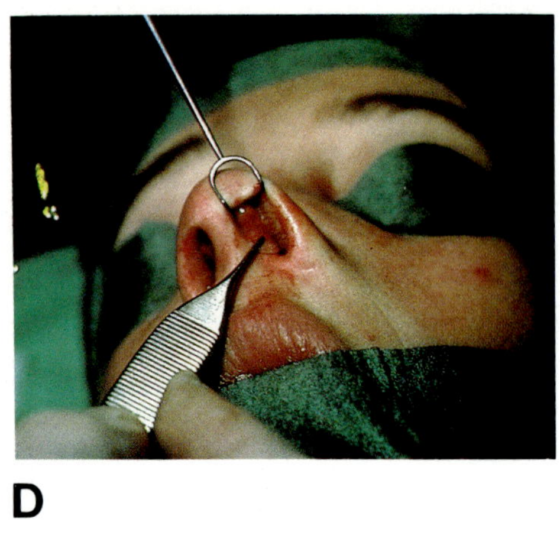

D

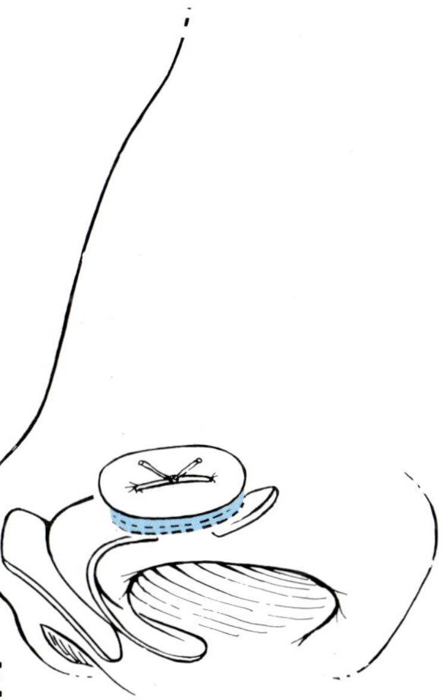

E

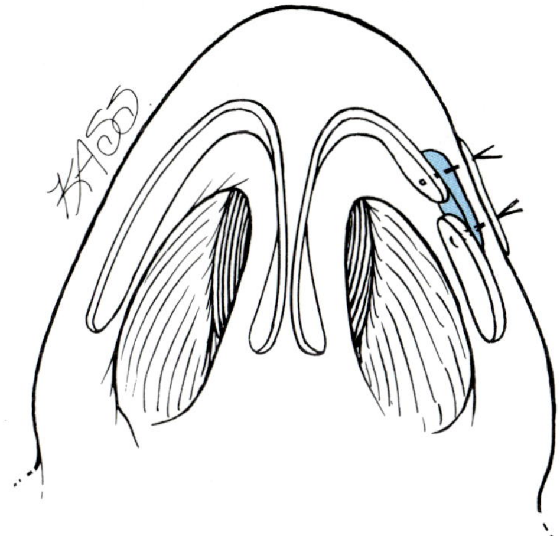

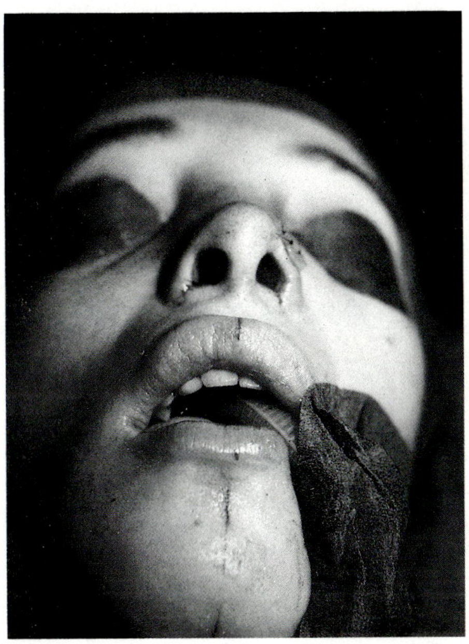

F

Fig. 84. Unilateral pinched nose with loss of lower lateral cartilage in the lateral crus area (A). Is corrected with apposition of a discoid cartilage graft from the septum, slightly carved on one side and fixed with transalar sutures. (B) Young girl with analog unilateral pinched nostril. (C, D, and E) Insertion of a septal cartilage graft into the nostril through the intercartilaginous incision. (F) End of the secondary operation with equilibrated nostrils and transalar mattress suture in place tied over a plastic sheet. At the same time the floor of the vestibule has been narrowed.

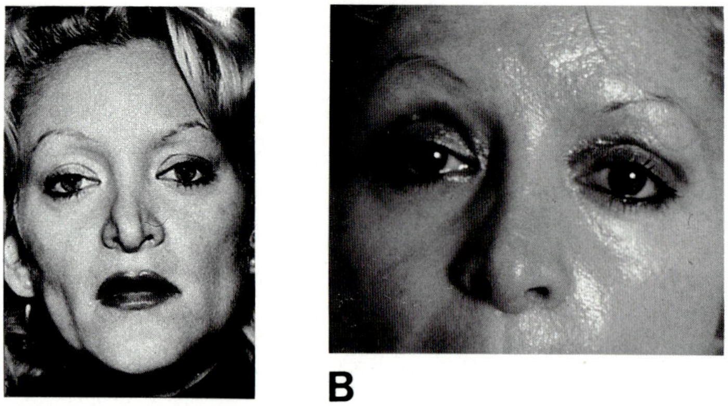

B

A

Fig. 85. Pinched nose in a 31-year-old lady after resection of nearly the whole lateral crus of the lower lateral cartilages. Carved cartilage grafts from the septum had to be inserted into both nostrils. (A) Preoperative and (B) postoperative view.

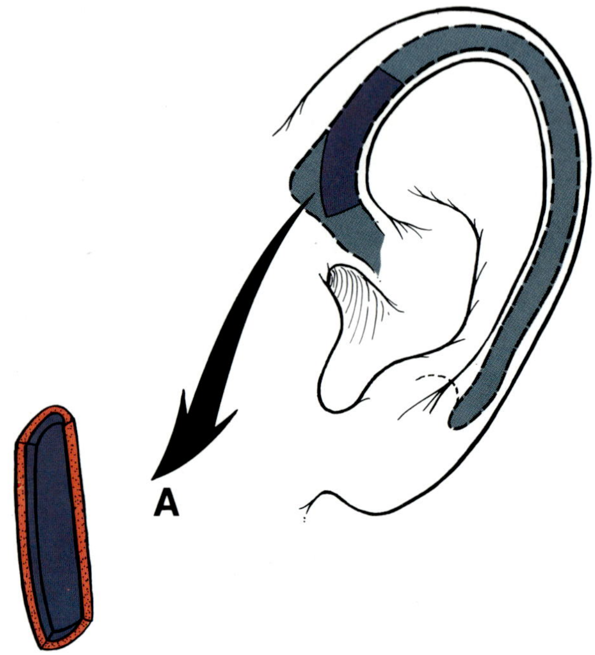

A

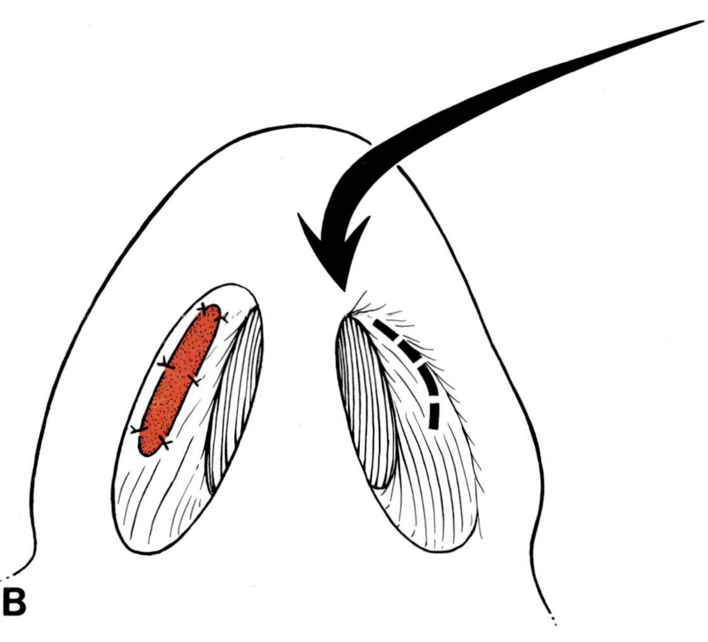

B

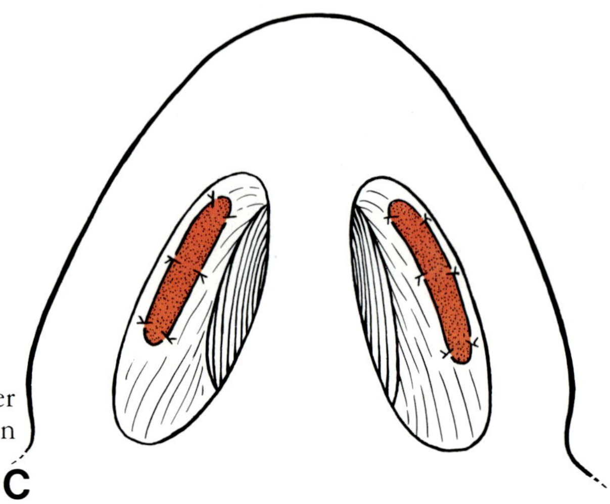

Fig. 86. Bilateral use of composite graft from the inner side of the crus helicis with skin and cartilage for expansion of the lateral vestibular wall. (A, B, and C,)

C

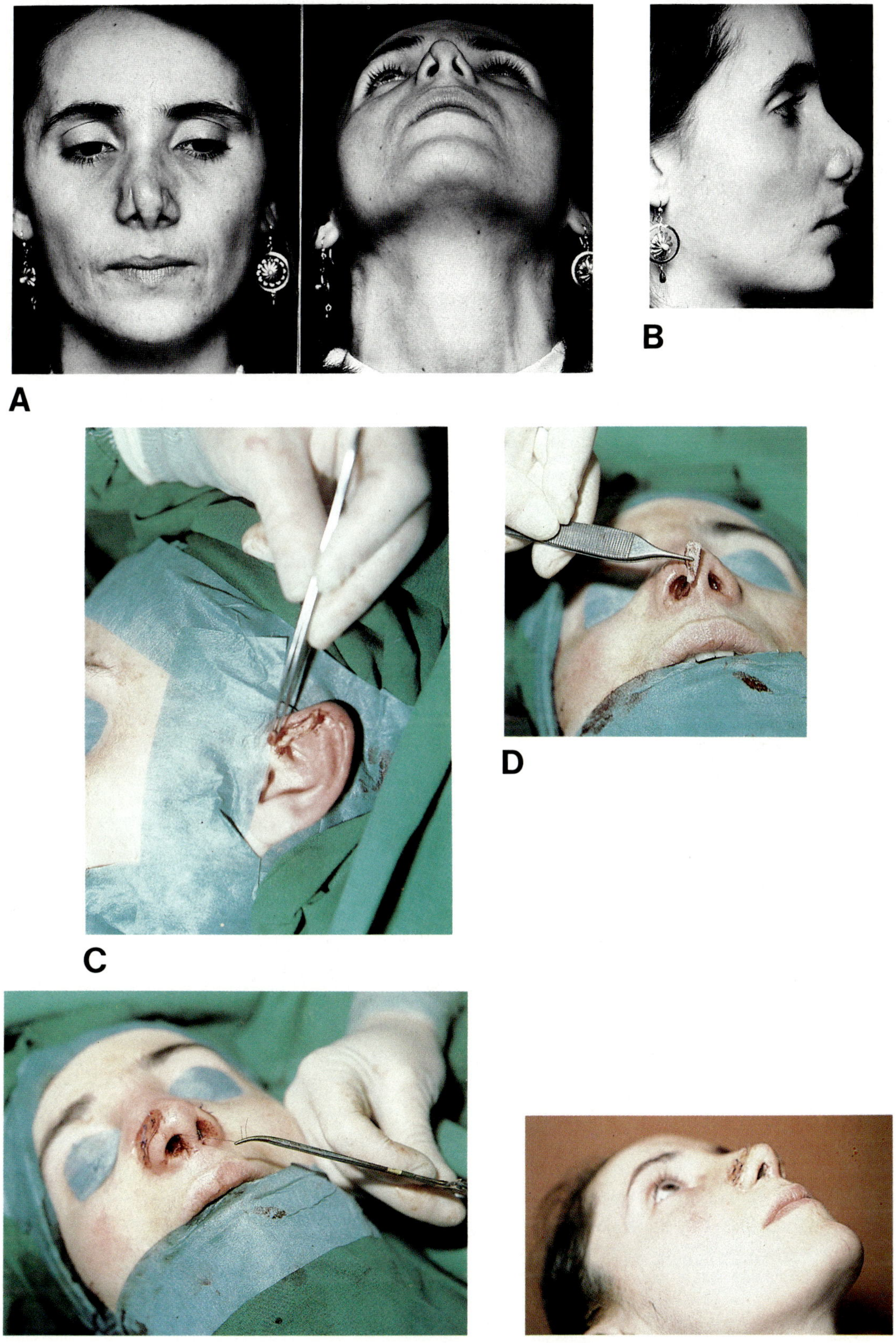

Fig. 87. continues.

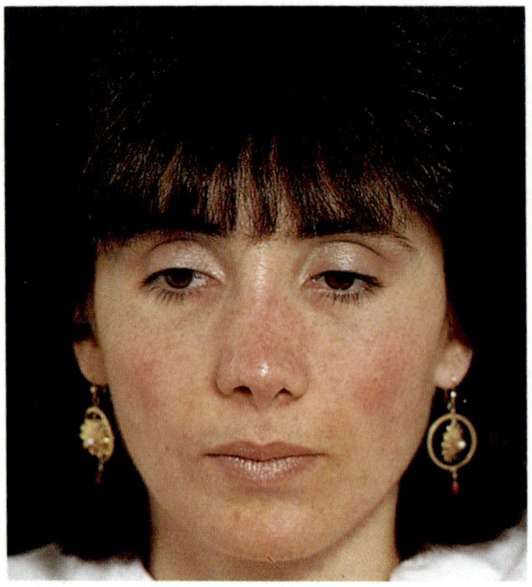

G

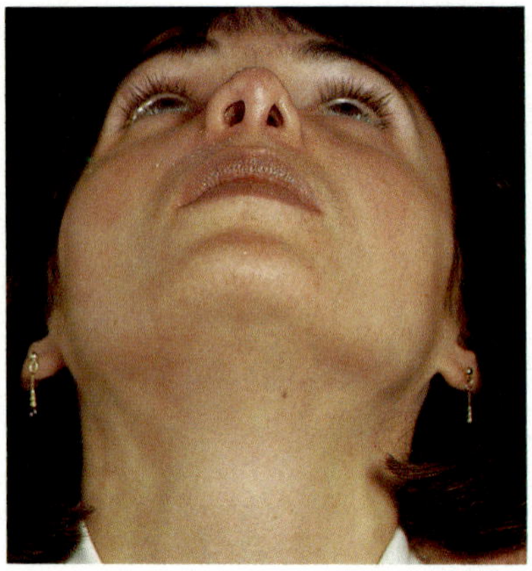

H

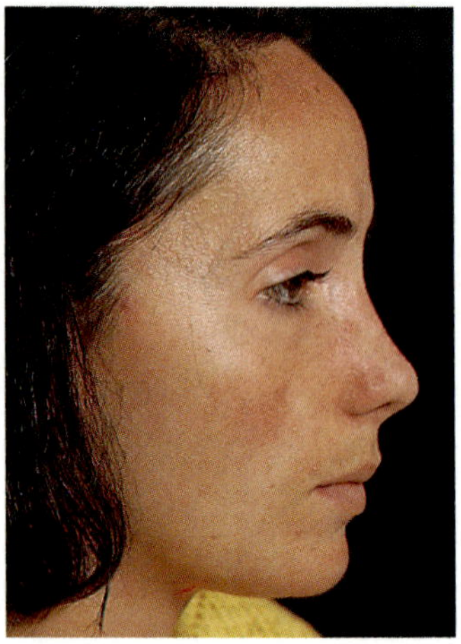

I

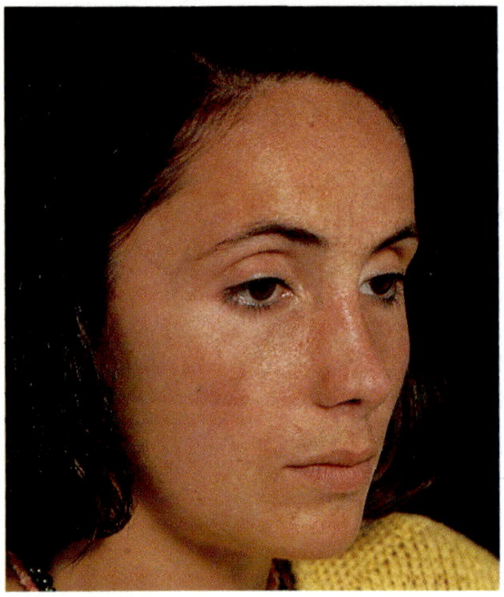

J

Fig. 87. In a severe case of pinched nose with cicatricial retraction of the nostril, a simple cartilage graft is not sufficient. There is a need for a composite graft from the inner side of the crus helicis with skin and cartilage for lining the scarred vestibular wall. Such a graft is used in this case on the right side after removal of scar tissue in the tip and alar area and spreading the intracartilaginous incision. It is then sutured into the gap of this incision with transalar mattress sutures tied over a plastic sheet. (A and B) Preoperative views. (C) Composite graft is taken from the crus helicis leaving the external skin intact. (D) A cartilage graft from the septum is used as columellar batten. (E) End of the secondary procedure with transalar mattress sutures in place. (F) Mattress sutures are taken off two weeks later. (G, H, I, and J) Late result of the revision.

Short Nose, Pig Snout Nose

For lengthening the whole nose, the external skin can usually be stretched downward and forward much more easily than the mucosa of the nasal cavity and the skin of the vestibule. Thus, it is rather difficult to lengthen a nose that has been previously overshortened. A cartilage graft can correct the obtuse nasolabial angle.

Rogers (1972) pointed out the importance of an extensive dissection of the dorsal skin for moving it downward as much as possible. He stated:

> The pig's snout nose must be completely taken down and the entire nose freed from the glabella or root of the nose to the nasolabial fold. In most cases this manoeuver permits the surgeon to stretch the degloved nose downward so that the entire nasal skin coverage can be fixed at a lower position with imbricating sutures to the most caudal and inferior margin of the cartilaginous septum in the region of the apex of the nasolabial angle. It is protected and held in place in the new position by prolonged splinting.

However, Rogers did not mention the difficulty that is often encountered when one tries to advance the mucosa downward to the same degree as the external coverage. Thus, an inner degloving maneuver has to be added to the external one. This procedure can be combined with the correction of the tethered upper lip by removal or reduction of the usually too prominent nasal spine, section or reduction of the depressor septi nasi muscle, and by freeing the upper lip and the gingiva from the anterior surface of the maxilla between the spine and the teeth.

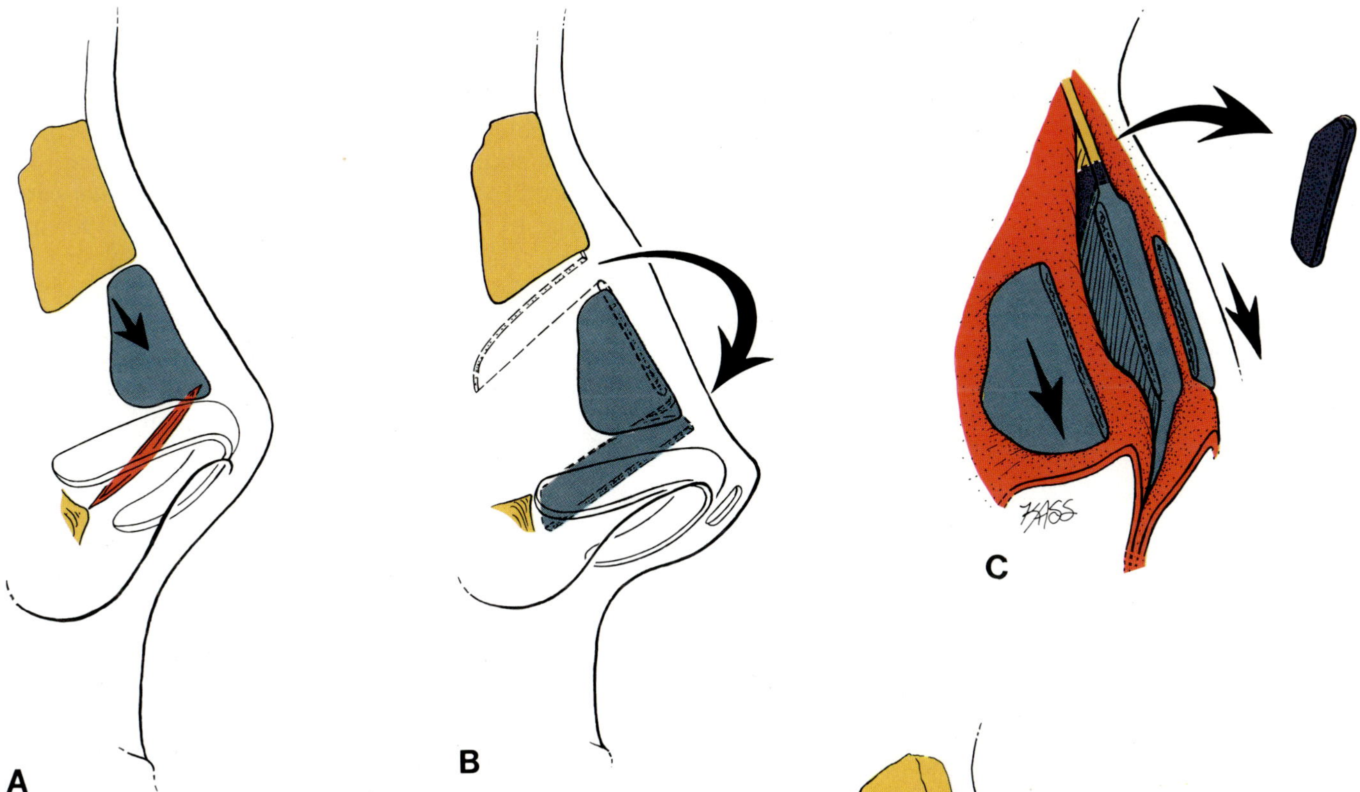

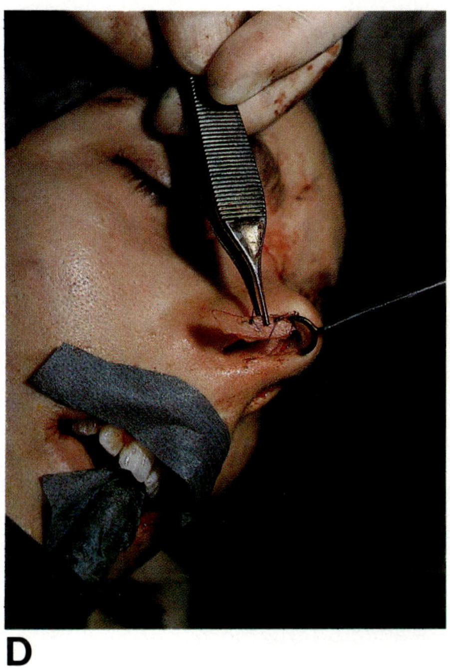

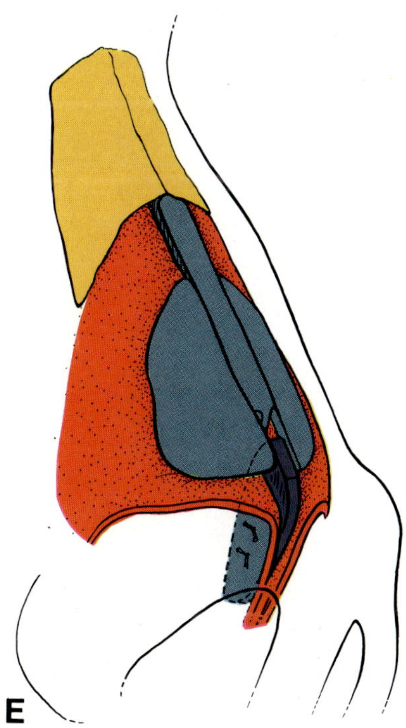

Fig. 88. (A and B) Lengthening of the nose by extramucosal technique transferring a strip of cartilage from the posterior part of the septum to the anterior border. At the dorsal ridge of the donor area the graft is cut very narrow in order to prevent a saddling at that level. (C and D) Double cartilage graft ready to be inserted. (E) Double cartilage graft inserted.

Depending on the degree of shortness of the nose, we can apply different techniques. If a moderate lengthening is required we do not need any graft. Once the mucoperichondrial vault is brought downward and forward using the extramucosal technique, the two flaps are sutured together in their new position by several mattress sutures. In more difficult cases of an overly "retrousse" or short nose deformity in which there is loss of septal membrane, more lining as well as a cartilage spacer must be provided to adequately lengthen the septum and with it, the whole nose.

Addition of a caudal septal or columellar autogenous cartilage graft in congenitally short nose when the membranes are adequate, unscarred, and elastic can suffice. The cartilage can be obtained from the posterior part of the septum as a straight or L-shaped graft (Fig. 87) and sutured to the anterior border of the septal cartilage by mattress sutures (Figs. 88, 89, 90, and 91).

Kamer (1980) expressed the fear that the cartilage removal at the bone-cartilage junction would create a postoperative depression in this area, but we have never observed such a complication. The cartilaginous batten can also be introduced through a small incision at the columella base (Fig. 92).

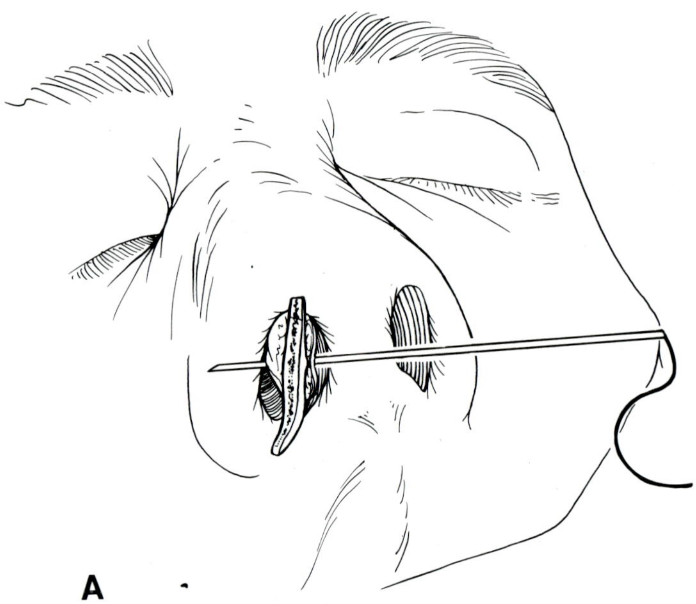
A

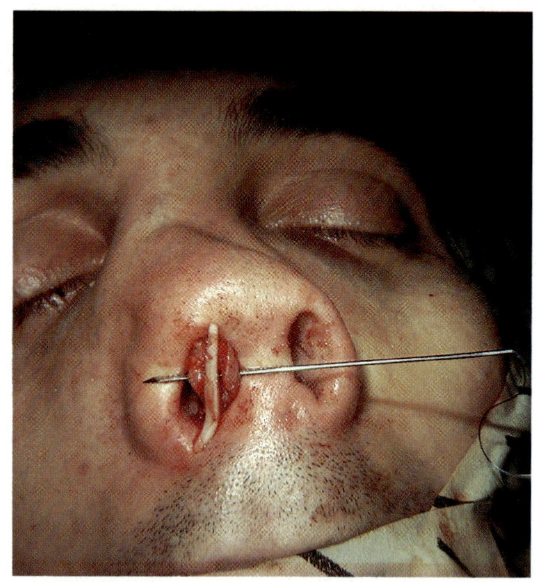
B

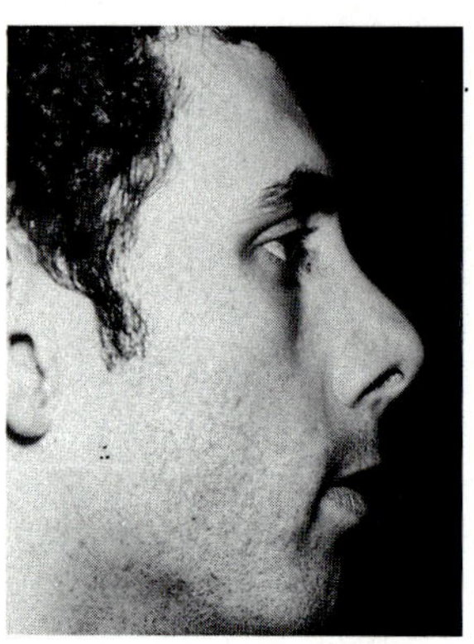
C

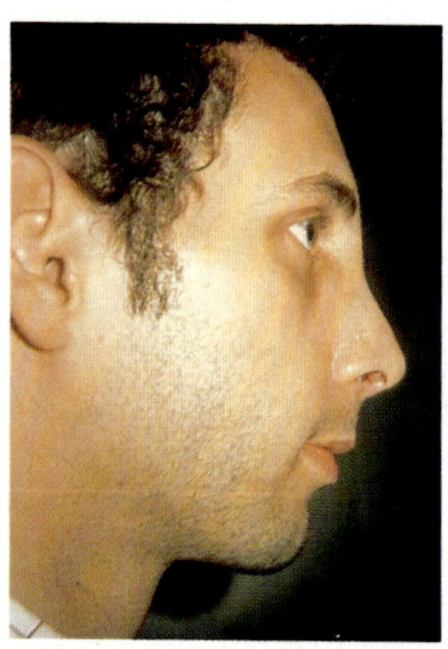
D

Fig. 89. (A and B) The posterior septal graft is anchored to the anterior-inferior border of the septum with a mattress suture passing through both advanced mucoperichondrial leaves. (C) Same patient before secondary elongating rhinoplasty. (D) Patient 2 weeks after revision with cartilage grafting. The graft can be harvested in the posterior part of the septum on a straight (E) or an L-shaped (F) form.

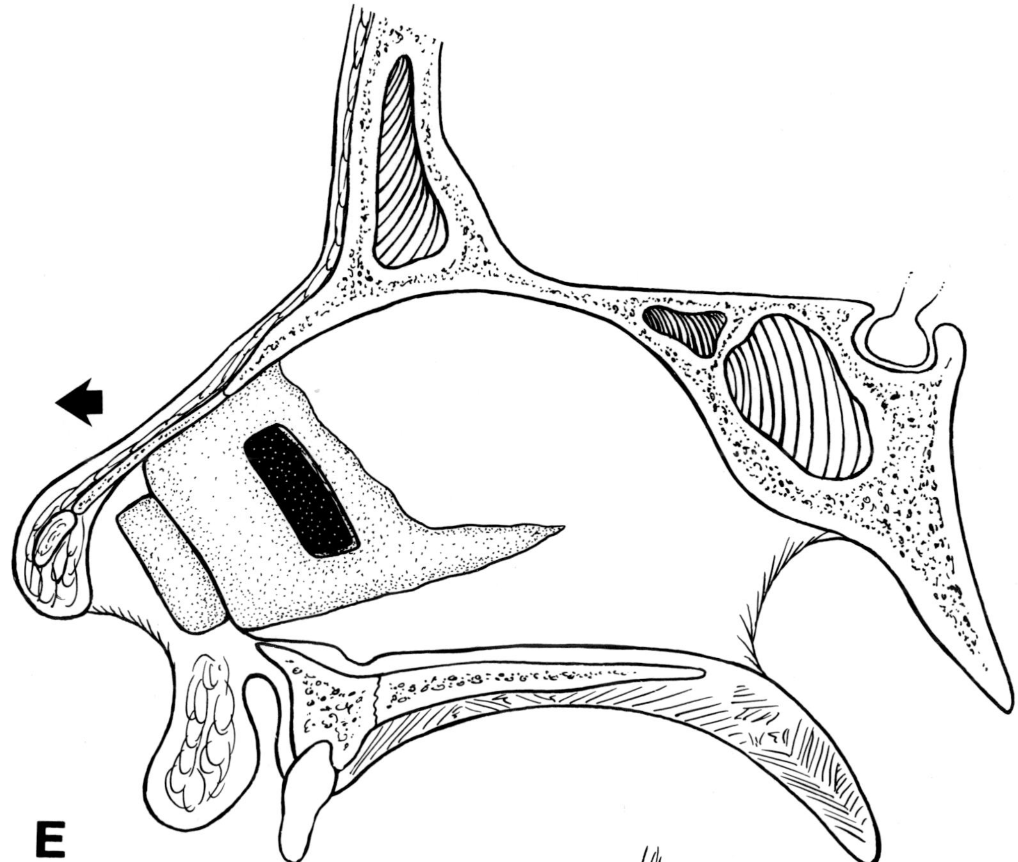

E

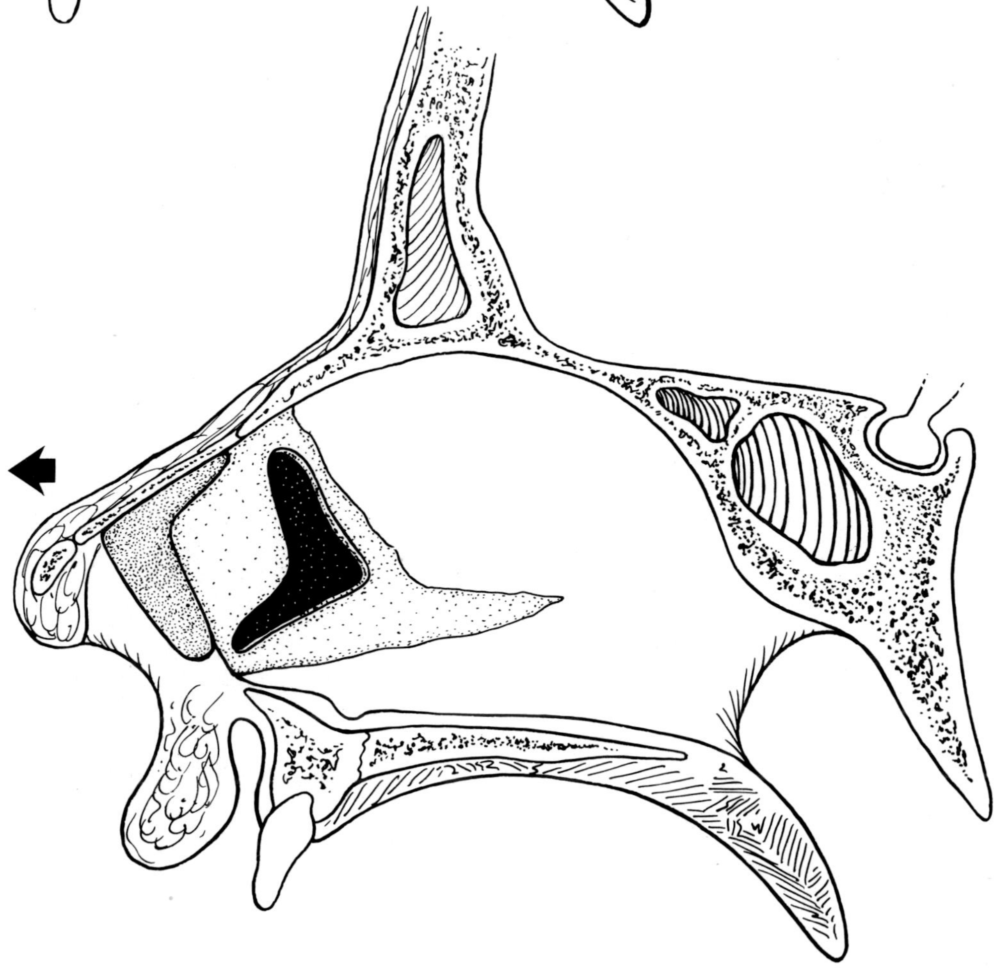

F

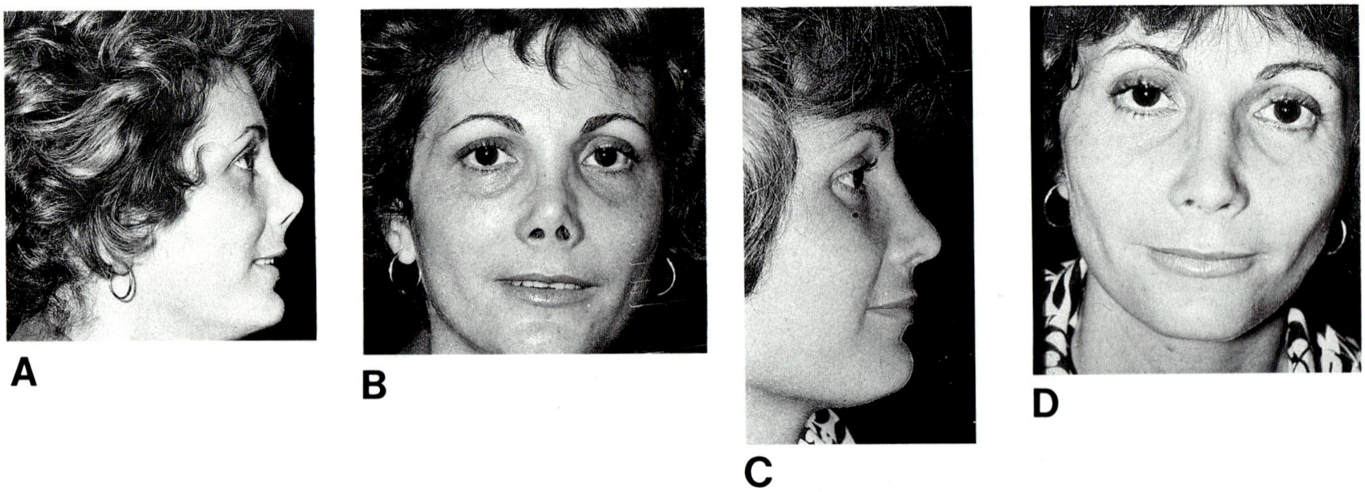

Fig. 90. Overshortened pig-snout nose corrected with the technique of Figure 88 (extramucosal dissection, advancement of both mucoperichondrial vaults and transfer of a cartilage graft from the posterior to the anterior part of septum). (A and B) Preoperative views. (C and D) Postoperative views.

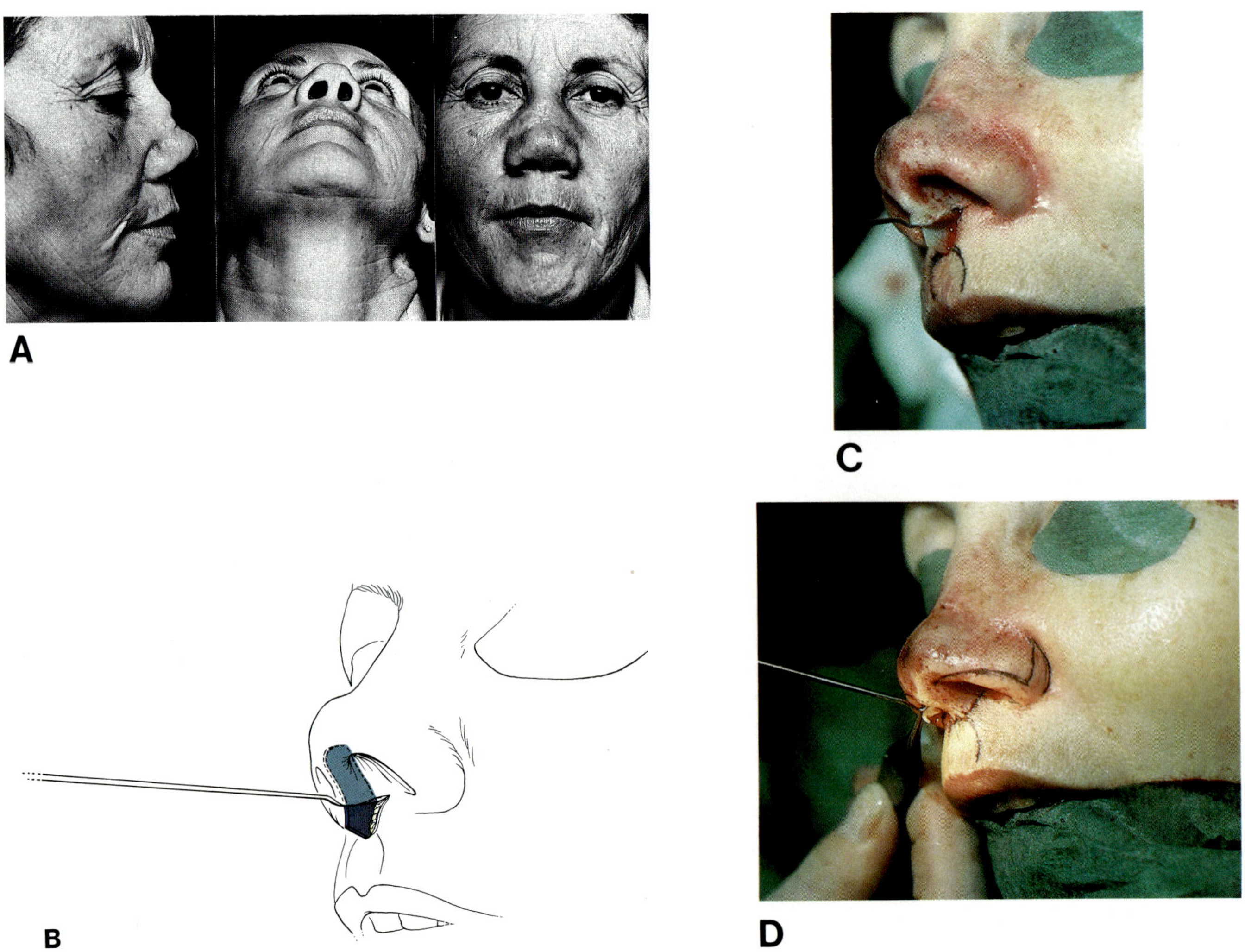

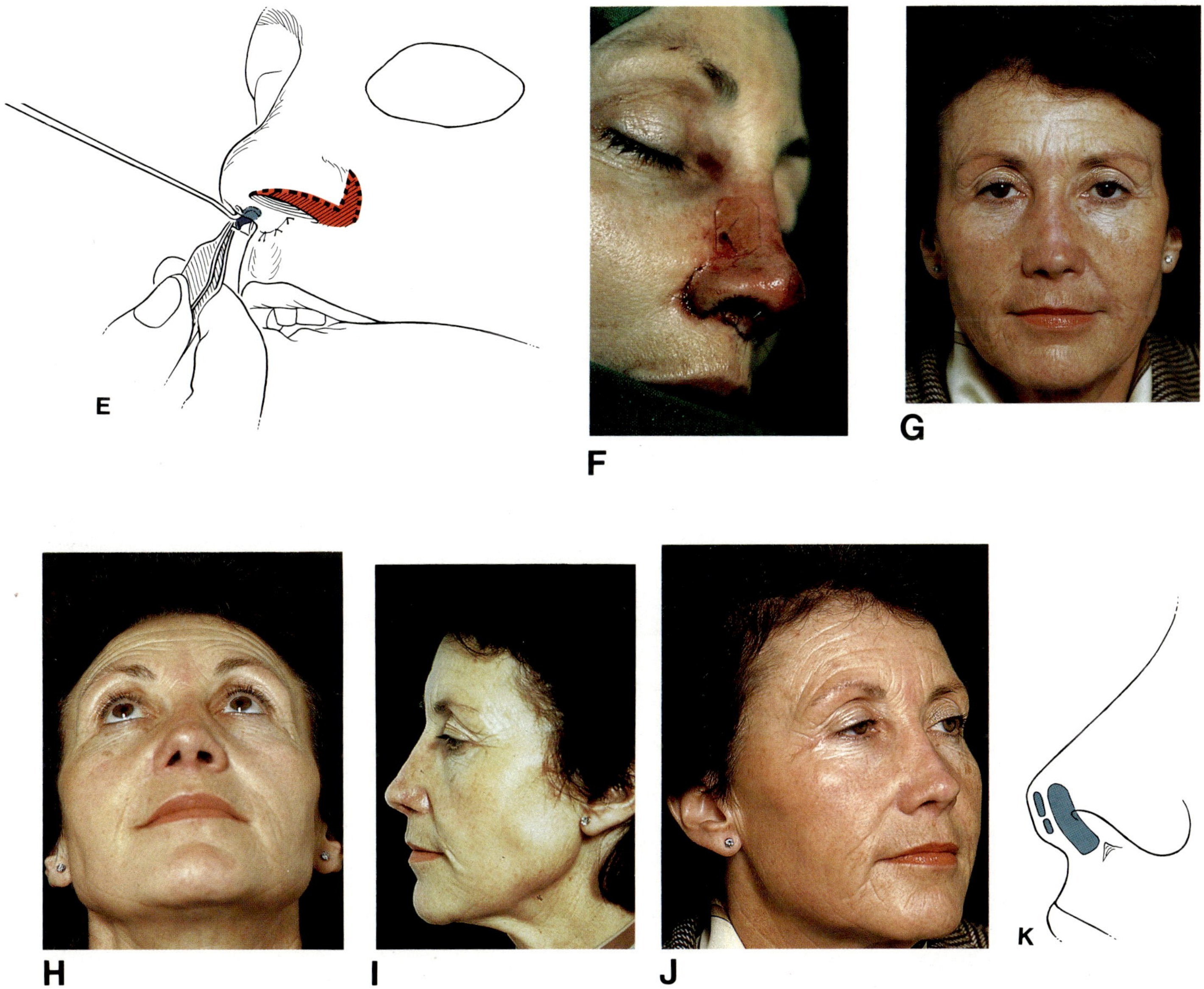

Fig. 91. In this middle-aged woman a similar secondary procedure has been used for elongation of the nose. After osteotomies and narrowing of the bony and cartilaginous pyramid a strut of cartilage from the posterior portion of the septum has been inserted into the tip-columella complex through an incision at the columellar base. Another smaller cartilage graft has been inserted into the columella in order to accentuate the double angle in the profile. For finishing of alar sculpturing a marginal alar and alar base resection was performed. The narrowed skeleton has been kept in place by transnasal sutures. (A) Preoperative views, (B and C) introduction of cartilage strut, (D, E, and F) insertion of the columellar onlay and outline of marginal and basal alar resection, and (G, H, I, J, and K) late result.

For the more difficult cases this procedure is not sufficient, such as in short noses with pig's snout tips with a fair amount of scar tissue at the valve. For these we prefer to compensate for the loss of lining (filling in, at the same time, the dorsal depression) by the interposition of a cutaneo-cartilaginous composite graft from the ear concha between the spread borders of the intercartilaginous incisions, as suggested by Dingman and Walter (1969) (Fig. 92 and 93). A strip of skin in the middle of the concave cutaneous side of the graft is de-epithelialized in order

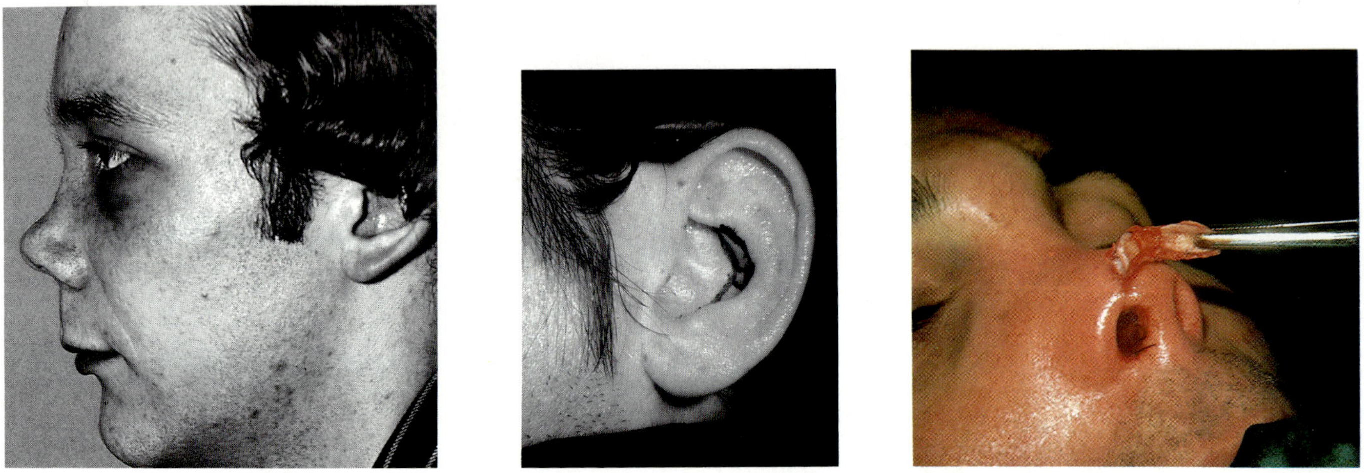

A **B** **C**

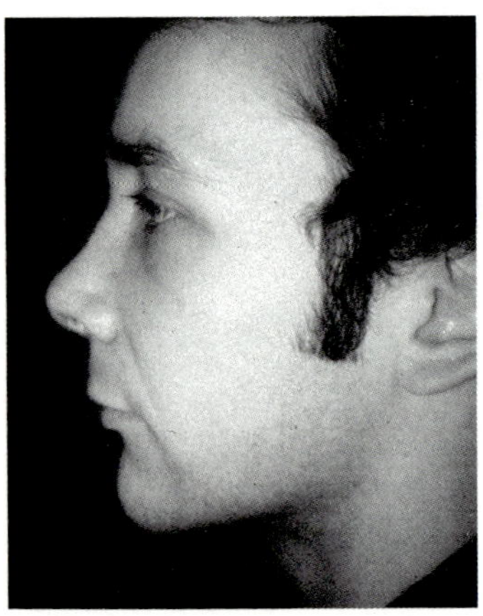

D

Fig. 92. Another method for lengthening the nose, particularly for augmenting the retracted scarred lining, is the interposition of an auricular composite graft at the site of the two intercartilaginous incisions (Dingman and Walter 1969). The donor area of the graft is the ear concha. The chondrocutaneous graft has to ride on the dorsal ridge of the septum. For that purpose, a median strip of its skin has to be deepithelialized. (A) Short saddle nose of a young man after too generous septoplasty. (B) Donor area of the concha (C) Composite graft with deepithelialized strip. (D) Corrected nose after 6 months.

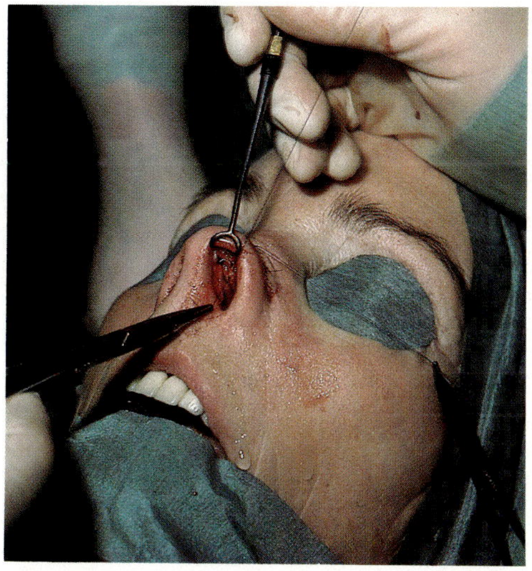

A

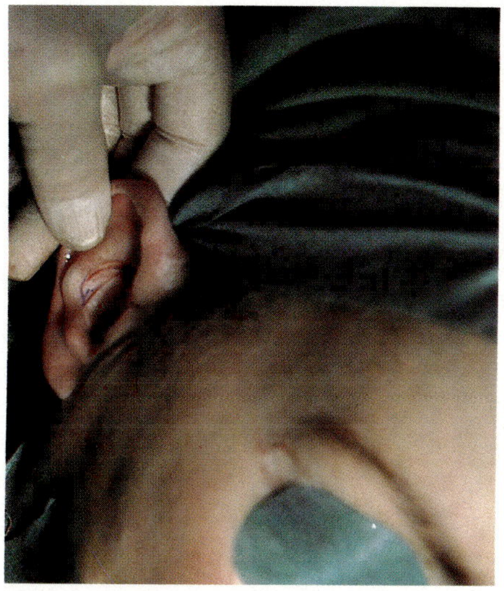

B

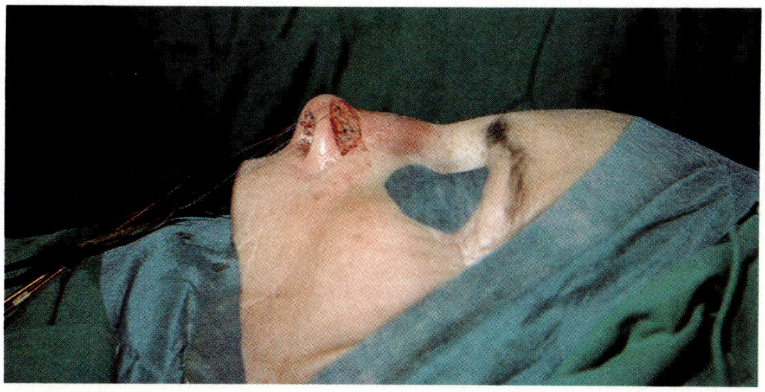

C

Fig. 93. Same procedure in a similar case of short nose. (A) Auricular donor area. (B) The graft is inserted. One of the two skin patches is sutured to the wound edges of the intercartilaginous incision. (C) The graft is furthermore adapted to the defect with transcutaneous sutures tied over plastic sheet.

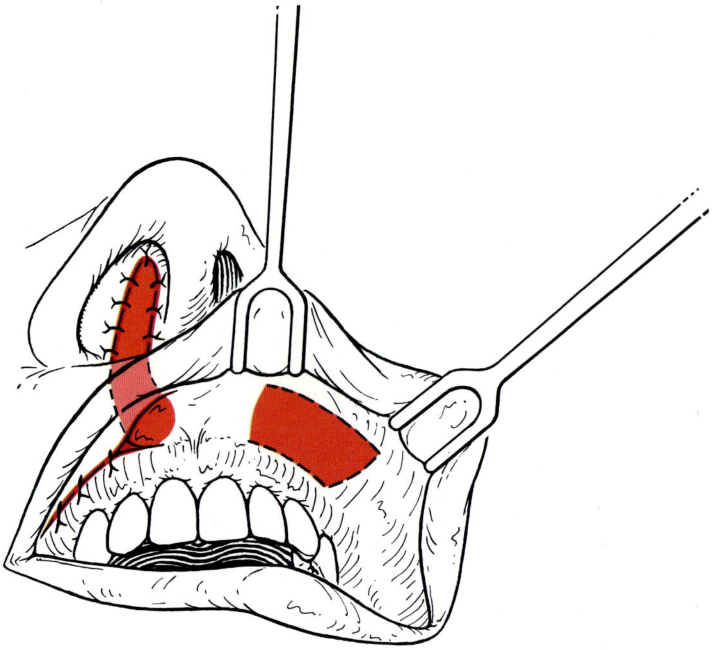

Fig. 94. Two labial mucosa flaps are transferred through a tunnel to the nose for enlarging the membranous septum in order to correct the retrusion of tip and columella in the pig snout nose. The same flaps are used for closure of septal perforations (Figs. 134 and 135).

to allow the graft to ride on the dorsal septal ridge. The skin borders of the graft are meticulously sutured to the edge of the vestibular skin and to the mucosa of the cavity at the expanded intercartilaginous incision on both sides. The convex cartilaginous part of the graft replaces the lost amount of both upper lateral cartilages.

Aiache (1982) increases the height of the septum with a wedge-shaped graft that is interposed and wedged into a spread horizontal incision in the membranous septum and columella, and not placed at the antero-inferior border of the septum as we do. The septal mucoperichondrial flaps, which are lengthened by extramucosal dissection and by traction, are then attached with transfixing mattress sutures (Fig. 94). Aiach also uses the posterior relaxing incision in the mucoperiosteal vault, as we advocated in 1977 (Meyer and Kesselring) and as shown in Figure 102.

We used to utilize a small chondromucosal flap of the wall of the nasal cavity just behind the valve, including a part of the upper lateral cartilage. The flap is turned at its base at the level of the valve and transferred to the septal wall to fill the dehiscence of the lining and to overcome the compression of the septocolumellar region. In 1972, we (Meyer, in Goldwyn) published the same flap as we used it for the closure of a perforation in the upper anterior part of the septum. For the purpose of correcting the pig's snout tips this flap is only suitable if the fold of the valve is not excessively scarred.

A similar flap was advocated in 1972 by Millard for the correction of a bulbous and snub tip. It consists of a lateral vestibular chondromucosal flap based on the septum and transposed into a releasing membranous septal incision, thus achieving simultaneous reduction of the tip, shaping and shortening of the sidewalls, and correction of the retracted columella. Apparently this flap includes the upper portion of the lower lateral cartilage and helps in this manner to correct the bulbous tip.

This technique is quite useful but shortens the nostril, which is, in many cases of short nose, already retracted. The shortening of the ala is not always desirable, especially when alar cartilage reduction has been performed previously. For exceptional retrusion of tip of the tip-columella complex we have used a bilateral gingivo-labial flap, and it is shown also in Chapter 14 in the section on septal perforation. Each flap has its base in a paramedian area near the frenulum and is carried into the vestibule through a tunnel beside the anterior nasal spine, joining the dehiscence in the membranous septum and covering if possible a forward displaced pillar of septal cartilage, or a cartilaginous graft. The two flaps complete the membranous septum on both sides (Fig. 95). The same flap can be employed for closure of septal perforations as advocated by Tipton (1970) and Hinderer (1973). We use it in special cases of perforation in combination with the extra mucosal flaps (see Chapter 14) (Figs. 134 and 135). After release of the entire inferior septo-columellar unit, Pers (1973) and Kamer (1980) fill the remaining gap with a composite graft from the ear concha. On one side the mucoperichondrial flap is only incised and released so that a strip of bare cartilage appears. On the other side, the skin of the composite graft completes the released mucoperichondrial incision. Thus, the risk of perforation or graft failure is greatly reduced due to the rich blood supply of the septal mucoperichondrium, which provides nutrition to the cartilaginous surface. The denuded cartilage of the normal septum superiorly is left to heal by secondary intention.

The postauricular skin is rather loosely attached to the cartilage. These attachments should not be disturbed in suturing the graft in place. In a few cases we have used such composite grafts from the crus helicis of the ear, as we do for lowering the ala (see Chapter 16) or for lining the alar-columellar commissure (see Chapter 17). The attachment of the skin to the cartilage is quite firm in this area of the auricle, which is an important advantage in these composite grafts. A Russian author advocated a complete three-layered conchal composite graft for the same purpose without graft failure.

In pig's snout tips with upward scar retraction, however, one encounters the same difficulty in finding enough tissue for the flap as we have in our procedure using the sidewall composite flap, which includes the upper lateral cartilages. In these cases there is already so much scar tissue at the valve that it would be nearly impossible to cut a flap without producing a stenosis. We believe that when tissue is removed from the anterior vestibular side of the valve, this may be more dangerous in producing secondary web-stenosis than when the excision is carried out behind the intercartilaginous incision on the cavity side.

In any event, all the local flaps possible we can harvest from the floor (Converse, (1964), Cinelli, (1966)) or sidewalls of the vestibule or nasal cavity can not achieve the same advantage we have experienced with the extramucosal dissection and forward advancement of the mucoperichondrial flap. Furthermore, skin grafts, mu-

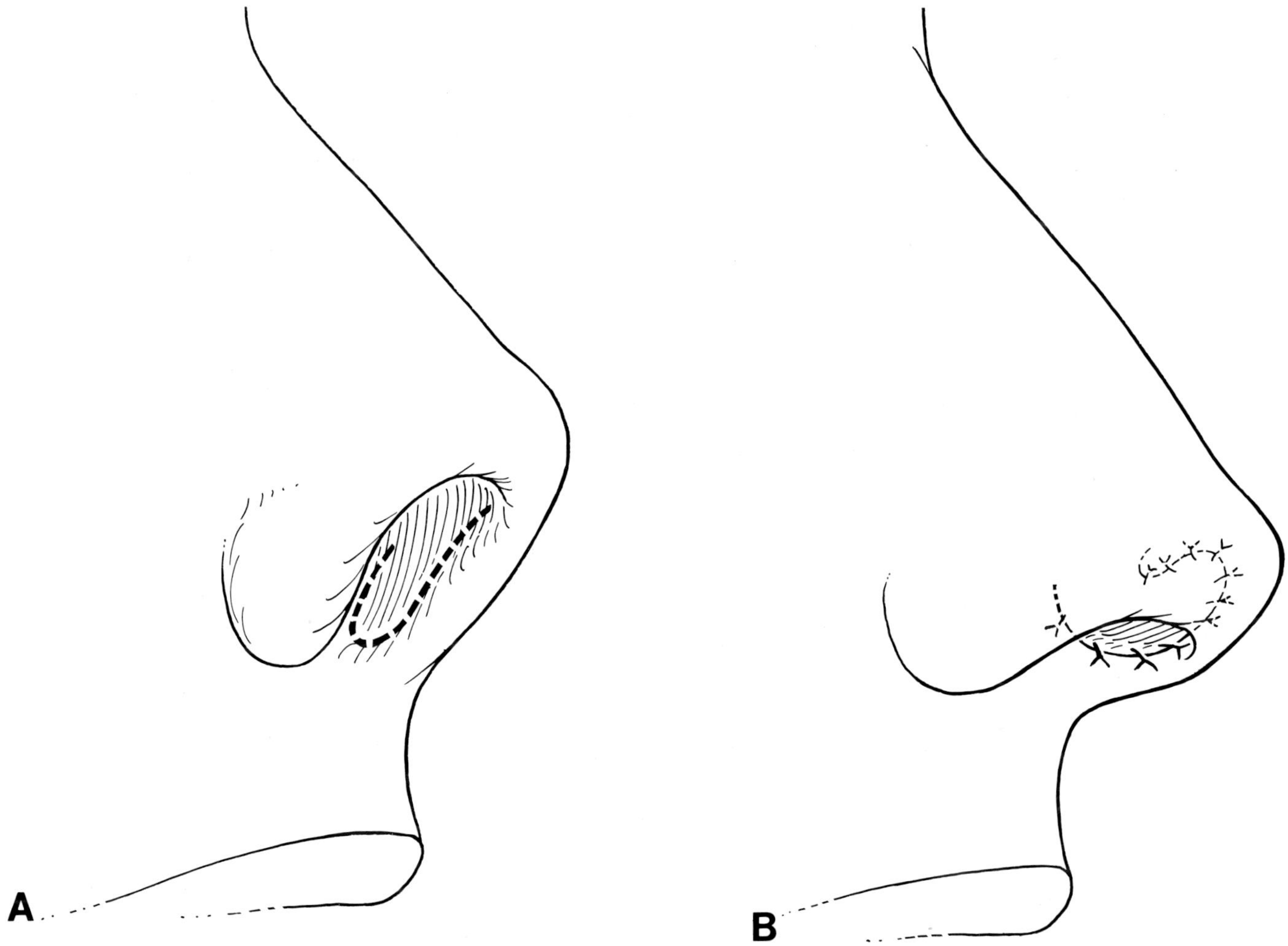

Fig. 95. (A and B) Bilateral transposition flap of Aiach for elongation of the nose. The flap includes a strip of cartilage from the anterior border of the septum. By this transposition, the tip of the nose is pushed forward and downward and the base of the columella is pulled backward.

cosal, or composite grafts would not work well for completing the lining, since we cannot put them in contact with the septocolumellar part of an L-shaped graft cartilage or with any other septocolumellar batten of cartilage or bone. We can, of course, implant a simple cartilage or bone graft to the dorsal profile and use composite auricular grafts to replace the missing membranous septum as proposed by Rogers (1976).

In our experience, when a severe pig's snout tip is combined with a true or false saddle deformity, a strong cartilaginous or bony support as provided by an L-shaped cartilage graft or a separate septocolumellar pillar is indispensable. The maximally shortened noses with pig's snout or bulldog deformity require an augmentation procedure corresponding in analogy to the ones used for correction of saddle noses. We proceed in these cases as for saddle nose deformities with the usual osteotomies (lateral, paramedian, and transverse) in order to narrow the base of the nasal pyramid and to advance the bony structures that are then fixed by transnasal mattress sutures. The latter should be tied at the end of the procedure once dorsal grafting has been completed. Upon the already elevated ridge we place either an L-shaped rib cartilage graft or an iliac crest, bone graft which then must be accompanied by a septocolumellar cartilage graft.

To correct extreme cases of pig's snout or bulldog deformities we prefer L-shaped rib cartilage grafts from the 8th and 9th rib (Figs. 96, 97, and 98). In contrast to the insertion of the graft in the saddle nose by an open roof procedure, we choose to gain access through the use of transfixion and the intercartilaginous incisions. The residual arch of the lower lateral cartilages can, if required, be modeled using the eversion (retrograde) technique. The bed for the cartilage graft at the dorsum is already formed by the approximated and elevated nasal bones with the untied transnasal sutures in place.

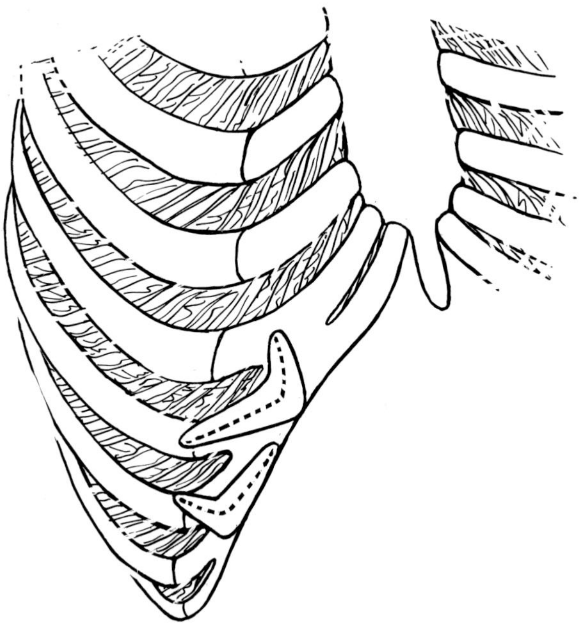

Fig. 96. The donor sites for L-shaped rib cartilage grafts are outlined at cartilaginous costal arch at the 8th and 9th rib.

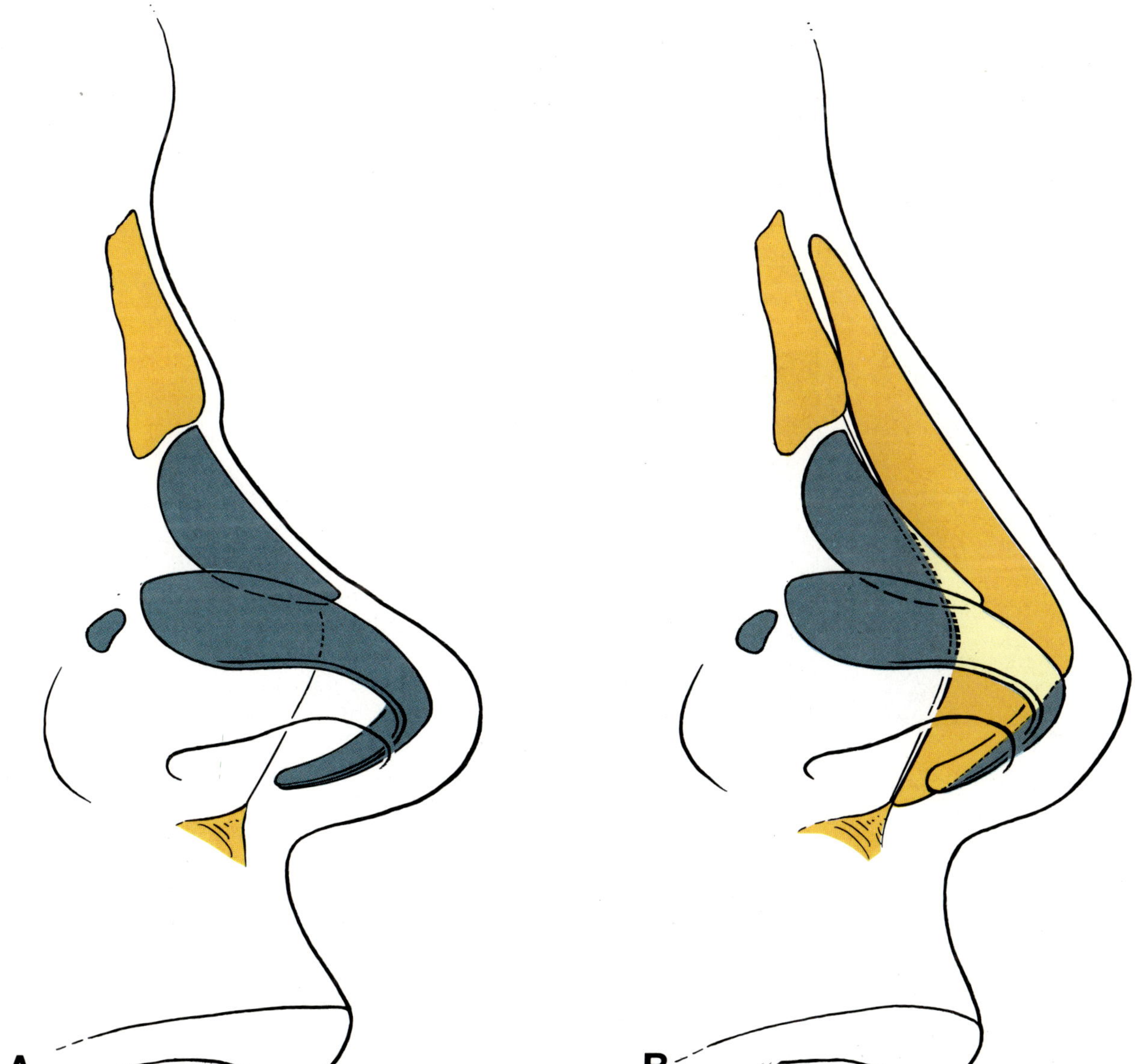

Fig. 97. Saddle nose corrected with L-shaped rib graft. (A) Before and (B) after grafting.

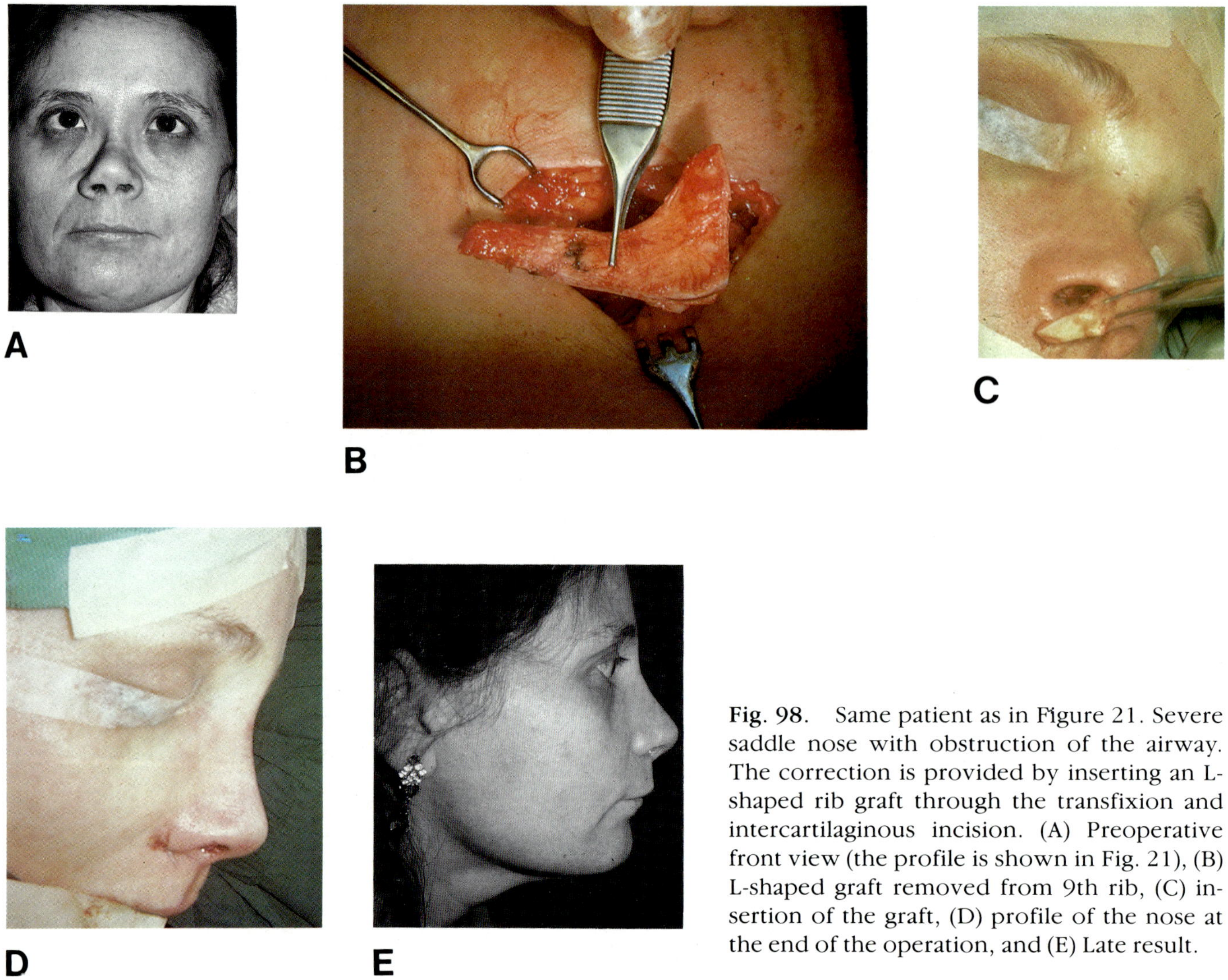

Fig. 98. Same patient as in Figure 21. Severe saddle nose with obstruction of the airway. The correction is provided by inserting an L-shaped rib graft through the transfixion and intercartilaginous incision. (A) Preoperative front view (the profile is shown in Fig. 21), (B) L-shaped graft removed from 9th rib, (C) insertion of the graft, (D) profile of the nose at the end of the operation, and (E) Late result.

The dorsal part of the graft may be short, resting on the bony vault, or long, ending at the glabella, where a hole drilled into the bones serves as an anchoring point. The columellar part of the L-shaped graft sits behind or between the medial crura of the lower lateral cartilage, which are spread via the transfixion incision. Using sharp or blunt dissection, we form a pocket extending to the anterior nasal spine, to the columellar skin in the midline, and to the skin of the tip between the two domes or their postsurgical remnants superiorly. All cicatricial tissue is removed in this area in order to soften the rigid columella-tip complex, which can then be pulled forward and downward using blunt scissors and elevators to free up the skin envelope. The carefully carved costal cartilage graft is then introduced (Fig. 98). To avoid later postoperative bending and distortion of the graft and to compensate for the inherent tensions, described by Gibson and Davis (1958), we make several longitudinal relieving incisions bilaterally into the graft and add on either side a narrow strut in apposition to the dorsal component of the graft, to counteract any tendencies toward curling. When the main graft is positioned exactly in the midline and is well shaped and the volume of the supplementary grafts is made symmetrical we can then proceed to tie over plastic sheet bolsters the two transcutaneous, transmucous, and transseptal mattress sutures, which pass through the osteotomy lines and also through the upper lateral cartilages (Figs. 99–101).

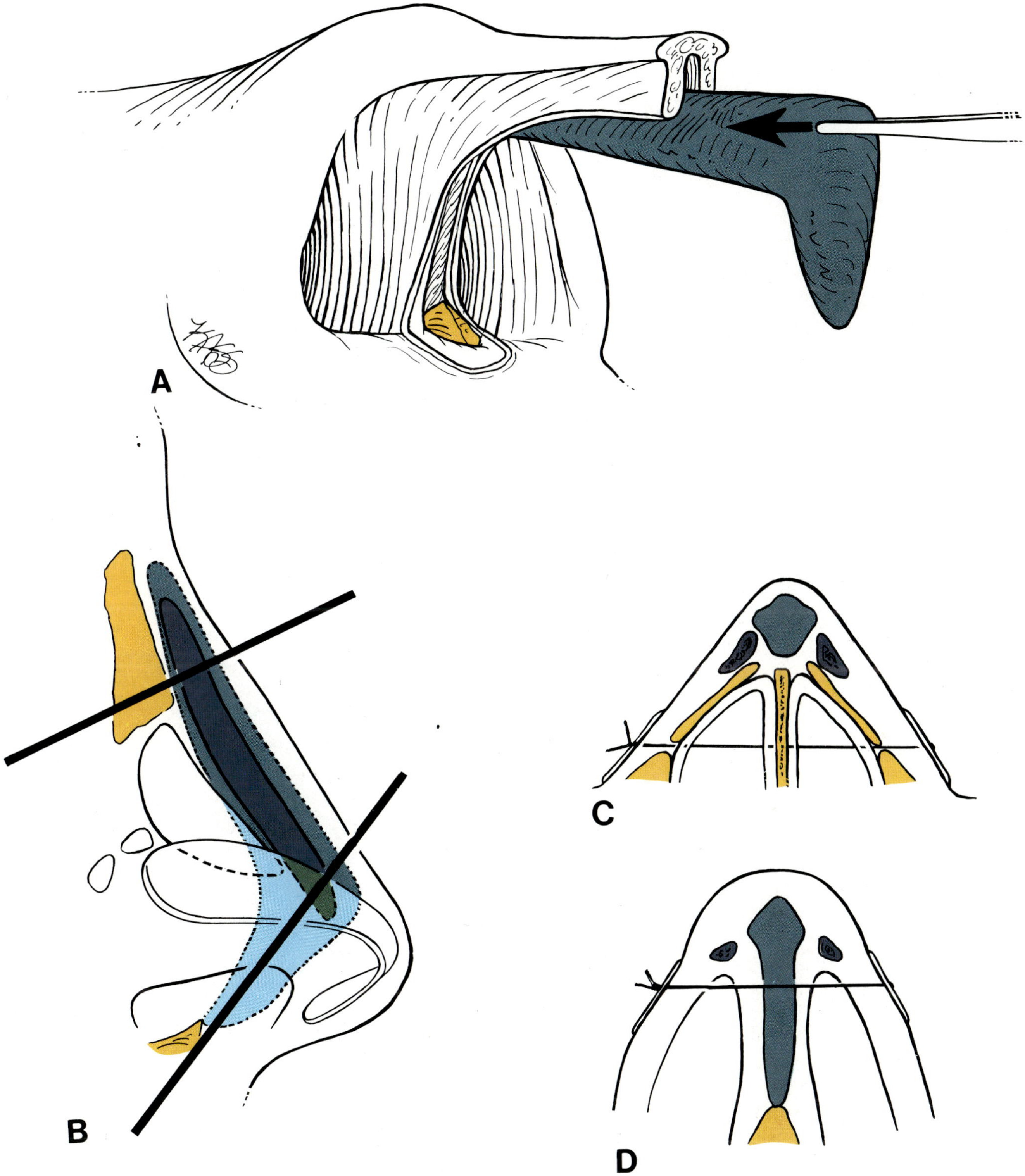

Fig. 99. continues.

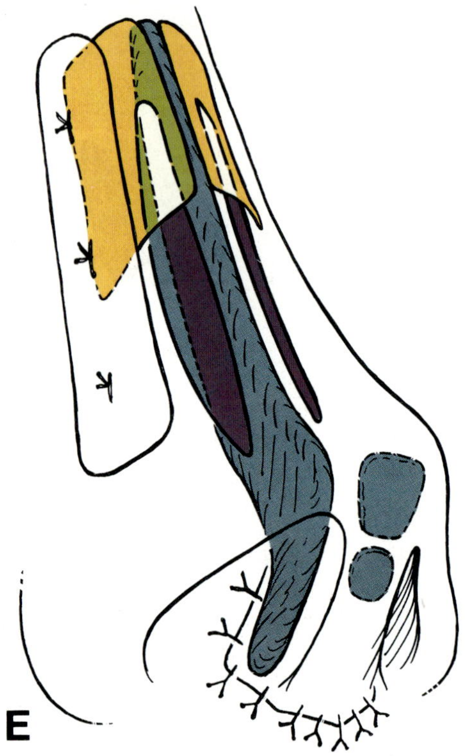

Fig. 99. Open procedure for inserting an L-shaped rib cartilage graft. The columella is sectioned at its base and separated from the membranous septum. The mucoperichondrium is dissected on both sides from the septal cartilage with the extramucosal technique and the skin is elevated from the depressed bony and cartilaginous pyramid in order to prepare the recipient bed for the grafts. Lateral, paramedian and transverse osteotomies are performed. A transnasal mattress suture passes through skin, osteotomy dehiscence and septum. (A) The graft is pushed into the dorsal bed. (B, C, and D) Cross sections show the situation of the median main graft and of two bilateral apposition grafts, which model the side wall of the nose. (E) End situation with columellar and lobular onlays, sutures at the columellar base and transnasal mattress sutures.

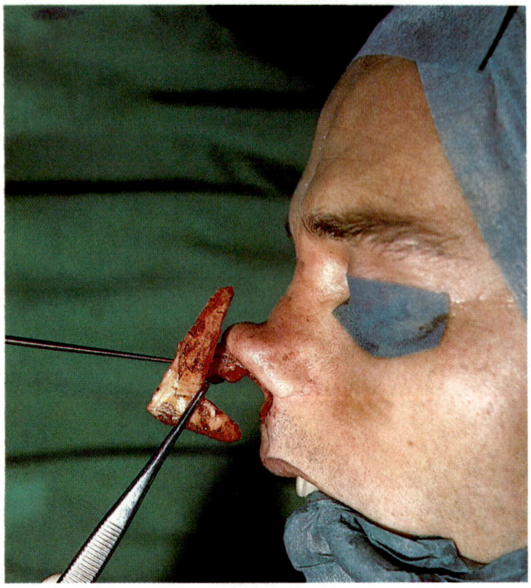

A

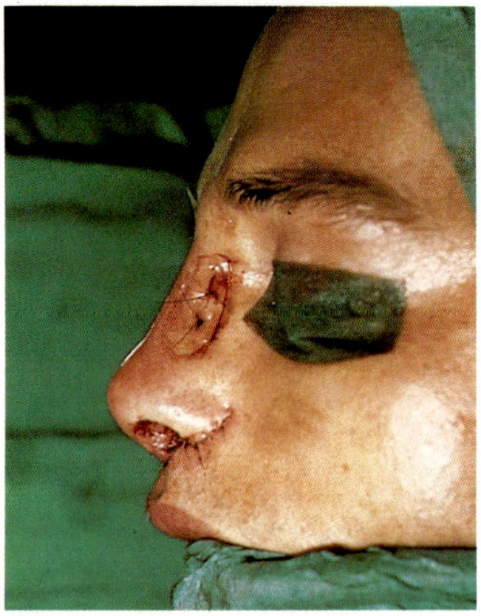

B

Fig. 100. Introduction of the L-shaped rib graft into a saddle nose with the open procedure (A) and fixation with two transnasal mattress sutures tied over plastic sheets (B).

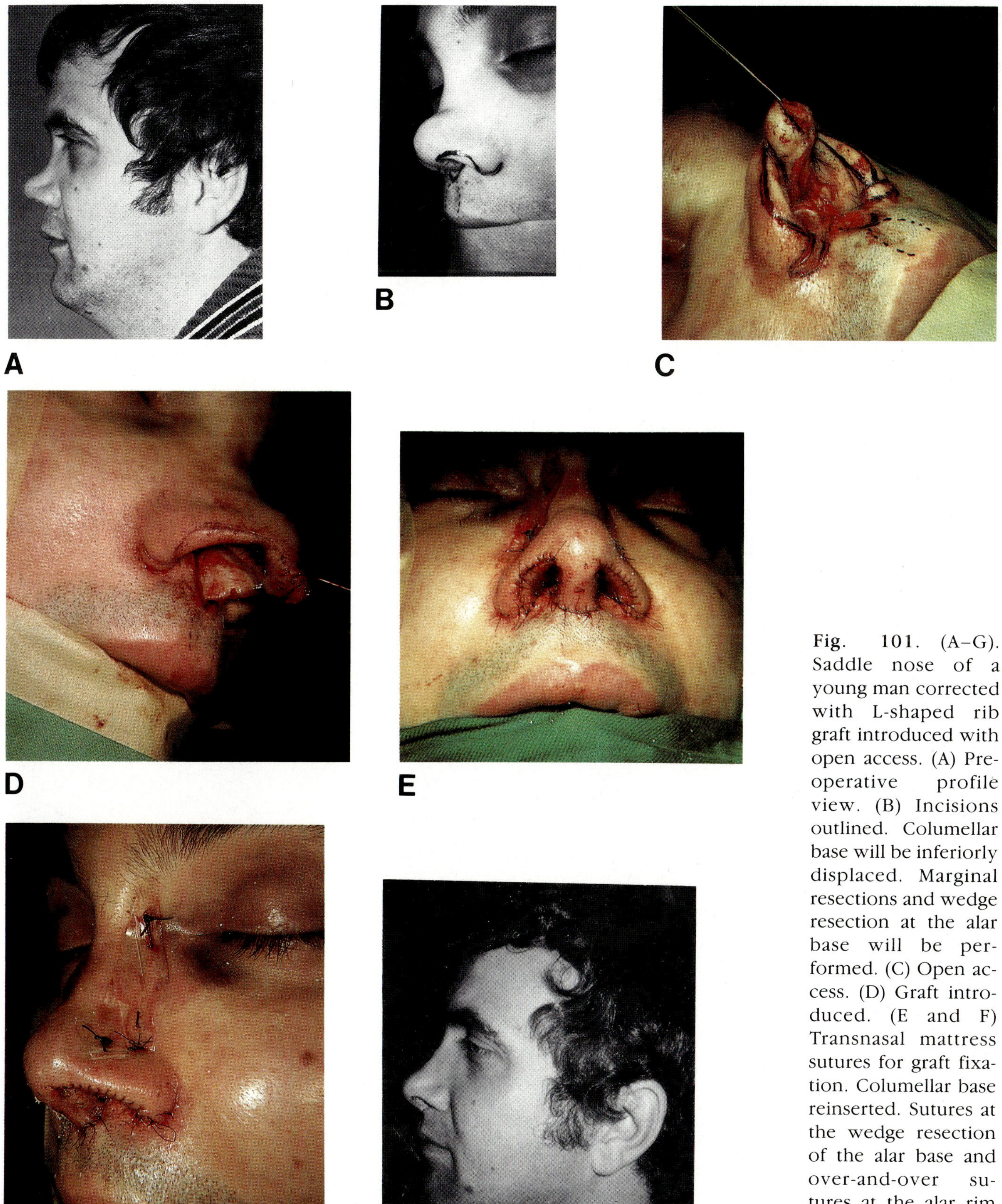

Fig. 101. (A–G). Saddle nose of a young man corrected with L-shaped rib graft introduced with open access. (A) Preoperative profile view. (B) Incisions outlined. Columellar base will be inferiorly displaced. Marginal resections and wedge resection at the alar base will be performed. (C) Open access. (D) Graft introduced. (E and F) Transnasal mattress sutures for graft fixation. Columellar base reinserted. Sutures at the wedge resection of the alar base and over-and-over sutures at the alar rim resection line. (G) Result.

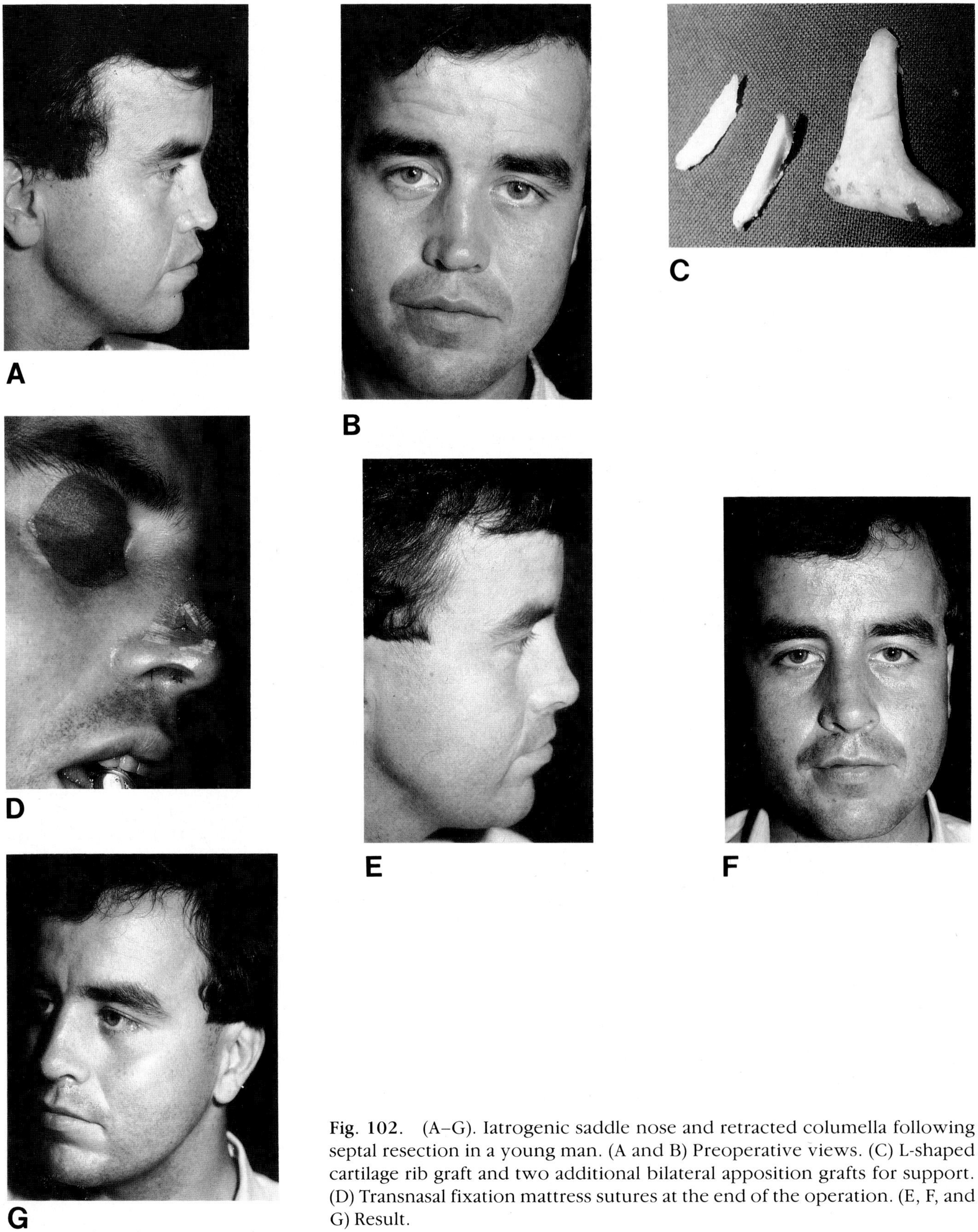

Fig. 102. (A–G). Iatrogenic saddle nose and retracted columella following septal resection in a young man. (A and B) Preoperative views. (C) L-shaped cartilage rib graft and two additional bilateral apposition grafts for support. (D) Transnasal fixation mattress sutures at the end of the operation. (E, F, and G) Result.

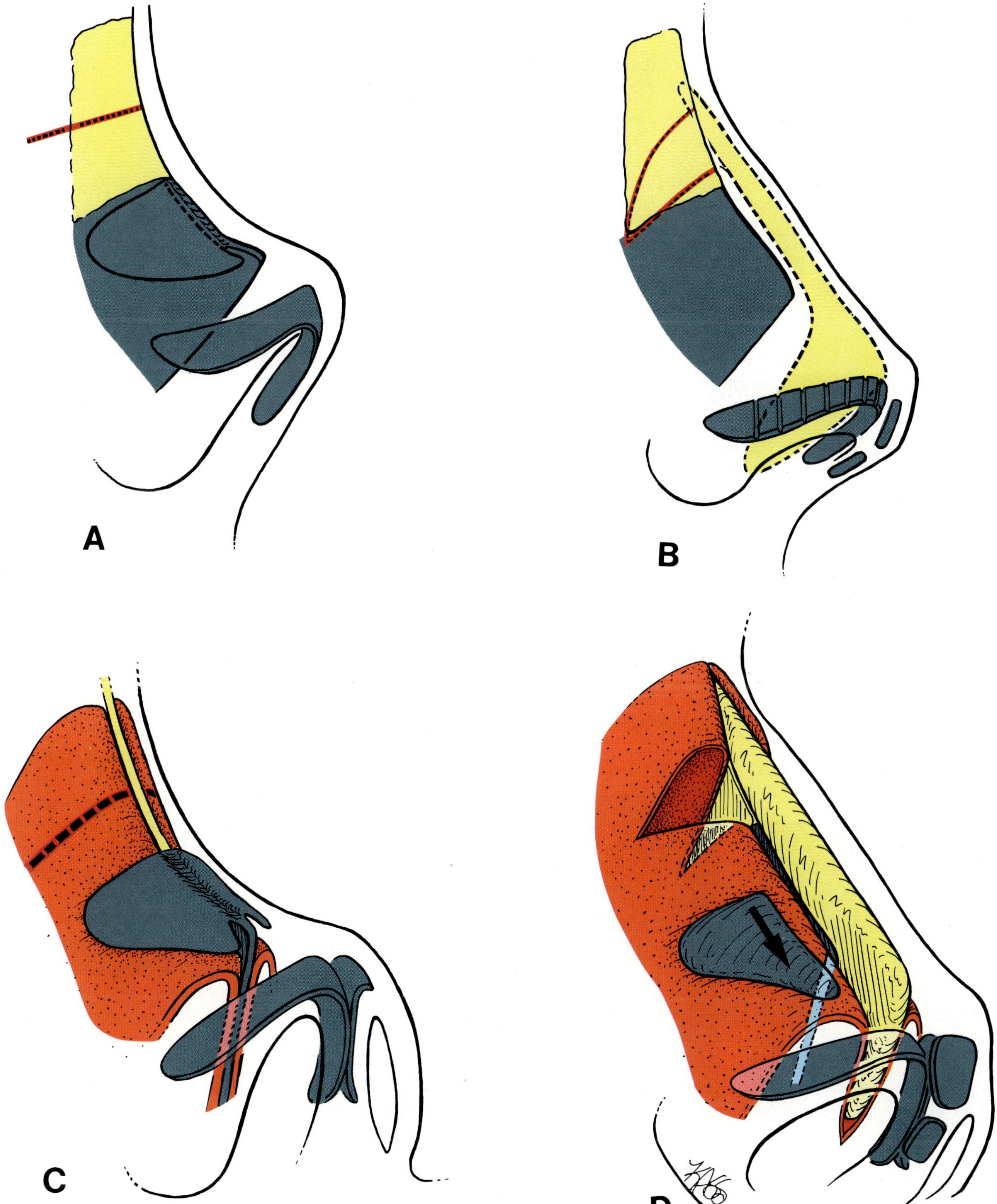

Fig. 103. To allow the mucoperichondrial and mucoperiosteal flaps to cover the supporting septocolumellar part of the L-shaped rib graft a release incision can be made in the posterior periosteal part. (A and C) Preoperative situation. (B) Release incision displayed. (D) As in B with increased advancement of the mucoperichondrium and graft in place.

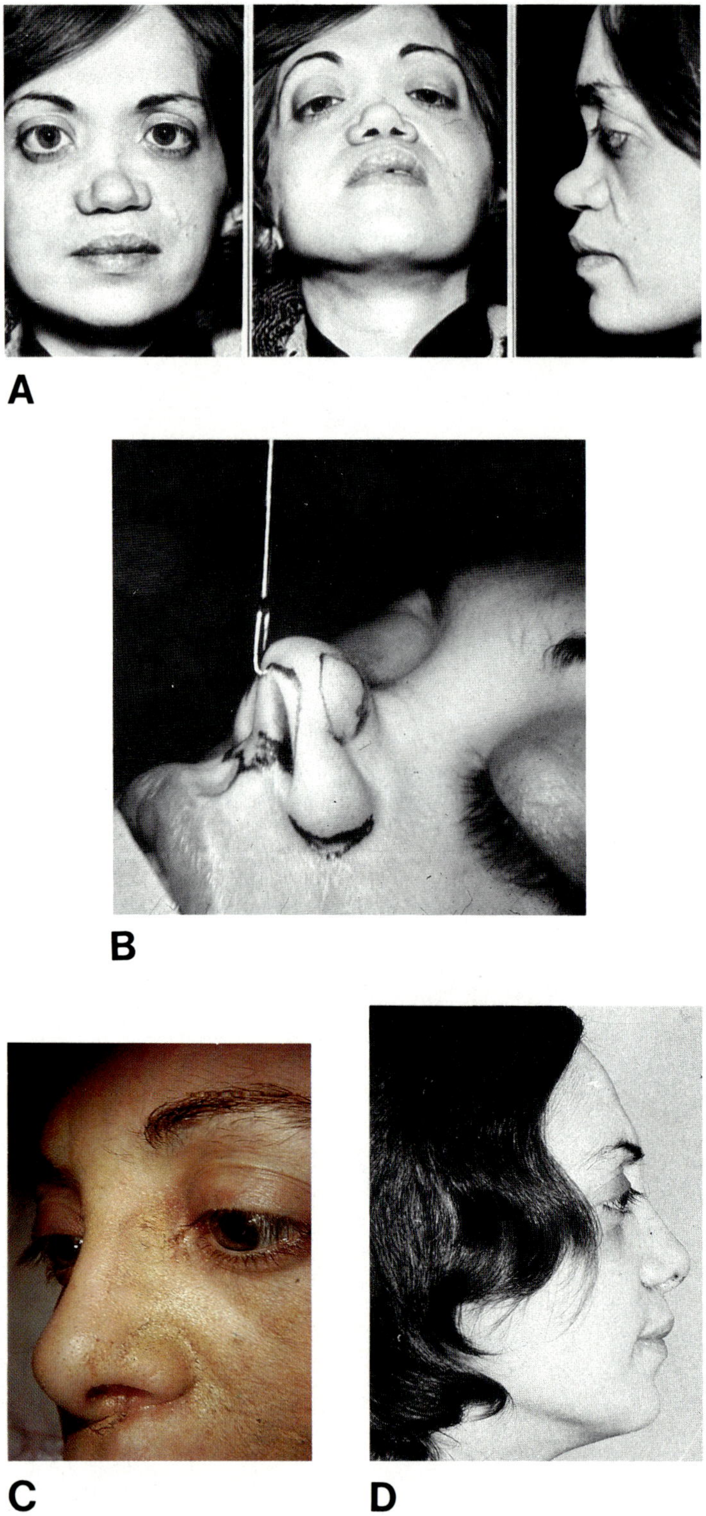

Fig. 104. In the case of this girl a release incision in the mucoperiosteal vault had to be performed on both sides in order to permit enough advancement of the periosteoperichondrial flap. (A) Preoperative views. (B) Outline of the incisions and excisions. (C) Result 2 weeks after the secondary procedure. (D) Result after 3 weeks.

Before packing, taping, and splinting, we have to check if the tip-columella profile is already properly defined by the graft. If not, an additional cartilage graft from the septum can be introduced into the lobule-tip area through a small marginal incision in order to accentuate the tip and the double angle in the tip columella profile. We close the transfixion and the intercartilaginous incisions with interrupted 4-0 Dermalon sutures or with absorbable sutures. At this point, we can usually see that the incision can be approximated without tension thanks to the advantages provided by the extramucosal technique, creating enough relaxation of the mucoperichondrial vault to permit forward advancement.

The elevation of the mucoperichondrial and mucoperiosteal flap can in special cases even be extended to the vestibular floor and the lateral wall. We use this same technique for closure of septal perforations. Furthermore, if the mucoperichondrial envelope cannot be pulled forward and downward enough to embrace the columellar part of the L-shaped graft, we incise vertically the very posterior aspect of the mucoperiosteal flap at the bony septum, resulting in a releasing gap (Figs. 102 and 103). We can make this releasing incision on both sides at that most posterior level, leaving the perpendicular plate in that triangular gap-area uncovered without risk of producing a septal perforation or a stenotic web.

Many surgeons, like Hellmich (1972) as well as other German, English, and especially Oriental surgeons, prefer Silicone block implants inserted into a separate pocket. Regarding the use of foreign material such as Silicone or Proplast in rhinoplasty, we still remain conservative and somewhat anxious. We are particularly afraid of utilizing alloplastic implants in excessively scarred noses with poor vascularity and thin skin coverage especially when this is used as a supporting pillar.

13

Residual Deformities of the Dorsum

SADDLE NOSE

Saddle nose is one of the most common nasal deformities. The origin of saddle nose may be congenital, a familial or racial characteristic, or acquired. The acquired forms may be luetic, traumatic, or iatrogenic. Traffic accidents, boxing, gymnastics, ball games, and winter sports are primarily responsible for traumatic occurrences. Unfortunately, postoperative saddle noses are rather common. They occur after septal resection when cartilage support is poor underneath the weak triangle of Converse, at the lower end of the upper lateral cartilages. The most common cause of saddle nose following primary rhinoplasty is the weakening with subsequent collapse of the cartilaginous septum after an extensive septal resection.

In a saddle nose, either the nasal bones or cartilaginous septum, or both, lie at a level lower and closer to the face than the "normal profile line." This profile line of course varies according to the ethnic configuration of the patient's face.

There are two kinds of true saddle nose: those with (Fig. 105) and those without tip support. Some saddle noses result from too radical an infracturing of the nasal bones so that they literally drop into the piriform aperture. In general, the postrhinoplasty deformities that occur along the cartilaginous dorsum are extensions of similar defects in the bony framework. The saddle deformity may involve exclusively the bony or the cartilaginous structures.

The normally oval-shaped airway found at the valve area in the transition from nasal vestibule to the nasal cavity is flattened from above. This directs the air flow downward towards the inferior meatus where normal physiologic conditions direct the air flow upward to the middle meatus and the olfactory organ. This abnormal condition can be relieved by correction of the saddle nose so that a functional indication exists along with a cosmetic indication for repair in such cases.

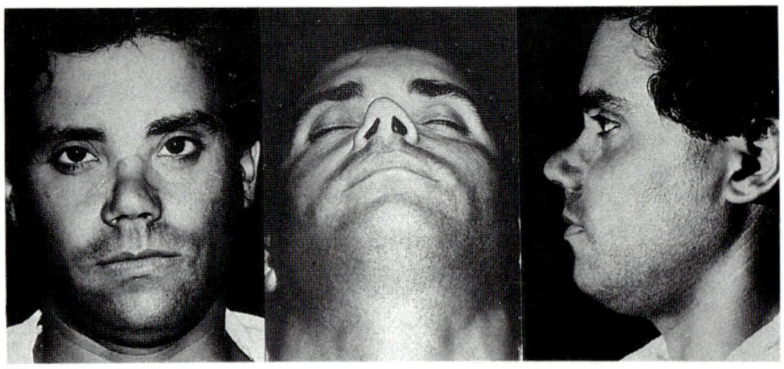

A

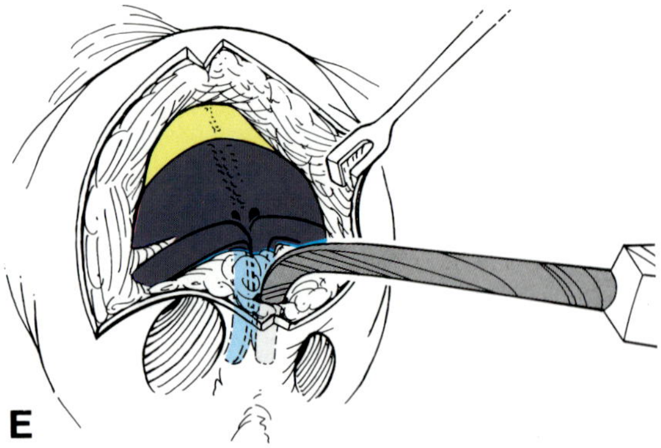

E

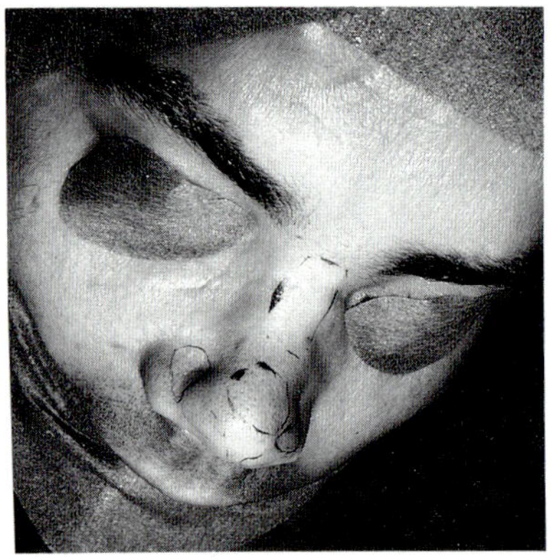

B

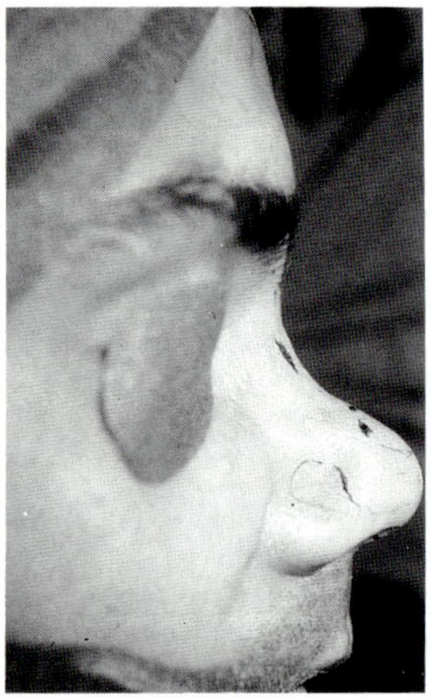

C

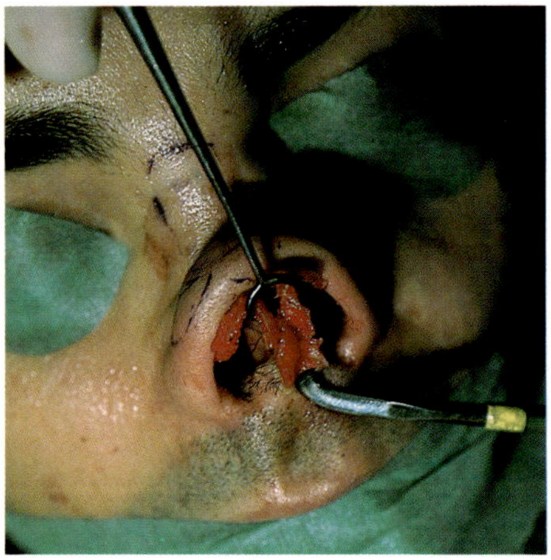

F

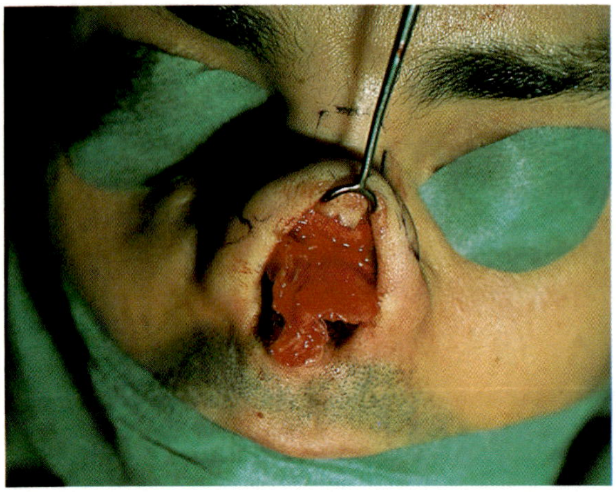

D

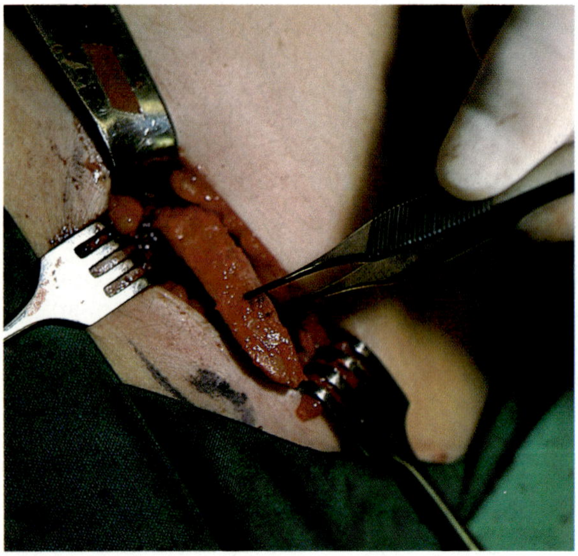

G

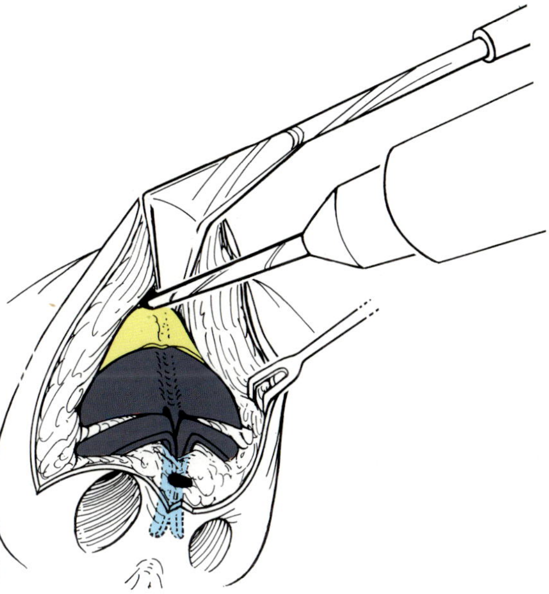

H

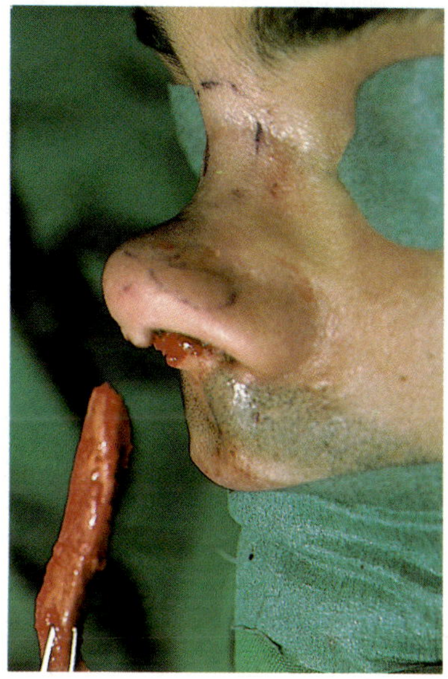

I

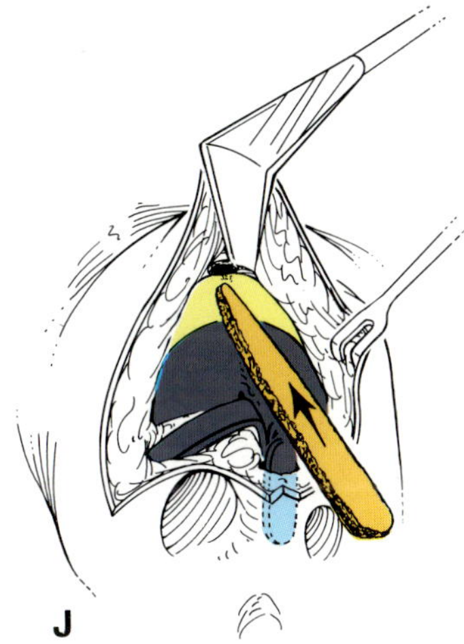

J

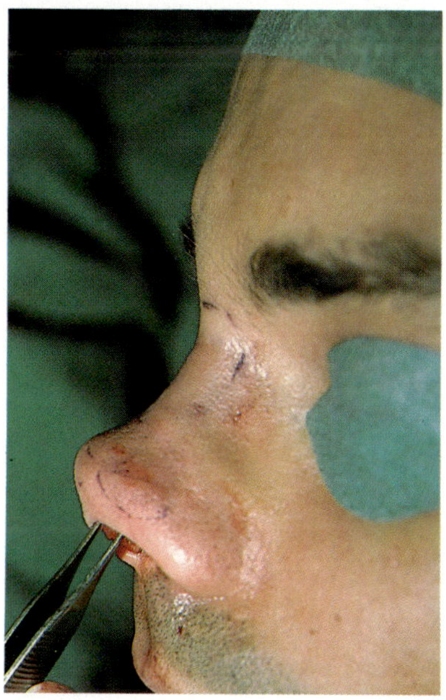

K

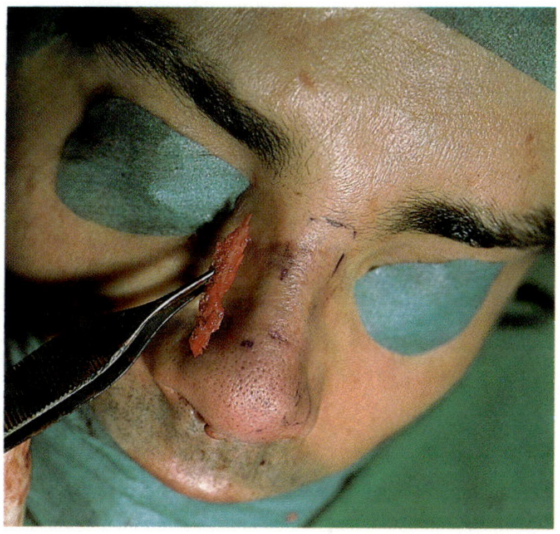

L

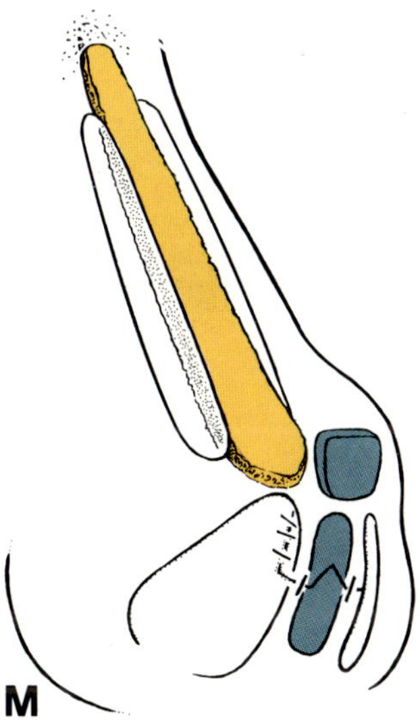

M

Fig. 105. In many cases of saddle nose with an already good support of the tip we only need a dorsal graft. For this purpose, we use bone grafts from the iliac crest. (A) Middle-aged man with posttraumatic saddling of the bony skeleton and bulbous tip and deep supra-alar groove. (B and C) Preoperative outline of the correction to be effected. (D) Rethi-Goodman incision for access. (E and F) Trelat elevator dissects a recipient bed for a columellar cartilaginous batten. (G) Harvesting iliac graft. (H) Drilling a recipient hole at the glabella (I, J, and K). Introduction of iliac bone graft. (L and M) On both sides a lateral apposition of fine supplementary graft is performed.

Fig. 105. continues.

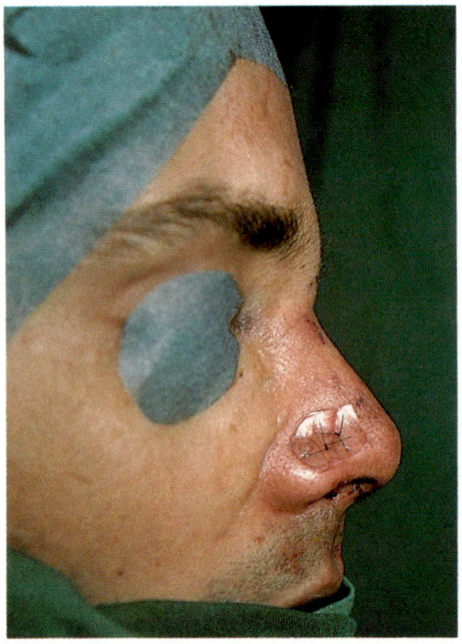

N

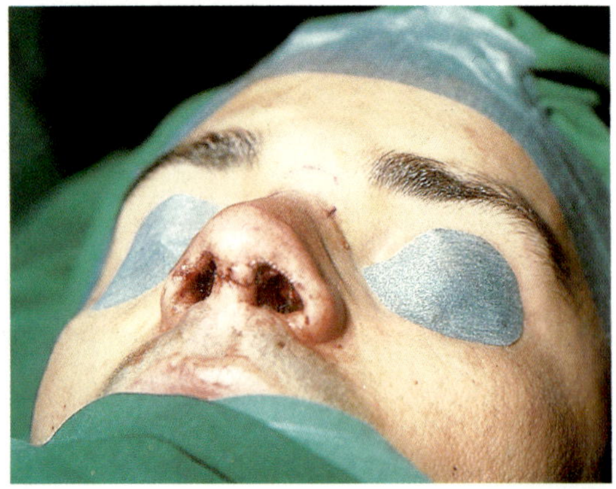

O

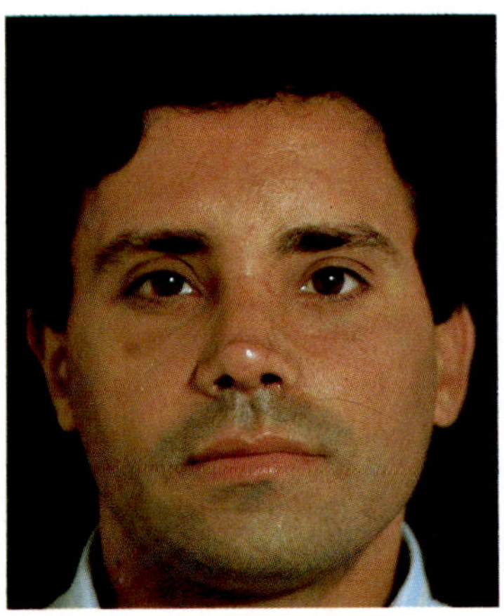

P

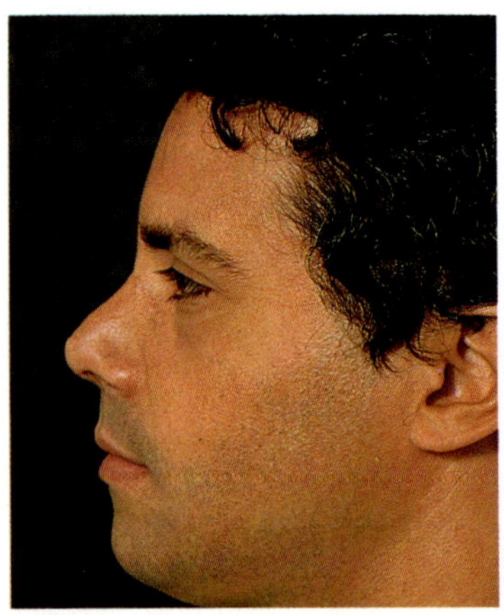

Q

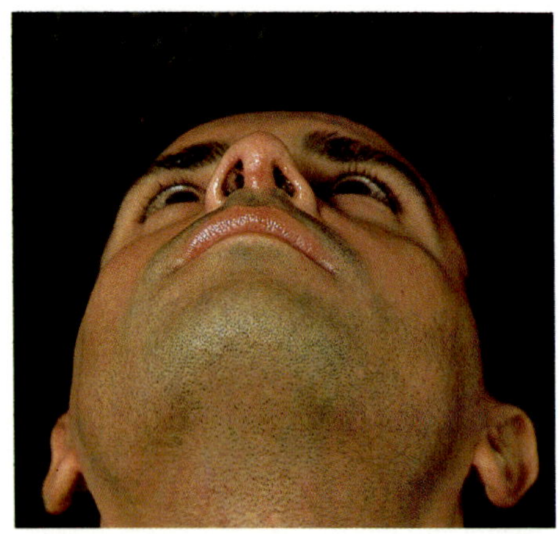

R

(N and O) End of the secondary operation. Rethi-Goodman incision is sutured. (P, Q, and R) Result.

The round or flat oval nare can especially be found in those postoperative saddle noses in which a hump removal has been performed after a submucous septal resection. If the strip of cartilage remaining at the dorsum after the septal resection is not high enough, then the subsequent hump removal leads to a depression of the vault, with the cicatricious contraction not being counteracted by any supporting force of the septum. Usually this deformity is composed of a depressed nasal dorsum involving the middle or the upper vault, or both, a real or apparent recession of the premaxilla with retruded nasal spine, an acute nasolabial angle, and bulbous tip that can either be sagging due to an absence of the caudal septum, or rotated cephalad due to the excessive depression of the middle third. The roof of the nasal cavities is low especially at the level of the valve where the depression causes an important narrowing of the airway. Thus many patients with saddle noses complain about nasal obstruction. As a rule it can be observed that the nasal cavity is patent and sufficiently wide, but that both vestibules are narrowed.

A saddle nose is difficult to correct in most cases because of the need to provide structural support for the nose while at the same time having to achieve a perfectly sculptured cosmetic result. There are also combinations of true and pseudo saddle noses in which the bony and cartilaginous dorsum are lowered too much and the tip is left extremely projected. A pseudo saddle nose, at times referred to as an "apparent" saddle, is usually the result of excessive projection of the nasal tip with what really is a fairly normal dorsal profile.

It is imperative to gain structural support of the nasal pyramid, enlarging the air passages at the valve for better function. This functional correction should not be carried out at the expense of giving an aesthetic definition to the nose. The correction of so-called pseudo saddle noses is easier. Such a nose may display an overly long and prominent tip with an otherwise normal dorsal structure, or have a slight bony hump together with a prominent nasal tip. In the first instance the tip should be reduced by resecting the lower part of the cartilaginous septum and by reshaping the lower lateral cartilages at the anterior angle. In the second instance the small bony hump should be removed with a rasp and the tip corrected as in the first case. If necessary, the nasal bones are repositioned toward the midline.

Beside the saddle nose other deformities need augmentation, these are: (1) congenital shortness in Caucasians; (2) racial shortness in non-Caucasians; (3) Binder's syndrome (maxillonasal dysplasia) with hypoplasia of the nasal floor, along with the apparent lack of length of the columella and often a degree of maxillary retrusion, adding to the general "dish-face" look (Fig. 106); (4) acquired shortness after fractures in childhood; (5) late acquired shortness after trauma, tumor resection, or illness; (6) iatrogenic deformity (pig snout nose); and (7) congenital deformity (hare lip nose, facial clefts etc.). The techniques of treatment are practically the same. If a true saddle nose is present, there are many ways to correct it. The choice of procedure depends first upon the degree of saddling and secondly on the grafting material available. Because of better "take," one should always strive to use autogenous tissue, best of all from the nose itself, and only in special cases should one resort to using foreign material. The correction of the slight saddle nose can by performed (1) with septal cartilage; (2) with lower lateral cartilage; (3) with upper lateral cartilage; (4) with ear cartilage; and (5) by narrowing the bony and cartilaginous vault.

The use of the upper part of the lower lateral cartilage as a flap, according to Kazanjian (1949), and the turn-up flaps from the upper lateral cartilage sutured together according to the method of Kazanjian (1949) and of Straith (1956) are examples of local tissue employed in the correction of the deformity. The alar swing operation appeared in Kazanjian's and Converse's textbook on Facial Injuries (1959) and has subsequently been referred to by Converse as Kazanjian's "flying wing" operation (Converse, 1976). The entire lateral crus is swung in a cephalad direction to be sutured one to another at the nasal root by means of a suture passed subcutaneously. Dingman (1956) and Holmes (1958) subsequently refined the technique leaving the inferior margin of the lateral crus in its natural position. The book by Denecke and Meyer describes the original technique. The operation and its modifications are suitable in the correction of mild to moderate saddle nose deformities. We have abandoned using these techniques.

To correct depressions in the middle third of the dorsum we like to use a cartilage graft from the septum, cut in multiple fine strips that are then placed to fill the saddle defect. They are introduced with blunt forceps just before pack-

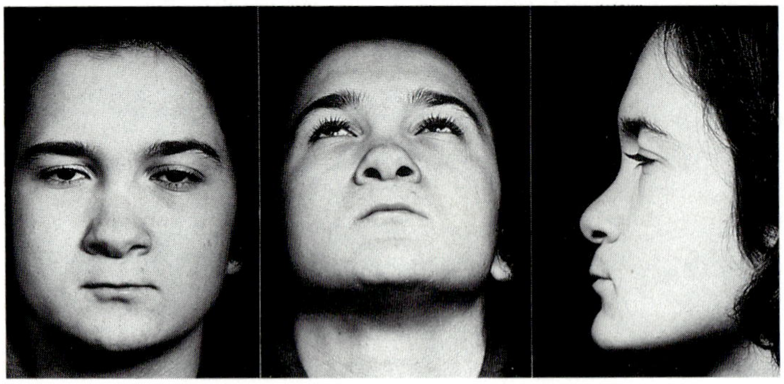

A

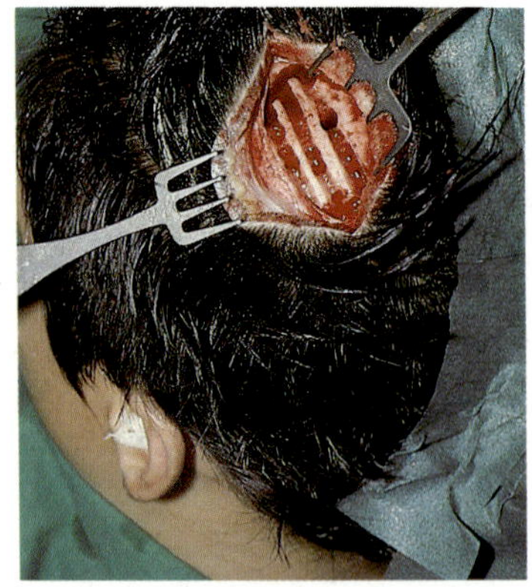

B

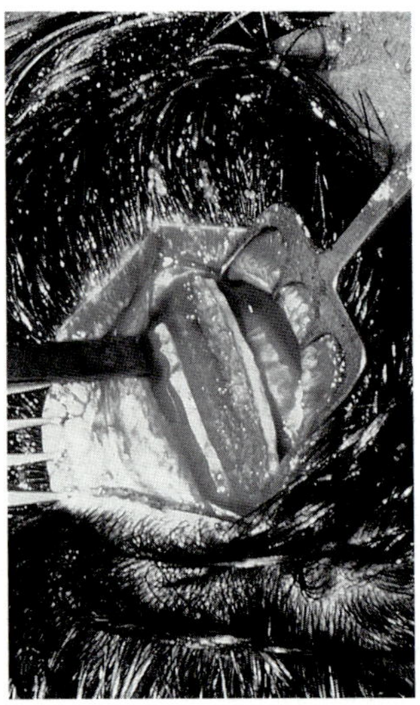

C

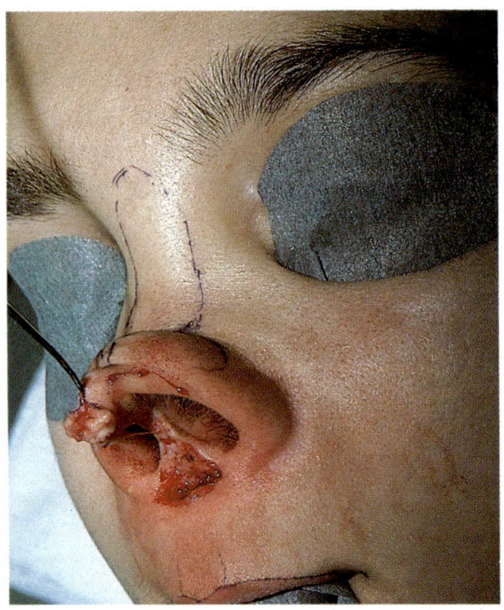

D

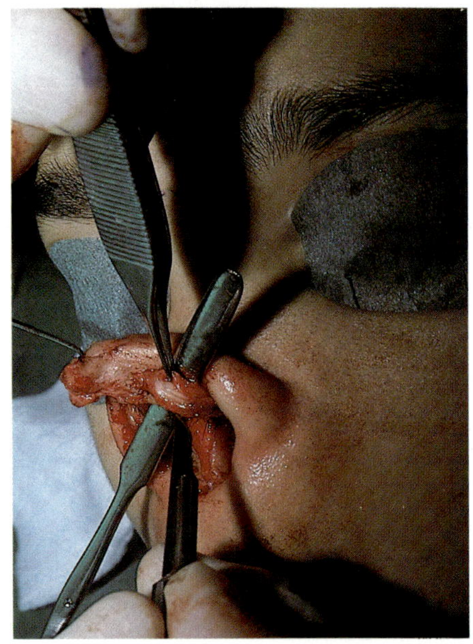

E

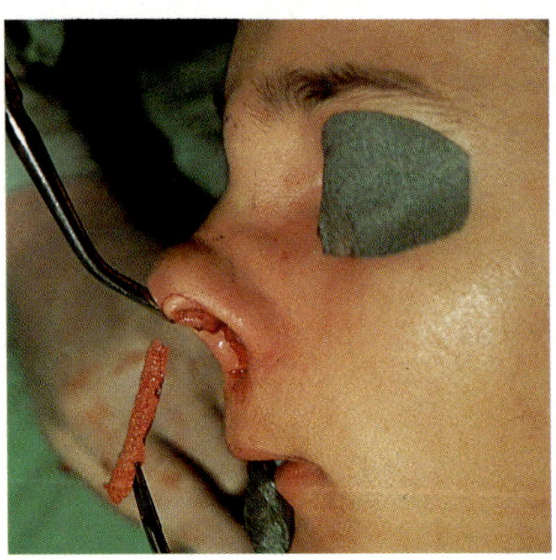

F

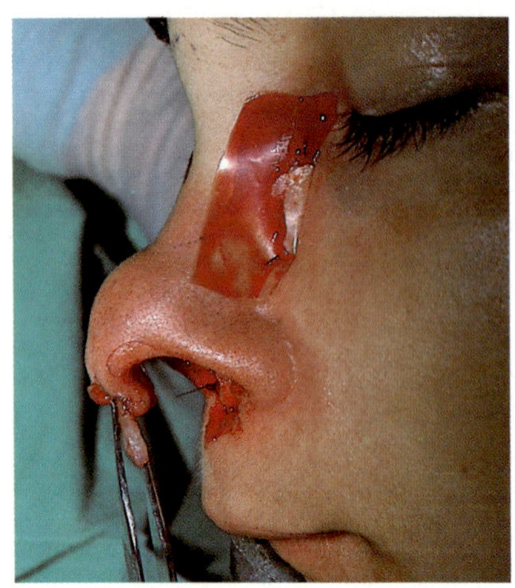

G

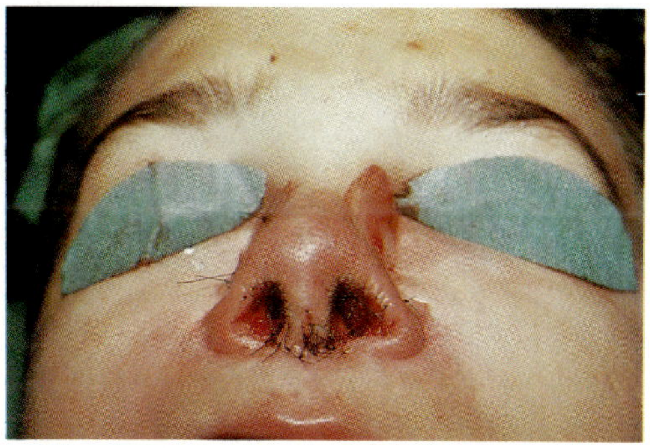

H

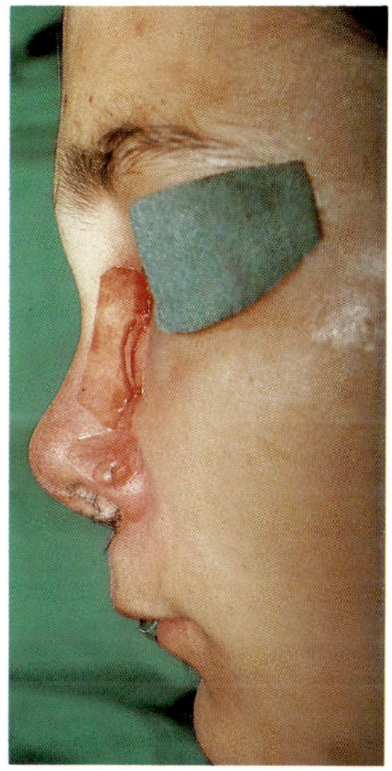

I

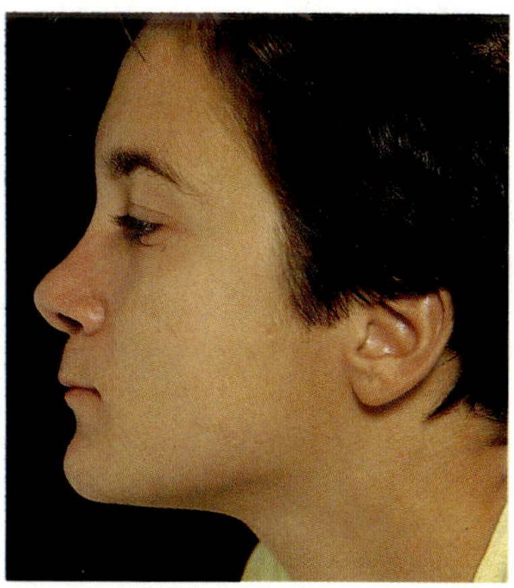

J

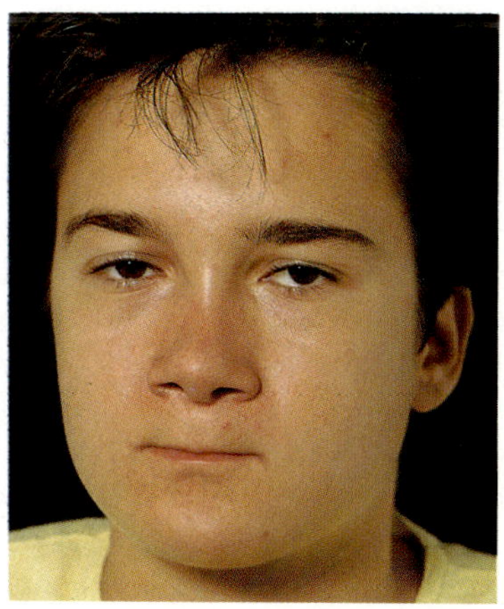

K

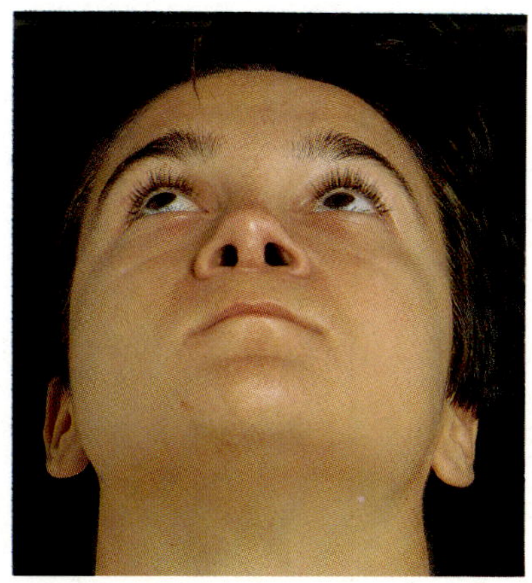

L

Fig. 106. In young female patients with a saddle nose when we want to leave a slightly curved dorsal line we utilize the skull graft of Tessier (1982). (A) Young girl with Binder's syndrome. (B) Preparing two bone grafts in the parietal area of the skull with the rotating burr. (C) The graft is removed from the skull. (D) Open access with section of the columellar base and at the transfixion incision. (E) Modeling of alar tip complex with luxation technique. (F) Insertion of the bone graft. (G) A cartilage strut from the septum is inserted into the columella. (H and I) End of the operation with elongation of the columella by V-Y technique, alar marginal resection, transnasal mattress sutures after osteotomies, and narrowing of the pyramid. (J, K, and L) Result.

ing the nasal cavities and the vestibule. Layers of temporalis fascia can further enhance augmentation in combination with autogenous cartilage. Usually, quadrangular cartilage segments provide the best grafting material for dorsal and columellar augmentation. They are harvested along the vomerine ridge.

Juri (1979) corrects slight dorsal depressions with two or three layers of ear concha grafts superimposed on one another, placed, and immobilized with transcutaneous sutures. He removes the thread one week later. Auricular cartilage has been used by many surgeons to correct smaller defects of the dorsum and columella. Muenker (1984) used this material for major saddle nose corrections. He described joining autogenous bilateral ear conchal grafts in a sandwich-like manner to obtain an L-shape. A three-layer graft to the dorsum and a two-layer graft to support the depressed columellar-tip area results in a more natural and elastic reconstruction of the nasal framework. The curved grafts are planed by "cross-hatching," fixed together with steel sutures to form an L-shape, and are immobilized in the recipient area by transcutaneous sutures. In severe saddle nose deformities a functional and aesthetic reconstruction of the entire nasal framework is necessary. These cases require larger cartilage grafts or bone grafting.

Cartilage Graft

Our personal experience and opinion is that cartilage is the relative first choice of all available materials to implant in the nose. Compared with all the other materials mentioned so far, cartilage has essential advantages. It possesses a consistency and elasticity that is physiologic for the nose; it is easily carved into the desired shape, the healing process is practically without problems, and it can be used equally well in all the very different kinds of recipient beds found in the nose.

Since autogenous cartilage has been favored as the graft of first choice for larger defects, until now we harvested L-shaped grafts from the rib (Fig. 96). The rib cartilage graft, both autologous and homologous, was enthusiastically advocated by Brown (1951), Salinger (1952), Gillies (1957), and others. O'Connor and Pierce (1938), Cottle, Quilty, and Buckingham (1953), Gibson, Davis, and Curran (1958), Mikelson (1962), Hellmich (1970), and many others prefer homologous to autogenous cartilage.

The question of whether autogenous rib cartilage is preferable to preserved homologous material is debatable. Both have biological as well as technical advantages and disadvantages that counterbalance each other. With reference to the main point of discussion—relating to the rate of resorption—it has been proven that under equal stress, autogenous cartilage will also show partial resorption, whether it is ear, rib, or septal cartilage.

Gerow, Stal, and Spira advocated in 1983 a so-called "totem pole" rib graft reconstruction resembling different parts of the anticipated reconstruction. The dorsal, the columellar, and the premaxillary parts are carved and kept articulated. The authors also recommend cutting a vertical incision at the nasion for clearing the soft tissue from the glabellar region and wiring the proximal end of the dorsal bone graft.

A second important question concerns the shape of the graft, should it be a single dorsal strut or L-shaped. If, in addition to the filling of the depression, support of the tip and columella is required we mostly use L-shaped grafts (see Figs. 96 and 97), which are taken from the eighth, ninth, or tenth ribs.

Made of one piece and being immobile in itself, the L-shape rib graft not only takes over the supporting function of a septal implant, but also the bridge function of a dorsal implant. Many authors, such as Hellmich (1970), believe that such a fragile construction will not be able to resist any great mechanical stress. Through our experience, we can prove that the resistance, in most cases, is perfectly adequate. In many cases, however, it is preferable either to reconstruct the septum and nasal dorsum with a stronger, boomerang-shaped septal graft or to choose to insert two separate grafts into the septum and the nasal dorsum (*see* Fig. 107).

We can introduce an L-shaped graft through the intercartilaginous and the transfixion incision (Fig. 98). The access for inserting the graft can be facilitated by the open approach procedure with sectioning of the columellar base, carrying the incision through the membranous septum and extending it into the vestibular intracartilaginous incision. The lower lateral cartilage can be modeled and trimmed in the usual way using the eversion technique. The bed for the graft at the dorsum as well as in the columella is prepared under direct vision (Figs. 99, 100 and

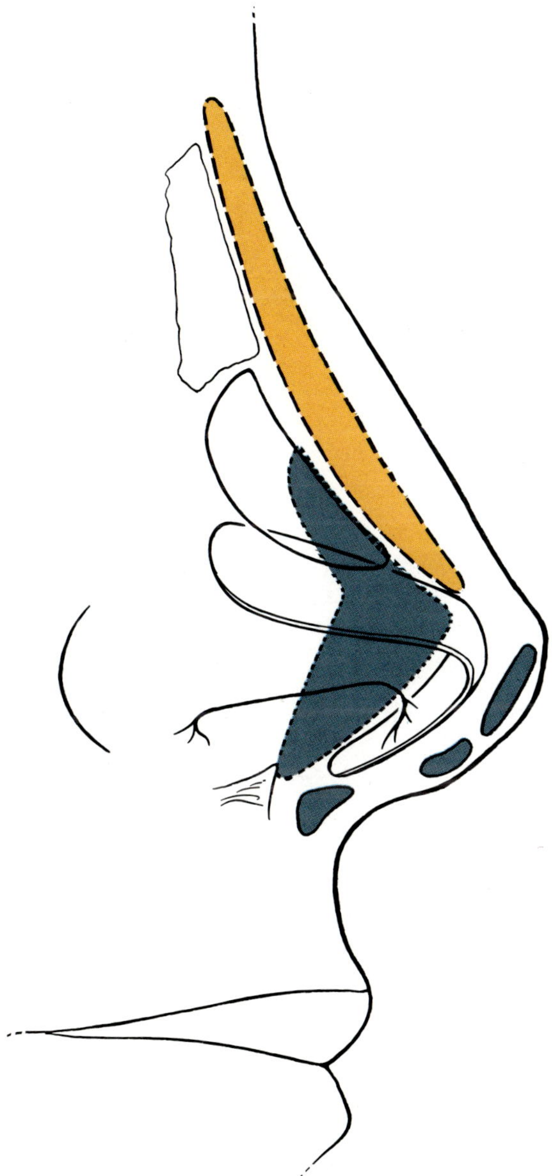

A

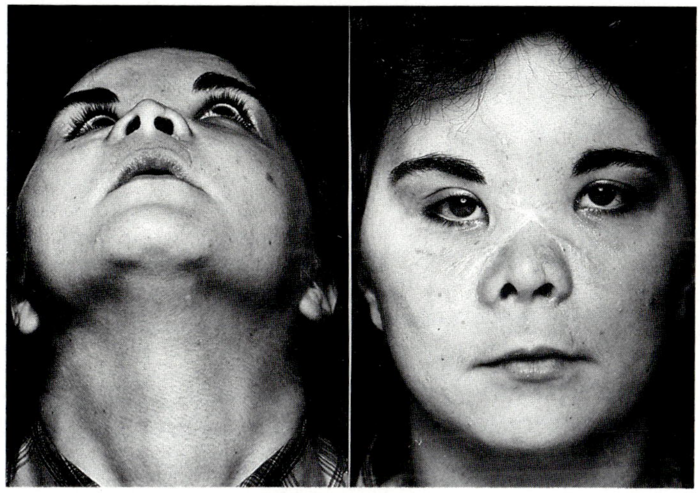

B

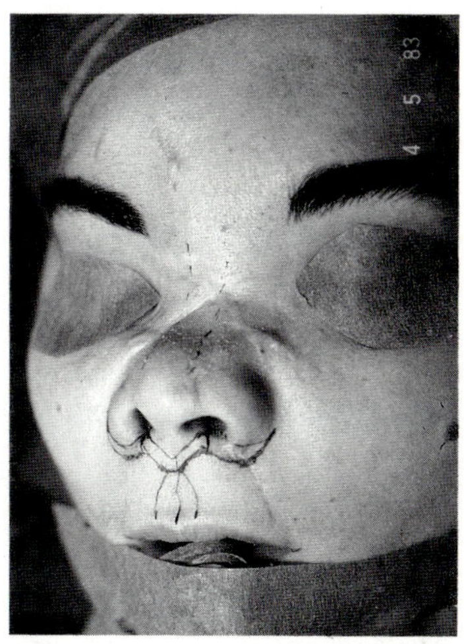

C

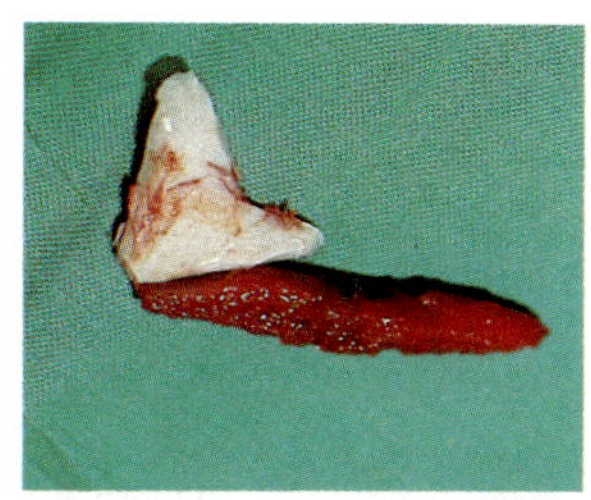

D

Fig. 107. (A) Occasionally when strong support of the tip-columella complex is needed we combine a straight dorsal bone graft from the iliac crest with a small L-shaped rib cartilage graft for tip, which is anchored at the nasal spine. In addition, we use onlay grafts in the lobule at the midcolumella level and the nasolabial angle. *(Fig. 107. continues.)*

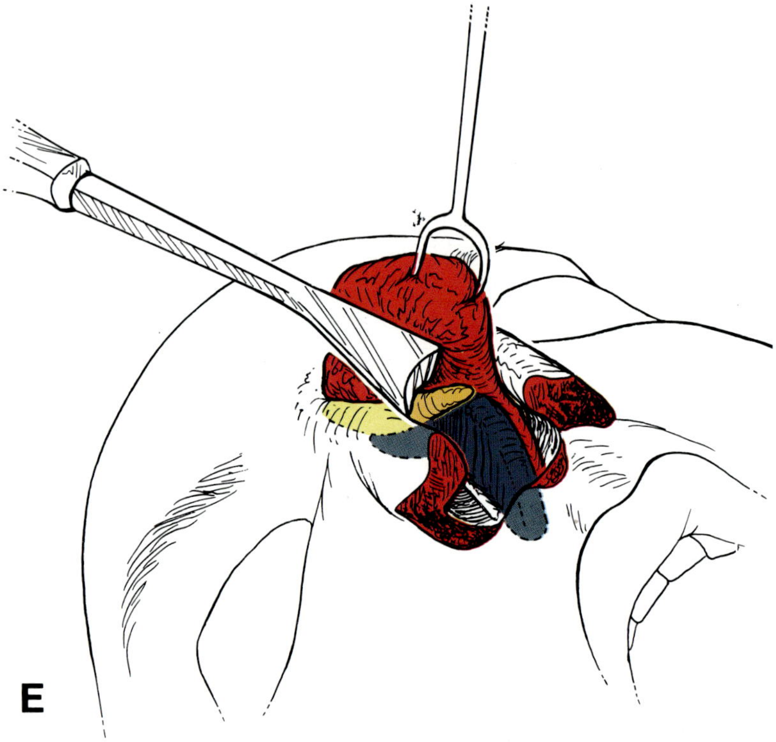

E

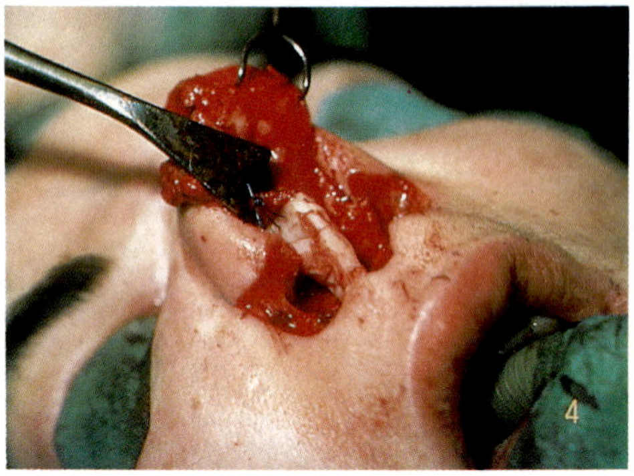

F

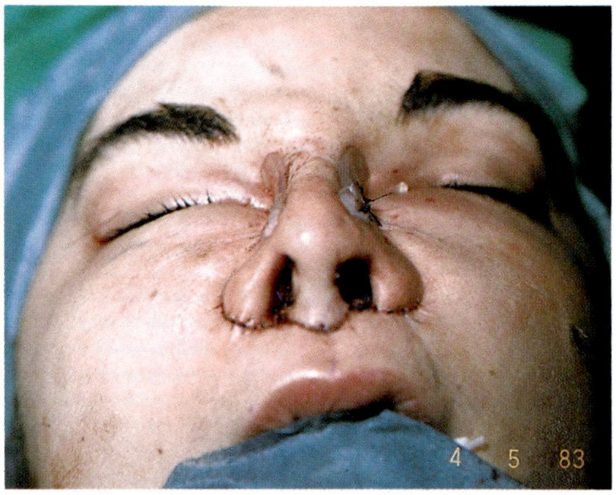

G

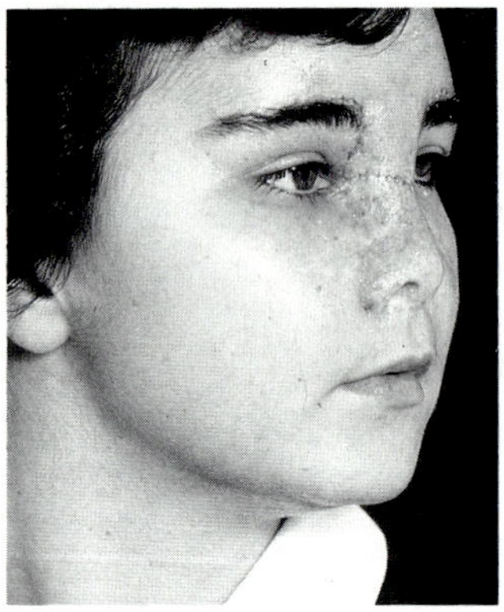

H

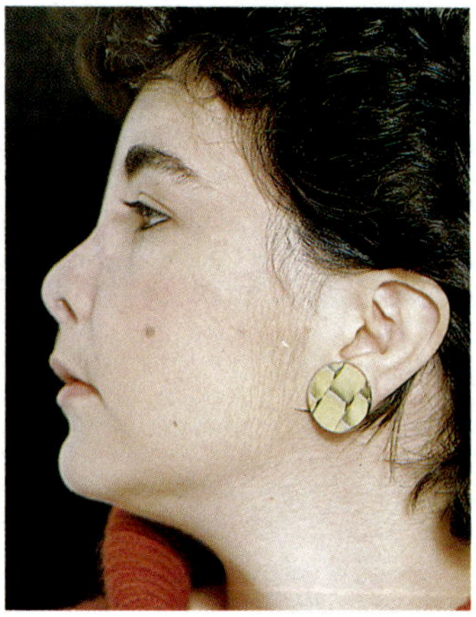

I

Fig. 107. (B) Young girl with posttraumatic severe saddle nose with airway obstruction after insufficient primary reposition. In the secondary operation the combined bone and cartilage grafts were applied. Situation after primary correction. (C) The placement of the dorsal graft and a buffalo-horn skin excision at the upper lip for lowering the columella and alar bases are outlined. (D) Bone graft and L-shaped cartilage costal graft are put together. (E and F) Insertion of both graft and fixation of each other with Mersilene suture. (G) End of the operation. (H) Early result. Glabellar scar corrected. (I) End of the operation with columella and alar bases sutured with transnasal mattress sutures after osteotomies.

101). On the dorsum it may be short, resting on the bony vault, or long, ending at the glabella where a hole drilled into the bone serves as a fixation point. The same anchoring hole is used for dorsal bone grafts from the iliac crest, which can be combined with a septocolumellar cartilage strut.

If we do not use an L-shaped cartilage graft and there is a need for support to the tip, we insert an accessory columellar graft for elongation and straightening of the columella. This graft can be a small L-shaped one of rib cartilage placed under the distal extremity of a bony bridge graft (Fig. 107), or a simple cartilaginous strut from the septum or from the ear concha.

As already mentioned in the section on pig snout nose (Chapter 12), we can correct the saddle nose together with the concomitant shortness of the dorsum. To provide sufficient lining to the cartilage without tension, we stretch the dissected mucoperichondrial and mucoperiosteal vault on both sides in a caudal direction, using an extramucosal technique after a posterior vertical releasing incision in the mucoperiosteum of the bony part of the septum (Meyer and Kesselring, 1977) (Figs. 102 and 103).

When there is extensive skin mutilation following trauma, such as following the resection of a deep burn as well as in congenital malformations, skin replacement is always done prior to support grafting. Should we wish to elongate the nose, the skin is usually elastic enough. However, the lining skin mucoperichondrium and mucoperiosteum are not as extensible, especially in revisionary cases of iatrogenic shortness where the lining surface is scarred. In these cases, again, the best way to adapt the lining to the new length of the nose is provided by the extramucous procedure. The elongated nose needs support tissue for advancing the nasal bridge, supporting the tip, maintaining the acquired length, or giving more "body" to the "flancs," as expressed by Tessier (1981, 1982). We obtain this lateral augmentation with additional bilateral grafts that are placed beside the main dorsal graft, or at the border of the piriform aperture.

Hellmich (1972) places a flat boomerang-shaped piece of banked rib cartilage into the septal pocket, supported below by the nasal spine, after mobilization of the scarred areas of the lower part of the nose to restore both the cartilaginous saddle formation and the function of the nose. Bruck (1981) also prefers the boomerang shaped graft. When we use an L-shaped cartilage graft as part of an augmentation rhinoplasty, the caudal portion situated in the membranous septum has to be pushed deeply towards the spine in order to prevent a projection of the supratip area, rather than of the tip itself by the angle of the graft. The latter should be slightly acute rather than obtuse to have the tip well defined and not amorphously round.

Some patients suffer from an increasing distortion and warping of cartilage graft in the nasal dorsum. This is very typical of this material. The solution to this problem is the strict adherence to the laws of the "balanced cross section," as stated by Gibson, Davis, and Curran (1958), by meticulous contouring, incising, and cross-hatching.

According to this principle we incise the rib graft longitudinally in multiple cuts with a No. 11 blade once the graft is already in place in the dorsum. When the recipient area is unevenly prepared or the bony framework is asymmetrically mobilized, distortion can occur, as the graft is unable to stand the mechanical stresses exacted on it by the nasal soft tissues.

Preserved homogenous costal cartilage can be irradiated with γ-rays with a minimal dose of 2 M rad for sterilization, according to Hellmich (1972). The usage of this material in rhinosurgery is increasing in Germany due to some advantage surgeons there feel preserved cartilage has as compared to other grafts. The problem of partial graft resorption has not yet been solved.

On a rib cartilage graft the perichondrium should not be left on one side. It should be removed on both sides. An infection in the recipient bed, as well as primary or secondary postoperative exposure of the graft can be rise for extensive resorption. Giving credence to Krizek's (1983) observation that the single most destructive event in implant surgery is infection, edema and hematoma in the recipient bed should be avoided, and subtle surgical technique as well as sufficient postoperative immobilization and protection with antibiotics are required. To prevent hematoma we inject fibrin adhesive into the dorsal bed around the graft (Fig. 109) (see Fibrin adhesive, Bleeding).

The high resistance of preserved homologous cartilage against infection has been proven by the bland "take" of grafts that have been inserted into the nasal septum directly after septal abscess draining (Masing, 1965; Masing and Hellmich, 1968; Huizing, 1970). The hazards to free cartilage transplantation in augmentation rhinoplasty depend on the kind of material chosen, the manner used to preserve the graft if it is not used immediately, the volume of the graft, the state of the recipient bed, the condition of the operated nose, the surgical technique used, and the postoperative mechanical stress that the graft is subjected to (for instance in sportsmen, especially boxers).

The main problems with grafts are: the possibility of partial resorption, risks of infection, and distortion of the grafted material. A nonobservance of a series of basic rules during the surgical procedure leads to mistakes that can cause or enhance the above-mentioned problems. In order to avoid partial resorption, which can affect both autogenous as well as homogenous cartilage, it is necessary to establish a recipient area free of stress by eliminating existing scar tissue that can produce contraction. Stress and strain represent the greatest postoperative hazards. With regard to the fate of a cartilage graft, it makes a great deal of difference whether the graft has been vitally transplanted or whether it has been preserved by heat, freezing, lyophilization, radiation, or through chemical means such as merthiolate or cialyt. In cases where banked cartilage is to be used, choosing preservation with merthiolate or cialyt has proven effective in our hands. The storing of homologous support material in a solution of cialyt (2-ethyl-mercury-mercapto-benoalzol-carbonacid-natruium) was introduced in Germany by Hauberg and Brucksen (1954) for bone graft. Schmelzle (1978), has used this solution to store bone, cartilage, and fascia (as do other German surgeons), in combination with intraoperative antibiotic prophylaxis since 1971. Actually, we use frozen and irradiated preserved costal cartilage for special cases of nasal reconstruction and paranasal augmentation. The paranasal grafting of the anterior aspect of the maxilla helps to correct any deformity due to the lack of bony projection in the mid-face area, such as in cases of congenital malformation with retromaxillism and short nose (see Fig. 108), or after telescoping traumatism (Figs. 110 and 111).

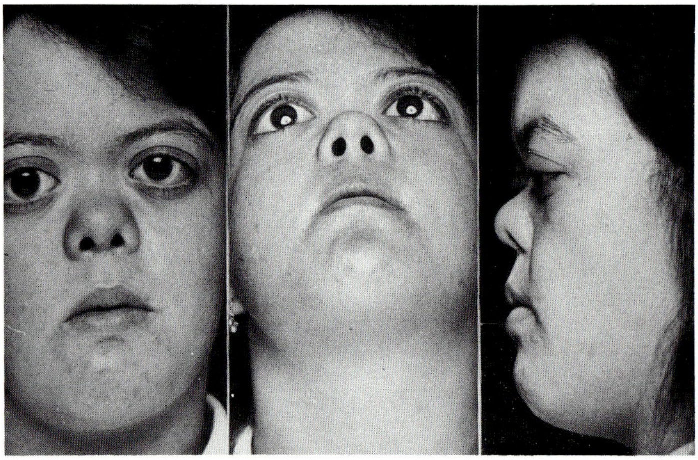

A

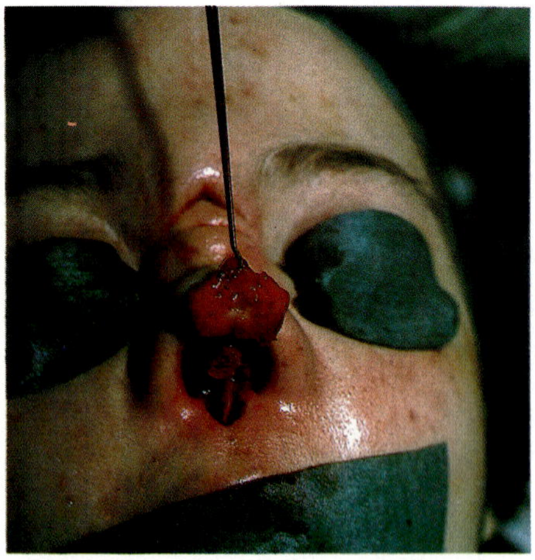

B

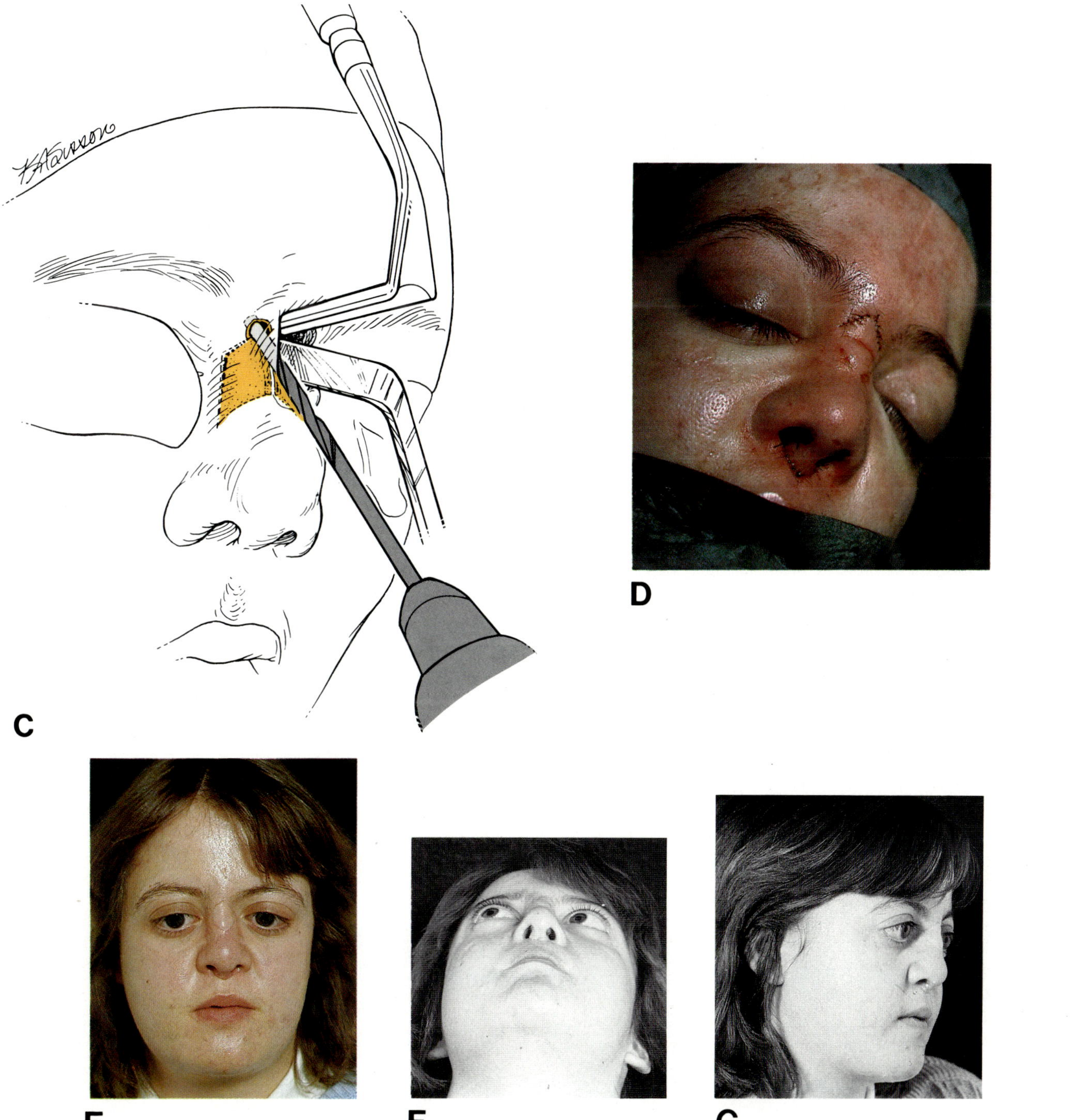

Fig. 108. Rarely we need additional skin for achieving enough expansion to allow a subcutaneous augmentation procedure. This is accomplished by grafting. In this young girl with exorbitism, retromaxillism and respiratory dysfunction we had to enlarge the upper dorsal skin surface with a free skin graft from the retroauricular region. A single bone graft from the iliac crest was used for the dorsum and a vomer graft was reinserted anteriorly to provide a tip-columellar support. The bone graft was anchored in a drilled hole at the glabella. For this purpose the rotating burr was introduced through a V-shaped incision at the margin of the free skin. (A) Patient before surgical treatment. (B) Open access. Vomer graft is inserted at the anterior nasal spine. A skin graft has already been transplanted to the glabellar region. (C) Carving a hole at the glabella with a drill through the glabellar skin incision. The upper extremity of the bone graft will be located and anchored in this glabellar hole. (D) Patient at the end of the operation with resutured columella base and glabellar incision. (E, F, and G) Result.

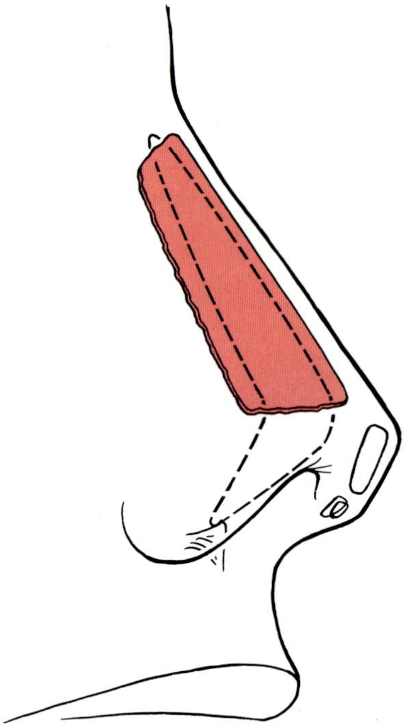

Fig. 109. If due to very thin skin the contour of the cartilage or bone graft is visible at the dorsum we have to smoothen it by means of subcutaneous interposition of a layer of dermis or temporal fascia graft.

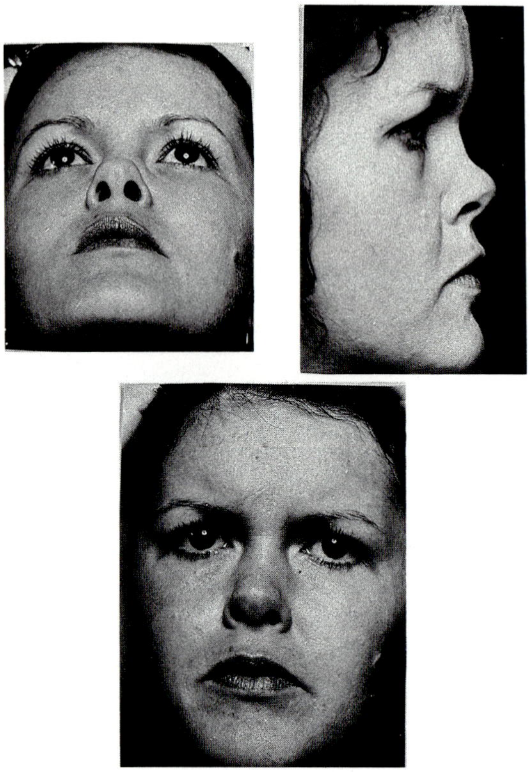

A

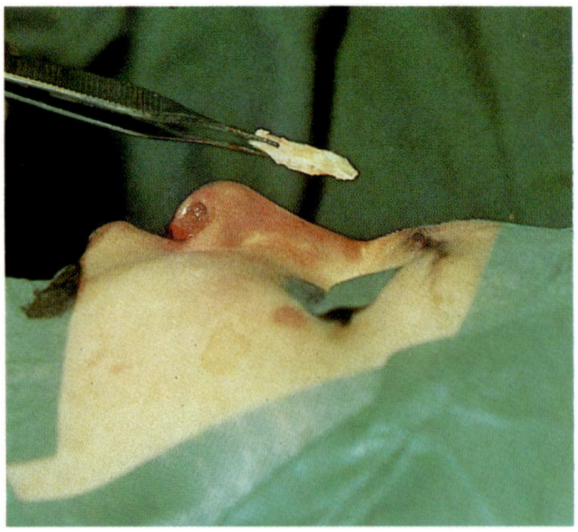

B

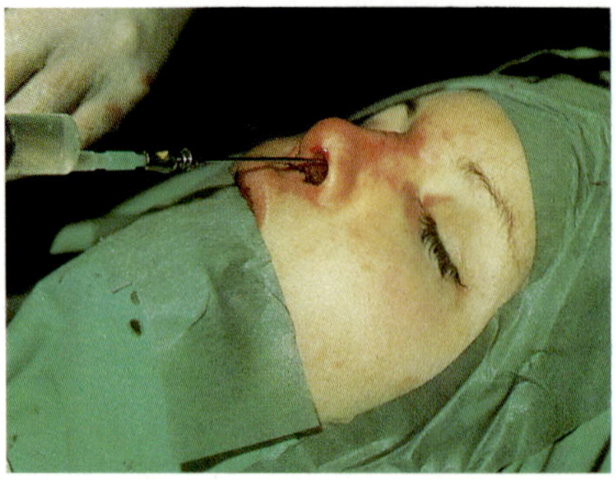

C

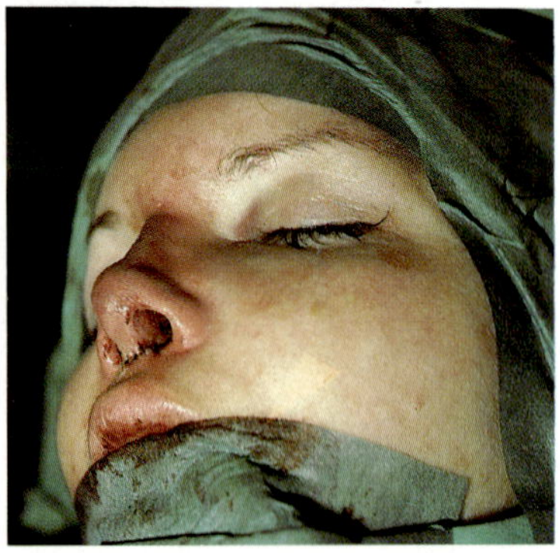

D

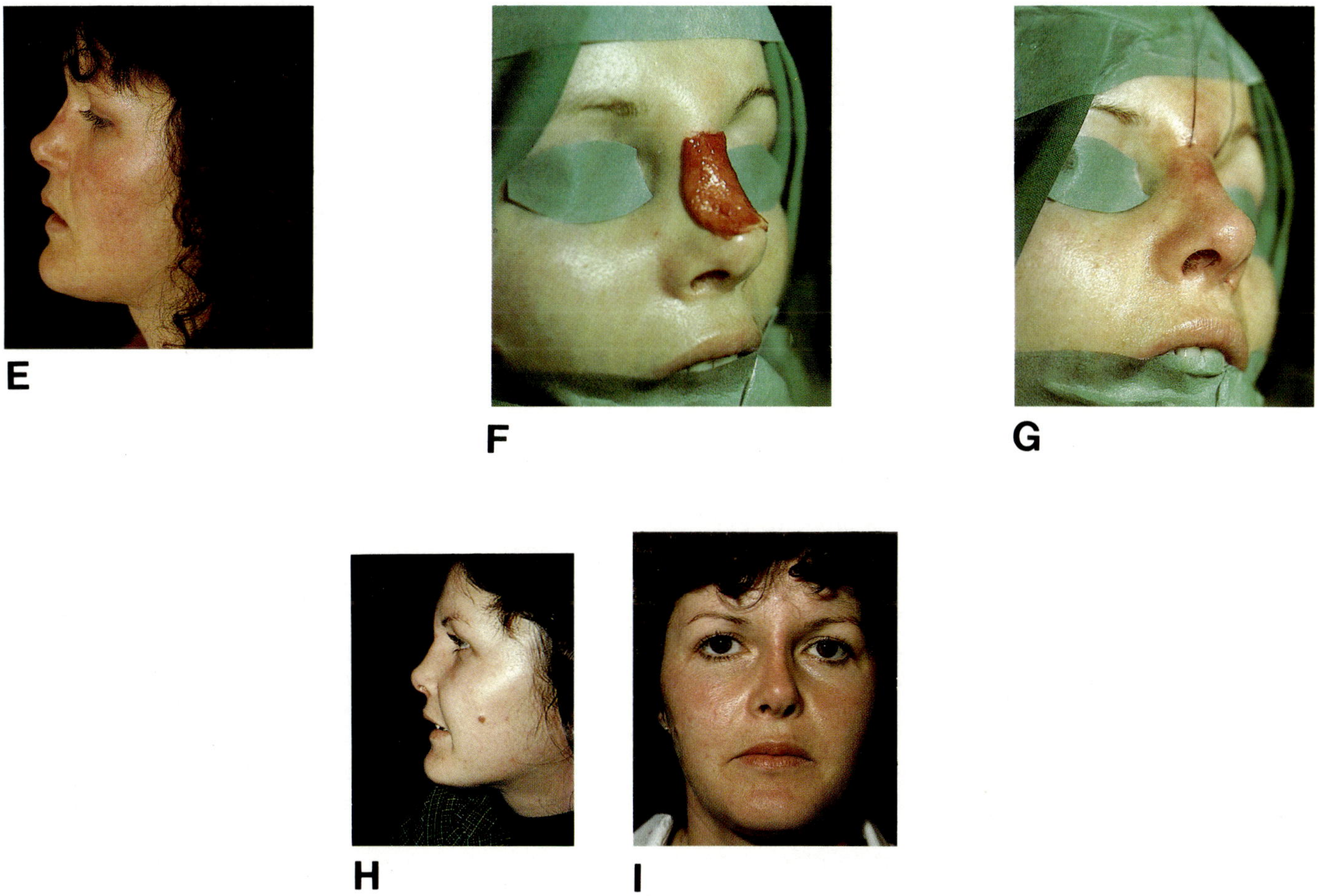

Fig. 110. The method of Fig. 109 has been applied in this case of a middle-aged woman with a posttraumatic telescoped middle third of the face. In a first stage the saddle nose and the maxillary retrusion were corrected and in a later revision smoothing of the dorsal contour was necessary. (A) Patient before augmentation surgery. (B) Anear cartilage graft is inserted into the dorsum. (C) The cartilage graft is glued in its recipient bed with fibrinogen tissue glue. (D) End of the first operation. (E) Acceptable result but visible edges of the dorsal graft. (F) Second revision. Dermis graft ready to be inserted through the intercartilaginous incision to the dorsum between the cartilage graft and the skin. (G) The superior extremity of the graft is passed under the skin by transcutaneous thread. (H and I) End result.

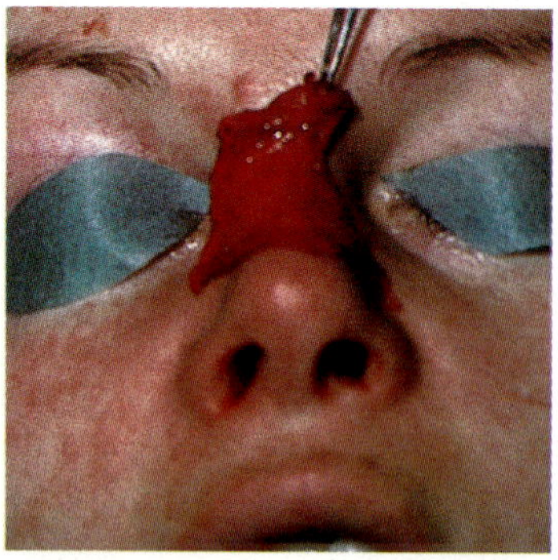

Fig. 111. Fascia from the temporal region can also be used for the same purpose.

In the surgical treatment of ozena we use irradiated or deep frozen homologous cartilage as a wedge to stabilize the displaced nasal wall (see ozena in Chapter 17). For minor nasal augmentation we store septal and auricular cartilage in simple saline solution as does Planas (1987).

Poor results can also be produced through a lack of appreciation of the risks found preoperatively, which would exclude for example the implantation of biological material in cases of severely predamaged recipient areas. In such cases a different solution has to be thought.

Hellmich (1972) believes that in such cases it may even become necessary to abstain from any surgical intervention. We think that in any case a surgical solution could be found. This can sometimes be by means of supplementary skin transfer with a flap. Then it becomes a true reconstructive procedure.

Ersek et al. reported in 1984 on the successful clinical use of processed bovine cartilage for nasal dorsal augmentation. They combined irradiation with a chemical processing to cross-link the bovine cartilage collagen, rendering it antigenically inert and dimensionally stable. The processing of the irradiated bovine cartilage (called Chondroplast) is done by genetic laboratories. In Europe, the material is especially utilized in Italy (Tassone, 1985).

In our opinion, homologous cartilage should be discouraged for secondary saddle nose correction, since it seems that with time, most of the implants are gradually resorbed or rejected. Exceptions to this generalization are certainly available but do not alter the concept that foreign living tissues should be avoided whenever possible in treating the patient with a secondary deformity who has already suffered enough from unsuccessful primary surgery.

As we do for the more important cartilage struts, we maintain the small grafts in their proper position with external mattress sutures tied over a fine plastic sheet, or just fixed externally with dressing tape.

Bone Graft

Many authors prefer to use bone grafts as a first choice. We like to insert bone grafts in special cases of saddle nose for simple dorsal augmentation when tip-columellar support is not necessary. In such cases a transcolumellar Rethi incision can provide good access, particularly for drilling a hole into the glabellar bone to act as an anchoring point for the straight bone graft (see Fig. 105, *see* p. 140–141).

We like to harvest the bone from the ileum, and in special circumstances, from the skull. We do not use tibial bone, as Farina does since 1948 (1983), or mastoid bone as other authors do. Italian authors advocate the use of bone grafts from the olecranon (Del Bene et al, 1985).

We also choose to "freshen" the nasal bones. A bone graft cannot take on soft tissues, scars, or even periosteum, since the lack of bony contact will cause instability of the graft and subsequent resorption. Therefore, we use the rasp or a chisel to freshen the nasal bones up to the frontonasal angle, which is also deepened. This creates a raw, recipient bed of spongeous bone that greatly increases the successful take of the bone graft.

The bone graft can be fixed at the glabella by drilling a hole in the bone, or by using transnasal metal or other nonabsorbable sutures. It has to be transplanted with meticulous care to permit its adherence and consolidation, if not, it will progressively resorb. The lateral dissection is carried out through the nasal or oral vestibule, and extends around the entire piriform aperture up to the medial canthal ligament. The dissection of the nasal mucosa is extended under the frontal process of the maxilla. Through intercartilaginous incisions, the dissection of the nasal mucosa is carried up under the medial part of the upper lateral cartilages to the nasal bones, where it joins the dissected area under the frontal process of the maxilla made through the vestibule. When the dissection of the mucosa is not sufficient, there is a major risk of secondary retraction, exposure of the bone graft, obstruction of the nostrils, and distortion of the alae. In the very rare cases of a short columella with an extremely scarred tip-columella complex we prefer a bony strut to a cartilaginous one to support the difficult protrusion of the tip.

We use a bone strut pegged into the nasal spine, as described by Tessier (1960), only as a provisional solution for giving enough protrusion to the tip in secondary scarred noses. In these cases it is later replaced with a cartilage strut, once the tip has maintained the required projection. By doing this, we avoid the late rigidity inherent with columellar bone struts. Tessier (1966) also suggests this changing of grafts, to be eventually performed after 1 year.

A split skull graft as described by Tessier (1982) and Jackson (1983) can be ideal for forming a nasal bridgeline. The curvature of such a skull graft may be less desirable in a man, but it is quite suitable for the nasal dorsum of a girl or woman (Fig. 106, *see* p. 144–145). In primary saddle noses of young females, for instance in cases of Binder's syndrome (see Fig. 106), and in many postrhinoplastic deformities these grafts are useful and can be preferable to other grafts. The approaches used for the insertion of the split skull graft may be intranasal, midcolumellar, and glabellar. The glabellar approach is preferred by Jackson (1983). We use the other two accesses.

The advantages of this over other conventional bone grafts include: donor site proximity to the nose; curvature of the graft, which can be varied as required; and the possibility of additional bone harvesting for bridgeline buildup or lateral bone grafting. Minimal pain and minimal scar complications are other advantages. Additionally, it would appear that membranous calvarial bone undergoes less resorption than bone harvested from other sites. As is Jackson, we have been impressed with the rapid healing and good results.

We combine a dorsal straight bone graft with a small L-shaped rib cartilage graft in severe traumatic or iatrogenically butchered noses in which the augmentation material has to be particularly strong (Fig. 107, *see* p. 147–148). The iliac bone graft can also be combined with a cartilaginous septocolumellar pillar from the posterior part of the septum, if available, or from the ear concha.

We place the distal end of the graft between the two domes of the lower lateral cartilages, which can be eventually fixed to the graft or to each other. The bony surface of the graft extremity should not reach the undersurface of the tip skin. In all cases we additionally perform a tipplasty with onlay cartilage grafts from the superior part of the alar cartilage or from the septum for accentuating the double break in the tip-columella profile and adding projection.

When discussing bone grafts, it has to be mentioned that they usually form a complete union with the osseous part of the nasal dorsum. As in the case of correctly implanted cartilage, these grafts are not mobile. Also, the incidence of primary infection is minimal.

Nevertheless, the disadvantage of bone grafts is their unnatural hardness and rigidity. Too often this can lead to thinning and perforation with loss of the graft on account of the mechanical stresses set in motion. The L-shaped bone graft is not easy to fabricate. Many surgeons find it far easier to project the main graft with a strut pegged into the nasal spine. Bone's hardness also excludes its practical use as a septal graft, and its brittleness has been the cause of often observed fractures of such grafts in the nasal dorsum. In zones of stress, bone behaves as badly as cartilage. It need hardly be added that due to too much resorption, homogenous bone should be avoided if possible.

The main complication is the displacement of the bone graft, according to Flageul and Grignon (1982), who are using two iliac crest grafts in the dorsal and retrocolumellar positions. Each of the two grafts is lodged in a deep recess and into either the frontal bone or the anterior nasal spine. The two grafts are blocked together at the tip by a mortice joint. It is important to respect the continuity of the mucosal lining.

In practically every case of saddle nose, in addition to the grafting procedure we narrow the base of the nose through lateral, paramedian, and transverse osteotomies in order to project the bony structures and increase the protrusion of the dorsum. The narrowed bones and the graft are held in place with transcutaneous, transmucous, and transseptal mattress sutures passing through the osteotomy lines and, if necessary, through the upper lateral cartilages. The contact of the dorsal graft with the bony dorsum has to be solid. When a separate dorsal graft is used, the intercartilaginous, transfixion, and Rethi incisions are appropriate for its introduction.

The separate columellar strut is positioned through either the transfixion incision or Rethi incision. The dorsal graft is maintained in its straight position by transnasal sutures of 4-0 nonabsorbable thread tied externally over pieces of plastic, while for the fixation of the columellar strut the transfixion sutures are sufficient. In general, it is not necessarily required to wire the graft, if we can fix it with mattress sutures.

Occasionally it is necessary to wire the graft to the nasal process of the frontal bone. This can be done according to Tessier (1966) and Jackson (1983) through three stab incisions, or through a transverse incision in the fold of the nasofrontal angle.

For fixation of a dorsal bone graft, Wheeler et al (1982) provide a good inset into the nasofrontal angle by using a special horizontal incision at the glabella and carving the glabellar bone with a burr. They contour the cancellous iliac bone, rib bone, or tibial crest bone grafts specifically to the defect with an air driven burr and fix the graft with two wires passed through transnasal drill holes. The bone graft is then anchored to the rest of the bony pyramid by means of a wire thread. Tape dressing and splinting with plaster of Paris is worn, as usual, for about 10 days.

As has been pointed out before, the main risk of human materials—whether bone or cartilage—is their tendency to partial resorption. In 1977, Gammert and Masing published their results after long-term observation. These results demonstrated that the rate of resorption depended on various different factors. In relation to the distribution of normal mechanical stress, the nose is divided into an upper zone of rest and a lower zone of stress and strain, where the resorptive processes take place. Gammert and Masing (1977) found a direct correlation between the rate of implant resorption to the extent of previously existing damage to the implant bed with its coexistent increases in pressure and traction stresses. This coincides with Hellmich's (1972) and our experience, that the rate of resorption of nasal grafts is largely independent of the type of biological material used, but rather dependent on the effects of mechanical stress. In our experience reabsorption of the bone graft is noted in practically every case but in no case has the reabsorption been to such an extent that a new saddle nose resulted.

The nasal skin can be lengthened or stretched to a sufficient extent without need of skin grafts or flaps. Only in extreme cases of congenital shortness, or in burn cases, iatrogenic loss or postinfectious loss, or tumoral loss of tissue is there a requirement for additional skin. Soft tissue augmentation has to be achieved prior to bone grafting. The marginal scar of the skin graft is revised and serves as the access site for carving the glabellar hole to be used as the anchoring point for the bone graft (Fig. 108, *see* p. 150–151).

Severe saddle deformity with a short nose requires a more reconstructive surgery with, in addition to a bone or cartilage graft, an elongation of the cutaneous cover. This can be achieved by inserting an elliptical skin graft from the postauricular area or through a V-Y procedure with a sliding flap from the glabellar or nasofrontal area as suggested by Gillies (1957), with his bishops mitre flap. Dupuis and Mainsdorf (1983) add four triangular flaps at the edges of the inter eyebrow sliding flap. They are transposed downward into two infraeyebrow and intracanthal lateral releasing incisions. The skin cover and the recipient raw surface are then enlarged for permitting the bone or cartilage graft to be covered without excessive tension.

We never had to provide additional skin by forehead flaps as shown by Millard in 1980. The dermal graft should be mentioned as another graft material. This is a free, full-thickness, skin graft with the most superficial layer, the epidermis, removed. In the donor site, an epidermal graft is removed. Then the dermal graft is removed from the deepithelialized skin area, consisting only of corium and subcutis. The fat must be carefully removed with scissors from the underside of the graft. According to the thickness necessary for the graft, two or three rectangular grafts can be laid one on the other. The graft is then handled with two nylon or silk pilot sutures. These sutures are passed into the prepared bed with a straight needle and drawn through the skin. The dermal graft can then slide into the subcutaneous pocket and be properly placed. The pilot sutures are removed, and the approach incision is closed. In figuring the size of the graft needed, one must add a little extra as is recommended with bone and cartilage grafts. With dermal grafts, one counts on an absorption of from 10–20 percent. This type of grafting was advocated by Straatma (1932) and Maliniac (1947, 1948), as shown in Denecke and Meyer's books (1964, 1967), and later developed by Reich (1983). We use it in secondary procedures after bone or cartilage grafting for saddle nose, if the contour of the dorsal graft is too conspicuous, producing an unnatural appearance to the dorsum. The dermal graft is then interposed between the dorsal skin and the bone or cartilage graft (Figs. 109 and 110, *see* p. 152–153).

Fascia from the temporal region can also be applied for the same purpose (Fig. 111). The fascia is harvested in the temporal or parietal region and introduced in the same manner as the dermal graft. Guerrerosantos (1984) envelopes the bone or cartilage graft with a leaf to fascia before inserting into nasal dorsum.

ALLOPLASTIC MATERIAL

The search for appropriate plastic materials has always found new stimulation. When hard and solid materials were used, the postoperative result was usually bad and would usually end in the total loss of the implant.

A large variety of alloplastic materials have been advocated by many surgeons, and nearly all have proven less suitable than autogenous material because of rejection, infection, and extrusion. Our experience continues to support the concept that autogenous cartilage and bone is the material of choice.

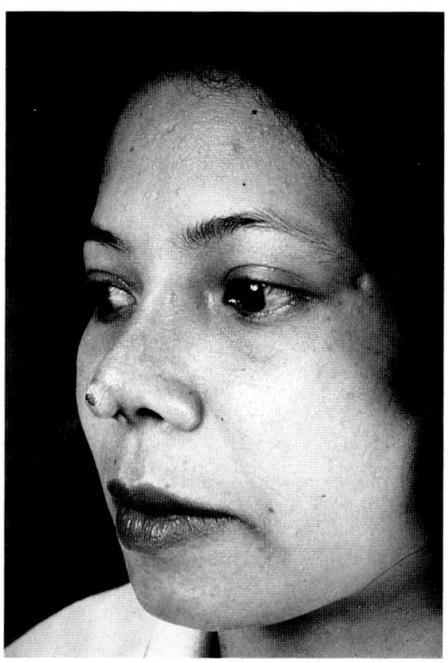

Fig. 112. Extrusion of silicone implant on a Japanese patient.

Despite the preference of some rhinoplastic surgeons for the use of solid implants or proplast implants in the treatment of saddle deformities, general experience suggests that rib cartilage grafts or iliac bone grafts are less likely to be extruded than alloplastic implants. Peer (1954) noted that most alloplastic implants were constantly being buried by one group of surgeons and then constantly being removed by another group of surgeons after varying periods of time.

Due to the continuous mechanical stress and minor trauma peculiar to the nose, a hard, rigid, and insufficiently elastic implant will cause microlesions of the recipient bed that, by way of edema, hematoma, ulceration, and necrosis, will lead to infection of the surrounding tissue and finally to its extrusion (Fig. 112). In most cases, at the end, there is nothing else to be done but to remove the plastic implant. Being foreign bodies, plastic implants present quite a number of further risks. They do not fuse, for instance, with their host's tissues and therefore usually remain mobile in their recipient bed. Apart from the aesthetic problems caused by this, the implant is frequently dislocated. Removal of the implant does not only become necessary due to recurrent inflammation, but also due to slippage of the implant in the nasal dorsum. In order to avoid the mobility of the plastic implants, many surgeons used and still use a method that consists of drilling holes into the plastic implants, believing that the ingrowing connective tissue will prevent the implant from slipping and remaining mobile. In case it then becomes necessary to remove the implant, the recipient bed will be severely traumatized, which, in case of a pre-existing infection, can even result in defects of the covering skin or mucosa. In addition, the perforations themselves can weaken the stability of the inelastic splints to such an extent that they will break even with minor trauma.

The search for the ideal implant led from softer, yet still hard, materials to injectable plastics (i.e., silicone and teflon). In a great number of cases, however, these materials show similar complications and difficulties. Circumscribed reactive tissue swelling often develops and considerable reactions of the covering skin may occur, which apparently are of an allergic origin.

Thus, there is a considerable choice of foreign materials available. It has to be chemically stable, heat stable for autoclaving purposes, and stable in shape. It has to exert a minimum of foreign body reaction and should not be cyto-

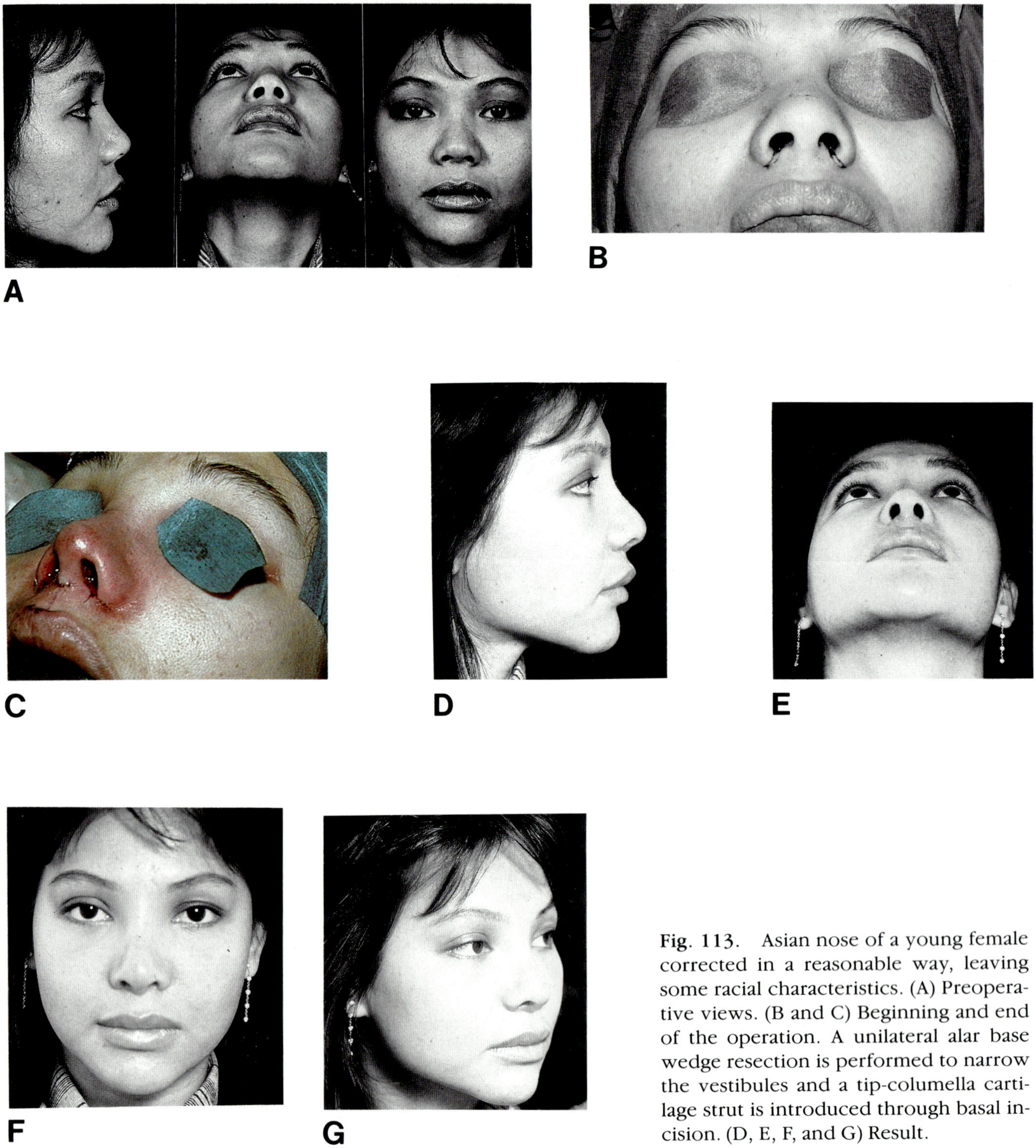

Fig. 113. Asian nose of a young female corrected in a reasonable way, leaving some racial characteristics. (A) Preoperative views. (B and C) Beginning and end of the operation. A unilateral alar base wedge resection is performed to narrow the vestibules and a tip-columella cartilage strut is introduced through basal incision. (D, E, F, and G) Result.

toxic, antigenic or carcinogenic. Some implant materials, such as Teflon® (Polytetrafluoroethylene—PTFE), Dacron® (Polyethylenterepthalate), Polyethylene, PVC (Polyvinylchloride), Nylon (Polyamide), Perlon (Polyurethan), and Ivalon (Polyvinylalcohol) have been abandoned.

In 1969 we published a case of platyrhynia with a short columella (Meyer and Flemming) corrected with a provisional L-shaped implant of Polyethylene. As we had done in other cases of maxillonasal dysplasia (Binder's syndrome), we changed the provisional alloplastic implant with an L-shaped rib cartilage graft at the age of 15 years. Two other cases of this same syndrome appearing in the same publication were treated only by means of tip-columellar grafting with septal and costal cartilage. Huizing (1986) is against the use of L-shaped implants (implant is the term for only alloplastic materials) or L-shaped grafts because he fears breathing impairment by the thickness of the implant or graft. It is obvious that they have to be sculptured very narrowly. In our opinion if a surgeon has poor results in correcting septum and columella in cases of Binder's syndrome or saddle noses following septal abscess, it is only because he or she has not the courage to use enough augmentation material. In those cases cosmetic improvement is at the same time a functional one. We have to be able to manage a septocolumellar correction as well as a septocolumellar reconstruction (see Chapter 14) with the appropriate material.

The most common polyamide mesh in use is well stabilized with fibrous connective tissue ingrowth; however, black dust-like particles are incorporated into histiocytes and giant cells around the implants. Polyamide mesh implants have been used by Beekhuis (1974) in the nasal dorsum in more than 150 patients for many years, apparently giving very gratifying results. The advantage of this filler material seems to be in its minimal foreign body reaction, good tensile strenth, elasticity, flexibility, and no observed long-term rejection phenomena. However, due to a felt-like ingrowth of subcutaneous tissue, the mesh is so firmly united to the skin that extraction, which might become necessary, results in defects of the covering skin. The disadvantage is that once infected, the removal of the implant is difficult due to the fibrous ingrowth. The author does not recommend the use of polyamide mesh as a filler in the columella or nasolabial angle or in the nasal lobule. If there is a loss of nasal tip projection and support and there is insufficient material available, the author resorts to the insertion of a Silastic (silicone) alar-columellar prosthesis. Berman (1975, 1980) also used polyamide mesh, but not in secondary procedures. T. Smith (1978) has abandoned this material in the correction of saddle noses.

Another common material that is available in block or preformed shapes is also well tolerated: Polytetrafluoroethylene-carbon (Proplast) stimulates an intense histiocytic and giant-cell reaction. Proplast I (black) is made of carbonized Teflon® and is very easy to carve with the knife. In contrast, the Proplast II (white), is an aluminum oxide-coated Teflon®, requiring multiple blade changes while carving because of the dulling effect of the aluminum oxide on blade sharpness. It is best used in reconstituting a simple nasal dorsal shape. Proplast must be sterilized with a slow wet steam (autoclave at 250 degrees) for 30 minutes. It should also be impregnated with antibiotic saline solution. Porous polyethylene (Plastic-Pore) implants induce only a mild response from histiocytes and giant cells.

Despite a continuous search, the ideal alloplastic material is still a sought-after objective. Today materials are either too fragile and of insufficient elasticity or too soft to serve as supporting structures. When using an alloplastic implant, the most common complication is infection. It must, therefore, be washed with an antibiotic solution before use. Usually infection is followed by extrusion. Lemperle (1985) reports a complication rate of about 22.9 percent. If extrusion occurs, it is sometimes very difficult and complicated to repair the loss of tissue produced, more complicated than for a secondary correction after bone or cartilage extrusion.

Only in limited cases of severely damaged and scarred nasal dorsum, does Hellmich (1983) use a silicone sponge to fill depressions, dimples, and furrows, cases in which we prefer to achieve correction with cartilage or fascia grafts or with collagen injection. Although silicone implants were very popular at one time, it is less so now because of the frequency of complications.

Nevertheless, silicone is actually the most common implant used in Eastern countries. Brown and McDowell were already using in 1965 a considerable number of silicone rubber nasal implants and had trouble with very few of them, fewer than they had with bone and cartilage. McDowell (1952, 1978) felt that many surgeons did not have the adequate experience in all the pitfalls of nasal augmentation and made mistakes, creating more trouble with synthetic implants than one would get with bone or autogenous cartilage. In his hands, implants were more prone to extrusion in the presence of scarring and mucosal deficits.

Regnault, reviewing in 1980 her 15 year experience with silicone implants, concluded that applying this concept has proven to be safer in reconstructive rhinoplasty than any other approaches. She has totally replaced bone or cartilage grafting in augmentation surgery with silicone implants. Silastic, medical-grade silicone rubber can be autoclaved without changing its physical properties and can be quickly adjusted by trimming.

In Japan, according to Shioya (1984), there is a very low rate of complications after silicone implant rhinoplasty. More problems and complications do arise from silicone injections. The following problems are connected with secondary rhinoplasty using silicone implants in Japan: displacement of the implant, improper size or shape, extrusion, a necessity for reduction of other structures of the nose, and a need to correct the nasolabial angle.

Shirakabe et al (1985) consider that since a Roman nose typifies a beautiful face in Japan, augmentation rhinoplasty represents an important interest for Japanese surgeons, encouraging them to develop methods using implants that generally lead to satisfactory results. In the multitude of operations performed also by inexperienced aesthetic surgeons, knowing nothing more than how to put an implant in a patient's nose, it is inevitable that some complications can and do arise. Many of the hard silicone implants pierce the skin easily and have to be removed. Shirakabe (1981) developed softer silicone-rubber prostheses, which can be adjusted by trimming. The authors classified the complications resulting from alloplastic augmentation rhinoplasty in Orientals into 6 types, according to the nasal area involved: type 1—involving the entire outer surface of the nose; type 2—involving the nasal root as a result of skin necrosis and perforation; type 3—dorsal depression due to a broken prosthesis; type 4—involving only the tip with localized congestion causing extrusion (see Fig. 112); type 5—in which inflammation of the columella leads to perforation through the surgical midcolumellar scar; and type 6—with extrusion of L-shaped implants at the columellar base cased by infection.

In Furukawa's (1974, 1984) augmentation rhinoplasties, 5–10 percent of postoperative deformities seen occurred with silicone dorsal implants. He uses a silicone prosthesis as an additional onlay over the nasal spine. His complications arise from the inadequate preparation and insertion of the implants. Reoperating with the placement of a newly prepared prosthesis following an adequate interval after the removal of the first one usually gives good results in his hands. If implant irritation of the surrounding tissue of the nose is observed, it is necessary to remove the implant as soon as possible. It then must be decided whether to give up the augmentation or to change the material, using an autograft.

Shioya (1984) employs the following methods for such secondary rhinoplasties: removal of the implant and replacement with another silicone implant, removal of implant and replacement with bone graft, and implementing ancillary procedures such as reduction of other parts of the nose. Lee (1983), from Singapore, is using similar prostheses and calls his operation "dynamic implant," stressing the importance of lateral flexibility. In Japan silicone augmentation is considered a relatively safe maneuver for routine augmentation rhinoplasty only if the surgeon knows its limitations. Thus, silicone implants should not be used in heavily scarred cases, especially those with a history of previous infections or fracture. If the previous operation was a simple aesthetic rhinoplasty using a silicone implant and the secondary rhinoplasty is for revision of shape, size, or displacement if the patient did not have infection, then implant removal with immediate silicone replacement is feasible. If the cause of the failure is an unstable recipient bed because of previous fracture or infection, bone grafting should be carried out as a secondary procedure.

When another correction is requested, such as remodeling of the tip or ala, the silicone implant can be left in place or eventually simultaneously replaced with a new one. If the patient needs a lateral osteotomy, the silicone implant should be removed and the osteotomy carried out followed by delayed bone grafting or silicone reimplantation.

Bull (1981, 1983, 1984) reports good results obtained with silastic material when the implant is inserted via a midline vertical columellar incision, and not via an intranasal or intraoral approach. There is much controversy as to whether silastic can be successfully used to correct saddle deformities of the nose. Some surgeons claim few problems with silastic while the experience of others is contrary to this. Silastic and other so-called inert artificial implants are, at best, successful only when inserted into a relatively unscarred recipient bed in which little or no overlying skin tension exists.

Silastic implants have the advantage of being readily available and are not associated with a painful donor site. But there is still the reputed high rate of infection and extrusion. Milward (1972) reviewed 76 cases in which silastic implants had been used, 27 of which were unsatisfactory. He did note, however, that no complications arose in 9 patients in whom silastic had been used to correct a submucosal resection deformity and in which the implant was inserted via a midline columellar incision. Rozner (1980) described 22 cases in which silastic implants were used and only 2 were lost because of extrusion, while Marvin (1980) reported 24 cases in which an "L-shaped" strut of silastic was used via a midline columellar incision with no cases of extrusion. MacKay and Bull (1981) have reviewed the fate of silastic implants used over the 10-year period from 1970 to 1980. Of 87 cases, the result was unfavorable in 12 (13.8 percent). The infection rate as reported by McKay and Bull corresponds to the rate seen with other kinds of silastic materials.

We have also observed unsatisfactory results after performing silastic nasal augmentation used only in Oriental patients, since they were accustomed to hearing about this procedure as it is popular in their country. Using implants carved from a medium-grade silastic block we have also seen infections or cases where the implant has been unstable.

Tricalciumphosphate ceramic has been used by Walter (1982) and Gammert (1984) as a bioactive implant in facial surgery and especially in nasal augmentation. Resorption of this material is variable, especially in soft tissue. Where there was broad contact of the implant with bony structures, strong fixation resulted by 4–6 weeks. No notable complications occurred.

Ferrari (1985) introduced the use of calcium hydroxyapatite for augmentation of the nasal dorsum and columella, as well as for cases of nasomaxillary retrusion in combination with fibrin adhesive glue.

In conclusion we agree with Steiss (1961) and Hellmich (1979) who state that the most common cause of complications after nasal augmentation with alloplastic material is actually an improper preoperative estimation of the risks of this kind of surgery. The analysis of the quality and quantity of the skin and mucous membrane forming the implant bed and covering the implant is one of the main problems. If the carefully established preoperative assessment of risks proves to be unfavorable, one should refrain from placing an implant and look for another way to correct a saddle nose with autogenous grafts. Summarily, in noses with atrophic thin skin or with scarred skin and subcutaneous tissue, and alloplastic implantation will generally lead to necrosis. The skin that has to be mobilized must be sufficient to cover the new volume of the nose after insertion of an implant, otherwise ischemia and subsequent necrosis occur.

THE NON-CAUCASIAN NOSE

Between black Africans and white Caucasians we find all grades of nasal characteristics with a melange in the brown nose. Rogers (1974) distinguished three basic racial nose types: the Caucasoid (white), Mongoloid (Oriental), and Negroid (black or African) nose. According to Farkas et al. (1986) the Negroid type is related to the nose of blacks and individuals of mixed African-Asian and/or Caucasian origin (e.g., the Latin American or Mestizo nose, the Brazilian Negroid nose, and the Caribbean "Chapta" nose). Like Caucasians, blacks and Orientals show many qualitative and quantitative differences in their noses. Compared with the Caucasoid nose, the characteristics of the Negroid nose are described as follows: shortness and flatness, wide and flat dorsum, wide and bulbous tip, flared and thick alae, short and wide columella, enlarged round and horizontally ovoid nostrils, obtuse nasofrontal angle, and acute nasolabial angle. A moderate amount of alar flare and moderately increased alar width is seen in Hispanic-mestizo, Asian, and Polynesian, as well as Negroid American.

The variations go from a saddle nose to a hump nose. The most frequently seen form in all non-Caucasian noses is the flat dorsum with broad base in a nose of poor bony and cartilaginous support. Maximal flare is encountered in the black African race, with no flare at all in the Caucasian. Flare can be defined as the extreme bow of the ala extending lateral to the alar attachment to the cheek. According to Matthews (1968) and Broadbent, the ideal nasal alignment in Caucasians is that lying within longitudinal lines drawn through the inner canthus. Corrections of flat non-Caucasian noses are more and more in demand in America, the Orient, and in black people in Europe, due to a trend where the ideal image of beauty is represented in the Caucasian-type nose. Common desires of non-Caucasian patients include narrowing the base of the nose, elevating the dorsum with a diminishing of the flare of the nares, reducing the thickness of the alae, adding more projection to the tip, and correcting the retracted nasolabial angle. The mestizo nose of Latino-American people has peculiar features. Framed by a wide face, the mestizo nose is relatively small. The dorsum is slightly convex with a minimal osteocartilaginous hump arising below the frontonasal groove. The base is wide, especially when compared with the limited forward projection of the tip. The nostrils are moderately large with a tendency toward horizontalization produced by the short columella and the wide nasal base. The nasolabial angle is small as a result of the prominence of the dental arches in front of the nasal spine and the downward projection of the nasal tip. The alar cartilages form a wide dome; the medial crura are not long and rarely prominent in the columella. This, associated with a short membranous septum, accounts for the fact that the columella may not protrude below the alar rim on the profile view. The nasal skin is moderately thick. The most striking feature is the presence of a layer of subcutaneous fat tissue covering the prominence of the osteocartilaginous framework, therefore adding to the general impression of thickness.

The usual correction of the non-Caucasian nose is provided by:

1. Narrowing the long and cartilaginous pyramid.
2. Narrowing of the base of the nose with interalar reduction.
3. Thinning of the alar cartilages.
4. Reverse V-Y plasty at the base of the columella with mediocolumella and transcolumellar mattress sutures according to Cronin (1958, 1983) and Avelar (1976, 1985).
5. Insertion of a septocolumellar support with augmentation of the retracted columella.
6. Narrowing of the lobule by marginal resection.
7. Insertion of a retrolabial cartilage or bone graft for correction of the nasolabial angle.
8. Marginal resection of the alae.

To conform with the current occidental standard of beauty, the objectives of the operation in the mestizo nose are about the same as those in a common non-Caucasian nose, with the addition of a few peculiar details, such as increasing of nasal protrusion. To decrease the width of the nasal base, wedge resections are performed on the nostril floor. As suggested by Falces (1970), it is convenient to resect the ala where it forms an angle with the facial skin, thus reducing the extra width produced in the lateral flaring. When reducing the flare of the nostril with basal Weir-resections, it is important that the resected strip of skin inside the vestibule be broader than the one at the outer surface of the alar base.

We find that to provide for the tip projection in the non-Caucasian nose, the same technical problems exist as in the bilateral cleft lip nose. The reverse V-Y plasty at the base of the nose as advocated by Cronin (1958, 1983) for the bilateral hare lip nose has been adapted by Avelar (1976, 1985) to the non-Caucasian nose for gaining tip projection, columellar length, and for correcting the transverse position of the nostrils into a more perpendicular oval (Fig. 113). In our experience this procedure is also very useful for reducing the alar flare and interalar distance without need of wedge resections at the sill and vestibular floor.

The overly sharp nasolabial angle becomes wider through projection with a retrolabial graft of cartilage from the septum, ear, or iliac bone (see Fig. 177). These grafts are inserted through the horizontal incision in front of the columellar base and vestibular threshold, which can also be the access for reinforcing the columella with cartilage (Fig. 113). It is particularly important to shape the columella and form the previously nonexistent double-angle in profile by inserting struts of alar or septal cartilage at the adequate level, the lobulo-columellar junction.

The continuity of the alar cartilage arch is left intact. However, if we have to narrow the base of the nares by additional alar base resections of Weir, we prefer to eliminate the spring of the cartilaginous arch by cutting through the lateral crura at the dome (see Fig. 57).

In the majority of non-Caucasian noses we perform a marginal resection of the nostrils, particularly in the lateral half of the border. When the sill is high we can combine its reduction (see Chapter 15) with a bilateral alar base rotation towards the columellar base, as described by Millard (1980). With regards to the correction of the dorsal saddling and flatness, we refer to the section on saddle nose.

One of the most important questions in converting a non-Caucasian nose into a Caucasian-like nose is to what degree should we attempt to change the features. Our opinion is to avoid an overcorrection, which can be the cause of unsatisfactory results.

According to Matory and Falces (1986), complications most peculiar to non-Caucasian rhinoplasty are (1) prolonged edema, (2) excess scarring, (3) racial incongruity, and (4) asymmetry. In our experience we have noted no special postoperative problems concerning prolonged edema as compared with those of Caucasian patients. The only scars we produced in these noses are at the nasolabial junction, the alar base, and the alar border. All of these have been minimal. In the non-Caucasian nose we would not perform any midcolumellar or transcolumellar incisions fearing that they could be more conspicuous than in Caucasian patients. We have not observed racial incongruity to the ethnic makeup of the patients nor disproportionate width of the upper bony skeleton and the lower cartilaginous framework. Neither did we have to perform any revisions for significant asymmetry.

Oriental Nose

The Orientals are the mesorrhines and the average breadth of their noses is intermediate between the Caucasian (leptorrhines) and the Negroid (plathyrrhines nose). In anthropology the length of the nose is the distance between the root and the naso-labial angle. The breadth is the distance between the two maximum points of the convexity of the alae. The nasal index is obtained by multiplying the breadth of the nose by 100 and then dividing the product by the length. The index indicates the form of the nose and varies from 40 to 120 according to the race of the individual. Thus, among the plathyrhinies the normal index exceeds 85, among the leptorrhines it is below 70, and among the mesorrhines it is between 70 and 85. Besides the plathyrrhinia and moderate flare, another characteristic of the Oriental nose is the short columella and the low alar rim. Rogers (1974) found that the Oriental nose differs from the Negroid nose as follows:

(1) nasal root width: smaller
(2) nasal root depth: shallower
(3) nasal bridge contour: concave
(4) nasal bridge inclination: smaller
(5) dorsum: narrower
(6) nasal tip: not bulbous
(7) tip protrusion: smaller
(8) nostril size: moderately wide
(9) alae: less flaring and thinner

According to Furukawa (1974, 1983), a variant medial crus of the lower lateral cartilage is sometimes found in an Omega shape, instead of being a slight curve. Considering the feature of the Oriental nose, the correction would include (1) dorsal augmentation with a graft or implant, (2) modification of the naso-labial angle with an onlay graft or silicone implant, or by sectioning the depressor septi muscle (Furukawa [1967]), and (3) decreasing the flare by medial displacement of the alar-fascial groove without any scarring in the groove itself, excising only an internal vestibular wedge of the alar base (Furukawa [1983]).

14

Residual Deformities of the Inner Part of the Nose

SEPTORHINOPLASTY

Septorhinoplasty is an operation that endeavors to improve both function and appearance of the nose. In 1905, Killian described the submucous resection operation in which, through an incision about 1 cm posterior and parallel to the caudal margin of the quadrilateral cartilage, a mucoperichondrial flap could be developed and preserved while still exposing the underlying septal anatomy. At approximately the same time, Freer (1902) described a similar approach, one in which the incision was made over the anterior leading edge of the septal cartilage at its junction with the membranous septum, again allowing dissection in the submucosal plane to reach and permit resection of deviations. Neither Freer's nor Killian's procedure, however, adequately dealt with the dorsal or caudal aspects of the often simultaneously deformed quadrilateral cartilage. These techniques, however, developed into and became known as the "classic" submucous resection operation, which, while preserving the intranasal mucosa, was limited to dealing with deformities localized in the central region of the septum.

Metzenbaum, in 1929, addressed the issue of the obstructing caudal septal "spur" by proposing the "swinging door" technique in which the caudal margin of the quadrilateral cartilage, if dislocated, subluxed, or overlapping onto the premaxilla, was trimmed at this junction to allow for the repositioning of the remaining septum into the midline. Subsequently, other techniques were described for dealing with deformities of both aspects of the dorsal-caudal strut fashioned during the "classic" submucous resection procedure, and altogether these developed into the general approach termed *septoplasty.* This technique then principally refers to the surgical repair and reconstitution of the dorsal-caudal aspect of the quadrilateral cartilage and of its junction with the premaxillary-maxillary-vomerine crest. From a primary dependence resting upon cartilage excision in the submucous resection procedure, the emphasis in septoplasty has shifted to the functional and cosmetic reconstitution of the septum while maintaining its structural integrity.

The septorhinoplasty is based on the principle that the entire nasal pyramid can be supported without risk of dorsal collapse by a minimal cartilaginous infrastructure. All one has to leave is an L-shaped osteocartilaginous strut of the upper and anterior part of the septum. If the upper ridge is crooked in an S-shaped and the lower edge protrudes into the nasal cavity, the whole osteocartilaginous septum can be removed in one piece (Planas, 1964) and replaced by strips of cartilage obtained from the resected septum itself. This new septum composed of cartilaginous strips is sufficient to support both the dorsum and the columella.

The majority of individuals with a distorted septum do not have airway obstruction, at least not subjectively. If these deviations appear before or during the operation, they have to be corrected to improve the nasal airway in these patients, who have no symptoms of obstruction but who are likely to get them postoperatively, or at a later age. For this reason it is important that young plastic surgeons develop skills in performing septal surgery.

Impaired nasal breathing is the reason for this operation. The prevention of a growth deformity can also be an indication for surgery (Huizing, 1966). Adolescents with a nasal deformity report that their nasal malformations developed very gradually. Thus, a slight septal deviation in childhood becomes increasingly deviated with growth, until adolescence. Since the septum determines the growth of the nose in its vertical and ventrodorsal dimensions, we can understand how a septal trauma in a child can influence further nasal growth. Fresh fractures, septal hematomas, and abscesses in children are also indications for surgery.

Septal surgery in children should be directed toward the respositioning of dislocated parts and should be as conservative as possible. Resections should be avoided unless they are required for proper repositioning (Huizing, 1966).

The operation should be restricted as much as possible to the cartilaginous septum in which the functional problems are mostly located. In extreme cases of fracture with bony deviations and hare lip noses, bony spurs and spines have to be corrected. Only small bony deviations are not to be repositioned.

Mosher (1971) had postulated two centers of growth found in the human septal cartilage after the age of 8, one to be just above the premaxillary wings and a second half way up its posterior border. Other authors state that a real center of growth is not known. The nasal skeleton is composed of 24 cartilaginous and bony elements, with full growth achieved by the end of puberty. Synchondroses and bony cartilaginous sutures are areas of varying growth potential. Chondrocyte activity in the quadrangular plate has been particularly detected, especially during different growth spurts until approximately age 16. Between the 20th and 35th year this activity slowly decreases, but in the supramaxillary region the septum continues to show some growing activity so that in this period the tip can become more protrusive.

According to Willemot and Pirsig (1984), septoplasty must preserve three zones, the anterior edge of the septum and suprapremaxillary region, and the central area. Vetter et al (1984) distinguished five different areas of growth in human septal cartilage from biopsies obtained during septoplasty. They are the anterior free edge of the septum, the supramaxillary area, the central area, the posterior area, and the caudal prolongation.

Vetter, Pirsig, and Heinze (1984) observed that regeneration of septal cartilage after septoplasty in late childhood may take place during puberty at the anterior border of the septal cartilage by appositional and interstitial growth. They showed that the anterior free end of the septum displays growth activity throughout life. Results of the studies of Vetter, Pirsig, and Heinze (1984) concluded that in the growing nose, the cartilaginous growth potential can be destroyed by resecting cartilage from the anterior free edge, from the central area, and from the suprapremaxillary area of the septum. Metabolic activity and proliferative capacity are highest in all areas during childhood. They decline with age but remain surprisingly high in the central area and in the anterior free edge, even in adults. The supramaxillary area displays its highest growth activity during prepuberty, undergoing thereafter a continuous decline during puberty and adulthood. A similar age dependent pattern in growth is found in the caudal prolongation of the septal cartilage. No age dependent variations could be detected in the posterior area of the septal cartilage. These findings may help the rhinosurgeon in making decisions about whether and where to resect or incise the septal cartilage in children.

Radical septal resection, according to Killian (1905) and Freer (1902), removes the central area of the septal cartilage, thus depriving the septum of one of its main generative centers in adulthood. In the adult, the resection of the anterior free border of the septal cartilage is advisable, together with other techniques, if one plans a nasal reduction.

Pirsig (1977) considers a septal intervention in the first 2 years of life dangerous. According to studies of this author (1977) there is no arrest of nasal growth after septoplasty and osteotomies if done later than 2 years.

Krieg (1900), Freer (1902), and Killian (1905) were among the first to perform septal surgery in children. The disadvantages of submucous septal resection, however, resulted in septal surgery in children being postponed until the age of 16. After Metzenbaum's description of a more conservative technique (1929), septal surgery in children was increasingly practiced.

Based on observations of a few children, Jennes (1964) demonstrated that no inhibition of nasal growth could be demonstrated some 8 years after septoplasty. His clinical observations have been supported by others such as Cottle (1939), Gray (1965), Huizing (1966), Farrior (1970), Masing (1971), and Pirsig et al (1974).

When nasal injury occurs in early childhood, cartilaginous regeneration may arise from the small torn pieces of perichondrium (Pirsig, 1979). Histologic examination has revealed cartilaginous regeneration at the borders of resected septal cartilage in cases in which a secondary rhinoplasty was necessary because of recurrent nasal obstruction. The regeneration of cartilage mainly arises from the perichondrium. When creating small cartilaginous defects during septoplasty it is important to preserve as much perichondrium as possible, to assure, to a certain extent, cartilaginous regeneration during the growth of the septum (Pirsig and Lehmann, 1975). In their experience, a secondary deviation in children after incomplete or imperfect primary septoplasty occurred in approximately 11 percent of cases needing a secondary intervention. The deviation is the result of histologically-proven undirectional growth of the septal cartilage due to unilateral dissection of the mucoperichondrium from the septal cartilage and to an incomplete sectioning of the septal cartilage. This is the reason why septoplasty in children is a most delicate procedure demanding some experience.

As previously mentioned, we perform more septorhinoplasties than simple rhinoplasties, especially as secondary procedures. We proceed to the correction of the septum at the beginning of the operation after separation of the stable part of the nose from the mobile part through the transfixion and intercartilaginous incisions. The transfixion incision is carried along the crest of the protruding caudal edge of the septal cartilage. Most of the members of the Academy of Facial Plastic Surgery prefer the hemitransfixion incision of Cottle (1960), while the majority of plastic surgeons use the transfixion incision. Kamer and Churukian (1984) advocate using a high septal hemitransfixion incision over the convexity of a caudal septal deflection with repositioning and fixation of the dislocated segment. They think that this access has superior versatility and reliability.

Through the transfixion incision we attend to the septum, beginning with hydrodissection, i.e. producing a swelling of the soft tissue at the caudal border of the septal cartilage by infiltration with saline solution containing epinephrine or POR (vasopressin) in order to facilitate the release of the mucoperichondrial borders. Using hydrodissection the subperichondrial dissection plane is easier to find with knife and elevator. This is especially important in secondary procedures where fibrous adhesions may be found in this area. The key to visualization, hemostasis, and the avoidance of mucosal tears, is to be in the right dissection plane. Often there is still one thin, almost invisible, perichondrial layer to get under before one is truly subperichondrial.

We now introduce a Nr 15 blade perpendicular to the cartilaginous surface and develop the perichondrial flap with a fine sharp elevator. If we are too superficial and do not recognize the grayish-blue surface of the cartilage, we again incise the perichondrium to develop the correct subperichondrial pocket. In secondary interventions this can be extremely laborious.

Then, we first dissect the convex obstructing side, beginning in the supero-anterior area near the origin of the upper lateral cartilage, lifting the mucoperichondrium from the cartilage and pushing it downward. We dissect all the way down over the convex midcartilaginous and inferior part of the septum. During dissection, one can feel the passage from the subperichondrial to the subperiosteal plane of the ethmoid plate and of the vomer. If we discover scar tissue in the basal junction, we find it best to continue the elevation carefully from the back, leaving, if necessary, a fine strip of cartilage and fibrous tissue attached to the dissected flap.

Many of the rhinoplastic surgeons with ENT background create tunnels, as described by Cottle (1953), one below the junction and one above. Elevating the mucoperichondrium to the roof of the nose and as far posteriorly as possible, Gorney (1984) also avoids dissecting directly over the septovomerine ridge. He then dissects an inferior pocket and the two spaces are then gradually joined from back to front. We prefer to form a single extended pocket on both sides, passing the elevator directly over the junction. We then proceed with the dissection of the concave, nonobstructing side, creating again a complete subperichondrial and subperiosteal pocket from the vault down to the floor of the concavity.

If an oblique facet of the anterior septum is present and touches the lateral wall of the nasal cavity or a turbinate, we proceed stepwise with maximal care. The summit of a very sharp angulation in the septum is always the limit of an easy dissection. At this point, we can remove a strip of cartilage and then, through the gap, we transsect the base, leaving the summit attached to one of the mucoperichondrial flaps. The elevation is then continued in the usual fashion.

Comminution and overlap of fractured cartilage occasionally causes the dissection plane to run out in the fibrous tissue at the fracture line. The dissection can proceed from above or below, allowing the cartilage to be bared from a different direction than from the front. We then extend the dissection to the vomerine crest and to the bony part of the septum. We know that the maxillary crest and vomer stay in a separate compartment from the septal cartilage. Both are wrapped in a separate envelope (see Chapter 5).

We can enter the inferior bone-containing compartment through the inferior end of the transfixion incision in the region of the nasal spine. The maxillary and vomerine crests are widely flared. By approaching these crests from below we gain the exposure required for chiseling off the flared part of the crest. They are repositioned or removed. Thus, the whole premaxilla can be bared with an elevator if necessary. From here the mucoperiosteum is raised from the medial part of the floor of the nose reaching to the vomerine crest where the elevation is more difficult because of fibrous attachments of the mucoperiosteum and mucoperichondrium. At their junction the dissection is easier posteriorly than in front and is sometimes best managed by coming at it in a retrograde fashion from the dissected layer first achieved posteriorly. The necessary exposure for the basal bony work is thus procured. Raising the mucoperiosteal flap, we transsect the connection between the flap and the incisive foramen, thus sectioning the sphenopalatine arteries, which run downward and forwards in the mucosa on their way to the incisive canal. This can result in some bleeding, occasionally necessitating cautious cauterization.

Any tears in the mucosa at the end of the operation require attention before closure. Small tears on only one side are not dangerous; they can prevent septal hematomas. Large tears can be closed by advancement of the mucosa from the nasal floor. Opposing tears cause perforations, vertical ones being worse than horizontal tears. In such cases we interpose pieces of cartilage, bone, or fascia from the temporal region, as we do in procedures for secondary septal perforation closure. For that reason it is best to dissect the convex side first. The dissection of the mucoperichondrium and the mucoperiosteum is completed on both sides posteriorly and inferiorly so that we can introduce a long speculum into the pockets. The base of the columella is detached, and the anterior nasal spine freed from the aponeurotic attachment of the fan shaped depressor septi muscle. In cases where we want to correct the nasolabial angle we cut through this depressor muscle (Fig. 114). When the spine is too prominent or extremely deviated, it is removed with a grasping forceps such as a

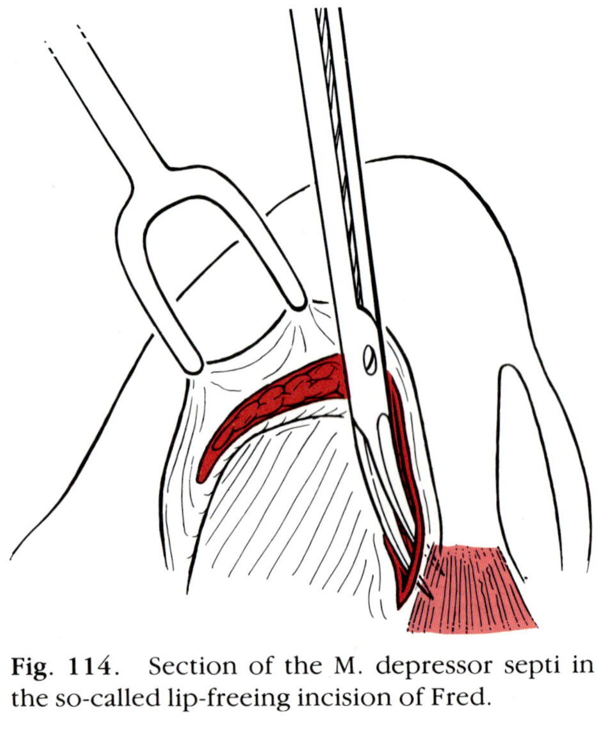

Fig. 114. Section of the M. depressor septi in the so-called lip-freeing incision of Fred.

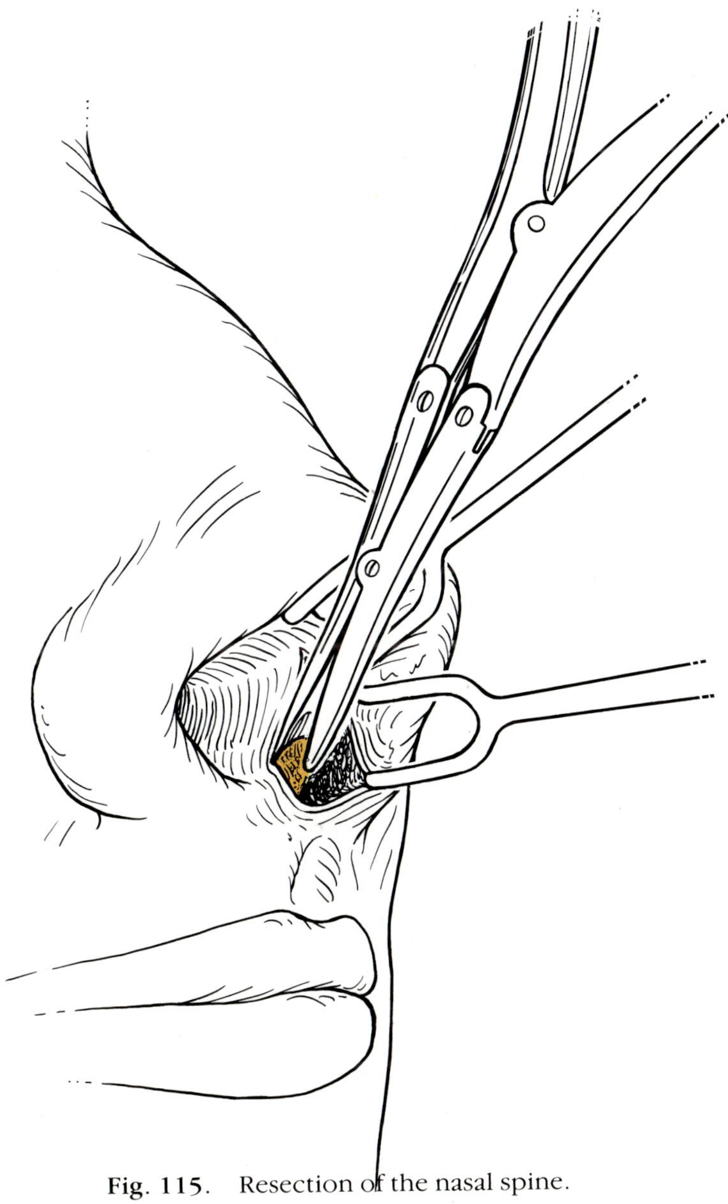

Levignac or a Luc forceps. In easier cases, it may be relocated in the midline with a fine osteotome (Fig. 115).

If the deviation reaches forward into the columella, presenting as a subluxation of the cartilaginous border at the anterior spine with retraction of the columella (Fig. 116 A and C), we choose the usual access through the transfixion incision and we carry out a wide bilateral dissection (Fig. 116). We remove or place into the midline the deviated basal crest of the vomer and resect a horizontal as well as one or two vertical strips of the quadrangular cartilage. Finally, we break or resect, if necessary, the lamina perpendicularis and insert several mattress sutures in order to hold the whole septal plate in a median position. With this, the columella is pushed forward eliminating the retraction (Fig. 116 B and E).

Fig. 115. Resection of the nasal spine.

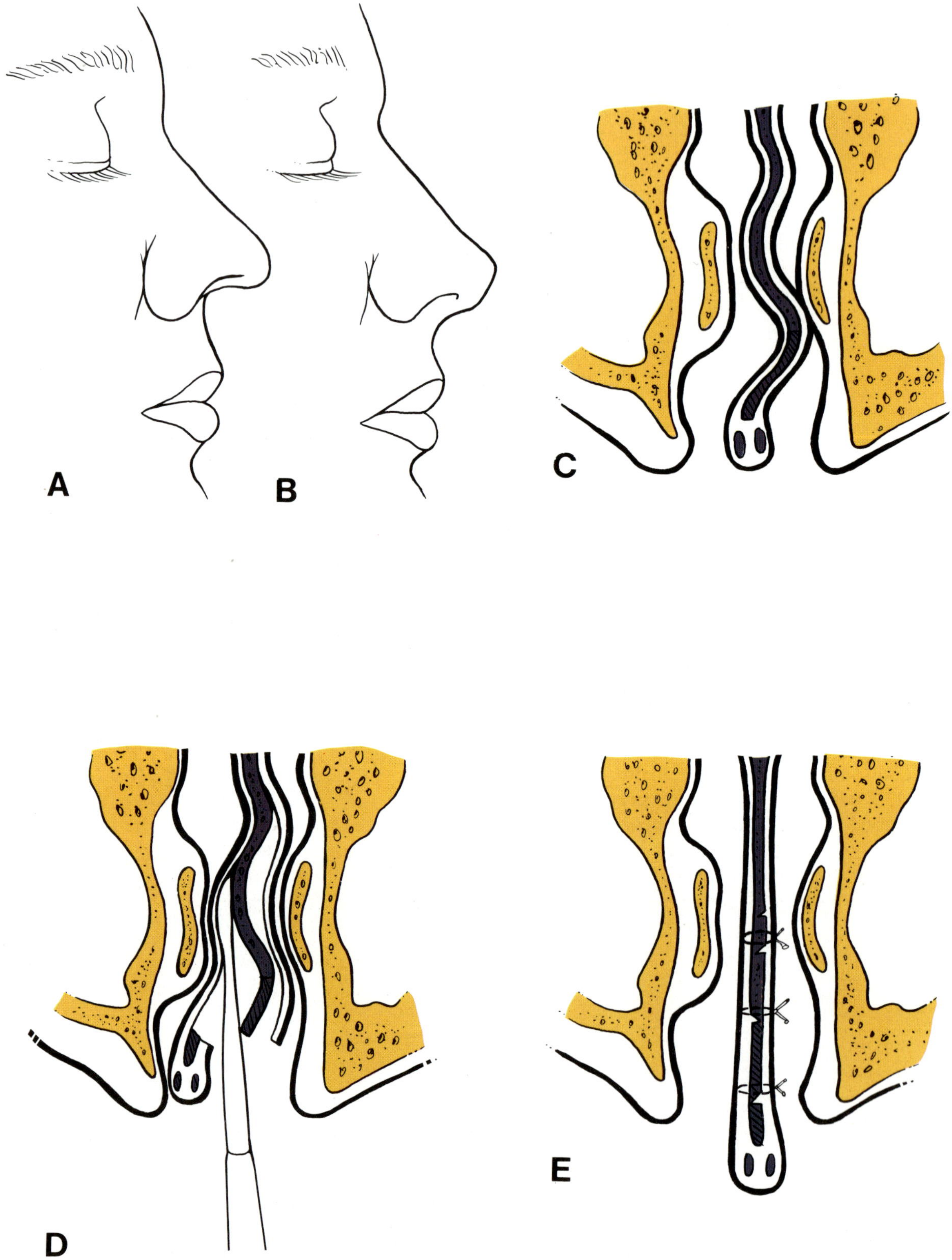

Fig. 116. A retraction of the columella (A) can be produced by a severe caudal anterior deviation of the septal cartilage (C). The wide dissection of mucoperichondrium and mucoperiosteum on both sides (D) and straightening with incision or if necessary with a swing-door method as well as with mattress sutures pushes forward the columella, thus eliminating the retraction (E and B).

In cases of subluxation of the septum at the caudal edge we can obtain the swinging-door effect of Metzenbaum (1936) and Seltzer (1944) with parallel vertical incisions. The whole vomer can be reset into the midline if protruding into the airway. If the vomer is deviated toward one side, creating with the septal cartilage a sharp S deformity in cross section, it may be resected. It is usually sufficient to move the vomer into its proper position and to remove a basal strip of cartilage (about 3 mm wide) where it overlaps with the vomer (Fig. 117A). This overriding inferior septal cartilage protruding into the airway with or without deviation of the vomerine groove is the most frequent septal deformity and can occur in various shapes and combinations.

When we remove the lower end of the septal cartilage, which is bent to one side out of the bony spur of the vomer, we create a gap between the two parts of the septal wall. Once both are rearranged in the midline, the bony part

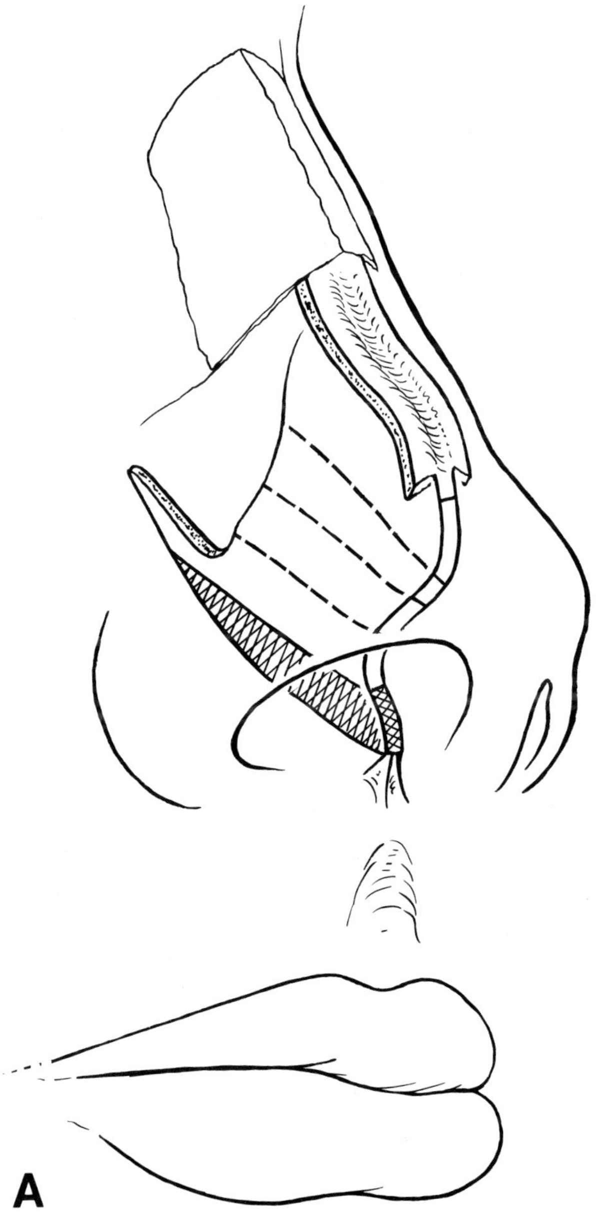

A

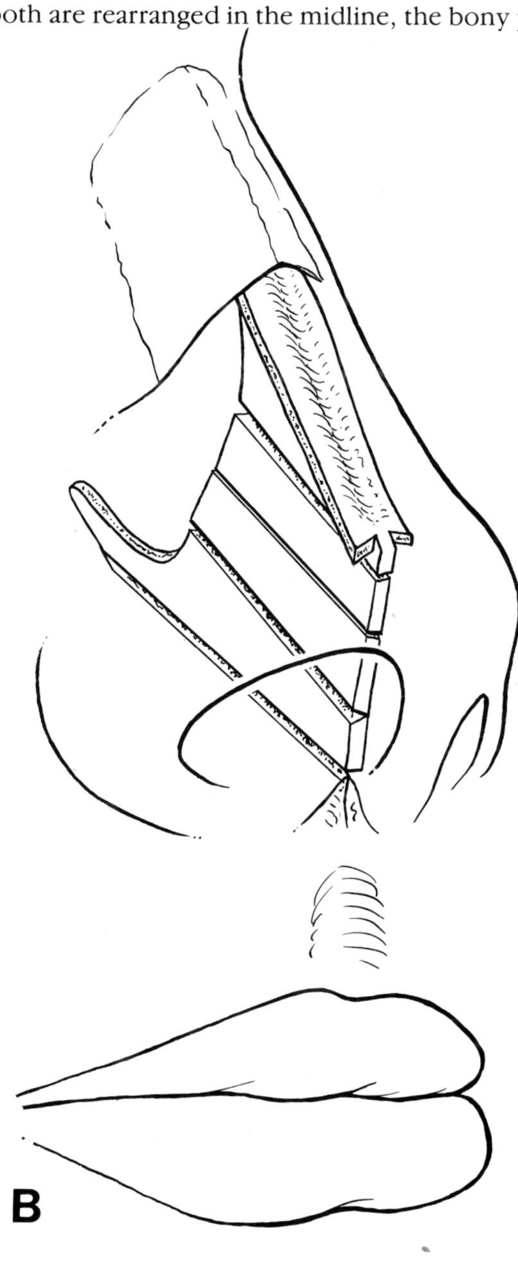

B

Fig. 117. In many cases a crooked nose is due to a deviation of the septal cartilage beginning at the junction with the vomer and contracting towards the roof with a C or S-shaped bending. The vomer is straight or also deviated. We usually resect a basal strip of cartilage (A), and eventually one between this and the root. The rest of the cartilage is scored or cross-hatched, repositioned (B) into the midline, and kept in this straight position by transseptal mattress sutures.

by repositioning and the cartilaginous by horizontal or vertical incisions (according to the shape of the deviation), the gap will be reduced to a slit (Fig. 117). The septum can be held in the midline by transseptal mattress sutures that include both mucoperichondrial leaves. By this resetting maneuver, the dorsum and the tip will be raised so that the dorsal line has to be reassessed. If there is an obstructing bulge in the septal cartilage or in the perpendicular plate of the ethmoid, this area is resected with a knife, angled scissors, or Craig rongeur while the mucoperichondrial and mucoperiosteal flaps are retracted with a long speculum (Fig. 118). For cutting strips of cartilage and bone we seldom use the Ballenger's swivel knife, and prefer the Craig forceps, which is used for the bony part as well as the cartilaginous resections.

Conservation of septal cartilage reduces intraseptal scar contraction to a minimum. Simple angulation of the central area can be flattened with excision of a strip at the site of the bend. The central area can be reduced to a number of islands or facets to allow flattening of the curved surface, as shown by Pearson and Goodmann (1973). All spring must be released to prevent recurrence of the septal deviation, as splints and plaster have no power in overcoming inadequate mobilization. We always check for a totally passive response to surgical displacement. Therefore, we sever the upper lateral cartilages at their insertion with the septum in all cases of septorhinoplasty, eliminating most of the attachments of the septum. Incisions, scoring, and cross-hatching on one side always produce a curvature of the cartilaginous septal plate to the opposite side.

We do not agree with the technique of Man (1981), who prefers to avoid routine elevation of the mucoperichondrium, making instead longi-

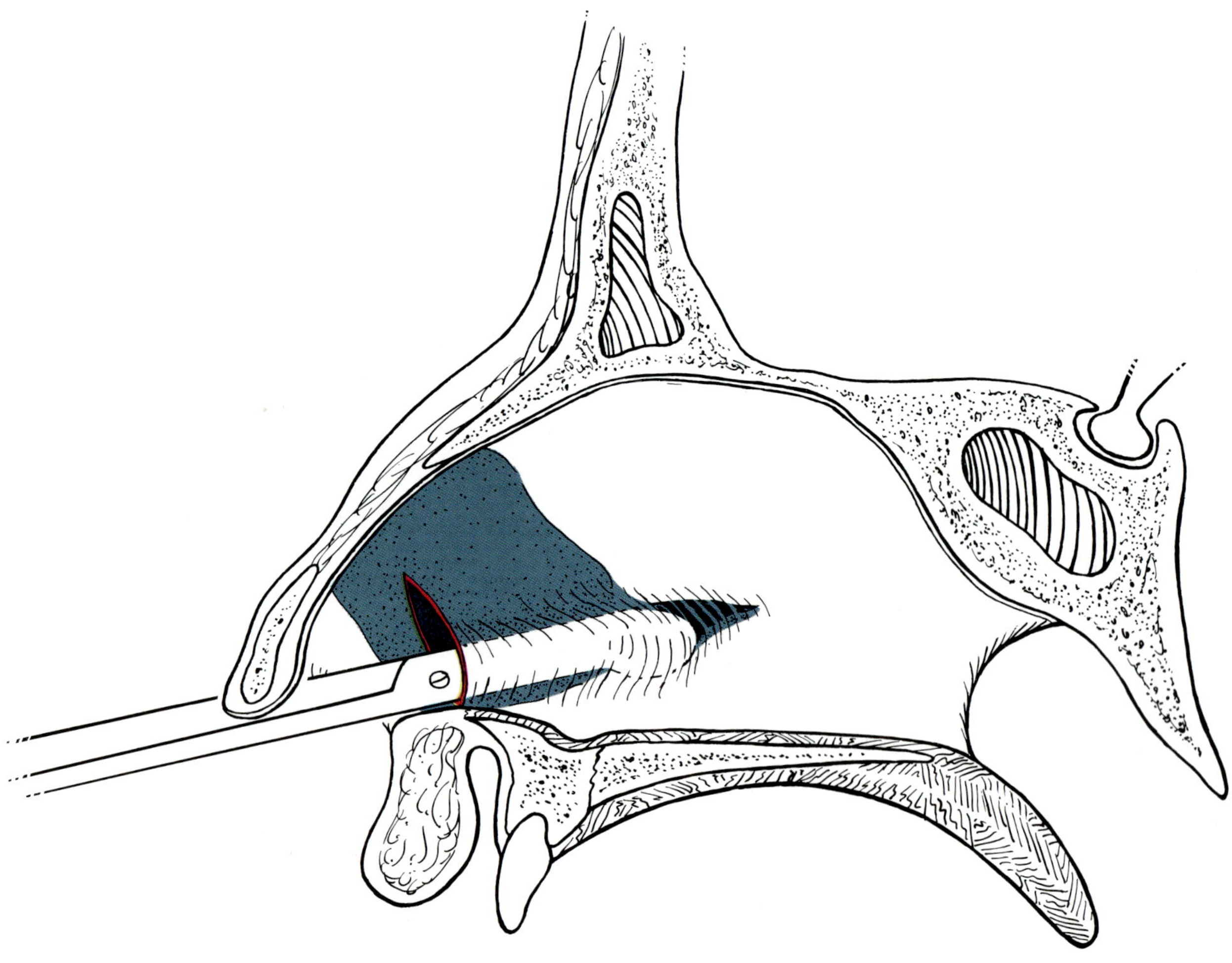

Fig. 118. The deviated vomer can be straightened with the Craig forceps. With the same instrument we can remove deviated portions of the perpendicular plate.

tudinal incisions through both the mucoperichondrium and cartilage over the most prominent part of the convex side of the deflection, leaving the mucoperichondrium on the concave side intact. Through one of these incisions he removes one or more cartilage strips without injuring the opposite mucous membrane. We believe incisions transsecting the septal mucoperichondrium completely on one side produces unnecessary bleeding. This technique also is certainly insufficient for huge deflections with angulations. In many cases the septal cartilage is displaced from its groove on the vomer and must be brought again into a median position. This is only possible with complete or at least partial dissection.

In some cases of secondary septorhinoplasty we find a defect in the cartilaginous and/or bony support of the septum when a more or less important amount of skeletal tissue has been removed in a primary operation. The extramucosal approach is particularly useful for the difficult dissection of either mucoperichondrium or the mucoperiosteum from each other and of the interstitial fibrous tissue at the site of cartilaginous and bony tissue. If one is able to achieve such a dissection, an interposition of a piece of cartilage, bone, or fascia at the weak site below the dorsal line could be advantageous. Occasionally in cases of revision septorhinoplasty where the anterior part of the septum is deprived of cartilage support, we transfer the perpendicular plate of the ethmoid bone to the caudal end of the septum, as Huizing (1984) does for primary cases. We glue the bony plate to the fibrous mucoperichondrial leaves on both sides. We would not recommend the replacement of septal cartilage by silicone sheeting as reported by some American authors (Patterson, 1966) and prefer, instead like Hellmich (1973), to place only cartilage, bone, or fascia between the elevated mucoperichondrial walls.

In dorsocolumellar deviations, the deviated support of the tip has to be centralized after partial resection of the quadrilateral plate. Separation of the columella from the nasal spine is sometimes sufficient to overcome the resistance. The remaining septum is then scored on its concave surface. If distortion persists, complete resection as advocated by Planas (1964) may be performed, removing the rest of the septal cartilage and reimplanting it as a free L-shaped graft. For that the whole osteocartilaginous plate can be cut off.

One must take care not to disturb the continuity of the remaining cartilage on the dorsal aspect of the nose with its ethmoid plate junction directly cephalad to it, particularly where they join, just below the nasal bones. Disturbances of this continuity can easily lead to a saddle nose with duck beak deformity, when healing and contracture occur. The resection of the central and lower parts of the septal cartilage should not extend to its upper border, leaving a strip at least 1 cm as a dorsal strut. If this is not present, a strip of cartilage harvested from the septal base has to be placed on both sides, or at least on one, at the end of the primary operation and, if necessary, fixed with mattress sutures in order to reinforce the dorsum and prevent bony saddling. We always recommend that novice surgeons reinforce the dorsal strip of cartilage with such appositions of cartilaginous struts immediately after an overzealous submucosal resection. In secondary cases, where there already is a slight dorsal depression present, we provide the same reinforcement with cartilage or bone. Dupont (1966), the first to describe such a dorsal reinforcement, used vomering bone. Planas (1964, 1977) advocated a strip of cartilage. Such appositions of cartilage with mattress suture fixation have also been described by Gornery (1976, 1984).

To prevent postoperative redeviation of the caudal third of the septum, Gorney (1976, 1984) also advocates the use of a straight batten taken from the septal cartilage and placed diagonally as a cross brace in the antero-superior corner of the septum and held in place with mattress sutures. In the event that the dorsal part of the support is curved or S-shaped, a bony piece from the vomer or the ethmoid is also used as a splint that can be fixed by transseptal mattress sutures, according to Dupont (1966).

Occasionally a traumatic, crushed septum may result in inadequate material to support the nose. A radical procedure of Planas (1977) can then be employed, and consists of a complete extirpation of the cartilaginous septum, the deviated portions of the vomer and ethmoidal plate, and inserting to support the anterior part of the nose a simple L-shaped bone graft from the iliac crest in the same shape as used for saddle nose correction. The insertion route is via the transfixion incision. Whenever possible, the supporting material should be harvested from either the cartilaginous or the bony part of the septum itself.

Maliniac advocated as early as 1948 the removal of the anterior dislocated septum and replacement of the fragment as a graft in the columella. Vilar-Sancho reported in 1984 a similar technique. Schuffenegger and Gubisch (1984) are also advocates of a total resection of the septum and reimplantation after having sutured plane pieces together, for cases of severe osteocartilaginous deformity.

We put some fibrinogen glue on both sides of the repositioned pieces of the septal plate and glue the mucoperichondrial and mucoperiosteal walls against it. In addition, we hold the whole straightened septum in the definitive position with transseptal mattress sutures (Fig. 119). Gammert (1985) makes a puzzle, gluing the pieces together to a plate with human biologic adhesive.

Rees (1986) is one of the first American surgeons to emphasize the importance of the extramucosal technique in such radical septoplasties involving resection and reinsertion of parts of the septum. This technique preserves the mucosal lining of the nose so that a sealed closure is possible, protecting the recipient sites and decreasing the risk of graft infection. The lining flap can be dropped like a curtain to the floor of the vestibule, providing access to the entire osteocartilaginous septum. As we do in severely twisted noses, Rees (1986) reinserts one or more struts of cartilage into the anterior part of the septum. These fragments of the quadrangular plate can be glued or sutured to each other. With the use of fibrin glue in nasal septal surgery, nasal packing can even be avoided or at least its use essentially shortened. This has also been confirmed by Wullstein (1979). As a result, she writes, nasal breathing is not interrupted and mucociliary clearance resumes at an early stage of healing. Staindl (1977) applied highly concentrated fibrinogen tissue adhesive for mucosa grafting at the septum in Osler's disease (Saunders plasty).

At the posterior choanal level, we occasionally find a staghorn-shaped part of the vomer that has to be extracted with the Craig forceps. Obstructing tilted deflected portions sometimes need to be removed with a straight or slightly curved chisel. An obstructing posterior segment of septum can be fractured and crushed to the midline by spreading the long speculum in the posterior cavity on both sides. In cases of excessive vomerine deformity, we remove the whole posterior portion without endangering septal support. In cases of persistent, prominent septal deformities involving the dorsal ridge of the septal cartilage, seen even after having sectioned the insertion of the upper lateral cartilage and removing a paramedian strip of this cartilage on both sides, one may perform 2–5 vertical incisions in this dorsal strip and align the cartilaginous portions in the midline (Fig. 119 D). For this purpose we sometimes use a Rubin's (1983) morselizer (Fig. 119 E). The straightened ridge may be reinforced with unilateral or bilateral apposition of cartilage taken from the inferior aspect of the septum. McCullough (1976) performs this ridge morselization through the Rethi incision as we also do (Fig. 119 E and F).

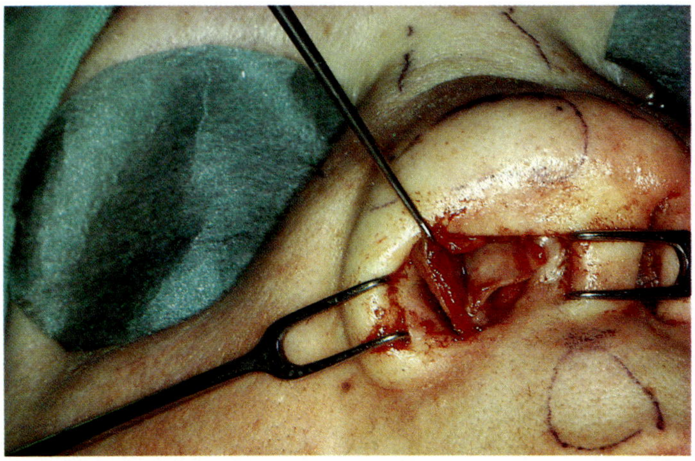

A

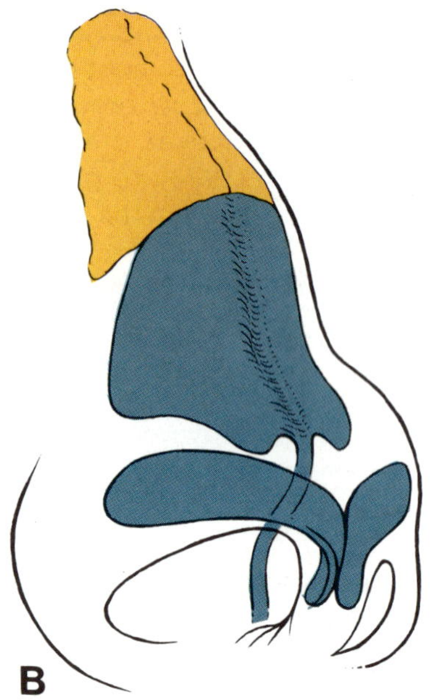

B

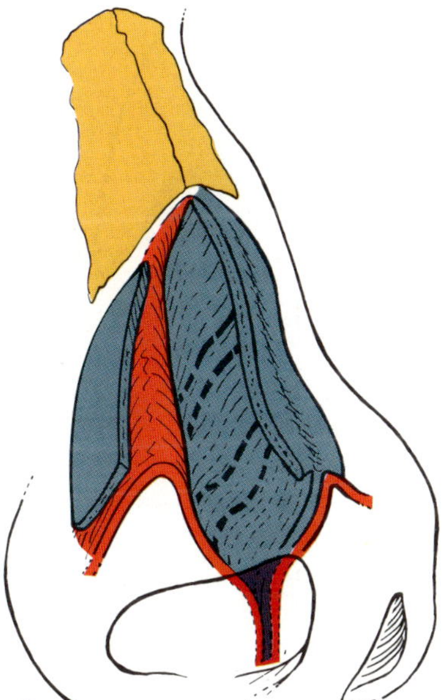

C

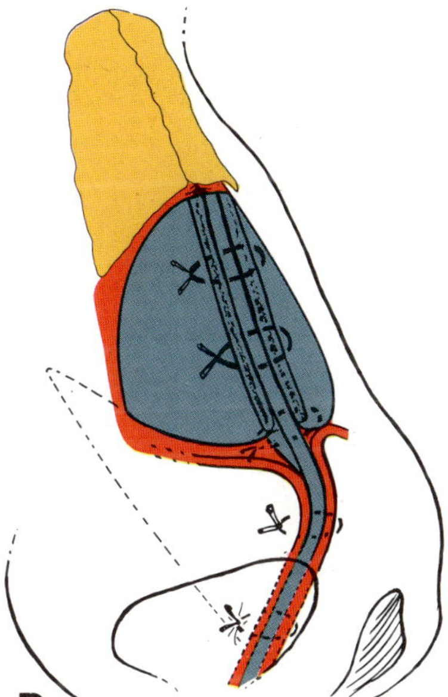

D

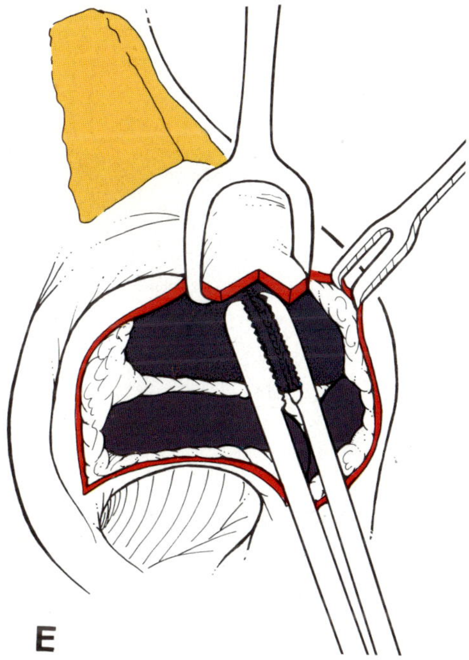

E

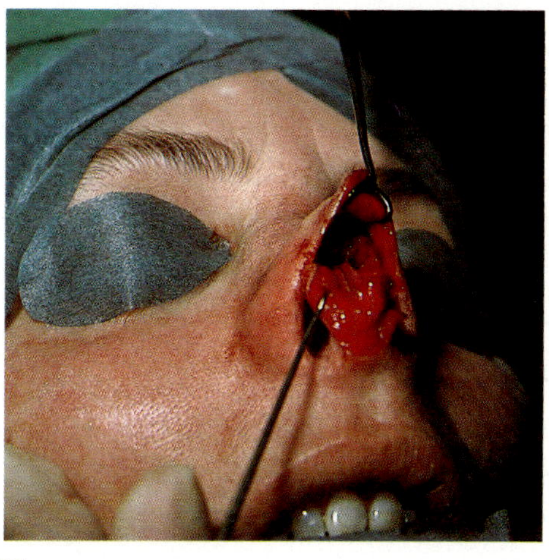

F

Fig. 119. After dissection according to the extramucosal technique (A and B) with section of the upper lateral cartilages (C) and straightening of the septum, the mucoperichondrial and mucoperiosteal leaves are pulled again to the cartilaginous and bony septal plate and fixed in the inferior portion with transseptal mattress sutures (D). In case of severe crooked dorsum, particularly when the external incision of Rethi is applied, the upper lateral cartilages are placed in a symmetrical position and sutured together and to the straightened septal ridge in the median line (E and F).
Fig. 119 continues

Fig. 119 continued

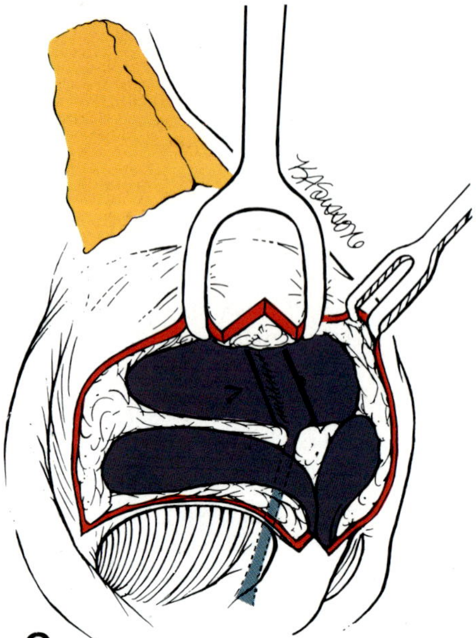

G

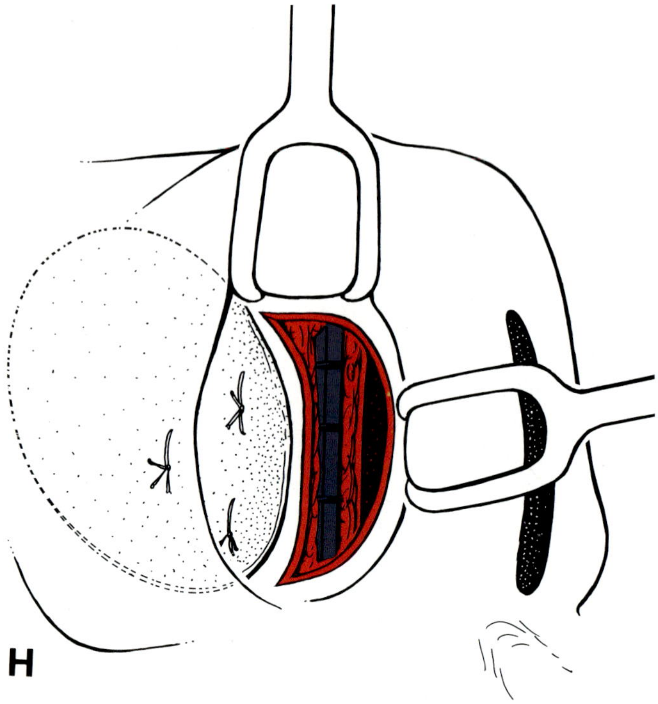

H

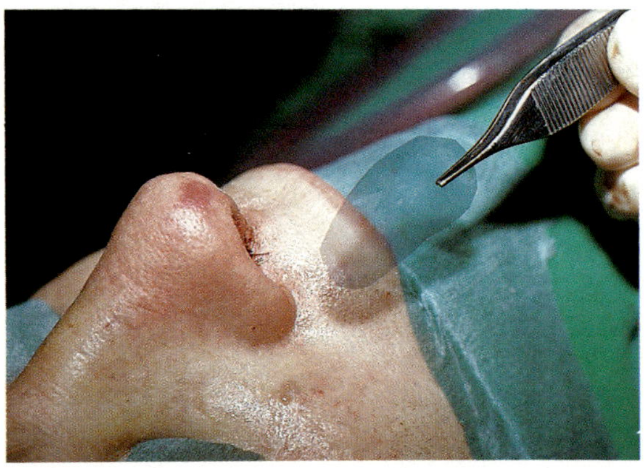

I

Diagram G shows in a preoperative view the sections of the upper lateral cartilages that have to be placed and fixed in the right position. For stabilization of the repositioned septal plate we occasionally use a plastic sheet in apposition unilaterally of bilaterally (H and I).

At the end of the septoplasty, one has to check if the airway is patent and unobstructed. In cases of severe preoperative deviation, we use a plastic sheet or small plates of x-ray film as a splint that can be placed on either side of the septum (Fig. 119 H and I). After revision of stenoses, we apply the custom-made Doyle airway silicone splint that provides a tube, open for breathing.

CROOKED DORSUM

External deviation of the nose after rhinoplasty may be due to deviations of the dorsal border of the septal cartilage, forming a C- or S-shaped curve. The severely twisted nose presents with pathology in two principal areas, the external vault and the septum.

We classify deflected noses as: (1) deformities restricted to the external nasal skeleton, (2) deformities of the inner skeleton, and (3) deformities affecting both. Usually, the deformities involving these structures are interrelated and have to be managed as one complex. This is the reason why the crooked nose should not be treated in a two-stage procedure. All three categories can be encountered as postseptorhinoplastic deformities. In the first and third categories it is necessary to bring the displaced nasal bones into normal position by means of the usual osteotomies and by a paramedian wedge resection on the side where the bony lateral wall is too wide.

The deflected nose can be combined with a residual hump. This hump has to be removed but asymmetrically so, resecting a broader strip of bone on the flatter side of the bony pyramid as we have previously shown. Along with the work on the external bone it is also important to perform adequate mobilization of the septum in the cartilaginous portions as well as in the bony part. This should be done with an extramucosal access with which we have treated all primary septum deviations and crooked dorsa since 1960 (Figs. 120 and 121). If the crooked nose is combined with a hump, there is a certain tension in the deviated septum that can be released by removing the strip of cartilage along the vomer, which we usually do. If the vomer presents a high grade deformity, as sometimes seen in unilateral hare lip noses, we have to reduce or re-

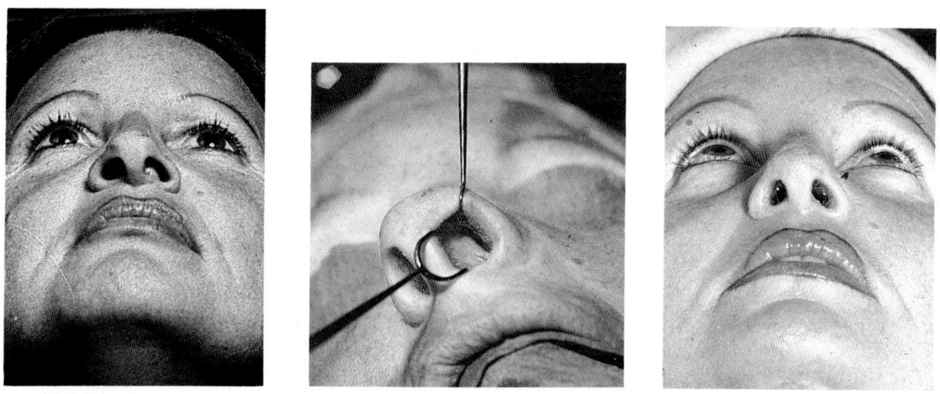

A B C

Fig. 120. A caudal anterior deviation corrected with extramucosal technique. (A and B) Preoperative view. (C) Postoperative view.

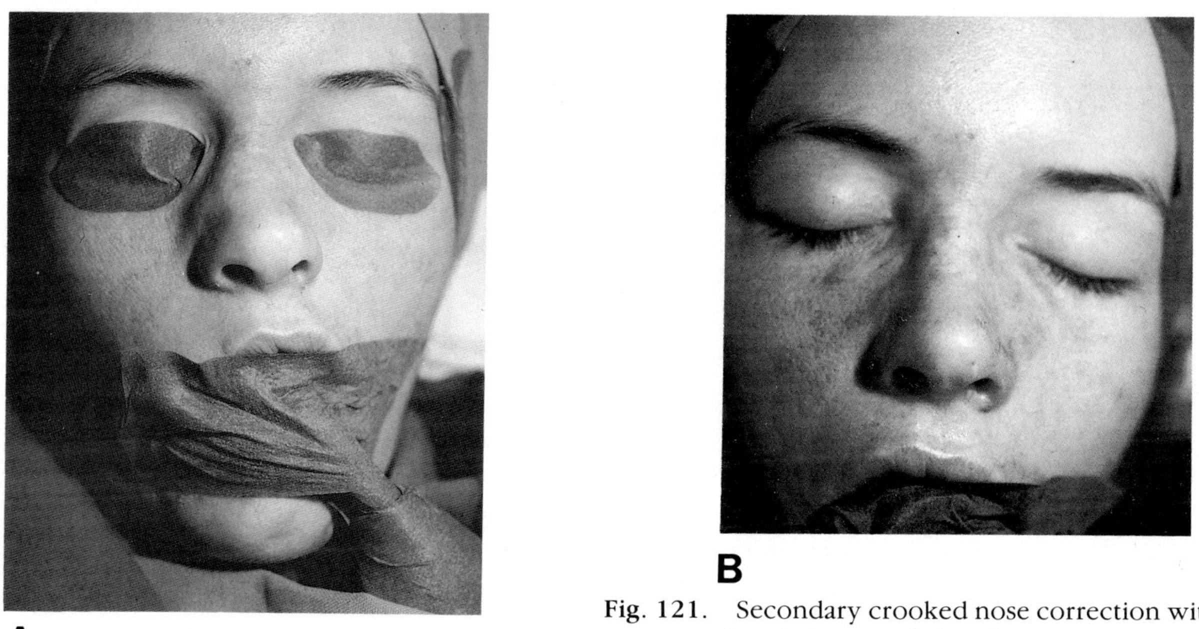

A B

Fig. 121. Secondary crooked nose correction with the extramucosal technique and dorsal mattress sutures. (A) Preoperative view. (B) Postoperative view.

move it unless a proper repositioning is possible (Figs. 122 and 123).

We do not agree with the rhinosurgeons who suggest that correcting a deviated nose in its bony portion by the simple removal of a strip of bone at the lateral osteotomy site, performing only a lateral osteotomy at the opposite side, and rotating the whole pyramid into the gap of bony resection without effecting any paramedian osteotomy will provide correction. For us, this push-to-side represents an incomplete work like the push-up and push-down procedures described by Cottle (1960). Bony strip resections are better applied in the dorsum and not at the site of the lateral osteotomy (see Bony deviations).

Of eminent importance is the stability of the septum, which can be achieved even if one resects a strip of cartilage along the vomer after having repositioned the latter. The continuity of the septal plate at the base is not absolutely necessary. By means of transseptal mattress sutures we provide the fixation of the scored and repositioned parts of the perpendicular bony plate and quadrangular cartilaginous plate. This is enough to stabilize the septum, even if a dehiscence in the osteocartilaginous wall is obtained.

If bone fragments have been completely mobilized they are reimplanted and kept in situ by packing, while reimplanted cartilaginous strips are held in place with transseptal mattress sutures. For this purpose we generally use nonabsorbable sutures on a straight or curved needle, stabilizing the reconstituted septum in the vertical position, and additionally reinforcing this with bilateral packing.

In cases of severe septal deflection, we pro-

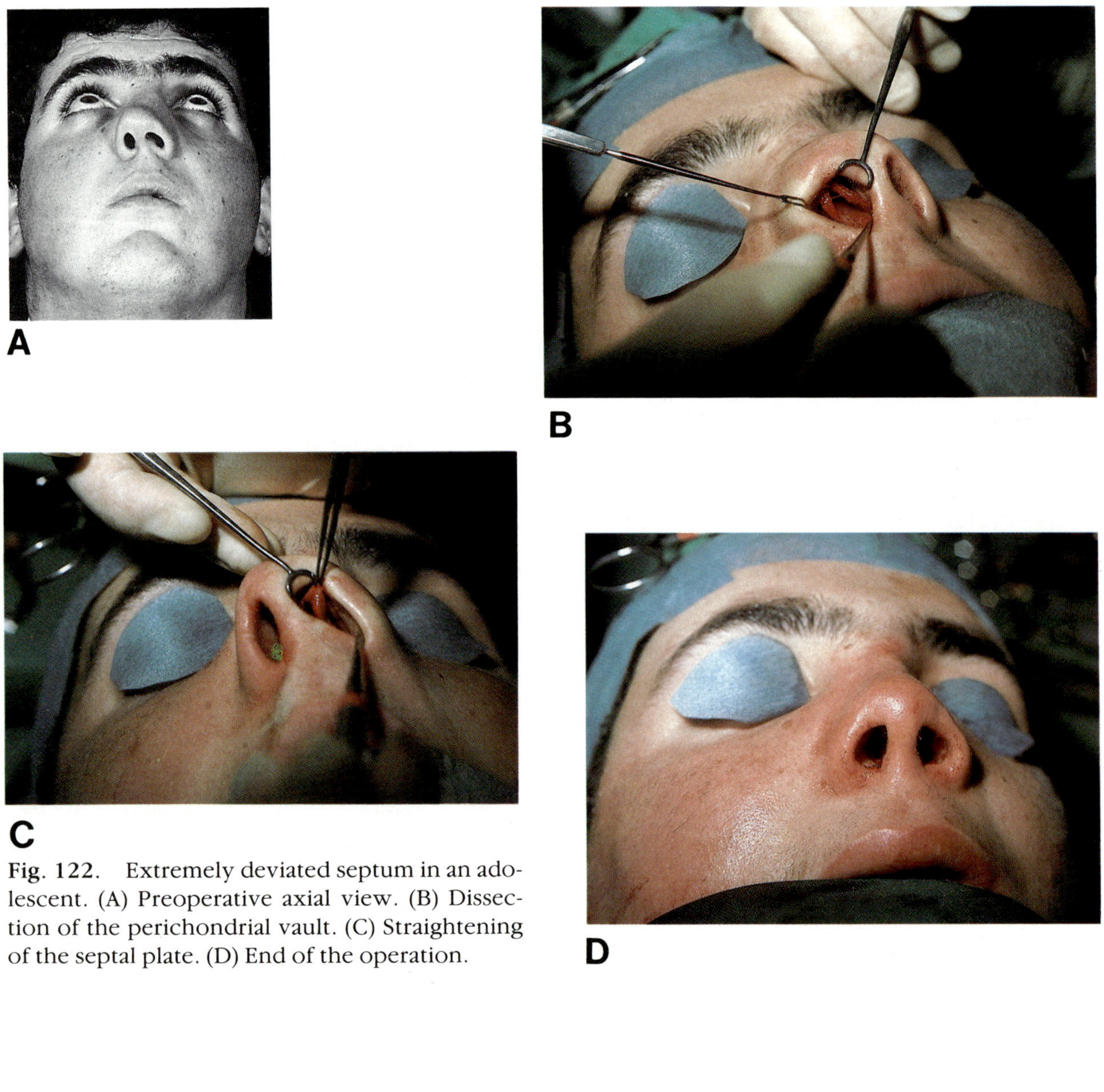

A B C D

Fig. 122. Extremely deviated septum in an adolescent. (A) Preoperative axial view. (B) Dissection of the perichondrial vault. (C) Straightening of the septal plate. (D) End of the operation.

ceed with an extramucosal technique using the open access of Rethi's (1934) method. This direct open approach facilitates the correction of septal deformities, repositioning of distorted and deviated structures, apposition and fixation of longitudinal straightening cartilaginous supports as well as suturing sectioned upper lateral cartilages (see Fig. 119).

At the end of a secondary correction of a crooked nose one has to check if all the osteotomies after incomplete or inadequate primary fracturing are complete and adequate on both sides and not "green stick" fractures with thick fibrous adhesions at all osteotomy lines—paramedian, lateral, and transverse (see Chapter 11). We have to make sure that the bony and cartilaginous septum no longer exerts unilateral pressure on the bony vault of the nose. More particularly, the paramedian osteotomy and the paramedian section of the upper lateral cartilages from the septum must be controlled because a failure to correct the dorsal cartilaginous and bony arch would again be the cause of a late recovering deviation with crookening of the dorsum, months after the revision procedure, even if the result on the operating table showed a symmetrical positioning of the bones.

For the same reason, the bony as well as the cartilaginous median transposition should be overcorrected, i.e., at the end of the operation the nasal dorsum has to deviate slightly to the opposite side because of the memory of the corrected structures. This dogma is more important in revision cases than in primary rhinoplasty. The overcorrected nose must be kept in the new position by dressing and splinting. The dressing and plaster should be left for at least 10 days or, even better, for 2 or 3 weeks. After the subsiding of skin edema, the plaster might have to be changed at 1 week or 10 days. The second splinting should then be less overcorrecting.

TURBINATE REDUCTION

With regard to septal surgery, one always has to evaluate the status of the turbinates. The first to describe the turbinate bones was Casserius in 1609. The inferior turbinate is considerably larger than the middle and the superior turbinates, being well endowed with erectile tissue. The bone is composed of lamellar bone and is completely surrounded by mucosa. The medul-

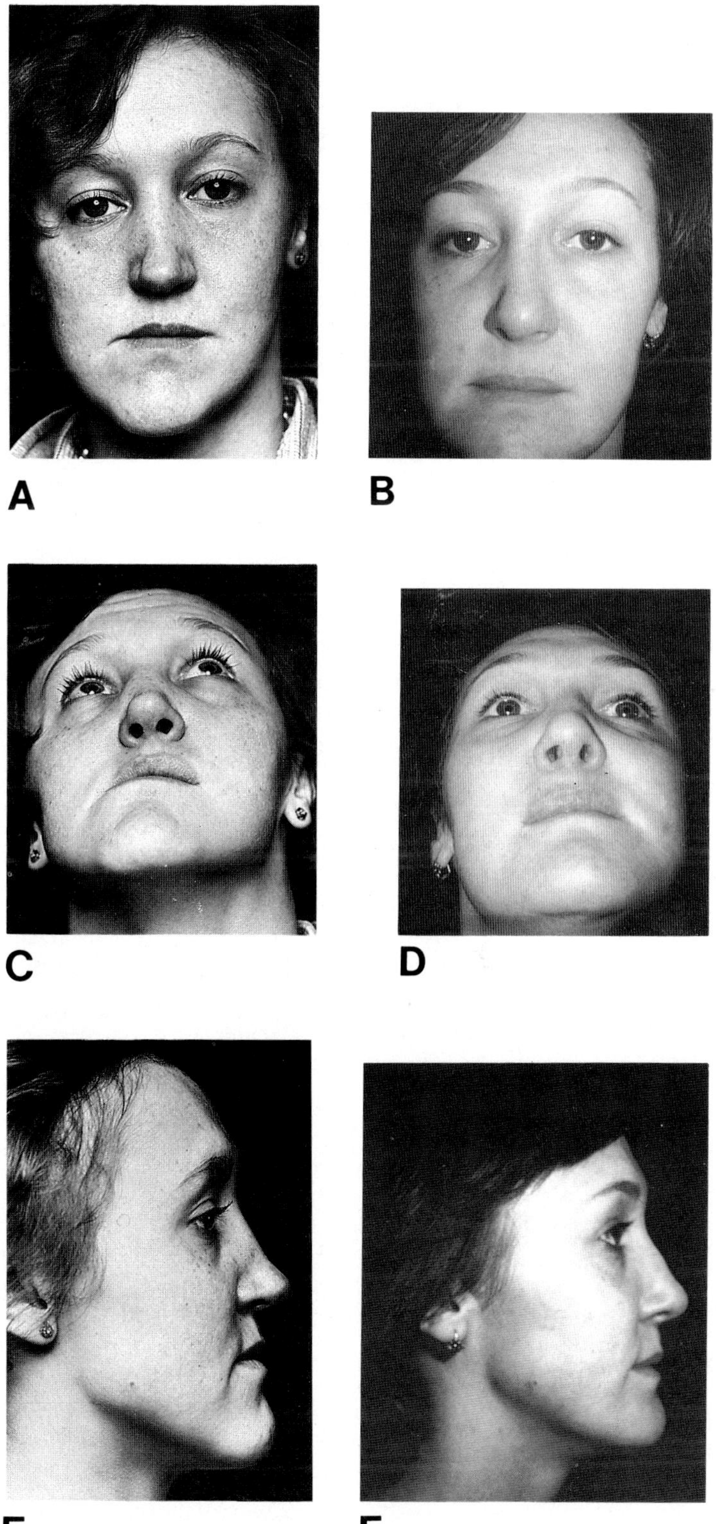

A B C D E F

Fig. 123. Straightening of a crooked nose combined with correction of mandibular deformity for equilibrating the facial features. (A, C, and E) Preoperative views. (B, D, and F) Postoperative views.

lar portion contains a loose fibro-connective tissues, matrix, and large arteries. It is lined by pseudo-stratified, ciliated columnar epithelium, containing numerous goblet cells, resting on a well defined thin basement membrane. The submucosa contains a large number of secretory glands of the serous and mucous variety, with a predominance of the serous type. Cavernous spaces characterize the submucosa. The mucosa has fewer glandular elements and more vascular spaces as compared to the rest of the lateral wall of the nasal cavity. The good vascularity of the inferior turbinates, derived from the lateral nasal artery, seems to be the basis for its valve-like function.

The filling and emptying of the vascular spaces regulates the airflow in the nasal cycle (see Chapter 6). Hypertrophy of the inferior turbinates is a common cause of nasal airway obstruction. It can be caused by chronic rhinitis, which is usually divided into two groups: allergic (extrinsic) and nonallergic (intrinsic, vasomotor). In both groups there is nasal congestion.

Turbinate enlargement in patients with allergic or vasomotor rhinitis is usually bilateral and is due to a thickening of the mucosa without hypertrophy of the underlying bone. In patients with anomalies of the nasal and sinus cavities, the inferior turbinates are also bilaterally enlarged. Turbinate hypertrophy may also be congenital or result from various causes such as dust, tobacco, hyperthyroidism, and pregnancy. In 1915, Pratt described the usual association of deviated septum and contralateral inferior turbinate enlargement. This association may be congenital, especially in cases of unilateral hare lip nose or the product of growth asymmetry, or the result of trauma. In the first two groups the unilateral hypertrophy involves mucosa and bone.

In 1983, Wespi reported that in cases of a septal spur with impacted hyperplastic turbinate with the septum and lateral nasal wall abutting, the patients often suffered from headaches, varying in localization and intensity. In 90 percent of the cases surgery leads to improvement in symptomatology. Schonsted-Madsen and Stocksted (1984) also showed that there is a significant association between operative resolution of nasal obstruction by septoplasty and cure of headaches.

Various surgical procedures aimed at this turbinate have been advocated, including resections of all or part of the turbinates, submucosal surgery, injections of submucosal sclerosants or corticosteroids, cryosurgery, and various forms of cautery. In spite of medical advances made in the treatment of rhinitis, particularly with the use of intranasal corticosteroid medications, surgery is frequently employed in treating the stuffy nose with engorgement of the inferior turbinate, with or without septal deformity.

Turbinectomy was first reported by Jones (1895) and later by Holmes (1900), Strandberg (1924), and Frey (1973). Hurd (1931) recommended electrocoagulation of the inferior turbinate mucosa as treatment for nasal obstruction. Failure to surgically reduce the size of the inferior turbinate at the time of septal correction may result in persistent airway obstruction (Pollock and Rohrich, 1984). House (1951), Tremble (1960), Goode (1977), Kressner and Kornmesser (1976), as well as Sheen (1978) and others have used inferior turbinate surgery in patients with nasal obstruction. Tonndorf (1958), reported that a turbinate cannot simply be removed to improve the nasal passage without there being any repercussions.

With outfracturing of the inferior turbinate, as advocated by Berman (1980) and others, we have obtained only poor results as Pollock and Rohrich (1984) and Curtiss (1983) also observed. We abandoned this technique and presently use electrocoagulation. Berman (1980) combines cauterization with outfracture.

Rather than excise parts of the inferior turbinate we are much more interested in preserving the mucosal surface. We use electrocoagulation in one or more areas, submucosally, linearly, along the turbinates. This produces a cicatricial shrinking of the turbinate and allows for a better airway flow.

Submucosal cauterizing has to be performed with minimal destruction of the surface epithelium in order to avoid postoperative synechiae. The shaft of the diathermy needle is isolated with a rubber protection sleeve to prevent burning of the vestibular skin. Inserted into the inferior turbinate, the exposed diathermy needle is placed against the turbinate bone. The engorged turbinate shrinks considerably, leaving an improved air passage in the nasal cavity with a substantial relief of symptoms in patients suffering from noninfective rhinitis.

In many patients we coagulate or resect bilaterally, especially when an allergic rhinitis accompanies the septal deviation and produces a bilateral enlargement. Unlike Pollock and Rohrich (1984) but more like Curtiss (1983), we operate on the mucosal hypertrophy in allergic and nonallergic cases. The treatment does not vary with the cause.

Lenz (1985) advocated the treatment of vasomotor rhinitis with Argon laser. The inferior turbinate is treated by laser strip carbonization over an area 3–5 cm long, 2 mm wide, and 1–3 mm deep, surrounded by a 2 mm coagulated border zone. Actually, laser treatment is performed also for many kinds of turbinate hypertrophy in many ENT Units, including the University Hospital of Lausanne. The advantage of the Argon laser carbonization is that it is a bloodless procedure, permitting excellent vision. The disadvantages are a longer healing period and temporary scab formation.

In 1978, Curtiss, Goldwyn, and O'Brien advocated partial resection of inferior turbinate hypertrophy causing nasal airway obstruction. There were no postoperative undesirable sequelae reported. A follow-up after 5 years confirmed the original recommendation, proving that this is a proper treatment for this indication. They did not observe any atrophic rhinitisia after resection, as feared by other authors. Only in severe cases do we choose to resect mucosa and bone.

Cryosurgery has been used in vasomotor and chronic rhinitis by Ozenberger (1970, 1973), Moore (1980), Bicknell (1979), and Puhakka and Rantanen (1977). Nyberg and Gammert (1983) who reported long-term benefits after cryosurgery in vasomotor rhinopathy recommended treating the entire length of the inferior turbinate. Half of the patients had complete relief of nasal symptoms.

Partial resection of turbinate mucosa, submucous turbinate resection, electrocautery, and outfracture of turbinates provide additional improvements to nasal airflow according to Martinez et al (1983) as well as to Protasevich (1983). For them a total turbinectomy does not seem to be a better therapy. Synechia between the cut edge of the turbinate and septum may occur. It can be prevented by judicious packing necessary particularly if simultaneous septal surgery has been carried out.

SEPTAL PERFORATION

Etiologies of Nasal Septal Perforation

Septal perforation is not a rare disorder in rhinology. While the overall frequency of perforations has decreased, the proportions of large defects has increased. Nowadays it seems that the most common cause of septum perforations is an inadequately performed submucous resection. In a statistic publication of Masing (1980), more than 60 percent of septal perforations had a iatrogenic cause.

During the last 20 years, literature on the subject of septal perforations (plastic surgical and otorhino-laryngological) has been rather scarce. There are many reasons for this scarcity: The abandoning of a too radical septal resection for septal deviation, according to Killian (1905, 1908), decreased the number of postoperative perforations of the septum. The difficult deviation of the septum is repaired by improved surgical techniques, as seen above. Prevention and adequate early treatment of nasal infections has also resulted in a decline of chronic untreated cases of rhinitis. Another reason for the scarcity in the literature on this subject is the fact that many septal perforations are asymptomatic. In addition, although the surgical interventions suggested for the repair of perforations were numerous, they usually gave, up until now, dubious results. Existing techniques were not tempting many operators, plastic surgeons, or ENT specialists because they demanded a particular skill and meticulous technique on the part of the surgeon.

The arterial supply in the region of the nasal septum is well defined. It consists of three arteries: anterior ethmoidal to the posterosuperior part, the posterior ethmoidal, and the sphenopalatine arteries, as well as branches of the palatine artery passing through the incisor foramen. In spite of the apparently sufficient vascularization by these arteries and the multiple anastomosis, the utmost caution is demanded regarding the mobilization of mucoperichondrial and mucoperiosteal flaps in this region. For the same reason multiple mucosal incisions in the posterosuperior area of the septum are not advised. Due to the rather small available surrounding surface, perforations of more than 1.5 cm in diameter are almost impossible to repair by transposition of local flaps only.

Various other iatrogenic measures may also result in perforations, including the ambitious use of transnasal tubes, as well as intranasal cryosurgery, and cautery for epistaxis, when performed bilaterally and simultaneously in corresponding septal areas. Nasal septal abscesses may also be the cause.

The consideration of associated systemic factors is also very important when a repair of the septum is undertaken. All the external factors that caused or favored the development of the perforation should both be avoided and treated: heat, dryness of the air, dust, toxic agents, etc. Any infection should be treated before surgery. Dryness of the nose with associated inflammation and sometimes a septal deviation provide the basic environment that can lead to a perforation. The triad is known as Hayek's disease. The current of inspired air causes further dryness and irritation on the convex side. There will be a loss of cilia, with scab formation. The mucosa continues to degenerate. Secondary infection then sets in, resulting in a chronic perichondritis and necrosis of the cartilage. The patient picks the scab and it reforms. Gradually the mucosa, then the perichondrium and lastly the cartilage, are eaten away. Usually the patient is unaware that an ulcer is forming. Finally, the opposite mucosal membrane is attacked and the result is perforation. The same pathophysiologic factors cause perforations of the septum in drug addicts, especially in cocaine abusers. Nose picking is a habit that may easily lead to ulceration and perforation of the septum, but it is rarely admitted by the patient.

Occupational causes where microtraumatic inorganic or toxic substances must be suspected are also possible. A wide variety of irritating substances have been indicated in the medical literature as causes of septal perforation. They cause damage primarily to the cartilaginous part of the septum. The process begins with nasal mucosal crusting, which usually tempts the patient to pick at his nose. Ulceration results, with loss of blood supply, ischemia of the cartilage, and, finally, perforation. Chrome can be mentioned as an example of the numerous substances that must be considered as a possible cause. Other chemical agents, like phosphor dusts, chromic acid fumes, calcium chloride paints, among others may result in perforation of the septum.

Cocaine, insufflated intranasally, injures the nasal septum by two mechanisms: first, it is a vasoconstrictor so it diminishes the blood supply available for the nutrition of the cartilage; second, it is rarely available in pure form for the recreational user, with the typical additives also acting as mucosal irritants (lactose, mannitol, lidocaine, caffeine, salicyclamide, heroin, amphetamines, flour, talc, or borax).

An undiagnosed septal hematoma may easily lead to a perforation. Extensive facial injuries with loss of soft tissue and comminuted fracture in the region of the midface may have the same unfortunate results. Perforations after treatment of nasal stenosis with intranasal tubes are occasionally observed.

The therapeutic measures applied to a "bleeding polyp" in Kiesselbach's area can easily lead to perforation. Systemic diseases, such as TB, diabetes, diphtheria, typhoid fever, and Wegener's granuloma have been reported as causes of septal perforation among the collagen diseases.

Carcinoma of the nasal septum is a very rare cause, but does occur. Due to its rather hidden location, it may reach a considerable size before attracting attention (see the last section in this Chapter).

Congenital defect of the nasal septum with perforation as an isolated deformity is very rare (Baıenger, 1943, Peer, 1937). More common are defects of the septum where we only find a lack of cartilage. A few cases of major deformities with complete lack of columella and of a part of the cartilaginous septum at birth are known. We had the opportunity to treat one case by operative reconstruction. The symptoms of perforation that lead the patient to ask for medical advice can be accounted in five points:

1. Aesthetic reasons: deformity of the anterior part of the nose, columella, and membranous septum.
2. Frequent epistaxis at the perforation level.
3. Excessive crust formation in chronic rhinitis sicca with offensive odor, uneasy breathing, and functional disturbances.
4. Pronounced whistling noises while nasal breathing (only seen in small perforations).
5. Headaches.

Nasal septal perforations, however small they may appear at the end of a submucous resection, are best repaired immediately; otherwise, the contraction that occurs in healing enlarges rather than closes the perforation. The formation of a perforation in the nasal septum after septal surgery usually follows a tear in the mucous membrane. The classic opinion was that if during dissection the mucosa on one side could be preserved then perforation would not occur. In a great number of cases this is so, but not in all. An untreated and nonsutured laceration of the membrane during surgery may cause secondary bleeding, infection, crusting, and perforation, even if the laceration of the mucous membrane was unilateral and the opposite surface of the septum intact.

Postoperative perforations may occur if dissection is carried on in the submucous and not in the subperichondrial layer. Such a dissection easily leads to mucosal lacerations with all its complications. The postoperative atrophy of the mucosa is rather common following such a dissection because of the secondary scarring that occurs at the vascular level of the mucous membrane.

Prevention of Iatrogenic Perforations

If a sharp septal spur deformity is encountered at the junction of the cartilage with the maxillary crest, we first dissect the perichondrium followed by the periosteum layer because laceration is more likely to occur in the plane of the subperichondrial dissection. At the junction between cartilage and bone special care has to be taken in the dissection on both sides in order to avoid a laceration that may yield a perforation. The edges of a one-sided laceration may be sufficiently well approximated with the packing material to result in healing, but a bilateral laceration requires suture closure with interposition of some thin, flat bone taken from the perpendicular plate of the ethmoid or the vomer. Bone is superior to cartilage for survival. It should be placed underneath the suture lines of the repaired mucosal laceration. Fascia is a good material too. Fibrin glue has proved to be helpful in fixation of the interposed autologous material.

Treatment of Septal Perforations

The indication for closure of septal perforations depends on the symptoms that trouble the patients. A hole in the posterior bony part of the septum can usually remain untreated because they do not cause any inconvenience. Today practically all septal perforations can be closed, in our hands by surgical means. Some surgeons still use obturators.

Treatment by Obturation

When the patient wishes an improvement without an operation, a two-layered obturator, as we advocated 20 years ago, may be used successfully. A button is modeled from a wax mold taken of the perforation. To introduce the obturator, at least one edge must be flexible. In small and medium-sized holes, the obturator can be made entirely of flexible material such as nylon or silicone. Silicone has proved to be better of the two. When we published this procedure on artificial closure in 1951, Link also proposed a similar obturator of Supramid. For closure of larger perforations, one layer of the obturator can be made of stiffer Acrylic or Teflon. This can be polymerized together with the other rubber-soft layer to form a disk with both a stiff and flexible edge. Soft nylon obturators become rigid after a few years, but silicone material remains soft and pliable (Fig. 124). For a very large perforation in which the nostril is too small for the insertion of the obturator, the alar base on one side or the columellar base must be cut. The columellar incision is extended to the perforation. Fixation of a large obturator is difficult and several have had to be removed. In our experience small and medium obturators are usually well tolerated. Occasionally, however, the perforation may increase in size due to irritation caused by the obturator itself, and this requires a larger implant. After Meyer (1951) and Link (1951), this method has also been recommended by Papangelou (1969), van Diesoek (1975), and Kern (1981). Actually we have completely abandoned this method in favor of surgical intervention that allows us to close all kinds and sizes of perforations.

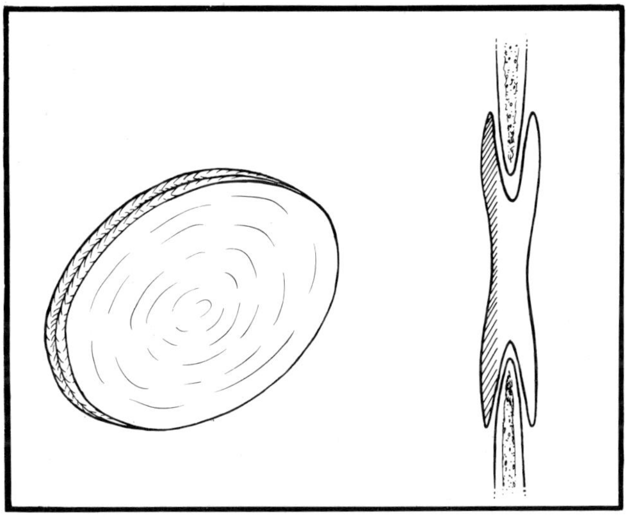

Fig. 124. Closure of a septal perforation with an alloplastic button (Meyer, Link).

Surgical Treatment

We have at our disposal several different surgical procedures for the closure of small perforation, middle size perforations, and large perforations, and for the reconstruction of septo-columellar defects. In cases with the previously mentioned clinical symptoms, a total closure of the septal perforation is always the goal to be strived for, and the surgical procedure chosen is partly determined by the size of the defect. Surgical techniques reported in the literature for closure of septal perforations are varied and ingenious.

While surgical techniques are described in the literature in considerable detail, the operative results are not. Often the number of cases is small, the follow-up period is brief, and the probability of success is not quantified. Advancement of viable tissue into a hole is, indeed, a difficult surgical challenge. Perforation often recurs as late as 1 year postoperatively. Pessimism regarding successful management is still common, and some practitioners give credence to the 1929 statement of Jackson and Coates: "Small perforations . . . are the most annoying to the patient and can always be converted into larger ones when it is inadvisable or impossible to close them." The annoyance they refer to is the accompanying whistling. With respect to the other annoyances of nasal crusting and bleeding, however, quite the contrary is true. Enlargement of perforations causes more crusting and bleeding and makes them more difficult to repair, since the availability of mucosa for repair is inversely proportional to the size of the perforation. It has been proved that this procedural dictum was wrong as it brought out other morbid symptoms. Nasal mucosal flaps should be based on the anatomic location of the blood supply. In 1968, Gollom reviewed the vascular supply of the nasal septum and proposed that flaps be designed to include branches of the anterior ethmoidal and sphenopalatine vessels in their pedicles.

Closure of Small Perforations

In 1965 we suggested the use of a rotating flap from the inferior turbinate, but symptomatic perforations are usually too anterior to the leading edge of the turbinate. An inferior turbinate flap requires a two stage technique, as Masing confirmed in 1980. The second stage is the transection of the flap base. This technique has the advantage of practically leaving the entire mucoperichondrium around the perforation intact. The effect of reduced turbinate size may contribute to a longer period of crusting than other procedures.

Ismail (1964) and McCullough (1976) recommend composite free grafts from the middle turbinate or the ear concha, but such free grafts survive only in the repair of small perforations (i.e., less than 1 cm in diameter). Trap door flaps of Seiffert (1922), in which mucosa from one side of the septum is everted toward the other, look interesting in the diagrams, but their pedicles are the scarred margins of the perforation where vascularity is compromised. Rettinger et al. (1986) also used septal mucosal rotating flap for small perforation.

Other methods that we accordingly abandoned about 8 years ago consisted in principle of mucoperichondrial flaps, one of which was cut from the area above the perforation and one from the opposite side in the area below the perforation, which were then pushed into place covering the hole.

The extramucosal technique is thereby so extraordinarily helpful that the procedures we adopted in previous years, in which local flaps (Fig. 125) were used for closure of small and medium-sized perforations, have been made superfluous. We now close small, as well as medium-sized and even large, perforations of the septum using variations of the extramucosal technique designed to fit the individual situation.

A similar, but less extensive, technique was proposed by Marino (Bari, Italy) in 1969. In closing small defects, it is sufficient to mobilize a large area of the mucoperichondrium coupled with the use of adaptation sutures free of tension on the perforation edges. In order to make this possible, the transfixion incision is first extended downwards and laterally, running parallel to the edge of the piriform aperture along the floor of the nose to the inferior nasal meatus and then upward somewhat under the inferior concha on the lateral nasal wall. An extension of the transfixion toward the dorsum leads beneath the roof of the nose to the lower edge of the upper lateral cartilage and then along the latter to the level of the limen nasi, so that this part of the incision corresponds to the intercartilaginous incision.

At the beginning, proceeding from this inci-

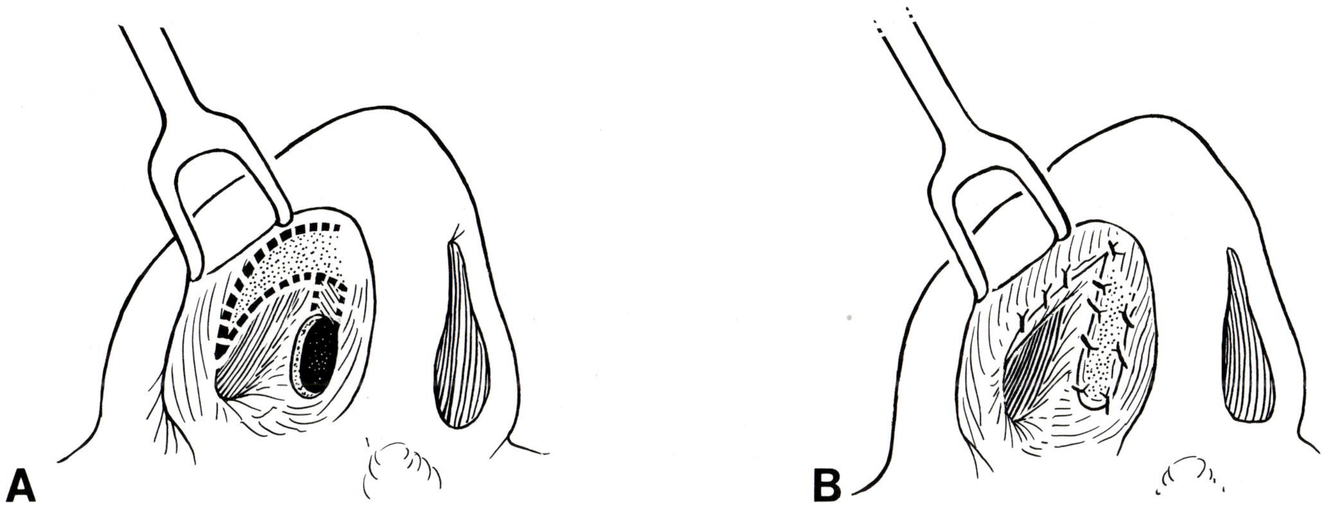

Fig. 125. (A and B) Former method (Meyer) with chondrocutaneous transposition flap from the lateral wall of the valve including either the cephalic part of the lower lateral cartilage or the caudal part of the upper lateral cartilage.

sion, the mucoperichondrium is separated from the septal cartilage over a large area. Then, the mucoperiosteum of the nasal floor is also detached as far as the lower nasal meatus. Finally, the external skin over the upper lateral cartilage is mobilized. The latter can now be severed at its insertion in full length along the cartilaginous septum, so that the result of the procedure, up to this point, is a hose-like structure consisting of mucoperiosteum and mucoperichondrium with the attached upper lateral cartilage. The perforation located therein has collapsed due to the elimination of tension. The round or oval hole becomes a slit (Fig. 126).

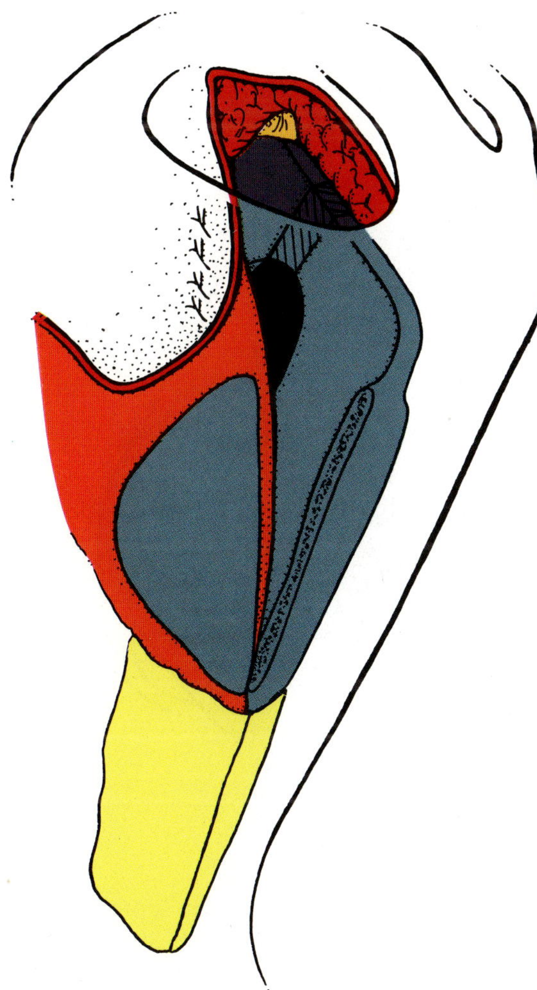

Fig. 126. Closure of small and middle size septal perforations. Sutures of the oval or round hole that has become a slit in the mucoperichondrial flap on the left side.

The same principle is followed in the other vestibule and nasal cavity. To mobilize the mucoperiosteum, an incision can be made along the lower edge of the lateral nasal wall extending deep into the bony cavity. Now, the loosely adjoining edges of the perforations in the mucoperiosteum can be freshened and, following approximation, sutured. To reduce the size of the actual cartilage defect in the lamina quadrangularis, we use two basically different methods, depending on the location and nature of the perforation. If the hole does not lie too far posteriorly, below, and with its greatest diameter perpendicular to an imaginary line of the floor of the nose, we perform resections of cartilage strips above and below the edges of the perforation parallel to its largest diameter (Figs. 127 and 128). As a result of this reduction, the lamina quandrangularis is divided into two parts: the caudal part can be fully mobilized and pushed backward and upward against the postero-superior part. This causes a decrease in the size of the perforation, which can be further closed by inserting a piece of the resected cartilage (Fig. 129), or a piece of temporal fascia. In order to avoid retraction of the columella, the removed strips of cartilage can then be reinserted at the caudal edge of the septum.

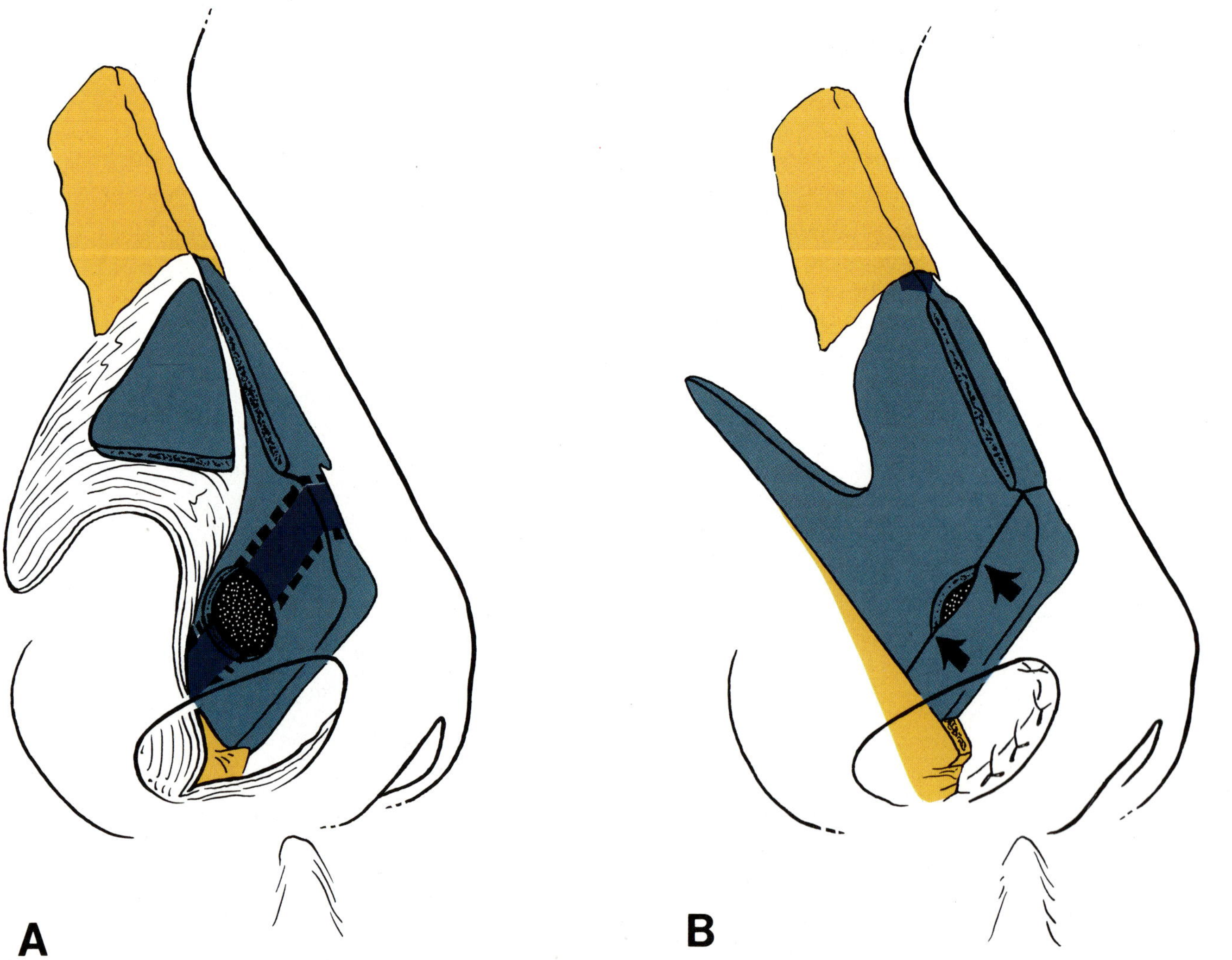

Fig. 127. Closure of small middle size septal perforations with extramucosal technique and push back maneuver for reducing the hole in the cartilage. (A) Strip of cartilage to be resected superior and inferior to septal perforation. (B) Anterior part of the septal cartilage pushed backward.

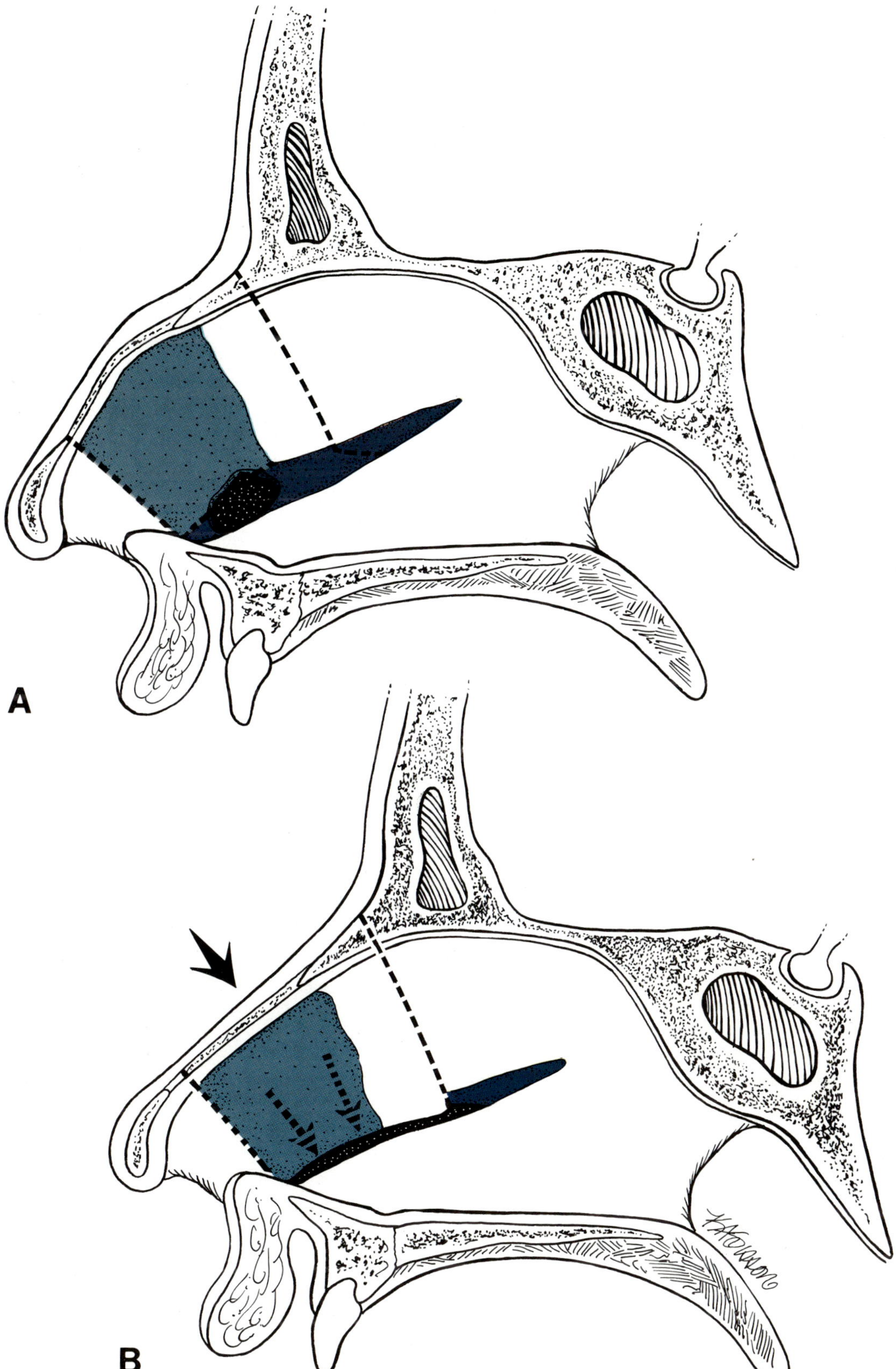

Fig. 128. Closure of small middle size septal perforation with extramucosal technique and push down maneuver for reducing the hole in the cartilaginous plate.

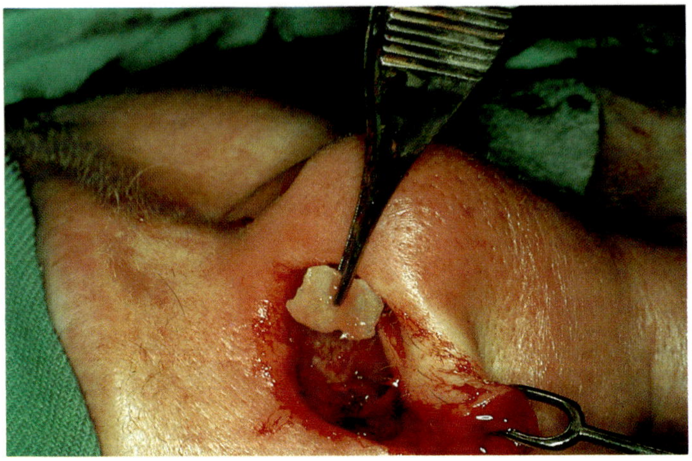

Fig. 129. Interposition of cartilage in the hole of the quadrangular plate.

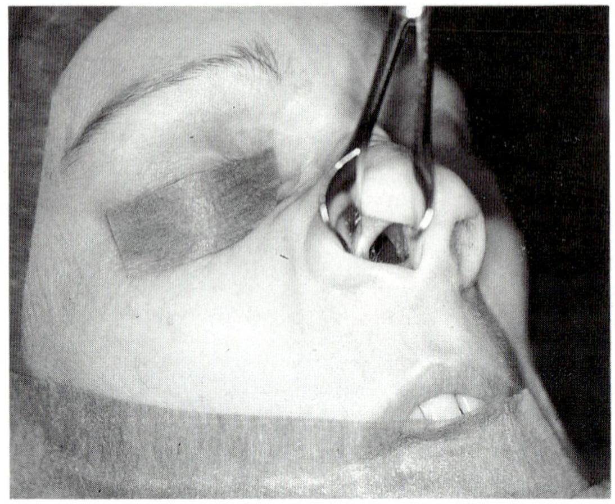

A

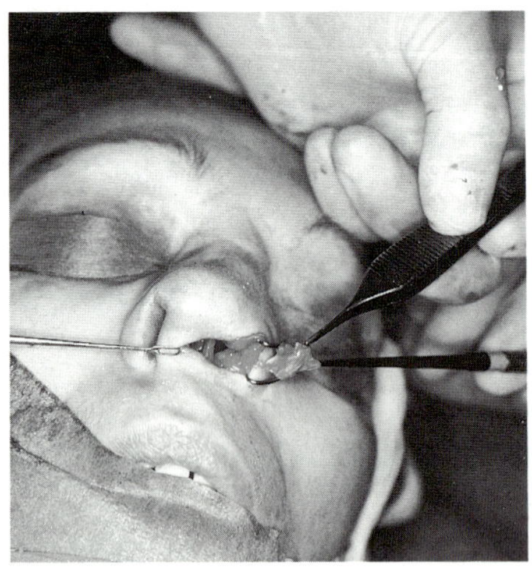

D

If the largest diameter of the perforation is parallel to the imaginary sagittal line at the floor of the nose, we perform horizontal cartilage strip resections in front of and behind the perforation. In this way, an antero-superior septal plate is separated from a postero-inferior septal plate. The upper plate can be pushed down onto the second half following mobilization at the dorsum of the nose in the same manner as it was taught by Cottle (1947) in his "push down" procedure for hump reduction (Fig. 130 and 131).

The perforation, which becomes smaller due to this maneuver, can now be further closed by inserting a strip of cartilage harvested in the very posterior part of the cartilaginous septum, as mentioned above (Fig. 129). This graft can be covered with temporal fascia, as proposed by Gollom (1968). We either interpose cartilage or fascia. Occasionally in this procedure it may be necessary to lower the bony framework of the nose, which means that the patient has to present with a slight hump nose and agree to a reduction of the dorsum. Suturing the mucoperichondrial perforation, a round Reverclin needle

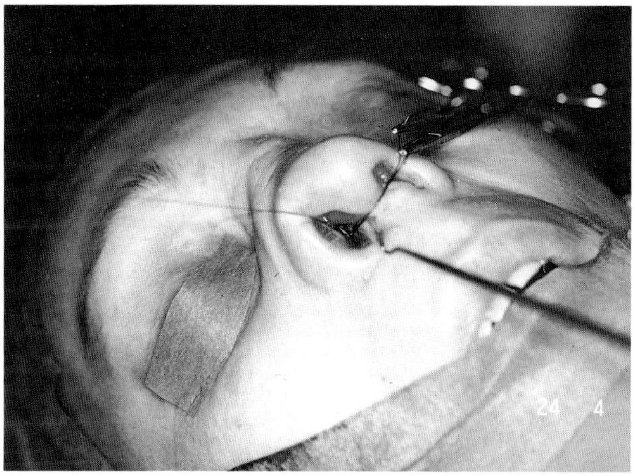

B

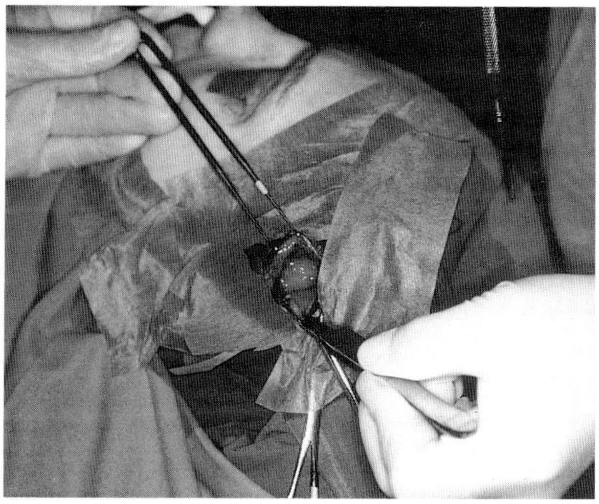

C

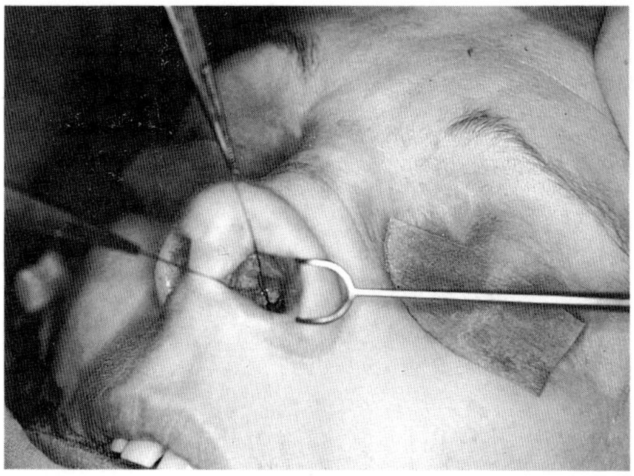

E

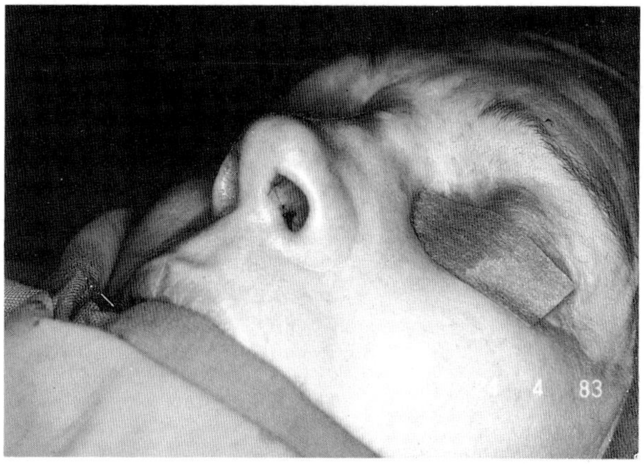

F

Fig. 130. Closure of antero-inferior middle size septal perforation with extramucosal procedure, push back of septal cartilage and interposition of temporal fascia. (A) Patient before operation. Perforation visible. (B) Perforation in the right mucoperichondrial flap sutured. (C) Temporal donor site for fascia graft. (D) Fascia graft is ready to be interposed between the two mucoperichondrial flaps at the perforation site. (E) Suture of the hole in the left mucoperichondrium. (F) Suture of the flap on the left side.

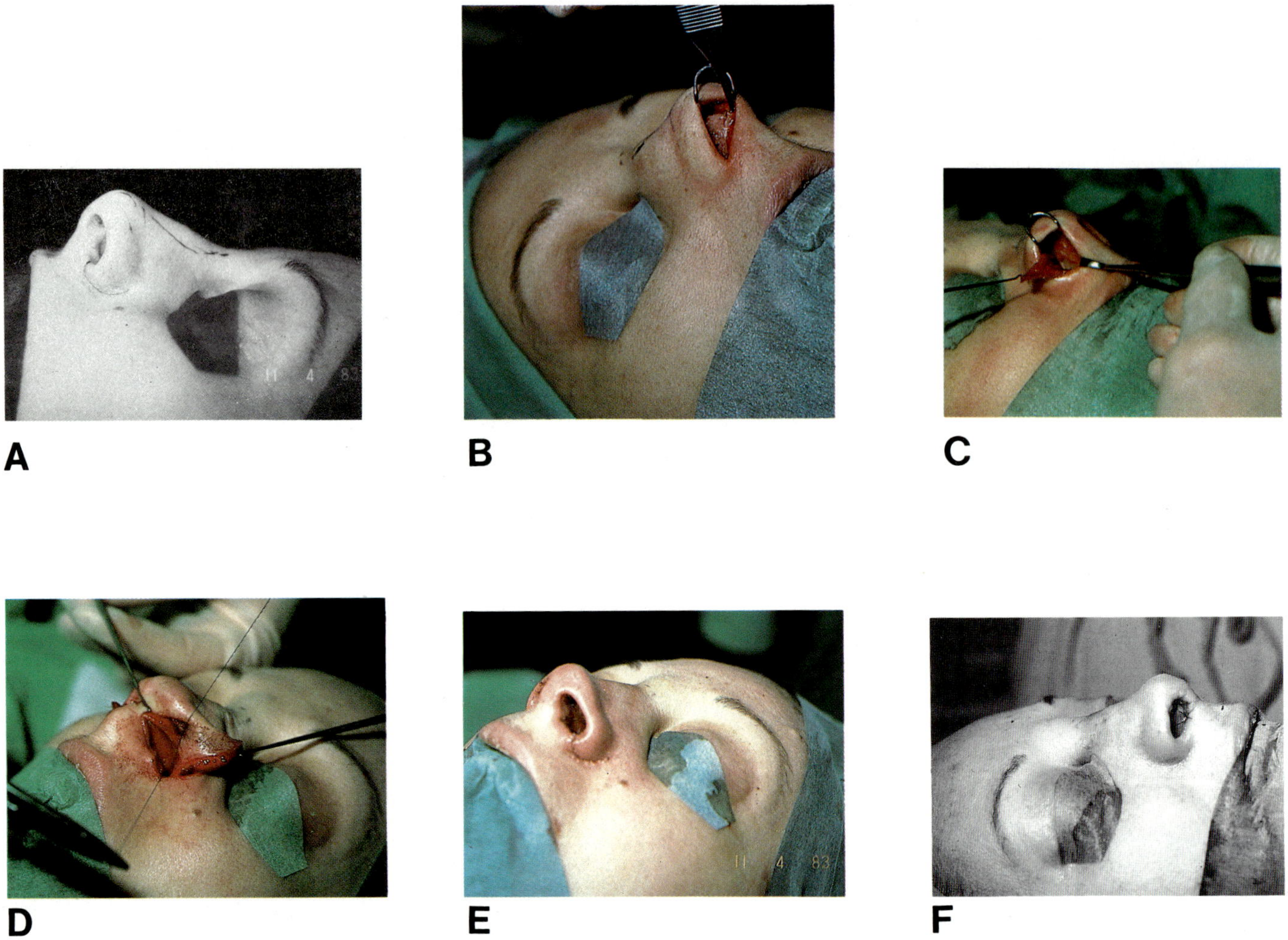

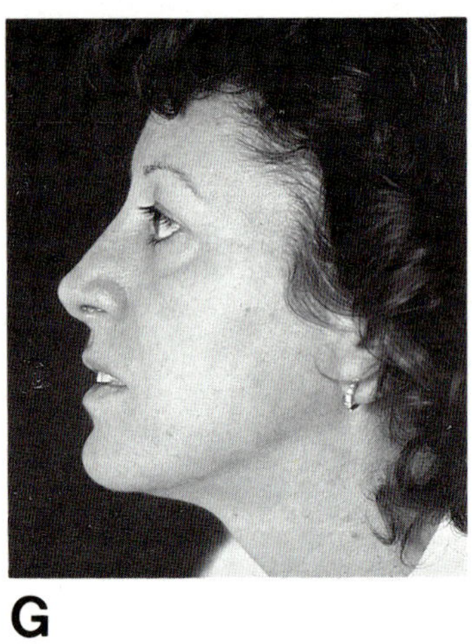

Fig. 131. Closure of middle size septal perforation with extramucosal procedure and push down of the hump. Thirty-five-year-old woman with hump nose and inferioposterior septal perforation (2 cm 0). (A) Alar base incision on the left side outlined. (B) Vestibular skin incision at the right columellar border. (C) Dissection of the mucoperichondrial flap on the right side. (D) Suture of left mucoperichondrial hole. (E) End of the operation. Suture of the left flap and of the alar base. (F) Suture of the right flap. (G) Patient with aesthetic result after push down of the hump.

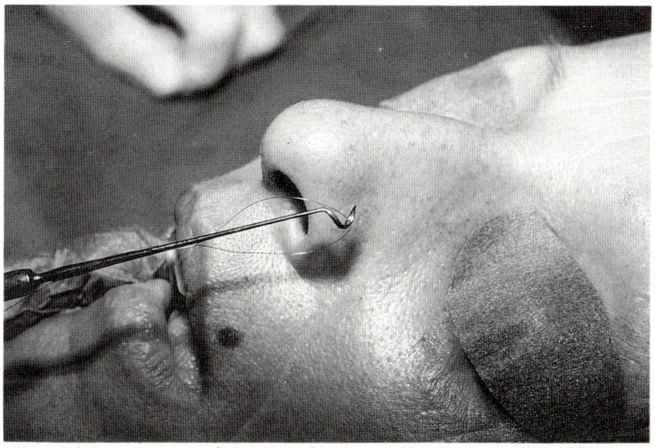

Fig. 132. Round Reverdin needle for suturing the perforation in the mucoperichondrial flaps.

can be very useful (Fig. 132). For the procedures mentioned, the access can be eased by sectioning one or both of the alar bases and if necessary the columella base too and folding them temporarily upwards and backwards (Fig. 133). This facilitates the suture of the perforation border, especially in cases of a posteriorly placed hole. At the end of the operation, the alae and the columella can be reset back down and sutured in place. If suturing is done carefully, the scars of such auxiliary incisions are practically not visible.

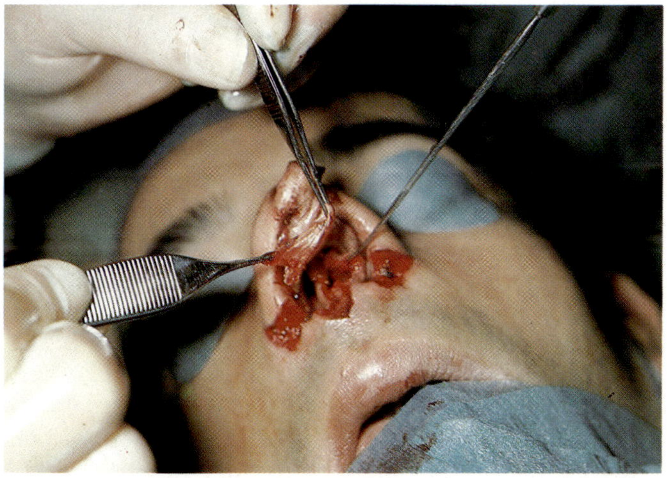

A

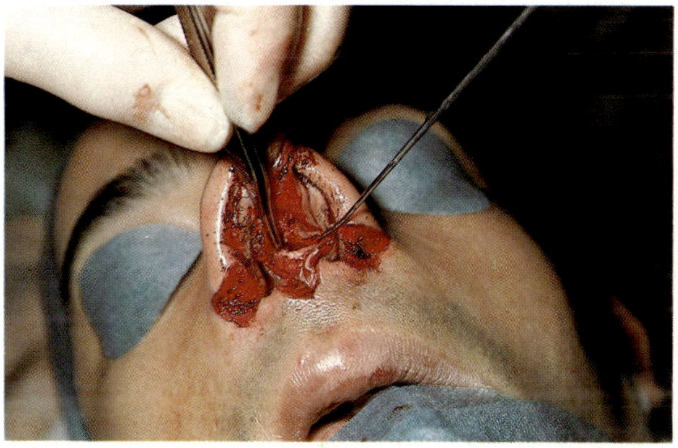

B

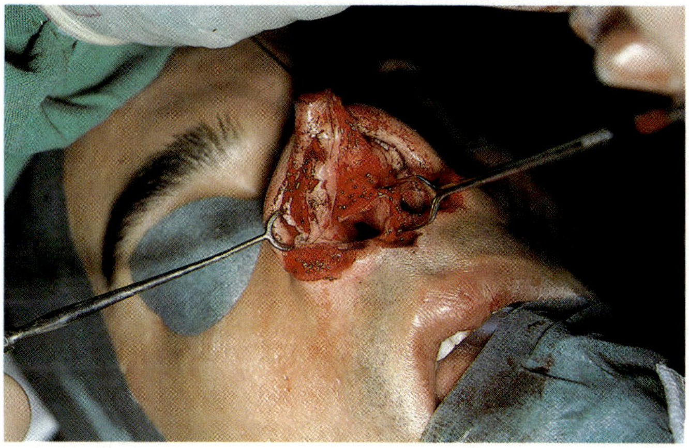

C

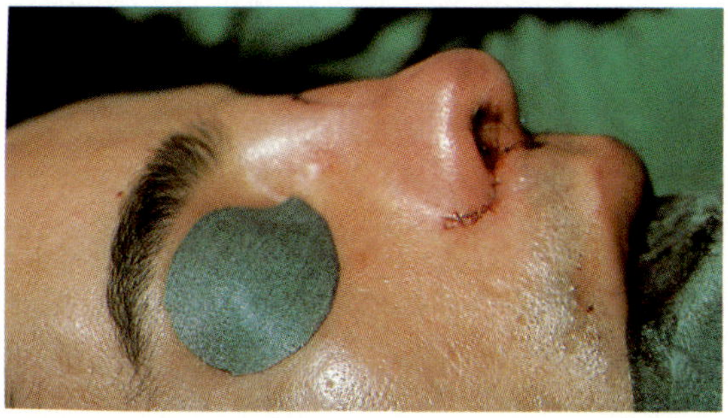

D

Fig. 133. Ideal open access for closure of septal perforation with entire columellar elevation by basal incision and transfixion. Two additional alotomies. Interposition of temporal fascia graft. (A) Perforation in the mucoperichondrial flaps are sutured. Fascia graft is ready for insertion. (B) Good visualization for interposition of a fascial leaf between. (C) Mucoperichondrial flaps are glued together after fascial grafting. (D) Wound of access sutured once the perforation is closed.

Closure of Middle Size Perforations

For perforations up to 2 cm in diameter that are in the central part of the septum, we formerly used the techniques of advancement of monopedicle or bipedicle flaps. After rather extensive undermining of the mucoperichondrial and mucoperiosteal layer on both sides of the septum, one incises the mucosa bilaterally along the lateral border of the nasal floor and at the inferior level of the perforation. One obtains two bipedicle antero-posterior flaps, which are displaced upwards reaching the superior level of the perforation. The raw area at the floor of the nose left by the upward sliding of the flaps is grafted on both sides with a skin or mucosal graft. The closure of perforations of similar size involving the caudal part of the septum demands a more extensive undermining of the mucoperichondrium and a mobilization of mucoperiosteum extending as far as the lateral walls of the lower meatus. As advocated by Climo (1956) and Kitajiama (1965), the mobilization of the mucoperichondrium can be performed anteriorly up to the superoanterior border of the septum, which is made visible by the transfixion of the membranous septum and dissection of the upper lateral cartilage from the septum.

For a few years we were closing septal perforations of this size, situated in the upper anterior part of the septum, by an original method (Meyer, 1972) differing from other techniques. It consisted of the using of the upper lateral cartilage of the nose. Through an intercartilaginous and posterolateral incision, we dissected and slid the upper lateral cartilage together with the adherent mucosa towards the perforation. The pedicle of this mucocartilaginous flap was slightly twisted at the dome of the nasal cavity and the raw surface was then carried into the perforation. The edge of the flap was sutured to the border of the perforation all around. On the opposite side, we either proceeded in a similar manner or covered the perforation by advancing a mucoperichondrial flap from behind. We abandoned this method 8 years ago in favor of the extramucosal procedure.

For closure of perforations ranging in size from 1.5 to 2.0 cm in diameter, McCollough (1976) uses an anterior superiorly based transposition flap, leaving a triangular part columellar defect that is filled by using a composite graft from the auricle. Composite grafts from the ear have also been utilized exclusively for closure of small perforations.

Georgi described in 1983 chondromucosal transposition flaps of the cranial borders of the lower lateral cartilages, anteriorly based, applied to one another, back to back, for closure of middle-sized septal perforations. This is a very similar procedure to our vestibular flap, including the utilization of the upper lateral cartilage. Both are indicated only for supero-anterior perforations not exceeding 2 cm in diameter, which are rather rare in our experience. Rettinger et al. (1986) diagrammed a similar small rotation flap. Since the blood supply is much better in a widely dissected flap of the whole septum, we actually prefer the extramucosal technique and this is the reason why we abandoned all methods of transposition flaps.

The extramucosal technique is especially valuable in the treatment of perforations up to 3 cm in diameter because it allows for their closure in a single stage. When considering the total number of septal defects, these middle-sized perforations have become relatively more common in the past decade. Therefore, it seemed of particular interest to work out a single-stage method to close them.

We begin the operation in these cases on one side with an incision, the course of which parallels to that of the hemitransfixion incision, but starts at a substantially greater distance anterior to the edge of the septal cartilage, so far forward in fact that it is located in the skin of the columella, only 1 mm behind the nasal orifice. The subsequent course of the incision then corresponds to that already described above, i.e., the incision is extended to the rear and upward as an intercartilaginous incision and at the floor of the nose, parallel to the lower edge of the piriform aperture extending to the lateral wall. Where the incision passes beneath the dome of the alar cartilage, care must be taken to avoid its damage.

Beginning by the incision at the edge of the columella, the lateral skin of the columella and the septum must be dissected with the utmost care and caution in order to avoid a perforation of cellulo-adipose tissue around and behind the medial crura of the alar cartilage. For this purpose, we recommend the use of magnifying glasses. When the dissection has reached the anterior edge of the septal cartilage, it can be carried deeper to the mucoperichondrium of the septum and of the vault under the roof around the perforation as well as to the mucoperiosteum of the floor and lateral wall. The upper lateral cartilage can be separated at its base from the septum, at which point the whole elevated flap is pulled forward and outward and the perforation located in the mucoperichondrium automatically narrows to a slit as the mucous membrane collapses as we mentioned above (Fig. 126). This slit is easy to close by continuous or separate sutures after freshening the borders.

The whole mucoperichondrial and mucoperiostal wall is then freed in the anterior two-thirds of the nasal cavity and vestibule (Fig. 126), extending more laterally in the floor and into the upper vault as for cases of smaller perforations.

On the other side the procedure is basically the same, with the difference being that the vertical course of the incision before the edge of the septum is found further posteriorly and corresponds to that of a transfixion incision. Thus, the two flaps come to reach a different level anteriorly. At these levels, special care must be taken not to create a defect connecting the two nasal vestibules. On this side too, the edges of the perforation in the mucoperichondrium collapse following extensive mobilization.

After freshening the edges of the defect in the cartilage, the hole can be reduced with the "push back" (Figs. 127 and 128) or "push down" (Figs. 130 and 131) procedure described in the previous section. Any remaining loss of cartilage at the site of the perforation is filled with a piece of cartilage (Fig. 129) or temporal fascia as has been explained.

The incisions in the mucoperichondrium and in the skin of the columella and vestibule are sewn with interrupted sutures of 4-0 or 5-0 nonabsorbable material. If dorsal displacement of the mucoperichondrium for suturing the defect would result in too much tension at the edge with the danger of producing a "hidden columella," the loss of skin, if necessary, can be compensated by a retroauricular skin graft.

Occasionally we facilitate the extended dissection of the two flaps and the suturing of the mucoperichondrial edges of the perforation on both sides by sectioning the columellar base, and, if necessary, one or both alar bases, as mentioned for small perforations (Fig. 131). They are sewn at the end of the operation by interrupted 5-0 sutures. Only in a few cases have we succeeded in effecting this technically difficult work without the aid of an alotomy or a columellar section.

In the last 5 years, we injected fibrin glue (solutions of fibrinogen, thrombin, aprotinin, and calcium) in order to improve the contact of the mucoperichondrial flaps with the septal cartilage and to hold in place the grafted cartilage or fascia used to fill the residual hole. Lippi et al. (1986) use the same sealant for perforation closure.

We do not think that the transcolumellar open access of Rethi is advantageous for this procedure because it is important to have direct access to the basal part of the septum and not to its anterosuperior part. The mucoperichondrial dissection carried around the perforation has to begin along the anterior border of the septum. For that purpose the best access is provided by the columellar base incision. If this is used the two flaps must not be at a different levels behind the columella, as mentioned above. The transfixion incision is the best choice. One must check at the end of the operation whether there has been any retrusion of the columella caused by the traction of the sutures, be it to the transfixion incision, columellar border, or columellar base incision.

Strelzow and Goodman (1978) are also using smaller flaps, interposing septal cartilage, vomerine bone, or perpendicular plate of ethmoid bone and even iliac crest bone into the cartilaginous dehiscence. Gonzales (1985) chose to use cortical bone interposed between smaller flaps. Gollom proposed in 1968 a method with limited dissection around the perforation that is hinged at the caudal end. Fairbanks also described in 1980 a similar but less extensive procedure involving the elevation of the septal mucoperichondrium and mucoperiosteum through two parallel incisions in the septum and with interposition of temporal fascia. This limited dissection does not allow the elevation of a sufficiently wide advancement flap for closing huge perforations. In the publication of his method Fairbanks (1981) stated that "breakdown occurred in cases in which large areas of the graft could not be covered on at least one side with mucosa. Consequently, very large perforations (4 cm or more) in which no conceivable flap could be expected to cover very much of the graft, may be inoperable." In our experience it should be possible to surgically manage practically every kind and every size of perforation and septal loss using our techniques of intranasal surgery. There are some extremely rare cases of septal perforation in which there is little space between the defect and the columella, so that when we dissect the mucoperichondrial flaps on both sides, the ante-

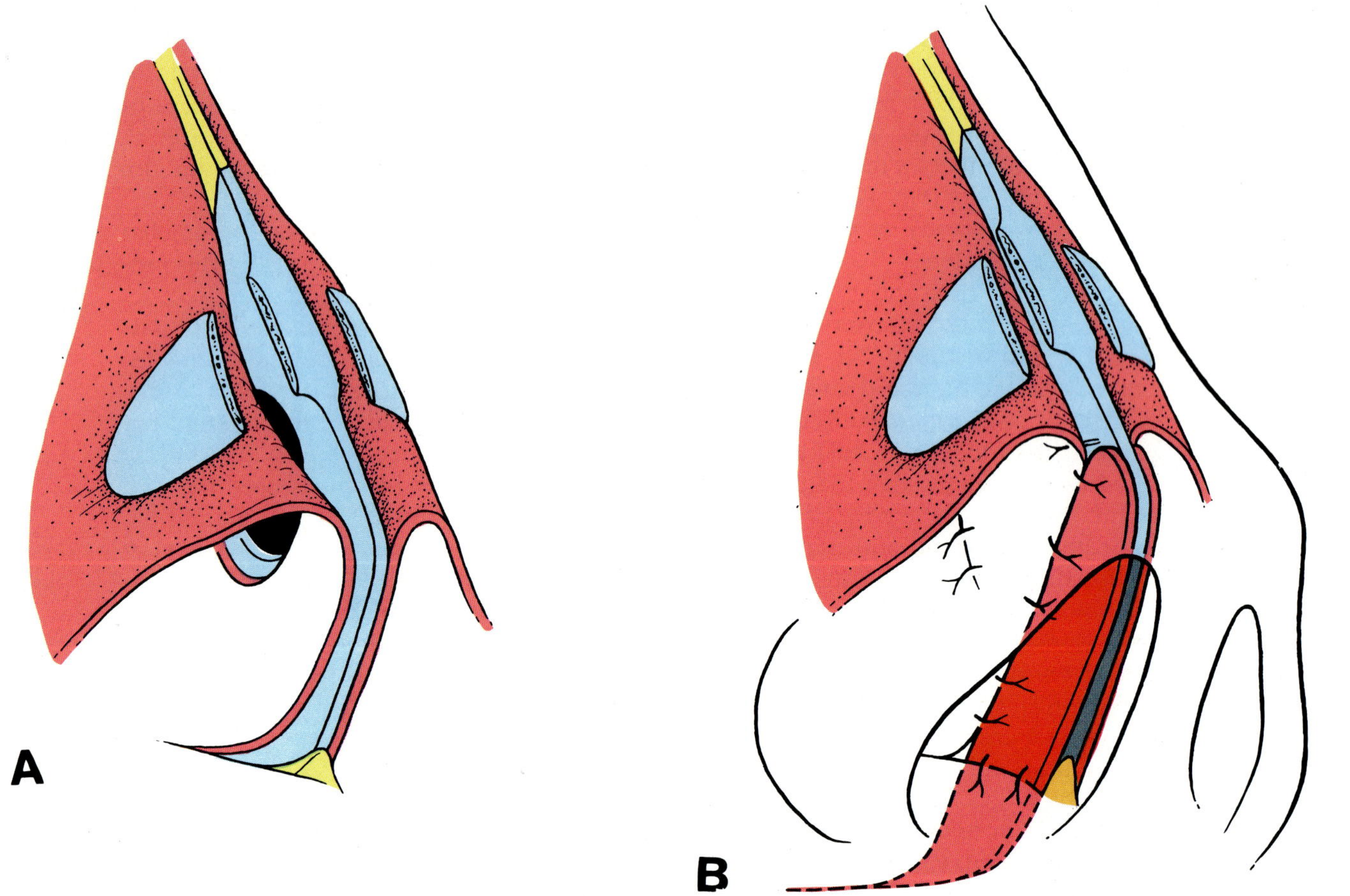

Fig. 134. In special cases of anterior perforation the extramucosal flaps cannot reach the septocolumellar pillar. We need then in addition the bilateral labial mucosa flap as shown in Fig. 94.

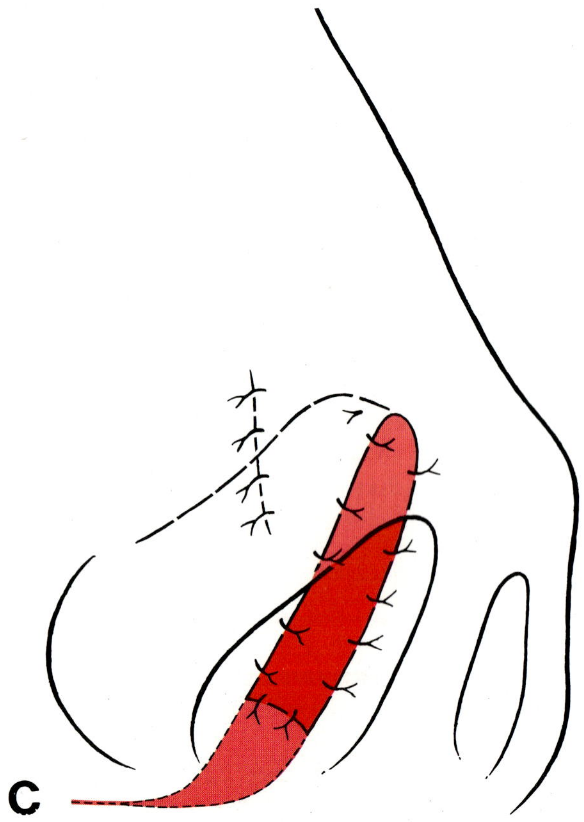

rior cartilaginous septal pillar remains deprived of mucosal covering. The bilateral flaps with the perforation closed and sutured sometimes cannot be advanced more than the caudal-most edge of the perforation in the cartilage. The anterior bare pillar then must be covered with skin or mucosa, either as a graft or transferred as a flap. When there is only a narrow strip of membranous septum to be covered just behind the columella we use a skin graft from the postauricular region. In more difficult cases we prefer the bilateral utilization of buccal flaps and apply in special cases the two simple gingivolabial flaps of Tipton (1970) and Hinderer (1973) without delay. In such cases we perform the closure of the perforation with extensive extramucosal dissection, as explained, and complete the covering of the septum anteriorly with two small gingivobuccal flaps (Fig. 135). For this complex proce-

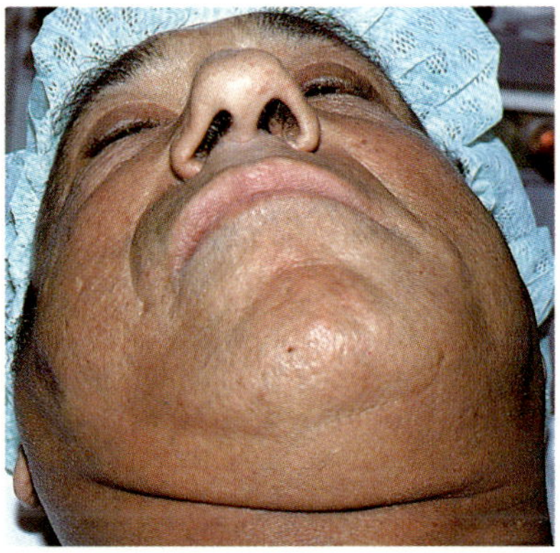

A

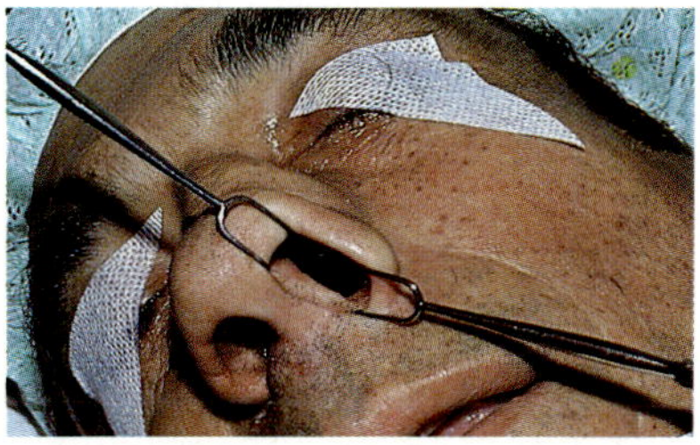

B

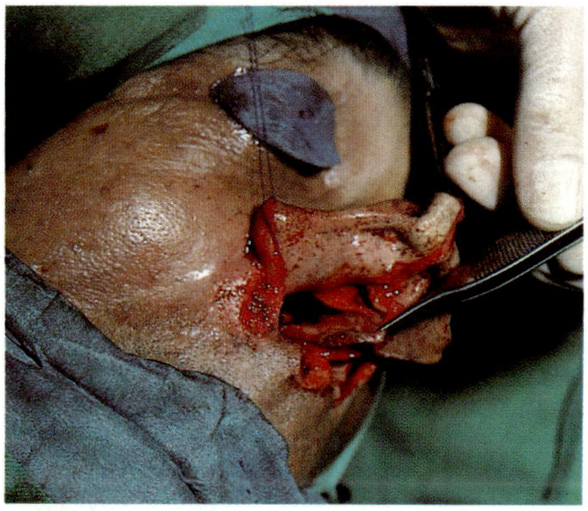

C

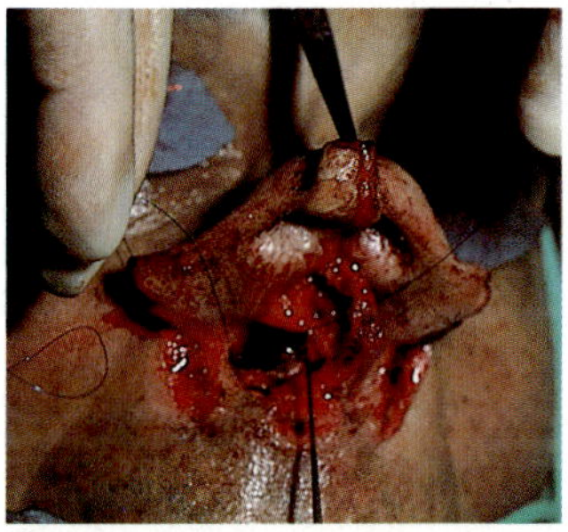

D

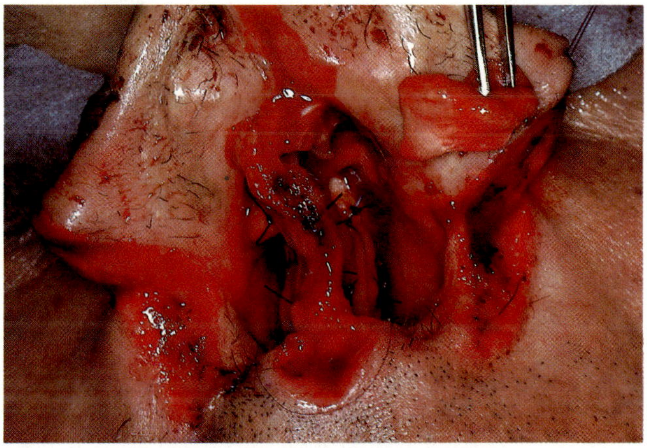

E

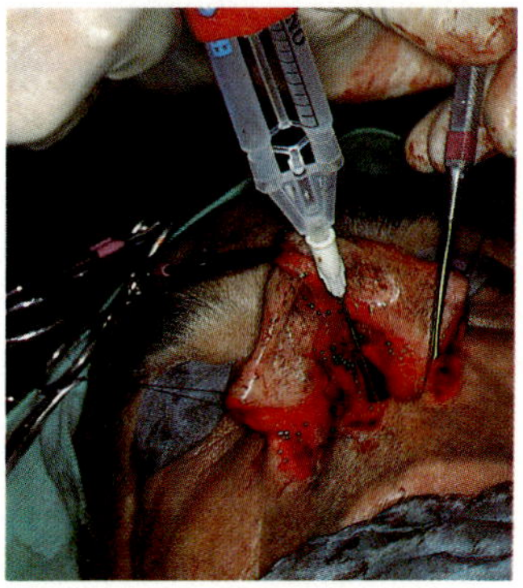

F

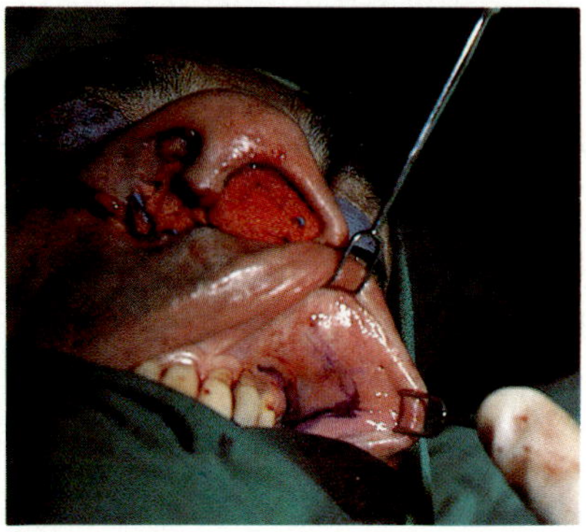

G

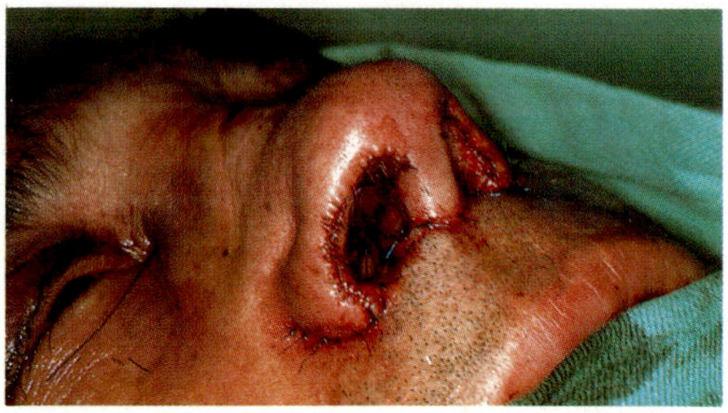

H

Fig. 135. Closure of septal perforation with extramucosal techinque combined with bilateral simple one layered buccal flaps. (A) Male patient with distorted nostrils before operation. (B) Big perforation visible. (C) Mucoperichondrial flap dissected on the right side. (D) Suture of the perforation in the right mucoperichondrial flaps. (E) Both flaps are closed by suture. A fascial leaf is ready to be interposed. The anterior fibrocartilaginous pillar has to be covered by labial mucosa flaps. (F) After interposition the mucoperichondrial and mucoperiosteal flaps are glued together with fibrin adhesive glue. (G) The left labial flaps are lifted. The buccal flaps are lifted into the nose to cover the anterior septal pillar. (H) End of the operation with alotomies, columella, and marginal alar resections sutured.

dure the open access method, incorporating at least the sectioning of the columellar base, becomes essential.

Actually, some authors, such as Kridel et al. (1986) propose the Rethi incision to obtain good access. This is true for these perforations of minor size, as they can be managed with Fairbank's (1980) method. We do not however, recommend this for closure of the larger holes where an extensive mucoperichondrial and mucoperiosteal dissection is necessary. For our extramucosal procedure the best external approach is the columellar base incision combined with a transfixion incision, because the difficult aspects of the dissection are usually encountered in the basal vestibular and cavity floor (Fig. 133).

Closure of Large Perforations

For closure of perforations greater than 4 cm in diameter, we advocate a composite buccal flap. This method was first presented at the Swiss ENT Congress in May 1968 by our assistant, Dirlewanger. We were happily surprised to read that a similar technique was shown by Akyildiz at the Rhinology Congress in Zagreb in September of the same year. In the following year, Hertig and Meyer published the procedure as Meyer's method. It was again described by us three years later (Meyer, 1972). In 1970, similar procedures were also adopted by Tipton and in 1971 Nagel, in 1973 by Hinderer, in 1977 by Tardy, in 1978 by Hirshowitz, Moscona, and Eliachar, in 1982 by Karlan, Ossof, and Christu, and in 1985 by Chalaye and Levignac. Tipton (1970) and Tardy (1977) have successfully closed perforations up to 2 cm with a shorter flap in one stage. A similar small flap had already been advocated by Filiberti (1965), but was not popularized. Hinderer (1973) proposed a similar two-stage procedure with bilateral small buccal flaps, one reinforced with a cartilage graft from the tragus. Like Hinderer (1973), Chalaye and Levignac (1985) used bilateral flaps transferred through tunnels on both sides of the spine but without reinforcement. The idea to transfer buccal mucosal flaps into the nose goes back to Jeschek, who used them in 1960 for treatment of ozaena. Ey (Denecke and Ey 1984) is still using this procedure bilaterally for this purpose. In an exceptional case, in which a buccal mucosal flap had previously been used unsuccessfully for the closure of a perforation, Matton and Beck had to resort (1985) to using an external, superiorly based, skin lined nasolabial flap. It is obvious, that mucosal flaps should be preferred for such a surgical treatment, if available.

Our method (1968) consists of a three-stage procedure in which a spoon-shaped flap from the oral vestibule with a piece of cartilage included is inserted into the perforation and then severed from its pedicle once its three-layered flap has taken to the septum. The surgical procedure consists of the following three steps. In the first stage we prepare the flap in the mucous membrane of the oral vestibule. The flap, which will later consist of a pedicle and an oval piece of cartilage covered on both sides with mucous membrane, is begun in the gingivobuccal fold of the oral vestibule, directly next to the frenulum above the upper row of teeth. A piece of cartilage is taken from the entire concha of the ear, without producing any substantial deformity of the pinna. It is then flattened by radial incisions and placed into a submucous pocket in the oral vestibule behind and below Stenson's duct. Next to this, another flap is cut in the mucous membrane towards the crista buccinatoria. This tiny flap retains an anterior pedicle and is folded under the already existing submucous pouch but in a deeper layer, not communicating with the pocket of the cartilage graft. The cartilaginous reinforcement is now situated between two walls of mucous membrane, one on the superficial oral side the other on the inner cheek side. The donor defect of the small posterior mucosal flap is closed by approximation. The pedicle of the whole buccal flap, beginning at the frenulum, is tubed by molding a longish horizontal roll of tissue using interrupted small incisions and mattress sutures.

After 3–5 weeks, during which time the cartilage and the accessory mucous membrane flap take, the spoon-shaped flap can be cut and fed into the nasal cavity to fill the septal defect through a tunnel running along side the anterior nasal spine. This is the second stage. The donor area is then closed by approximation. In order to facilitate the suturing of the mucous membranes of the buccal flap to the edges of the perforation, it is convenient to section the base of the columella and if necessary also of one or both alae. The columellar base incision extends backward to the anterior lower edge of the perforation so that the portion of the septum located in front of the defect can be raised along with the columella, thereby opening wide the perforation. If the mucous membrane on both sides of the flap is now sewn to the freshened edges of the perforation, the columella and the ventral portion of the septum are automatically brought back into their original position. Thereafter, the columellar base is again sutured to the philtrum and to the medial edge of the vestibule on both sides. The occasional alotomy is also sutured (Figs. 136–140).

The patient is left to heal for another 3–5 weeks. Then the third stage can be carried out on an outpatient basis. The division of the pedicle is performed under local anesthesia. At the same time, the three-layered flap in the septum can be thinned if necessary.

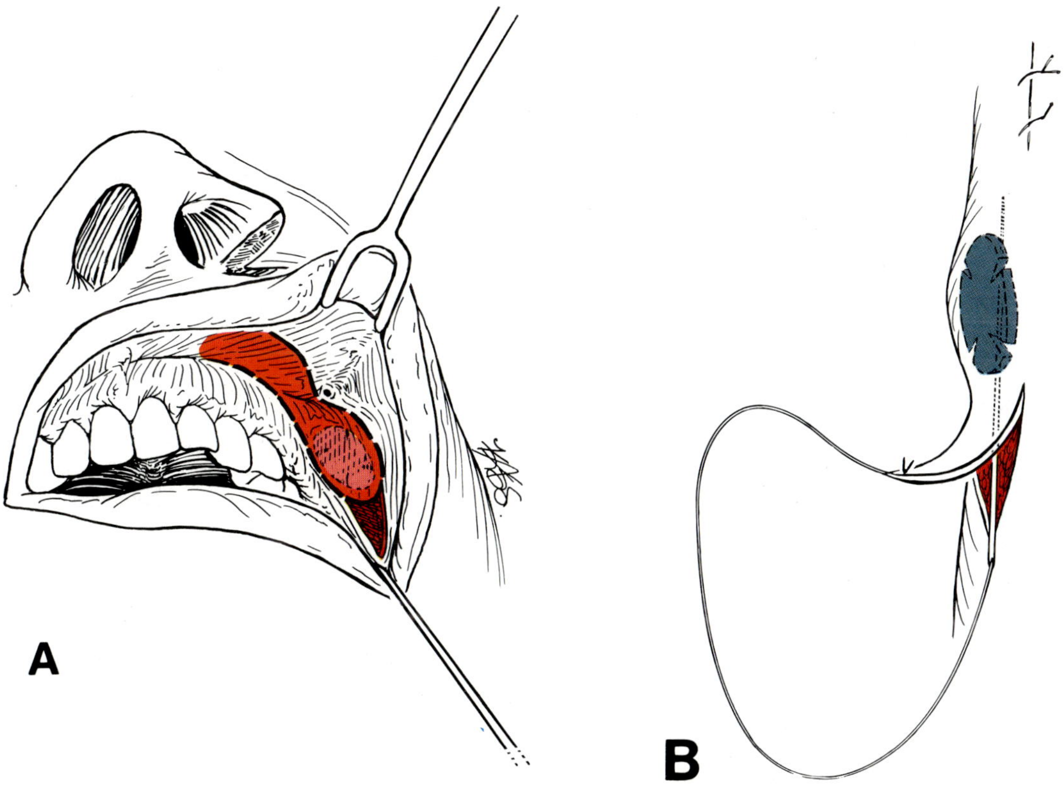

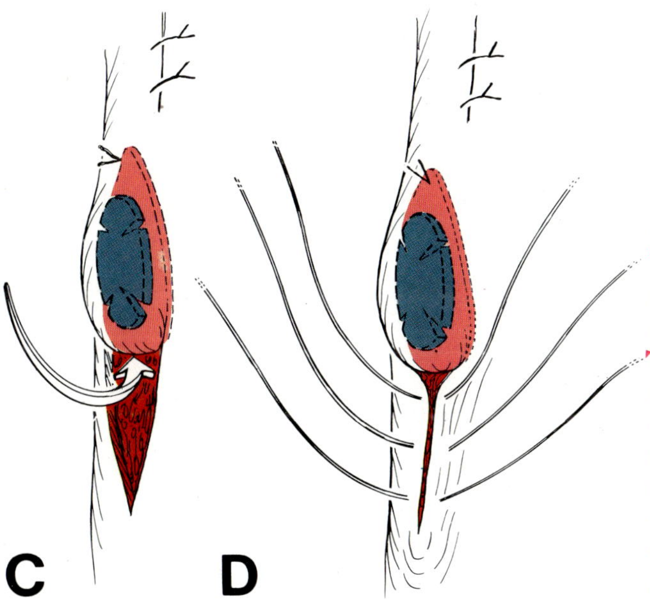

Fig. 136. Closure of large septal perforation in a three-stage procedure with gingivo-buccal flap. (A) First stage: The three-layered compound flap reinforced with ear cartilage is elevated at the buccal extremity. The incision for insertion of the cartilage graft is sutured. (B) The distal extent of the compound flap is cut in a "V" shape and is turned behind the cartilage graft in another deeper submucosal pocket. The conchal graft is spread and flattened and lies in a very superficial submucosal pocket. (C) The reverse flap is in place in the deep pocket and lines the cartilage graft. A transmucosal suture holds the flap extremity. (D) Closure of the donor area of the distal aspect of the flap. *(Fig. 136. continues.)*

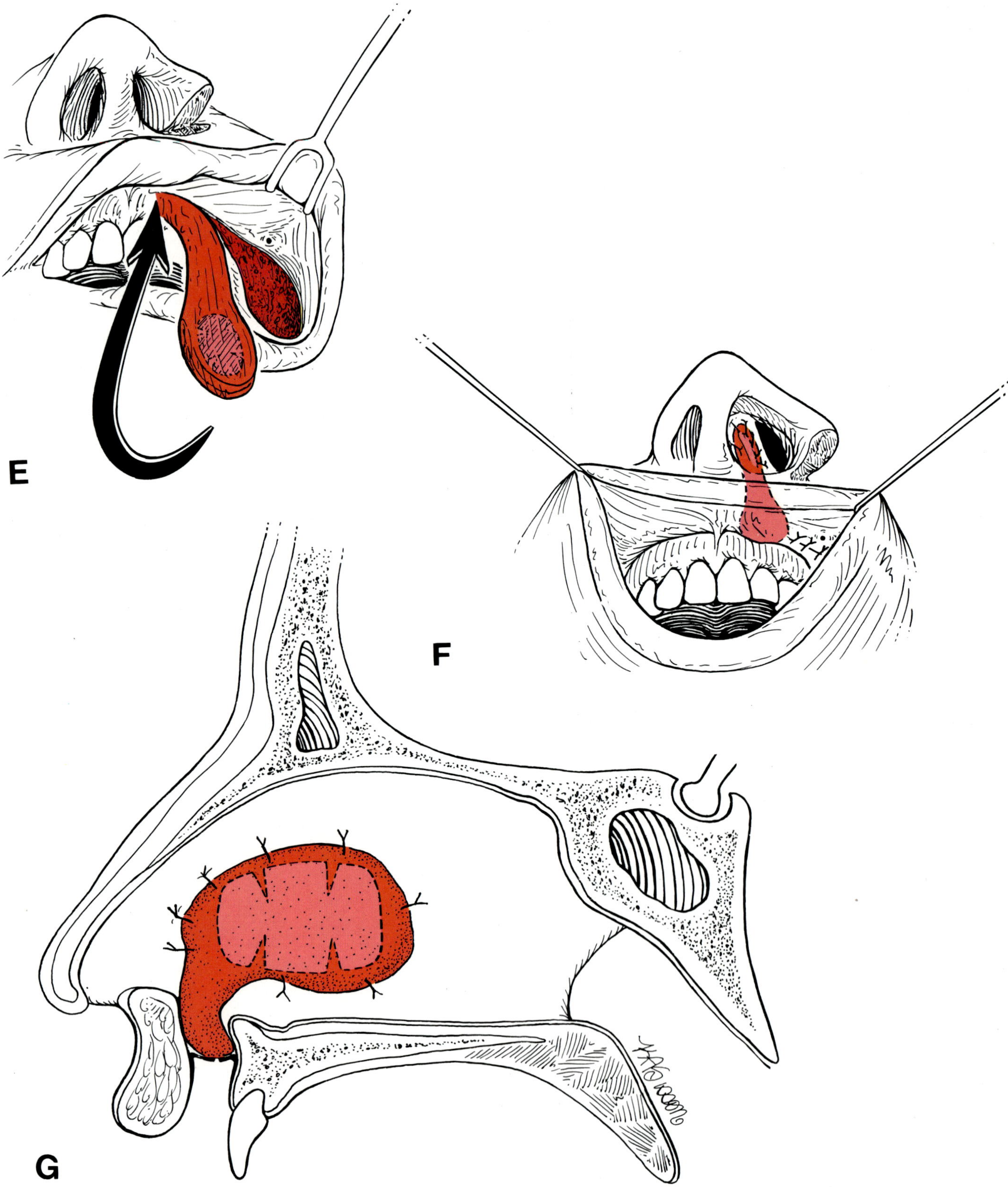

Fig. 136. *(continued)* (E) Second stage of the procedure: The compound flap is mobilized and ready to be introduced into the nasal cavity. (F) Transfer of the flap to the septal defect through a tunnel in the nasal spine. (G) Flap sutured into the septal defect. The pedicle can be discarded in the third stage.

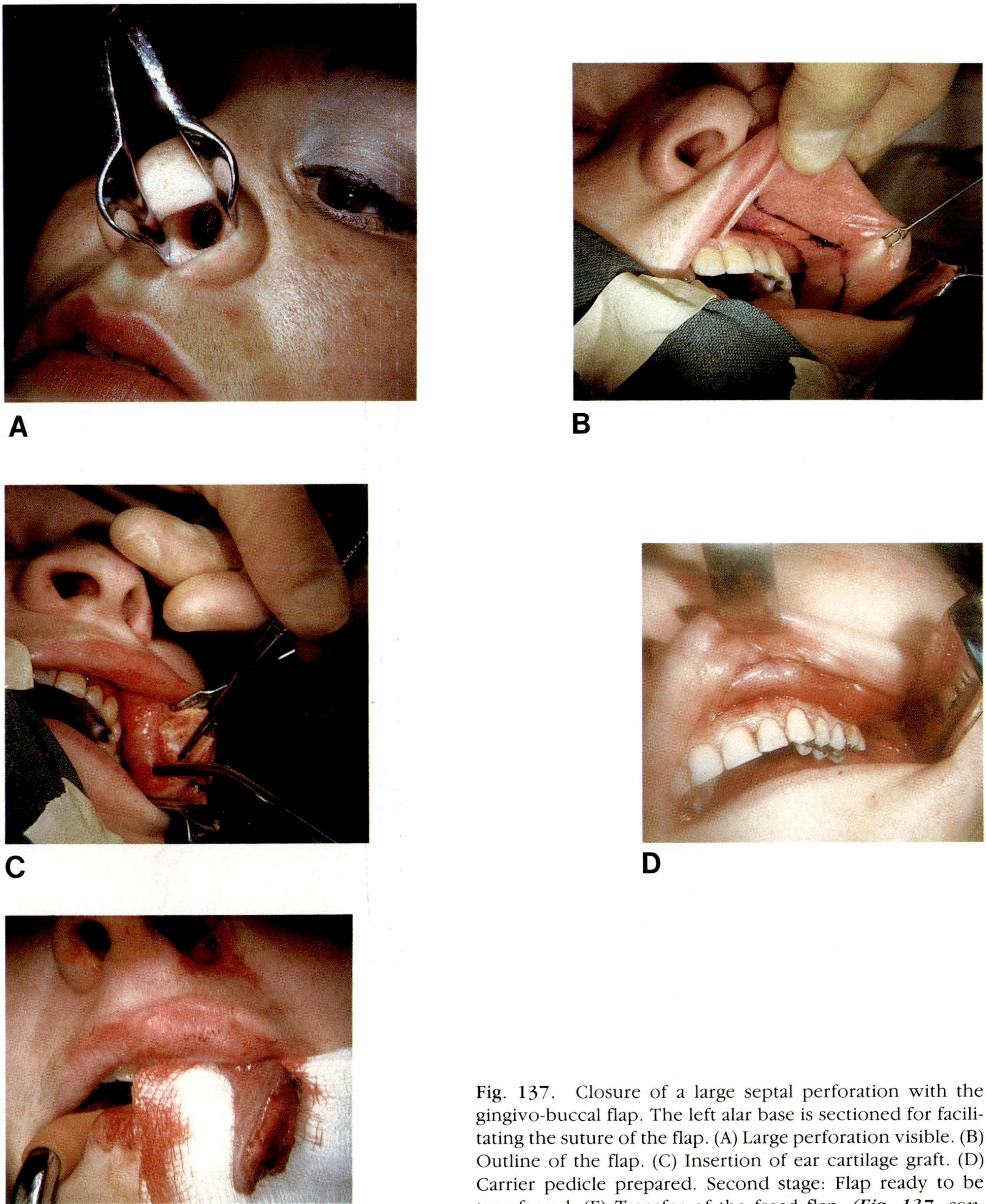

Fig. 137. Closure of a large septal perforation with the gingivo-buccal flap. The left alar base is sectioned for facilitating the suture of the flap. (A) Large perforation visible. (B) Outline of the flap. (C) Insertion of ear cartilage graft. (D) Carrier pedicle prepared. Second stage: Flap ready to be transferred. (E) Transfer of the freed flap. *(Fig. 137. continues.)*

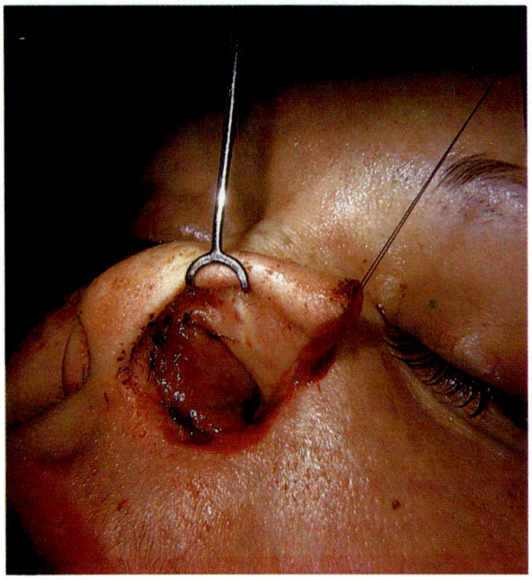

F

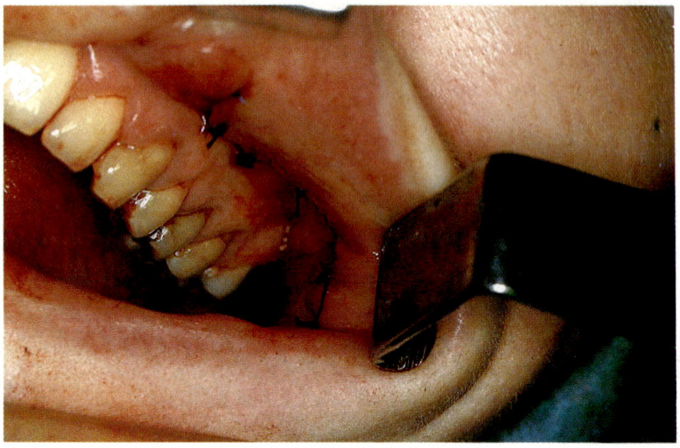

G

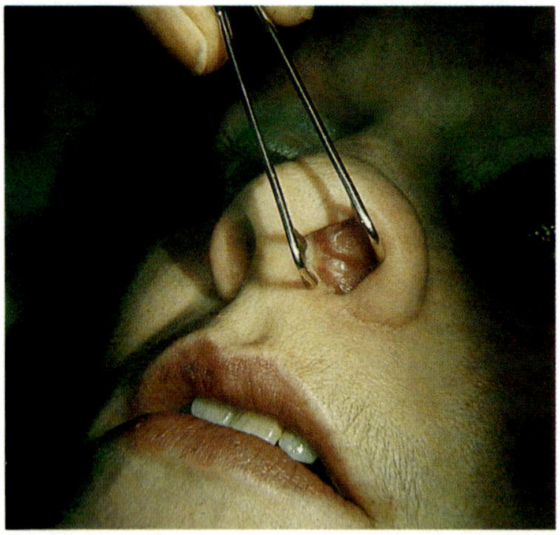

H

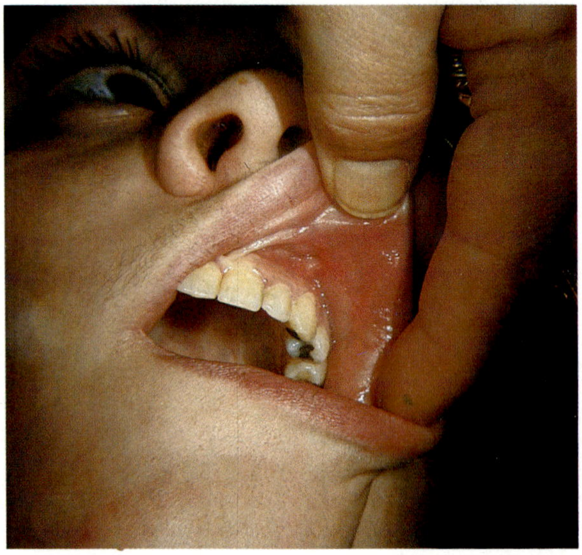

I

Fig. 137. *(continued)* (F) Flap sutured to the septal defect. (G) Base of the pedicle can be left in place. (H) Result after defatting of the flap. (I) Donor area without retraction of the upper lip.

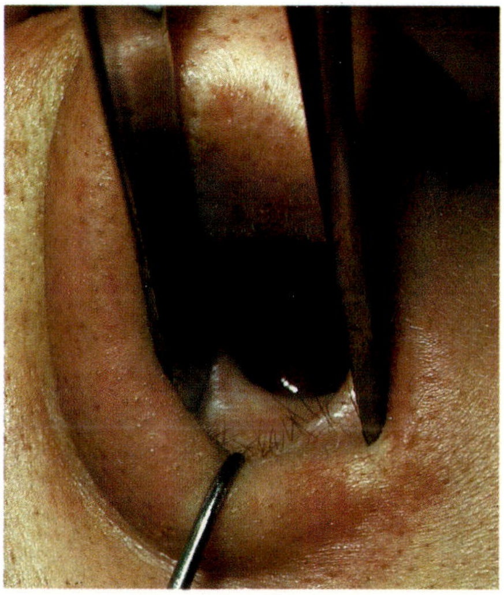

A

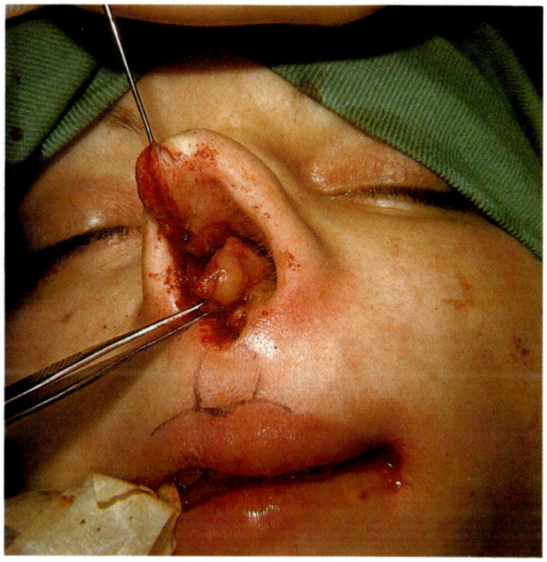

B

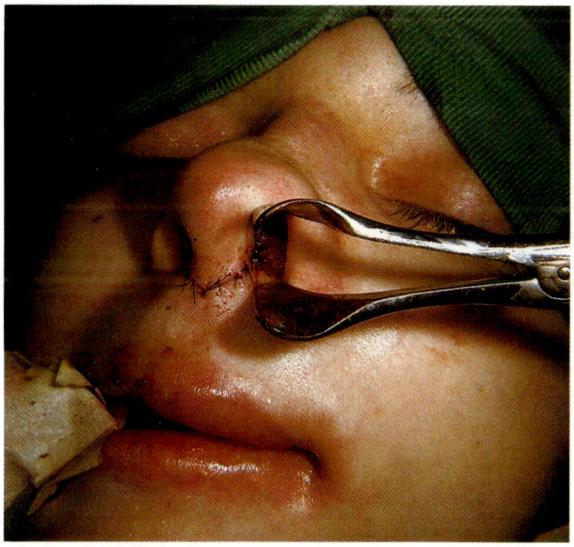

C

Fig. 138. Closure of a large septal perforation with the same flap. The columella and the anterior part of the septum are sectioned at the base until the perforation and elevated in order to provide an open access for suturing the flap into the perforation. (A) Perforation before closure. (B) Open procedure for suturing the flap into the anterior perforation. (C) Suture of the columella into the former position.

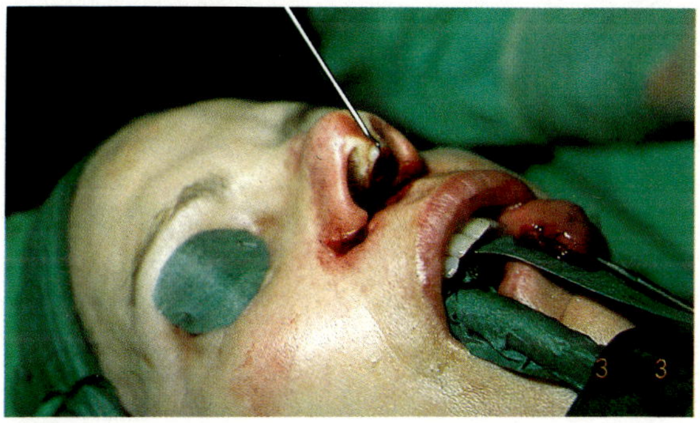

A

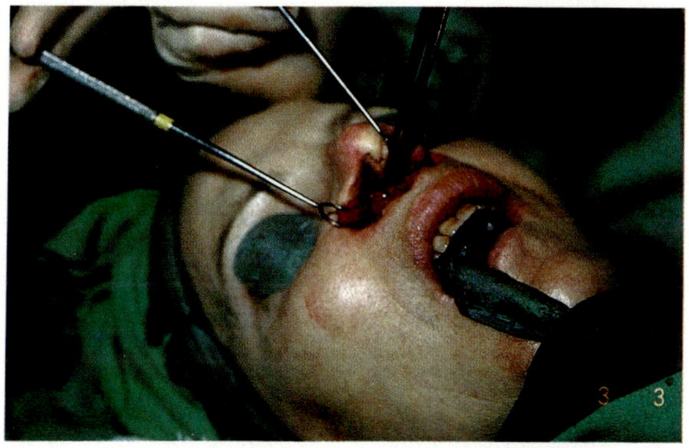

B

Fig. 139. For huge perforation and a corresponding large flap the access is consequently enlarged with columellar base section and bilateral alotomy. (A and B) Transfer of the flap.

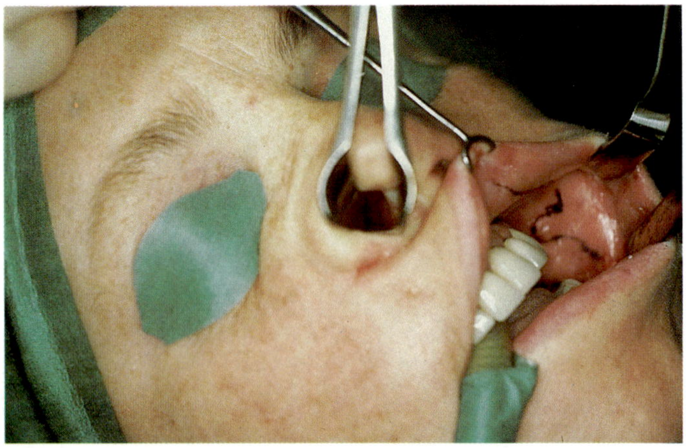
A

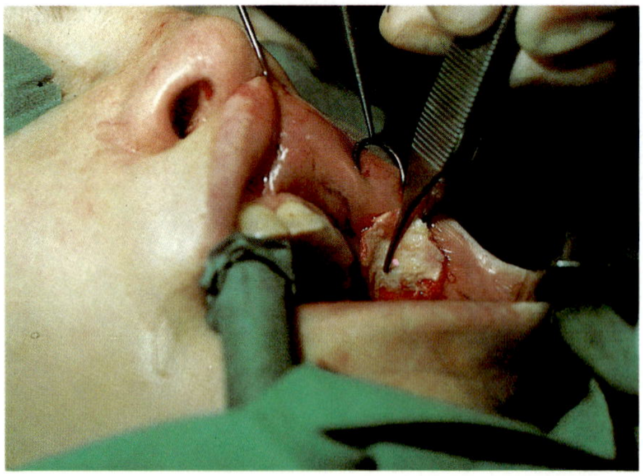
B

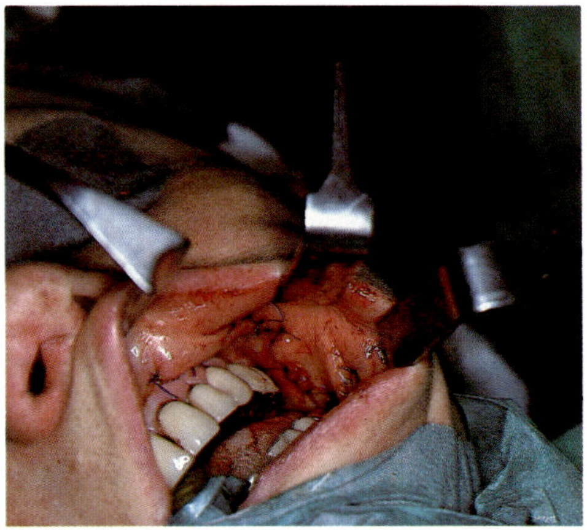
C

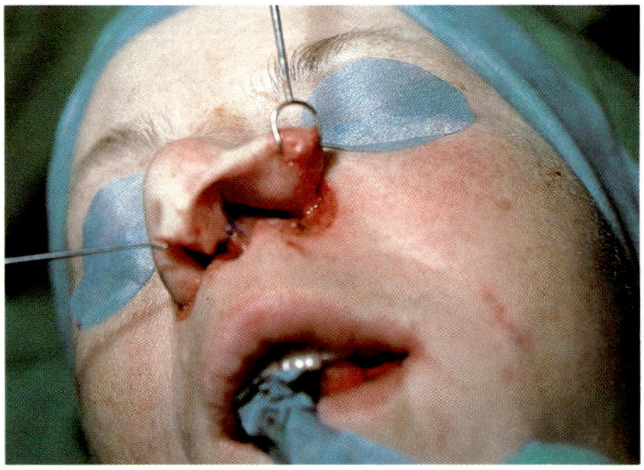
D

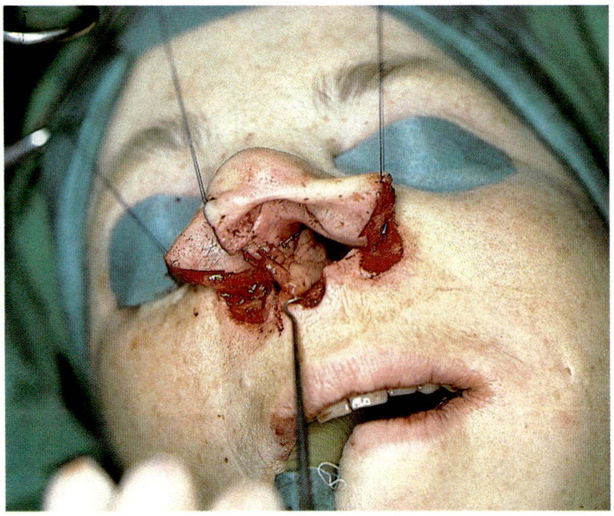
E

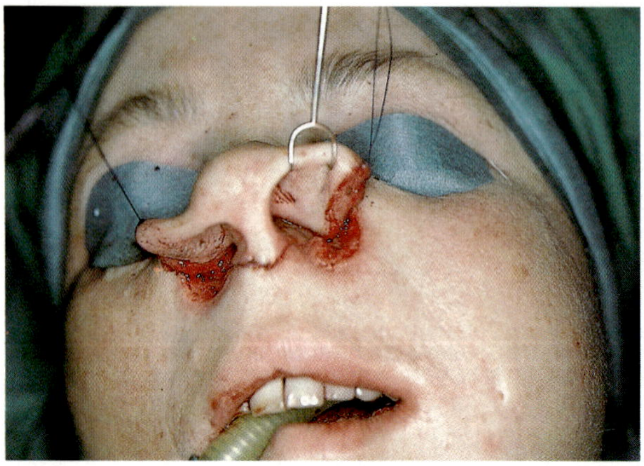
F

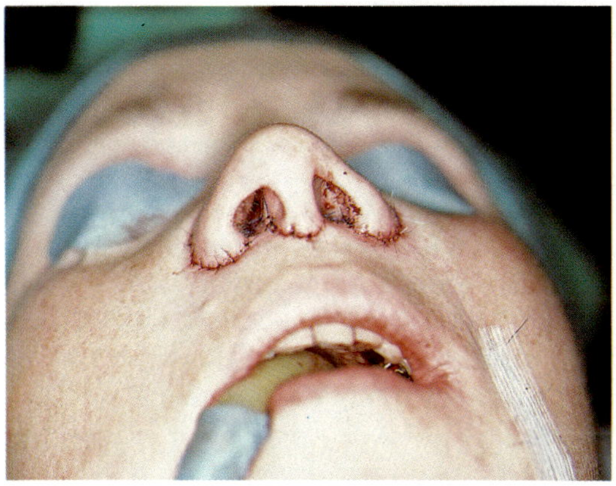

G

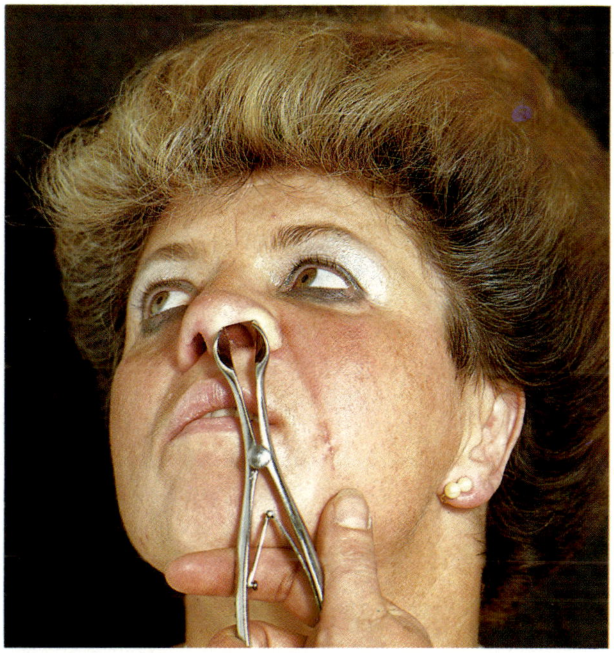

H

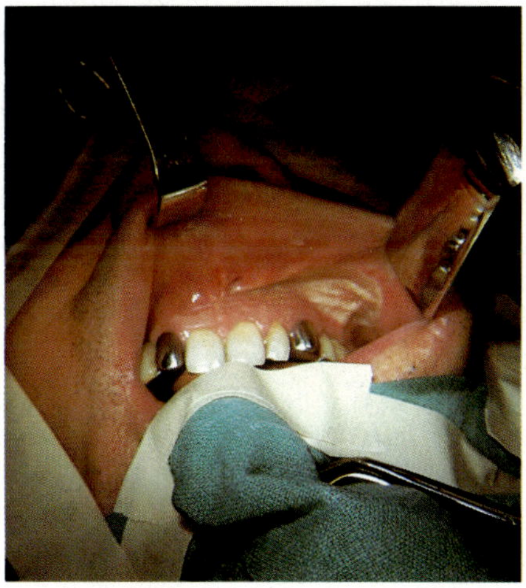

I

Fig. 140. Closure of an extremely large septal perforation including the whole cartilaginous portion and a great part of the bony septum. (A) Perforation before closure. (B) Large cartilage graft inserted into the jaw. (C) End of the first stage. Flap prepared and sutured in the gingivolabial area. (D) Transfer of the flap at the second stage. (E) The flap moves into the cavity to be sutured to the borders of the defect. (F) Closure of the alotomy wounds and suture of the septocolumellar pillar. (G) End of the second stage. (H) Closed perforation. (I) In exceptional cases the donor area can be covered by a split skin graft as shown here or by mucosal graft from the opposite buccal area.

In some cases the third stage has not been necessary due to the postoperative shrinking of the pedicle in and above the premaxillary tunnel. Karlan, Ossof, and Christu (1982) are using our buccal flap, recommending as well the transoral approach to the nose for mucoperichondrial dissection. This could be helpful for defects at the base of the septum, but, we believe it would not be sufficient for managing the meticulous dissection of the mucoperichondrium, in a more superoanteriorly placed large perforation. We prefer to open an oronasal tunnel only for passing the flap. There is practically no danger of oronasal fistula formation.

Hirshowitz et al (1978) successfully treated a case of Osler-Weber-Rendu disease with an anterior septal perforation of middle size and with epistaxis, using the bilateral buccal flap without cartilaginous reinforcement. The patient had already undergone several unsuccessful local interventions that included electrocauterization and silver nitrate applications and tamponade attempts, which are the common methods of conservative treatment for this hereditary systemic disorder. None of these methods cure this old disease, which is characterized by hemorrhages from epithelial telangiectasia, so recurrences and failures are reported frequently and in many cases septal perforation may result. A well-known surgical treatment is the replacement of the telangiectatic mucosa in the nasal cavity with split skin graft, after Saunders (1960). This has to be done before the cartilage begins to necrose. We have had the opportunity to apply a buccal mucosa graft to the area of Kiesselbach in cases of Osler disease. Fry (1967) has reported successful results using the Argon Laser.

In general, mucosa grafting into the nasal cavity is better tolerated than skin grafting because the skin tends to smell in a nose already affected with dryness. In some cases of endonasal reconstruction we have had to replace dry skin with a mucosal graft from the cheek.

SEPTOCOLUMELLAR RECONSTRUCTION

The term reconstruction should be applied only for real repair in case of tissue loss and not for reconstitution of a straight septum by septoplasty (see Chapter 13). For septal reconstruction our buccal flap can be used in conjunction with a frontotemporal flap for cases of subtotal loss of septum. The frontotemporal flap finds its best indication in septocolumellar repair. The columella and the septum are the most difficult parts of the nose to reconstruct. Cartilage supported tongue flaps (Schmid, 1976), arm flaps (Jacobs, 1984), and cheek flaps (Ellis and Le Liever, 1981; Matton and Beck, 1985) are not versatile and sophisticated enough to be modeled to conform to the fine shape of the apicocolumellar structures. For this purpose we advocated in 1968 the use of a frontotemporal flap that was already in use by us for other kinds of reconstructions ever since 1963 (Meyer 1963, 1964, 1972, 1977, and 1981). In our hands it gives very good aesthetic results in the partial and even subtotal repair of the nose and for orbital-palpebral reconstructions. It is particularly advised for the rebuilding of fine structures of the nose such as the tip and the alae (Fig. 120).

For those situations of septocolumellar loss of tissue we do not know of any other technique as valuable as the frontotemporal flap. The original technique described by Schmid and Widmajer (1961) for alar repair has been refined by us for special usage in apicocolumellar and septocolumellar reconstructions (Meyer and Kesselring 1981). The septocolumellar repair flap is cut in the frontotemporal region and is composed of a bipedicle carrier flap at the upper border of the eyebrow and a rectangular flap at the temple. This temporal component, which joins the lateral pedicle of the bridge flap, is lined by a mucosal graft and carries a cartilage graft from the ear concha. At the first stage the superciliary carrier flap is cut as a skin strip 5 mm in width with the incision beveled outward to include a greater width of subcutaneous tissue. This subcutaneous layer is backed by a strip of split skin that is carefully sutured to both the skin edges of the flap. The donor defect of the bipedicled limb is closed by pulling down the mobilized skin of the forehead. At the same time we form a superficial subcutaneous pocket in the temporal region through an incision at the lateral orbital rim and we place the auricular graft into the pocket. Through a second incision, near the temporal hair-bearing skin, we dissect a second pocket in a deeper subdermal layer of the skin. This pocket, which does not communicate with the first one, is partially lined with a mucosal graft from the cheek, leaving the deeper raw surface only covered with gauze. The edges of the graft are sutured to the incision. At a second stage 3–4 weeks later, the rectangular temporal flap composed of three layers, skin cartilage and mucosa, is transferred to the septocolumellar defect by means of the superciliary carrier flap (Figs. 141 and 142). To facilitate the suturing of the rectangular flap, and the modeling of the tip, columella, and septum in the proper position, we usually have to open the vestibule by using a wide basal alatomy or a paramedian dorsal incision. Both external layers of the flap, the muco-

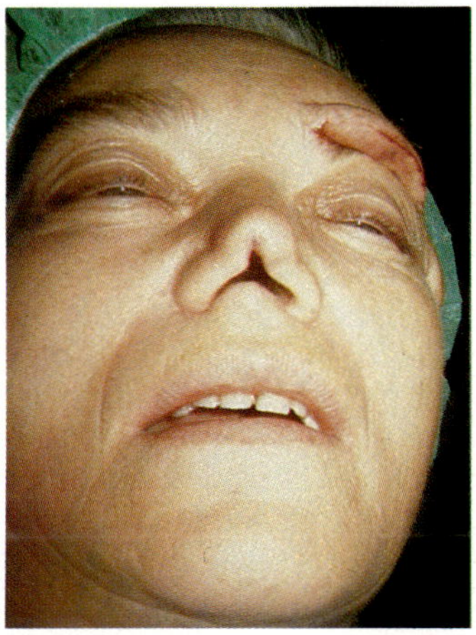

A

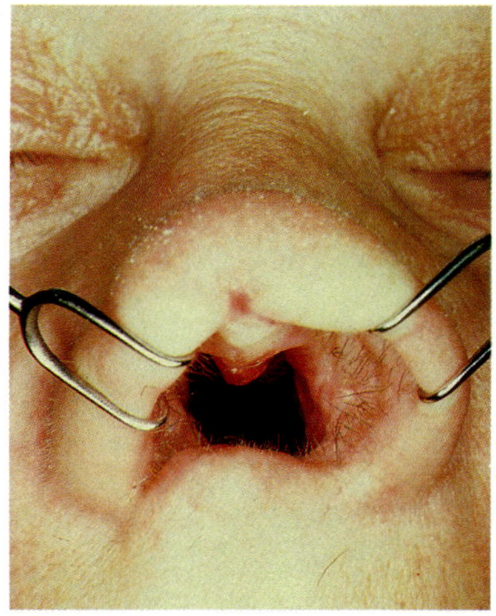

B

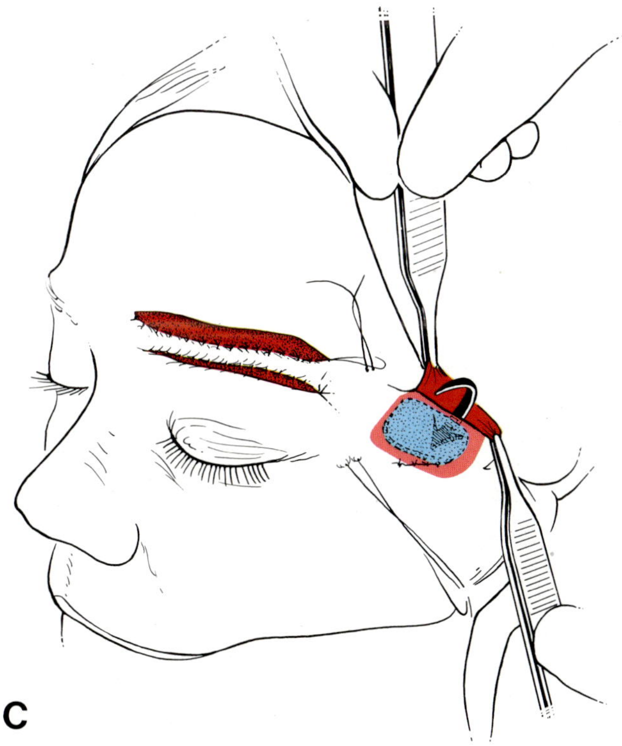

C

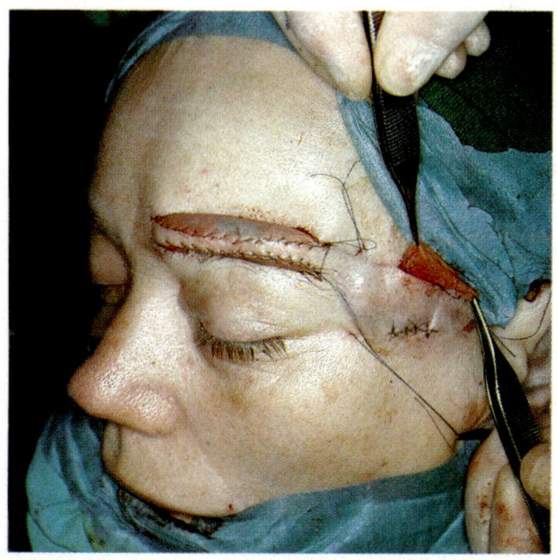

D

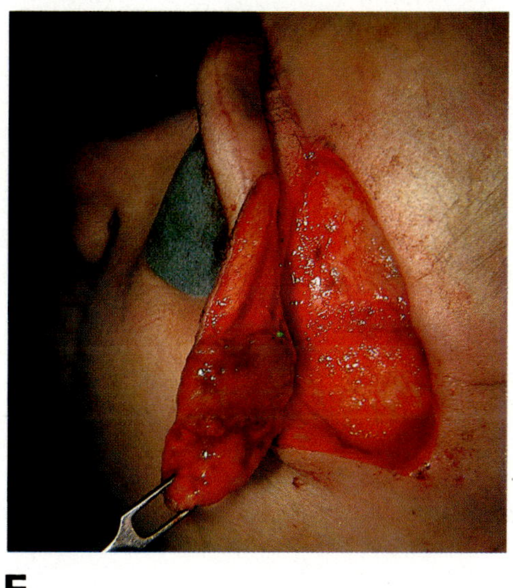

E

Fig. 141. Reconstruction of a septocolumellar defect with temporal flap. (A and B) Middle-aged woman after selfmutilation with a defect including the tip, the columella, and 2/3 of the septum. (C, D, and E) End of the first stage. The pedicle is formed at the supraorbital arch and covered with split thickness skin graft. A buccal mucosal graft is inserted into a deep pocket at the temporal compound extremity of the flap. A cartilage graft has already been introduced in a very superficial subcutaneous pocket. *(Fig. 141. continues.)*

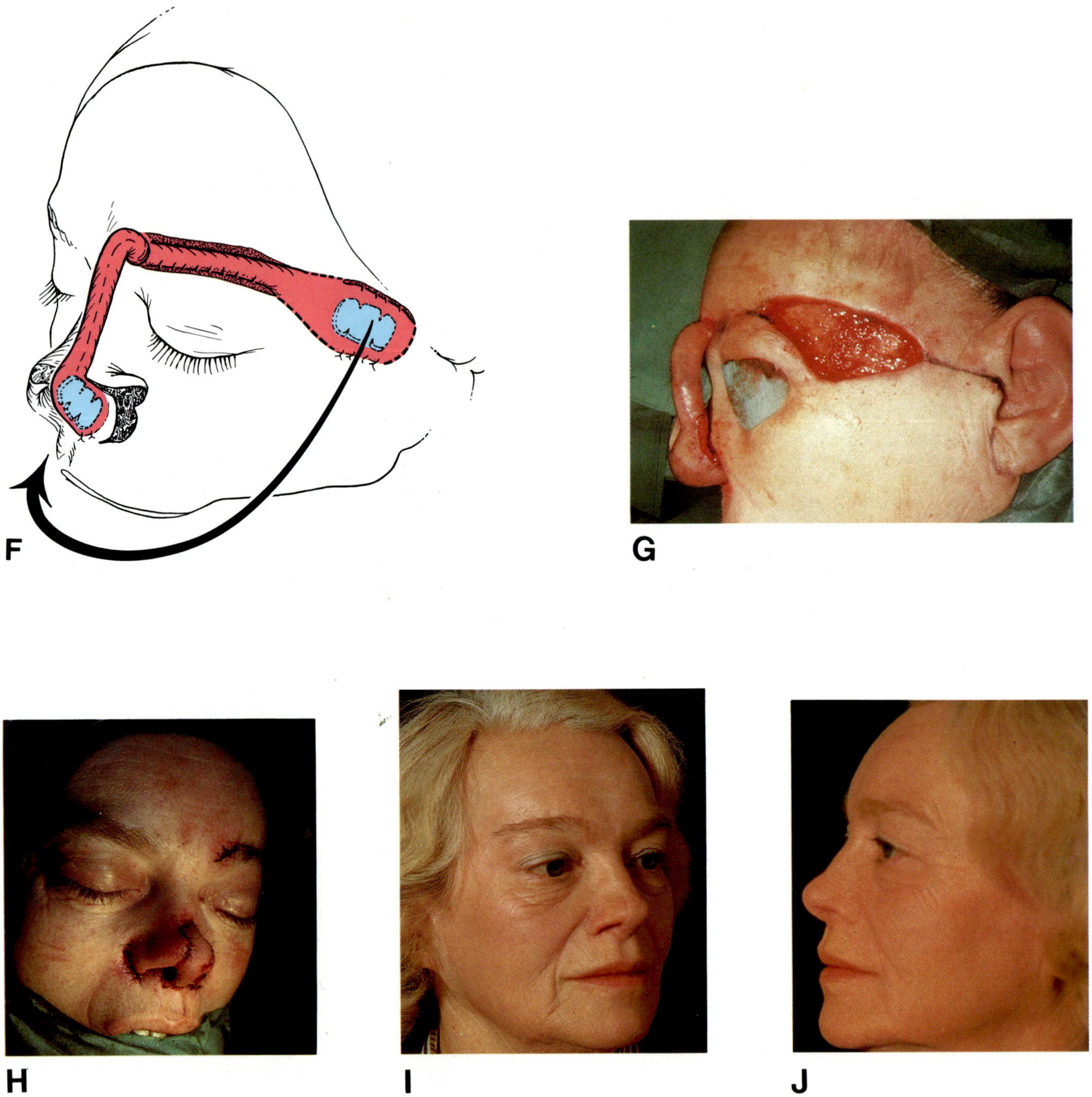

Fig. 141. *(continued)* (F and G) Second stage. Transfer of the flap into the septocolumellar defect for facilitating the sutures in the nasal cavity as the left alar base is sectioned. (H) End of the third stage after dissection of the carrier pedicle. (I and J) Final result after defatting of the flap in the nose and refinement at the alar border.

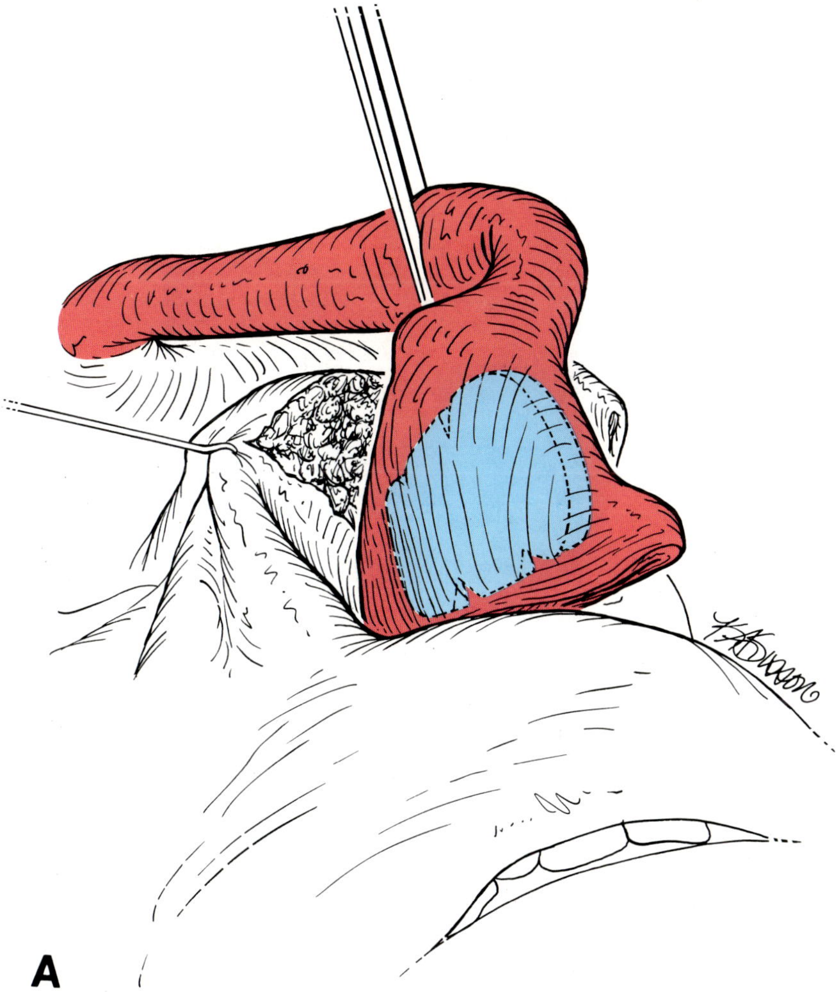

A

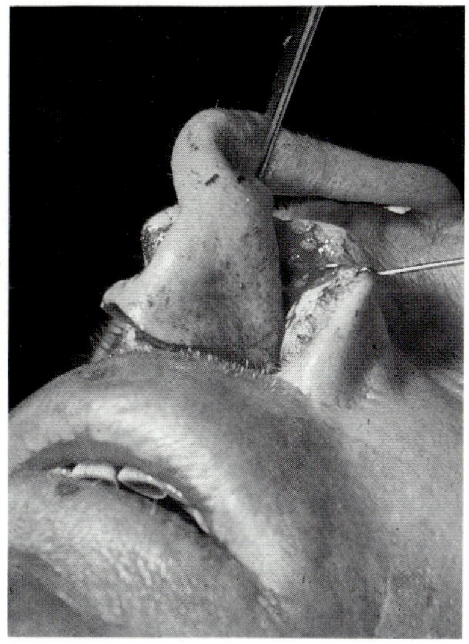

B

Fig. 142. (A and B) Transfer of a frontotemporal flap into a septocolumellar defect.

sal and the cutaneous, are meticulously sutured to the freshened edges of the internal septonasal defect. After another 3 or 4 weeks, at the third stage, the nourishing bridge flap is divided at its proximal and distal ends and the septal part of the inserted flap can be thinned. Using this procedure of the composite flap, we have been able to rebuild the anterior half of the septum together with the columella and at least a part of the tip in several traumatic cases (Fig. 141). One case concerned a congenital loss of the tip (Fig. 143), the columella, and the anterior third of the septum. A few cases of septal and septocolumellar reconstruction resulted after tumor extirpation (Figs. 144 and 145). Malignant tumors of the septum are rare, reflected by the few cases reported in the literature. Most of these tumors are epidermoid carcinomas: the second most common histologically being melanomas. Unless diagnosed and treated early, these tumors are lethal. The therapy is a wide surgical excision and postoperative irradiation. Surgical considerations must primarily include adequate excision of the tumor followed by functional and aesthetic restoration as has been stated by McGuirt and Thomson (1984).

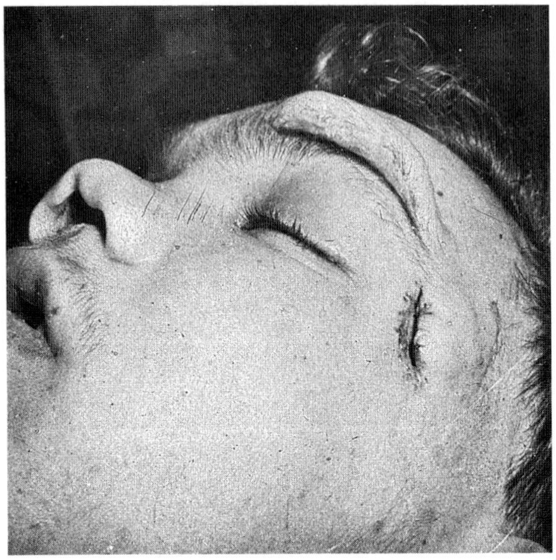

A

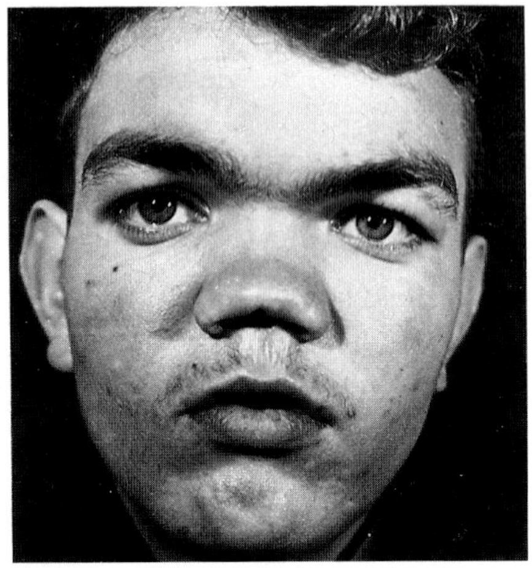

B

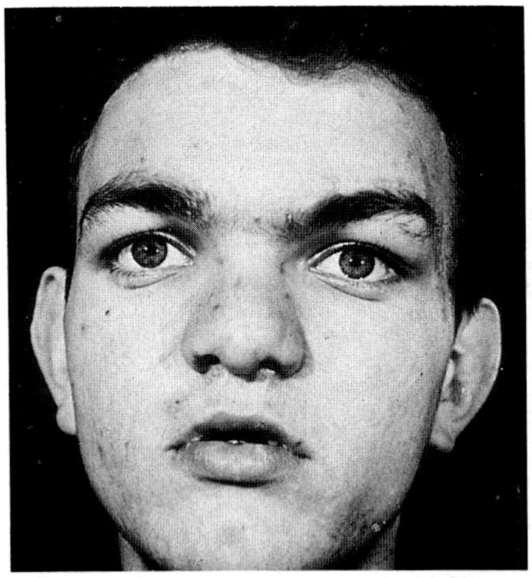

C

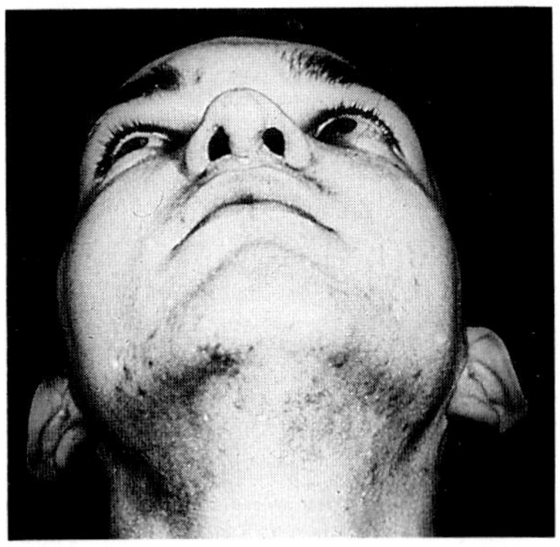

D

Fig. 143. Septocolumellar reconstruction with frontotemporal flap in a case of congenital loss of tip columella and anterior third of the septum. (A) Frontotemporal flap before second stage. (B) Preoperative front view. (C) Postoperative front view. (D) Postoperative axial view.

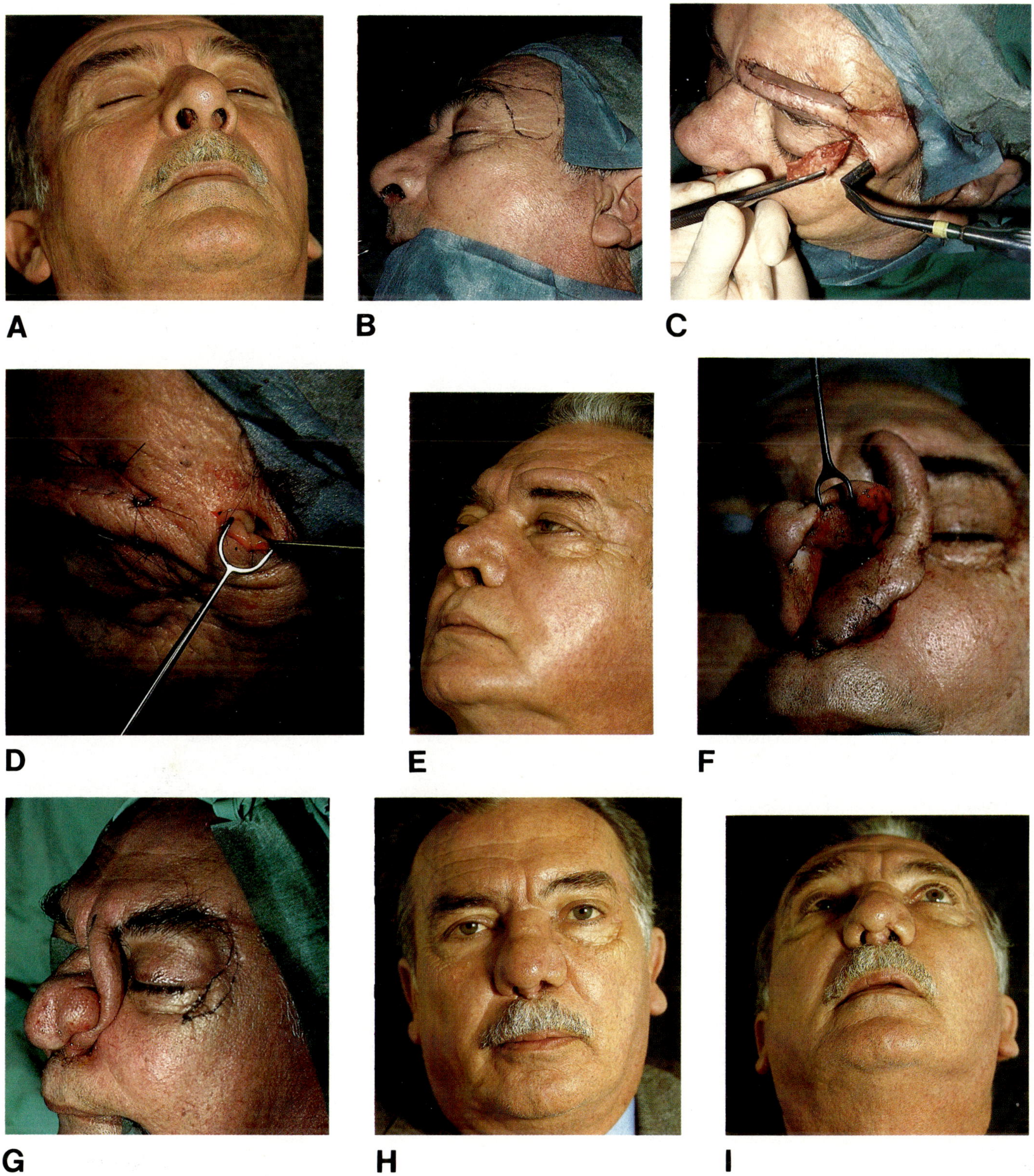

Fig. 144. Sixty-five-year-old man with carcinoma of septum. (A) Patient before removal of the entire septum. (B) First stage of septocolumellar reconstruction at the time of tumor removal. Outline of the flap. (C) Insertion of cartiliage graft in superficial pocket. (D) Deep pocket at the temple is lined with buccal mucosa. (E) Patient before second stage. Flap ready for transferring. (F) Second stage : transfer of the flap into the total septal defect. (G) Beginning of the third stage. The carrier flap will be removed. A secondary correction in the donor area is outlined. (H and I) Acceptable aesthetic and functional result.

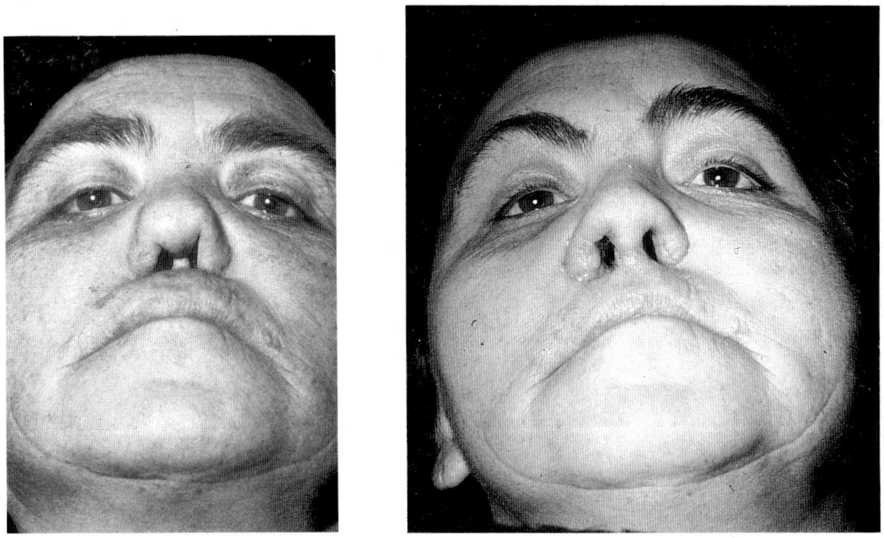

Fig. 145. Septocolumellar reconstruction with frontotemporal flap after tumor removal. (A) Preoperative axial view. (B) Postoperative axial view.

15

Residual Deformities of the Columella

GENERALITIES (BALANCED COLUMELLA, DOUBLE ANGLE)

Columellaplasty is an important procedure in rhinoplasty. We can alter the length, width, shape, and prominence of the columella as well as the angle between the nose and the upper lip. There are many structures involved, including the medial crura of the lower lateral cartilages, the septal cartilage, the anterior maxillary spine, the fibrous tissue supporting these cartilages, and finally the muscles of the base of the nose.

During rhinoplasty the nasal spine can be exposed and reshaped by carving with the Rowland or Kazanjian forceps by drilling, as Stocksted and Gutierrez (1982) have shown.

Residual deformities of the columella can be of varying degree and presenting varying challenges for their secondary surgical correction. The straight columella profile does not correspond to the aesthetic profile we wish. To reshape it in a more harmonious way, we have to create an obtuse angle between the anterosuperior third and the inferior two-thirds of the columella, by inserting a small graft of cartilage (Figs. 146 and 147). This onlay is made of one or more pieces of the lower lateral cartilage or of the septal cartilage, previously morselized to avoid sharp prominences. If one does not pay attention to the balance of the nose when performing a secondary rhinoplasty, previous disproportion can appear more evident postoperatively. It can happen that an attractive nose with a well-shaped tip shows too long a columella which remains after revision. To correct this resulting deformity and restore a well proportioned length we perform a horizontal basal resection instead of sculpturing once again the entire deep tip columella complex (Fig. 148). The sutures located at this new base of the columella are inconspicuous.

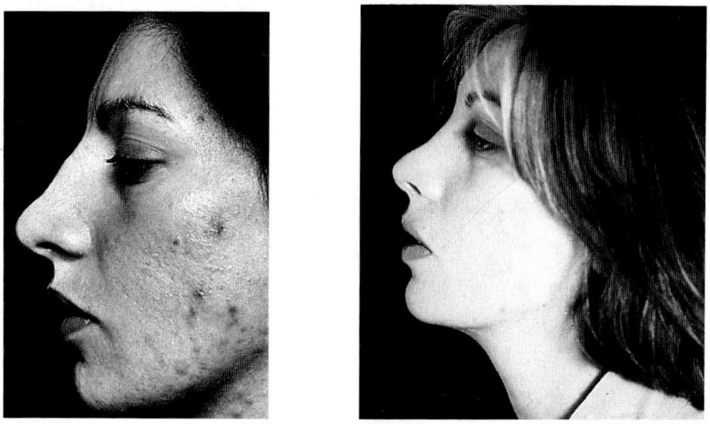

A B

Fig. 146. (A and B) Straight columella profile corrected with midcolumellar onlay.

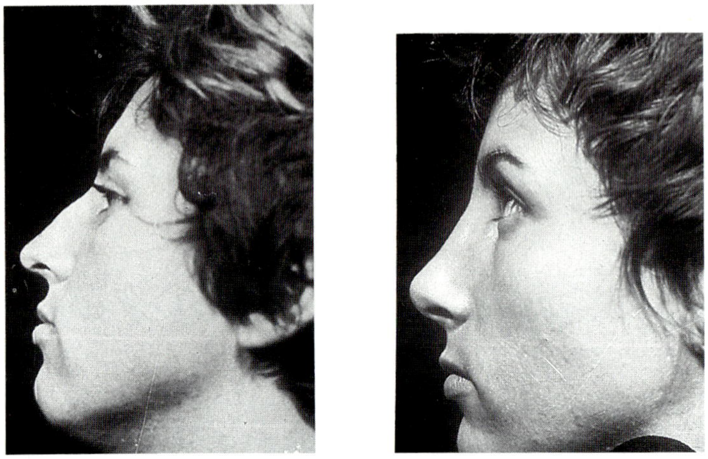

A B

Fig. 147. (A and B) Double-break formation in a similar case.

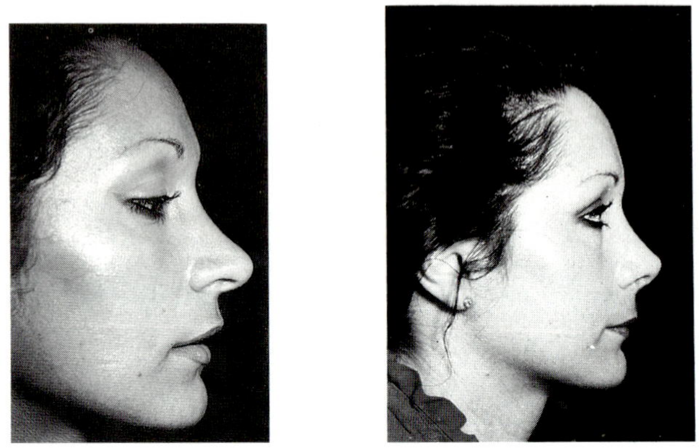

A B

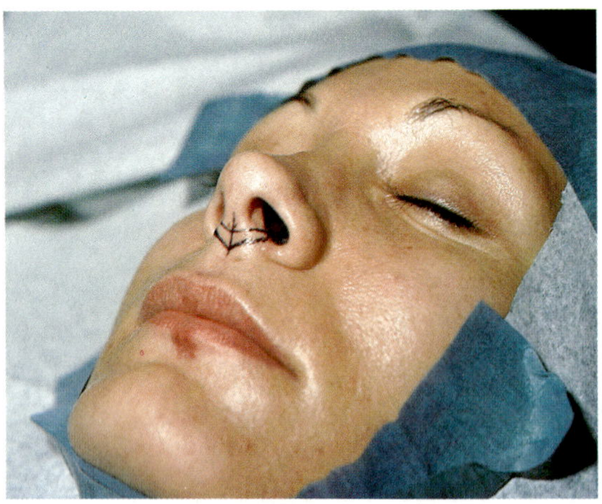

C

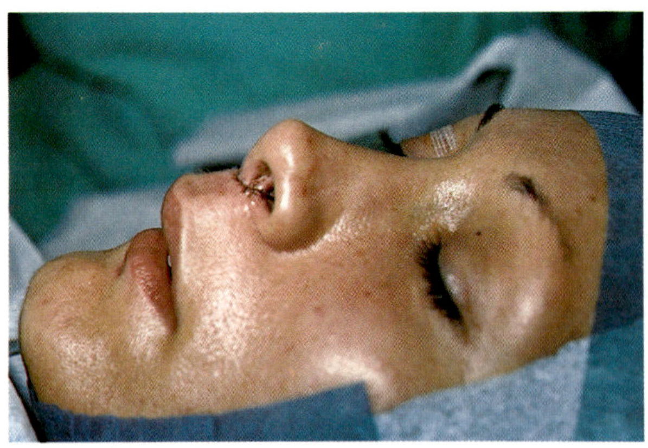

D

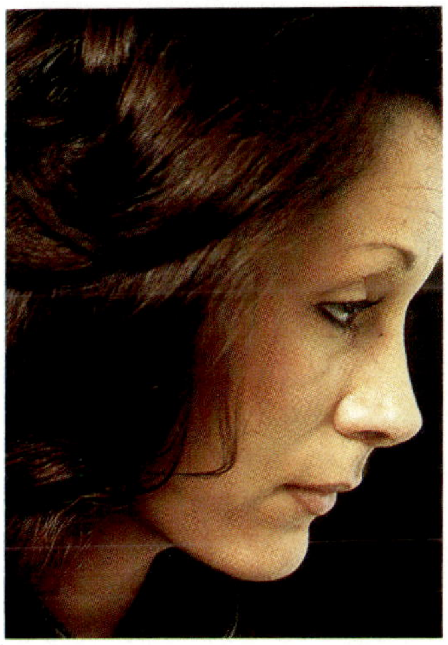

E

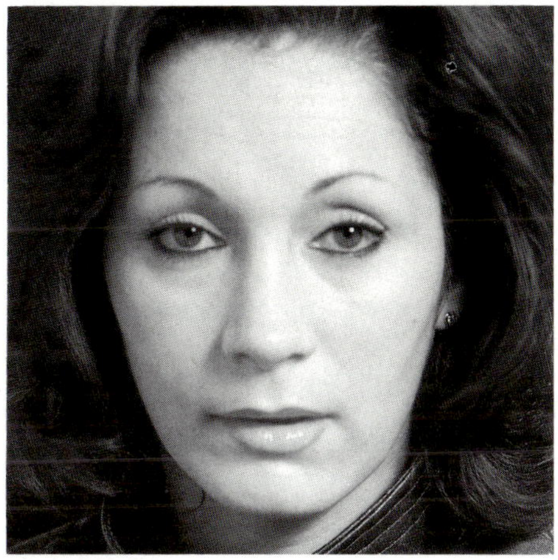

F

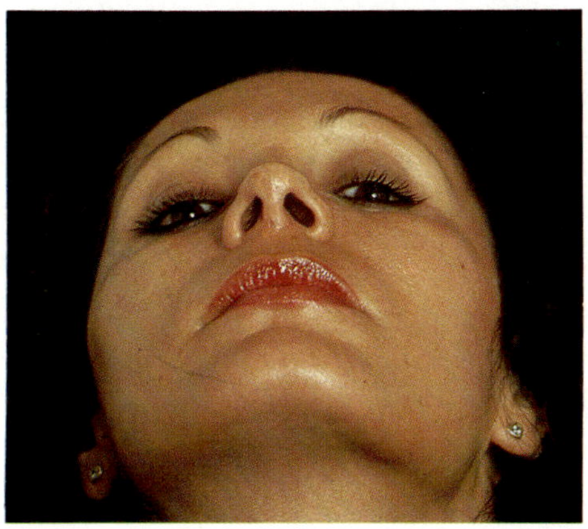

G

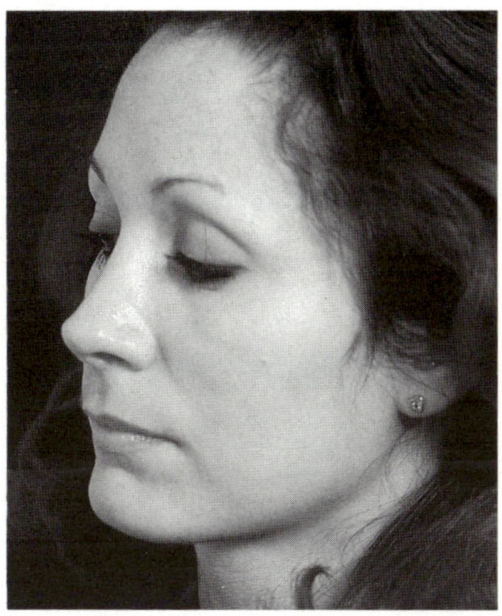

H

Fig. 148. Correction of a too long columella with a basal resection. (A) Young lady with too prominent tip. (B) After the primary reduction of the tip the columella appears too long. (C) Reduction of the columellar length with horizontal resection of a segment at the base, which is outlined. (D) End of the secondary reduction. (E, F, G, and H) Late result.

TOO SHORT COLUMELLA

The opposite situation, of too short columella, can also occur. For correcting this discrepancy one has to choose from several different procedures, depending on the degree and type of shortness. For the more simple cases, the appearance of a longer columella is given by bilateral marginal resection at the ala-columella commissure, at the level of Converse's soft triangle. Over and over sutures close the marginal wound after meticulous cauterization and commissure may result (Fig. 149). Additionally, basal and subvestibular mattress sutures sometimes help to maintain the achieved result (Fig. 150).

The correction of the flat broad nose can be achieved with the Berson's (1943, 1948) method or by using a V-Y advancement procedure. Berson's method consists of reestablishing a normal proportion between the length of the medial and lateral crura. Two mattress sutures, one at the base of the medial crura and the other at the level

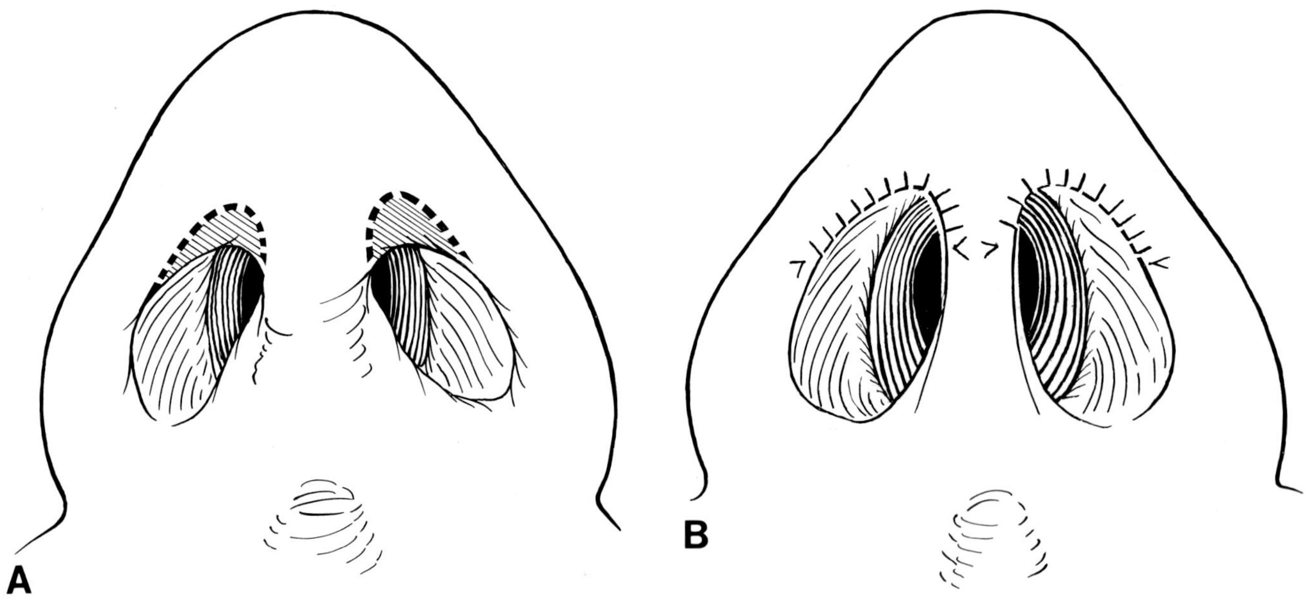

Fig. 149. Too short columella and too high lobule. Columellar elongation using bilateral marginal resection at the ala-columella commissure (soft triangle of Converse). (A) Outline of the resection. (B) Over-and-over suture.

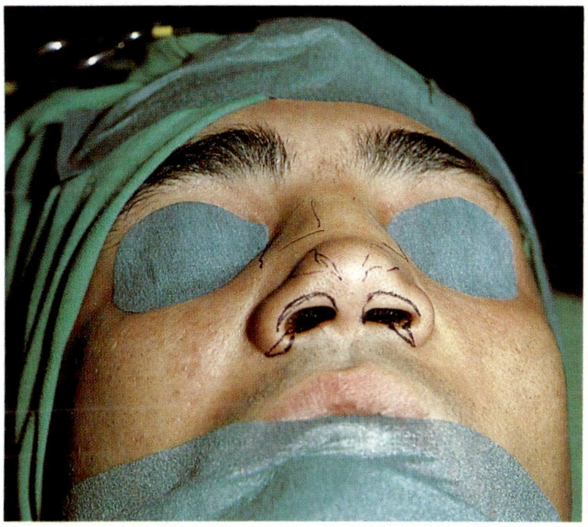

A

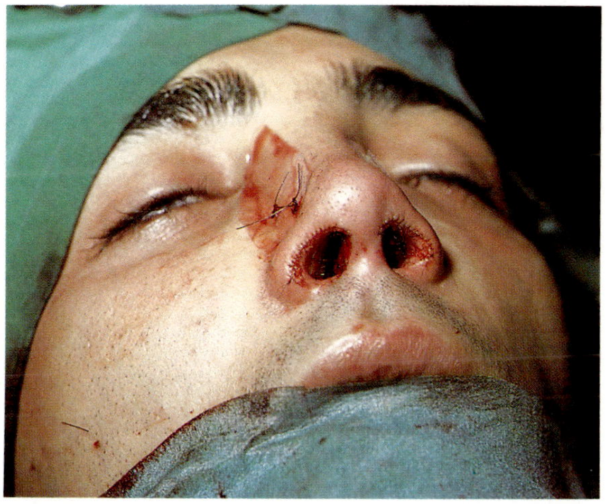

B

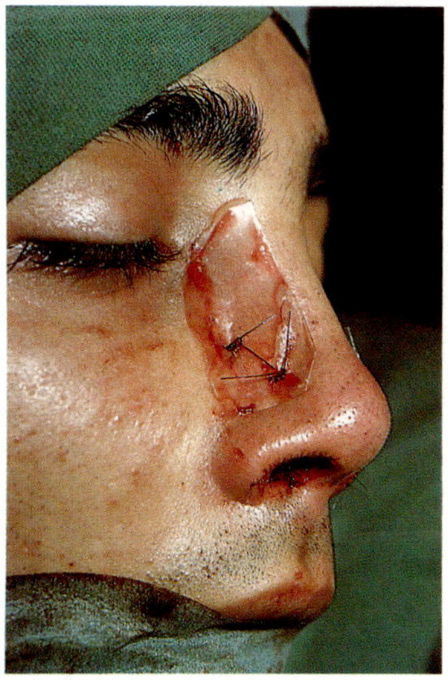

C

Fig. 150. Elongation of the columella by marginal resection as shown in Fig. 149, and by basal and subvestibular mattress sutures. (A) Resections outlined. Resection at the alar base was not necessary. (B and C) End of the operation with resection wound closed by over-and-over sutures. Transnasal mattress sutures in the bony area and middle third of the nose.

of the new dome (Figs. 151 and 152), elongate the columella and narrow the tip at the same time. The V-Y advancement flap at the base of the columella can also be used to increase its length (Fig. 153). In addition, narrowing mattress sutures at the superior part of the medial crura may be necessary for lengthening of the lobule and refining the tip. If this procedure is not sufficient in lengthening the columella, we can add a marginal resection (Fig. 154).

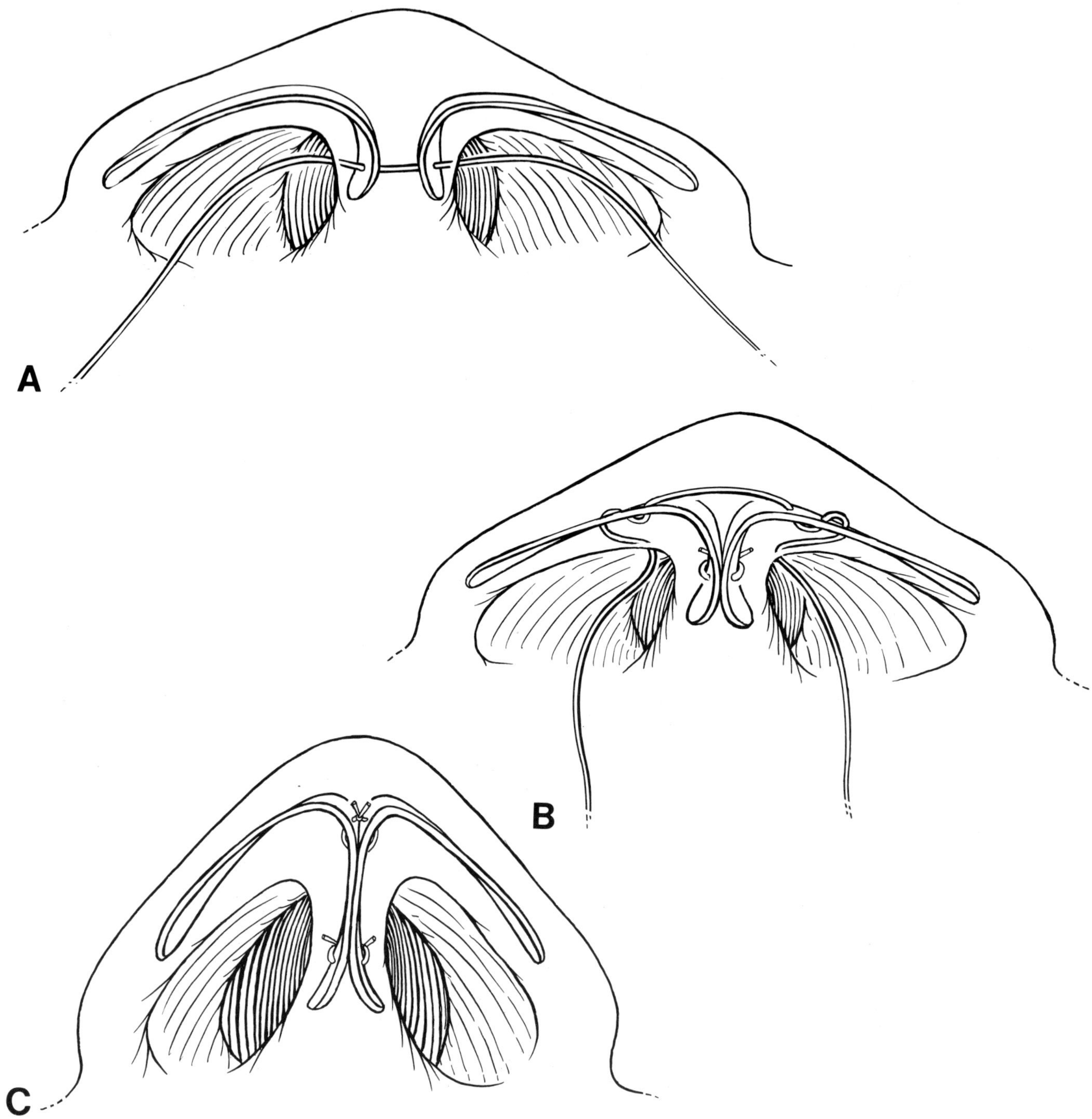

Fig. 151. Elongation of the columella with Berson's method. (A) Flat broad nose with short columella. First mattress sutured through the medial crura of the lower lateral cartilages. (B) Tip narrowing mattress suture elongating the medial crura. (C) Result with elongated columella and narrowed tip. The sutures are knitted under the skin.

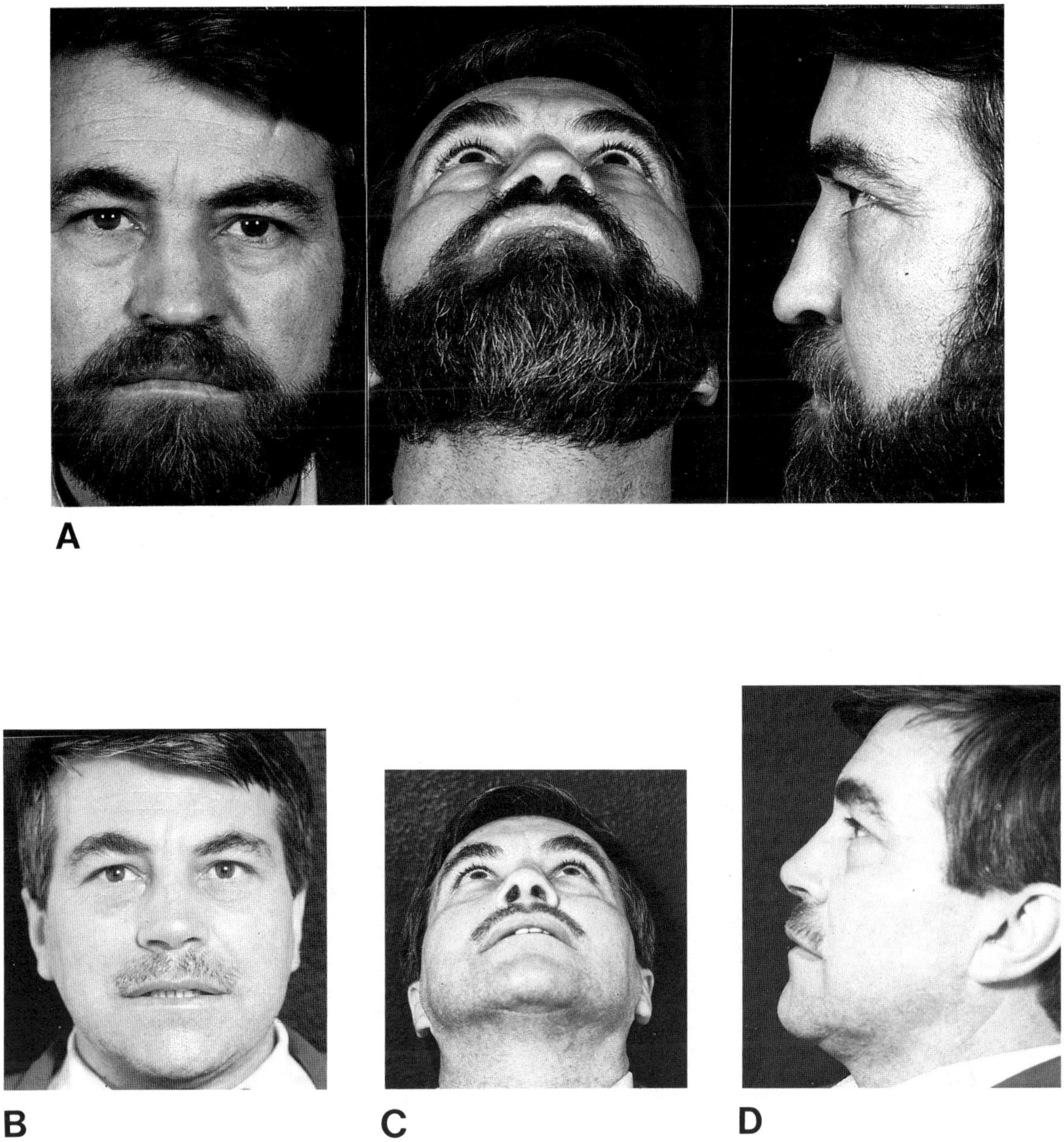

Fig. 152. Flat nose corrected with Berson's method. (A) before and (B, C, and D) after operation.

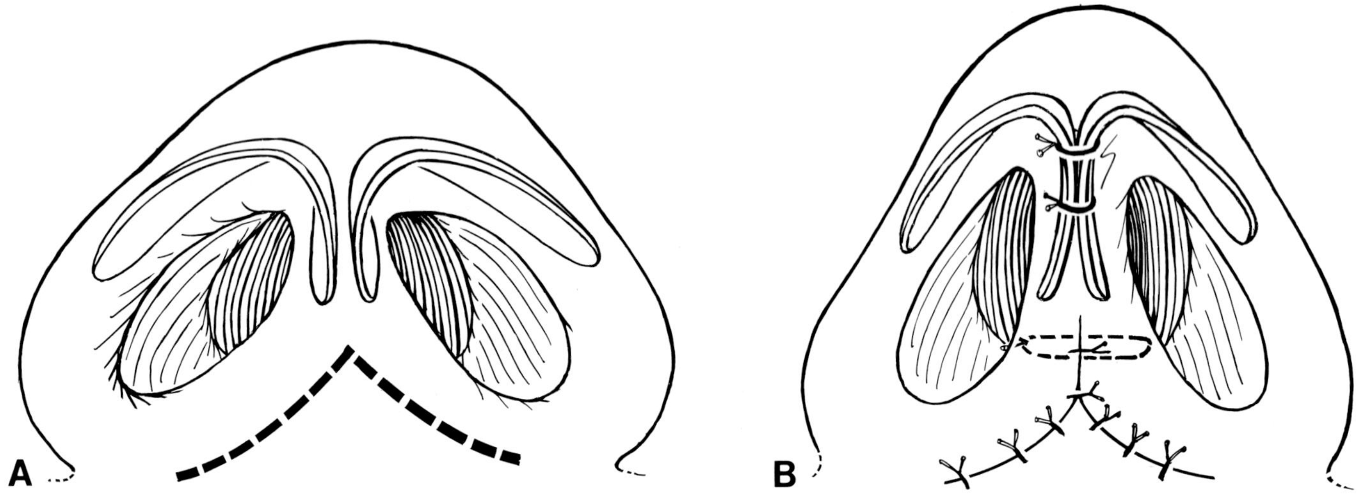

Fig. 153. Flat nose with short columella. Elongation of the columella with mattress sutures through the medial crura of the lower lateral cartilages and with V-Y procedure at the columellar base. (A) V outlined. (B) Y sutured. Transcolumellar mattress suture at the columellar base and narrowing mattress sutures through the anterior part of the medial crura thus lengthening the columella and narrowing the tip.

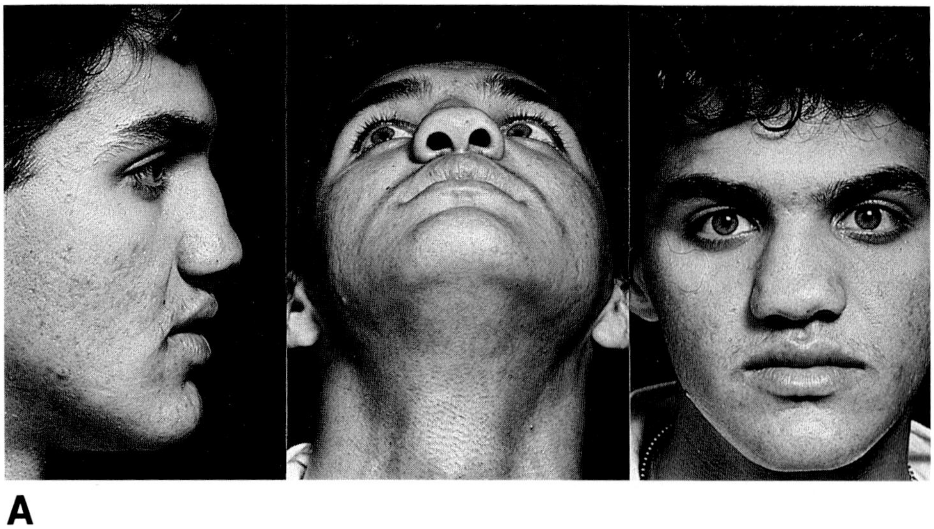

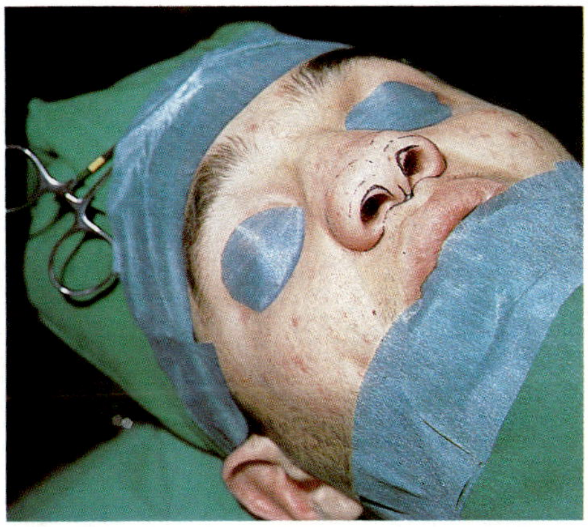

B

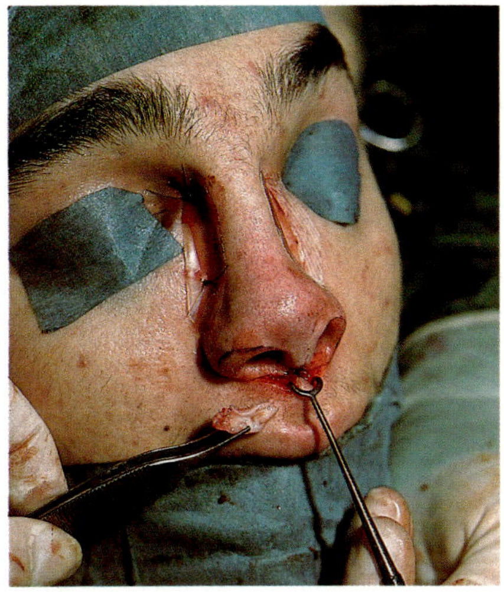

C

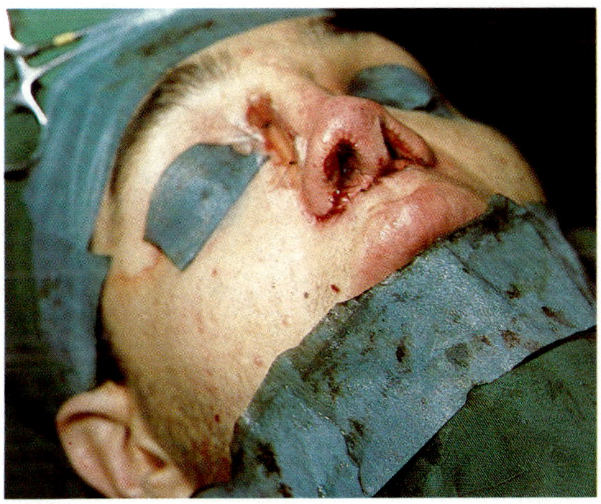

D

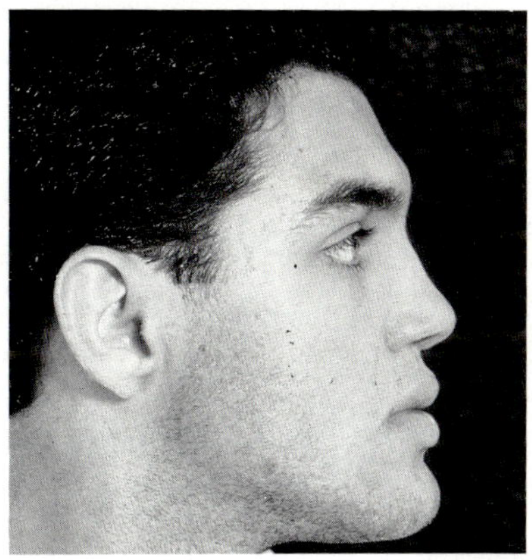

E

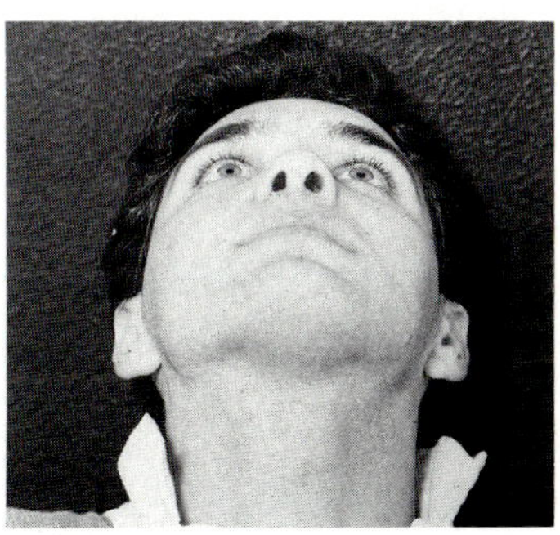

F

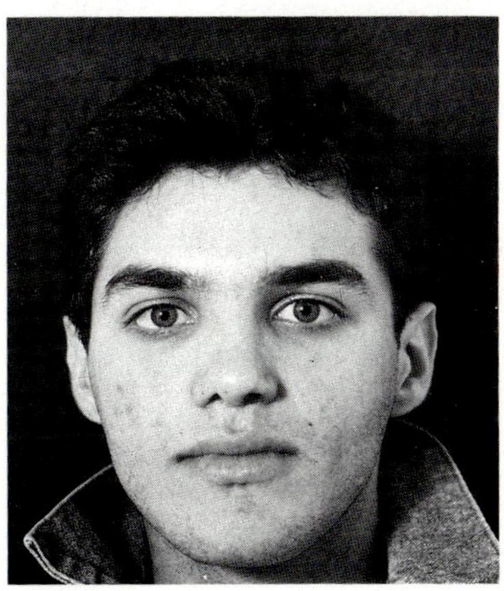

G

Fig. 154. Elongation of the columella in a young man with a thick broad tip and short columella. (A) Preoperative views. (B) Marginal resections at the ala-columellar junction and V-Y technique at the columellar base outlined. (C) Cartilage onlay from the ear concha is about to be inserted at the nasolabial angle. Transnasal mattress sutures for fixation of the narrowed pyramid are tied over plastic sheets. (D) End of the operation—V-Y procedure, columella alar border, and inner wedge resection at the alar base sutured. (E, F, and G) Result.

If there is no retrusion of the nasolabial angle we can provide additional length to the columella with a V-Y plasty at the upper part of the philtrum as was done for cases of Binder syndrome (Fig. 155). The lateral incisions of the small flaps outlined on both sides of the philtral crease join the transfixion incision bilaterally at the columellar base. The fish-tail shaped flap is elevated together with the anteriorly-superiorly based columella flap and then the two ends of the flaps are sutured together, obtaining a reverse Y. In this way, 3–5 mm of columellar length can be gained. However, by suturing the labial skin on both sides of the philtrum the lip tends to become narrowed and retracted at the nasolabial angle, so that this procedure is not indicated in cases where this angle is already retruded. An extension of this technique is the forked flap discussed on page 305 (see Fig. 252).

A further elongation procedure we use consists of transplanting an ear conchal composite graft (see Fig. 216). Only in exceptional cases the columella can be lengthened using an island flap from an abnormally broad dorsum as Edgerton advocated in 1967.

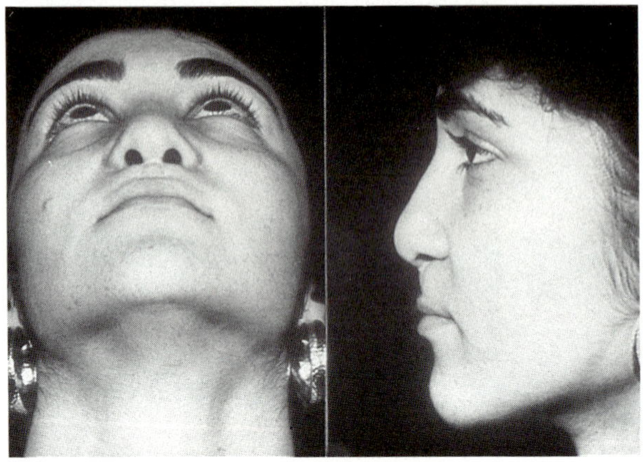

A

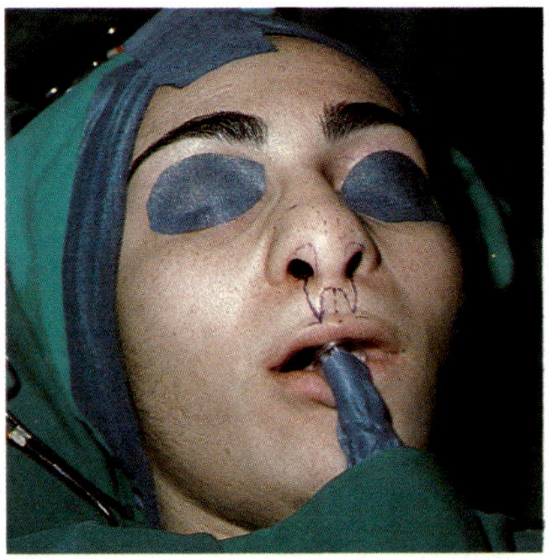

B

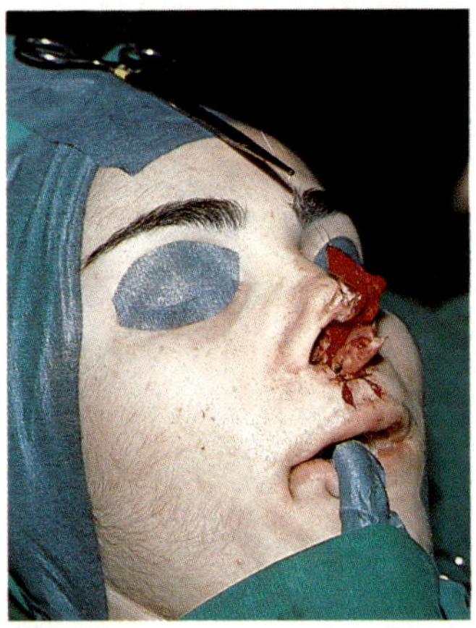

C

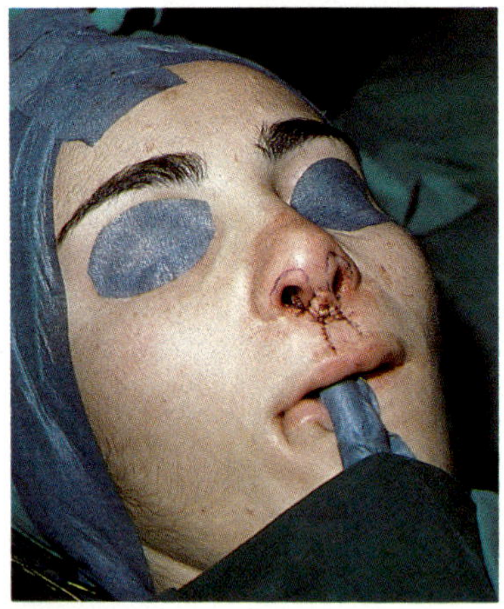

D

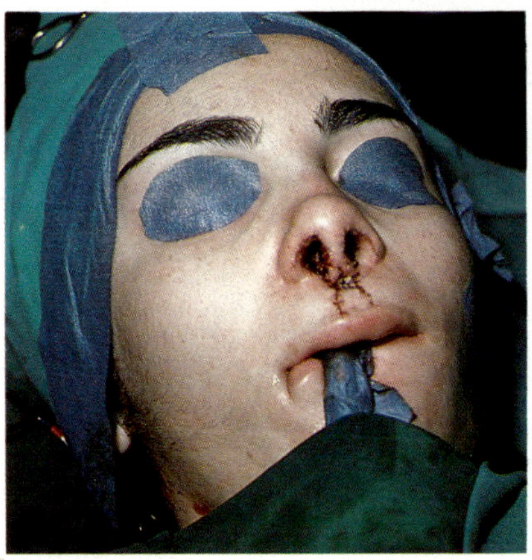

E

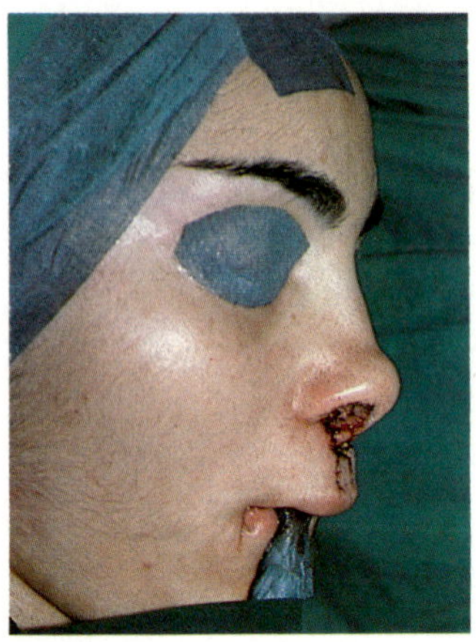

F

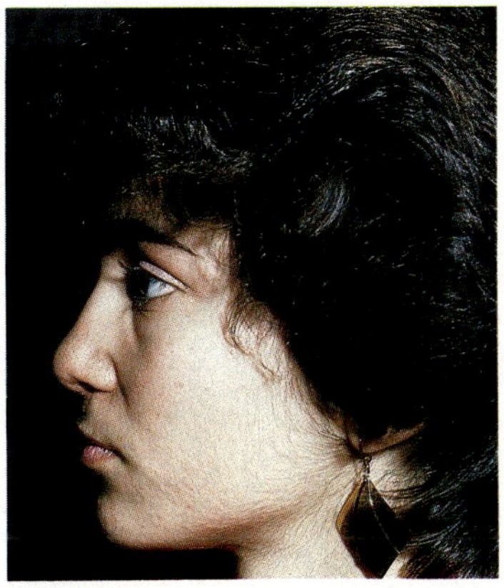

G

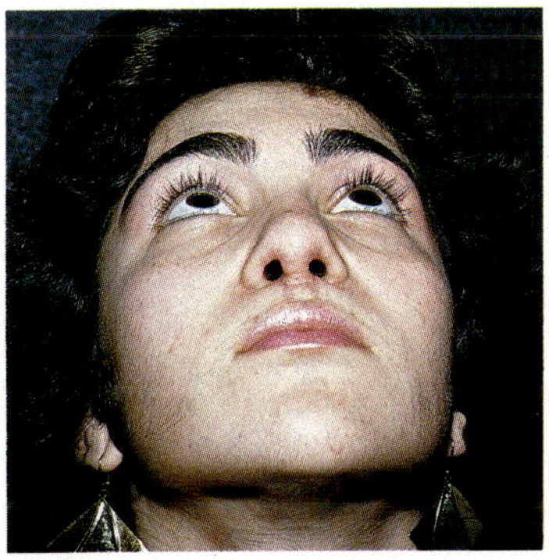

H

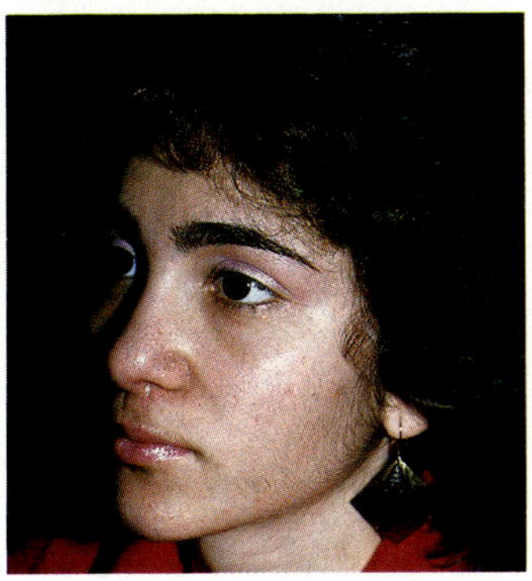

I

Fig. 155. Lengthening of the columella in a girl with Binder's syndrome. (A) Preoperative views. (B) Forked flap and columellar-alar commissure resection outlined. (C) Insertion of a rolled ear cartilage and of a plate of septal cartilage into the membranous septum and columella. (D) Forked flap sutured. (E) Marginal resection at the commissure sutured. (F) End of the operation. (G, H, and I) Result.

HIDDEN COLUMELLA

The hidden columella, following an overcorrection of the septal length, spoils the patient's profile. To correct the retraction of the whole columella we insert a cartilaginous strut, taken from the posterior part of the quadrangular cartilage. This graft, shaped as a batten, is inserted into the columella through the transfixion incision (Figs. 156 and 157). By inserting this

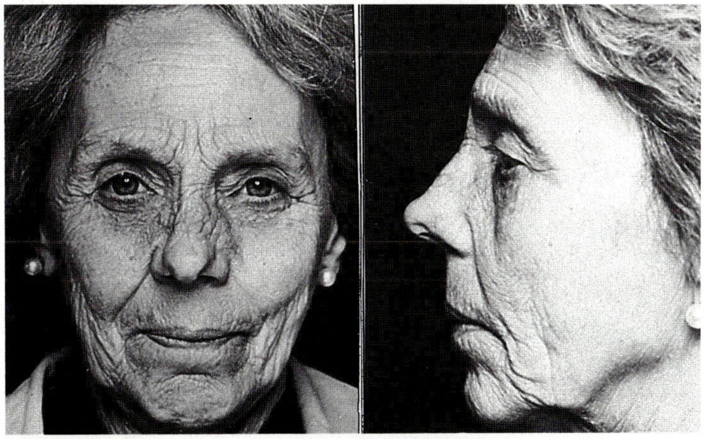

A

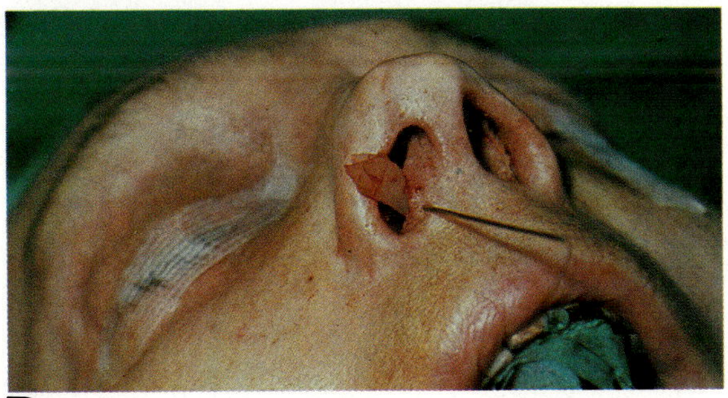

B

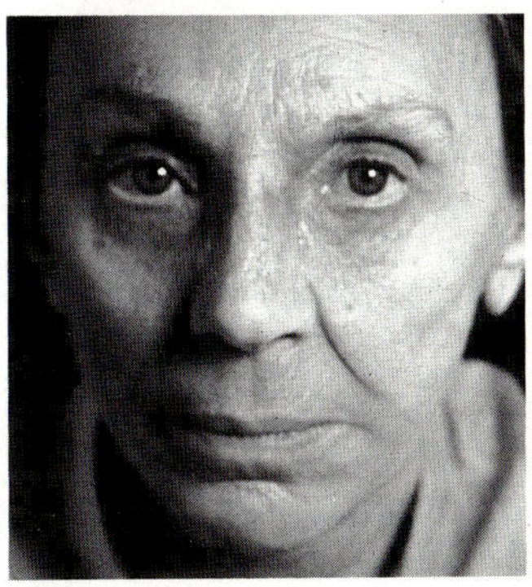

C

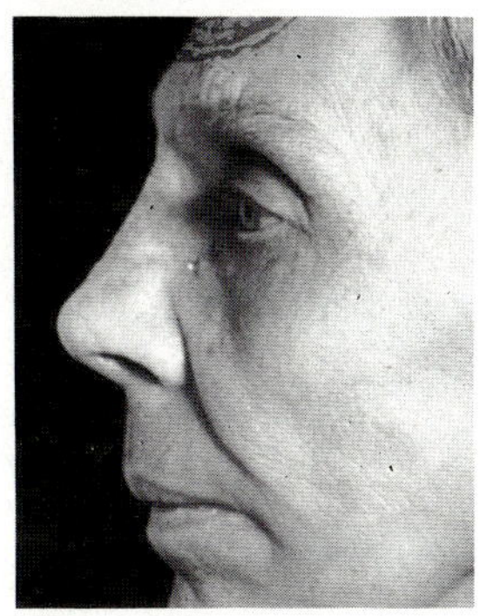

D

Fig. 156. Hidden columella corrected with cartilaginous strut from the septum. (A) Preoperative views of a middle-aged woman after overshortening of the septal cartilage. (B) Insertion of the cartilaginous batten at the transfixion incision. (C and D) Early result.

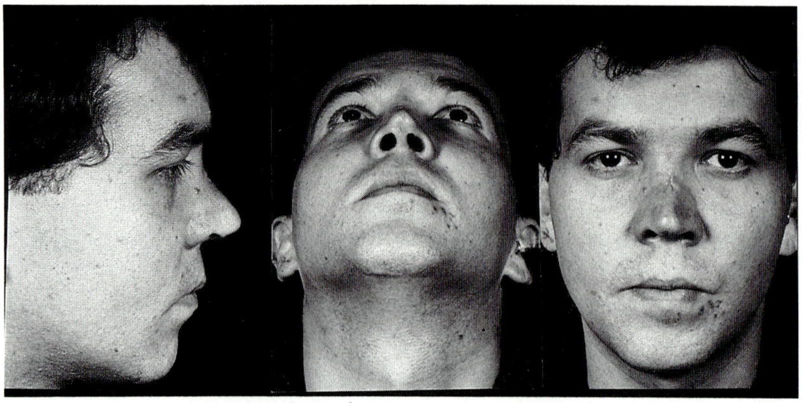

A

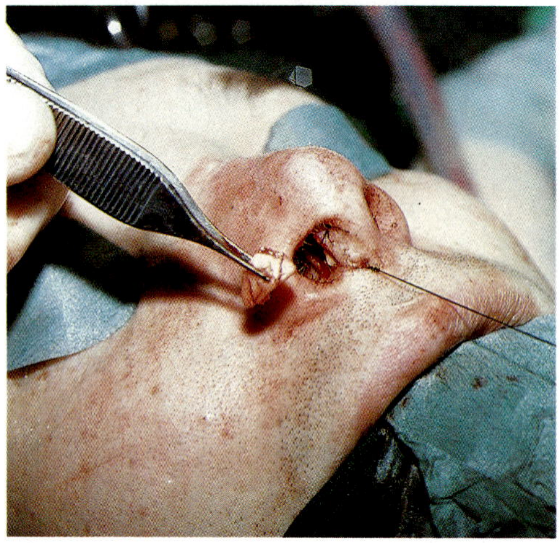

B

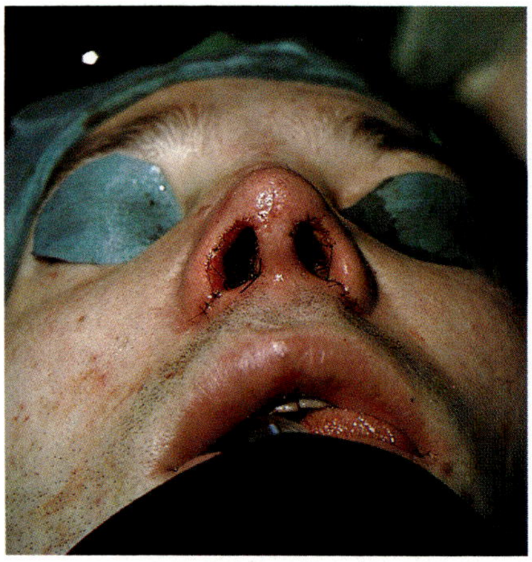

C

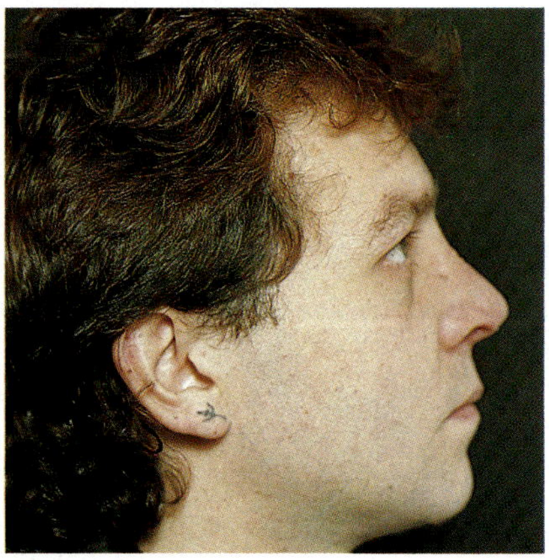

D

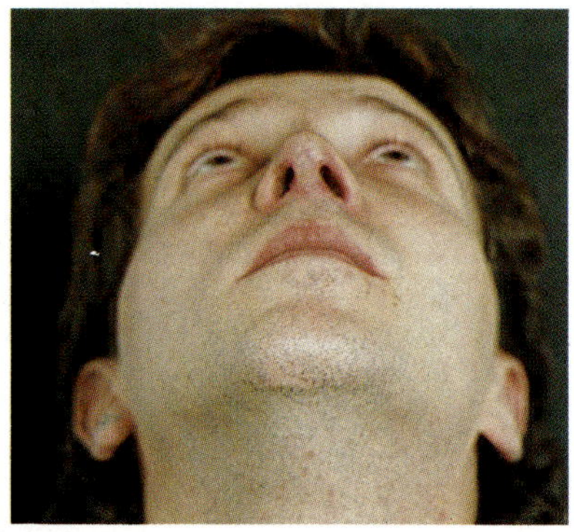

E

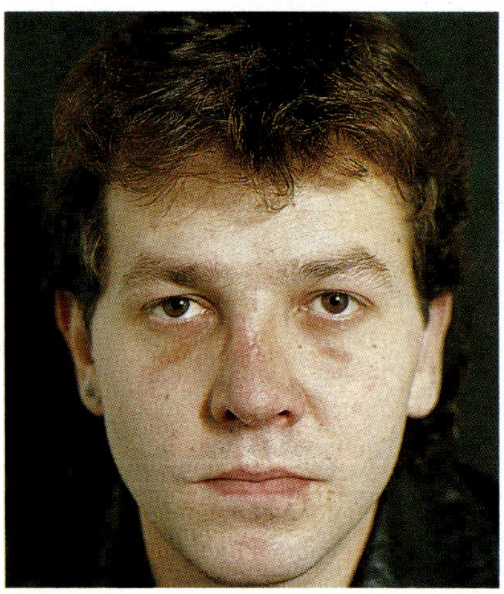

F

Fig. 157. Iatrogenic hidden columella following septoplasty. Secondary correction with cartilage struts from the septum. (A) Preoperative views. (B) Insertion of the grafts into the columella through the transfixion incision. (C) End of the operation. Additional alar marginal and alar base resections are sutured. (D, E, and F) Result.

septal graft we can restore the columellar projection, changing also the nasolabial angle (Fig. 158).

By losing its columellar support the tip of the nose collapses, inducing aesthetic and functional disturbances. The tip columellar support then has to be rebuilt by using a rolled conchal cartilage graft. This material is strong enough to sustain the tip yet soft enough to fill the columella without producing any unaesthetic spurs. The ear graft is rolled and sutured on itself before being transplanted into the columella. The recipient area of the graft is an anterior pocket of the columella, prepared through the transfixion incision (Fig. 159). Using this grafting method, flaccid, distorted, and unsupported columellae can be repaired with satisfactory results (Fig. 160).

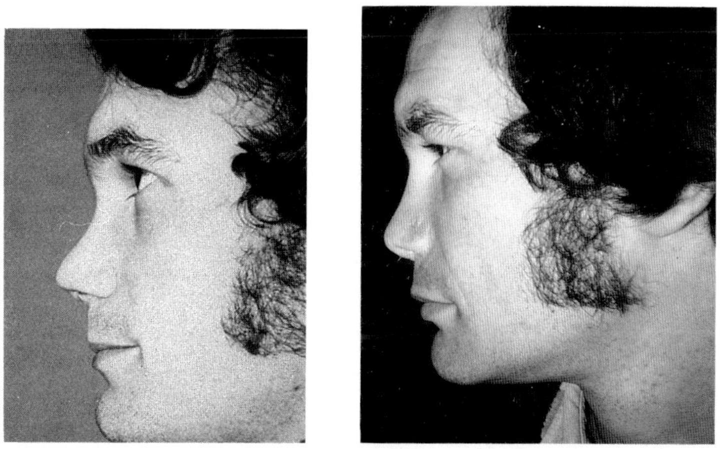

A B

Fig. 158. Retracted columella corrected with columellar strut. (A) Preoperative profile view in a young man after overcorrection of the tip-columella complex. (B) Profile after revisional procedure.

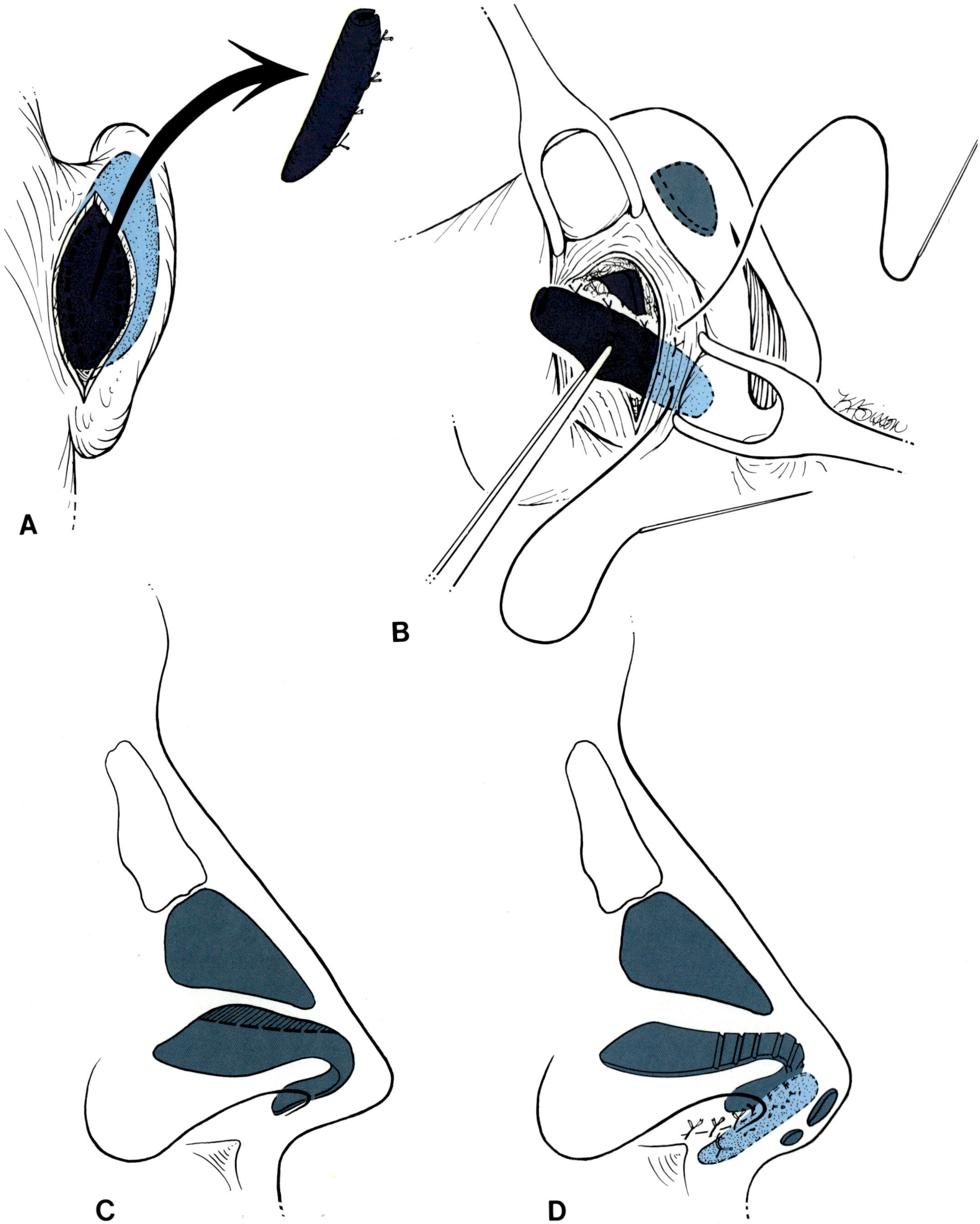

Fig. 159. Tip-columellar support with rolled ear cartilage. (A) Conchal cartilage as donor area. Cartilage is rolled and sutured ready for transplantation. (B) Ear graft is inserted into a pocket at the transfixion incision. (C) Profile before correction. (D) New profile with inserted rolled ear cartilage and lobular and mid-columellar onlay.

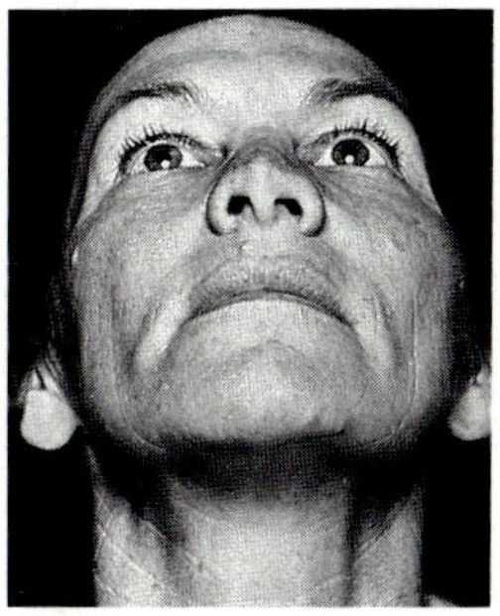

A

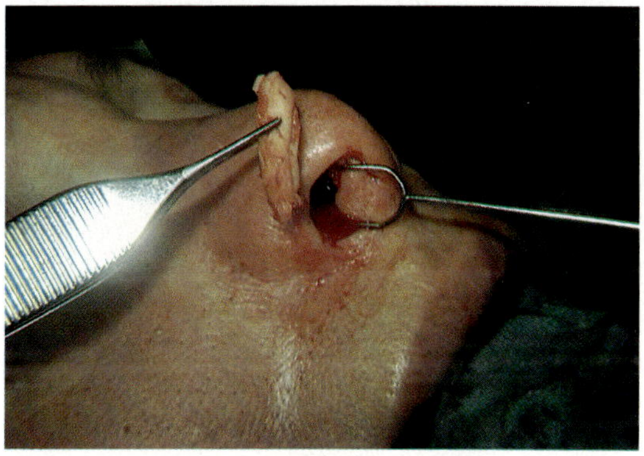

B

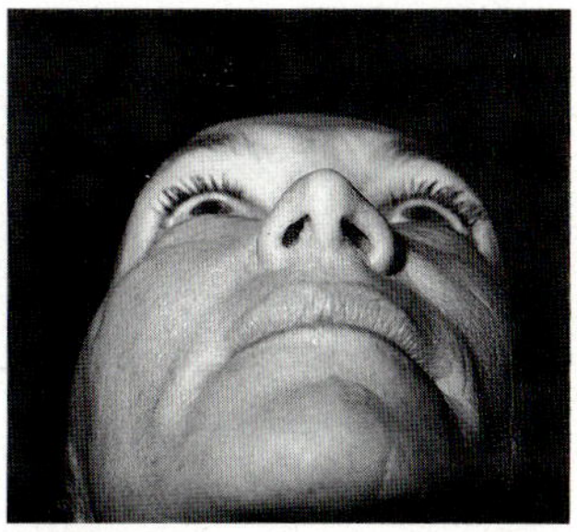

C

Fig. 160. Middle-aged woman with flaccid and distorted columella (A) requiring a tip-columella support with ear cartilage. (B) Insertion of the rolled ear cartilage. (C) Result.

In these types of columellar deformities an additional retraction of the columellar base occurs in most instances and necessitates concurrent correction. To do this, we open the columellar base through an external horizontal basal incision and undermine the skin with the the Trelat elevator forming a columellar pocket in front of the medial crura. The pocket will receive an ear cartilage onlay (Fig. 161). Some other types of flaccid columella can be reinforced with ear cartilage grafts inserted simply through the columellar base incision.

Another way to improve the tip support is to use an open approach. The side of the opening to be used in the columella depends on the type of construction needed. In the case of platyrhinia, with loss of tip support, we need to perform a dorsocolumellar augmentation. For this type of revision we have to open the columella at its base in order to be able to increase, at the same time, the tip support and the dorsal contour, without interrupting the columellar profile line (Fig. 162). When columellar support

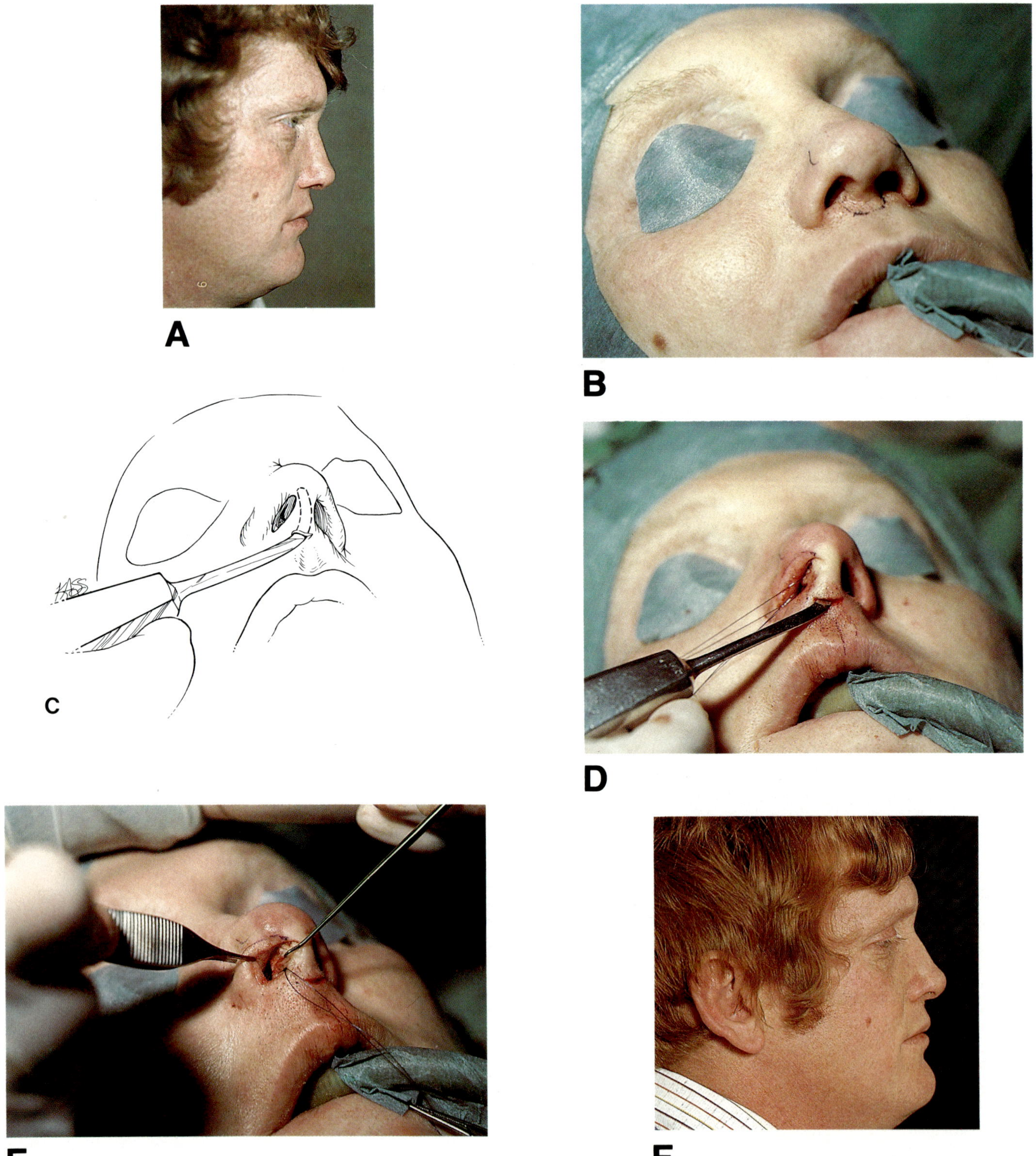

Fig. 161. Correction of retraction at the columellar base with ear cartilage strut at the transfixion incision and basal columellar onlay. (A) Preoperative view of a young man with secondary columellar retraction. (B) External incision at the columellar base outlined. (C and D) Columellar pocket formation with Trélat elevator for insertion of ear cartilage onlay. (E) Additional columellar augmentation with ear cartilage strut at the transfixion incision. (F) Late result.

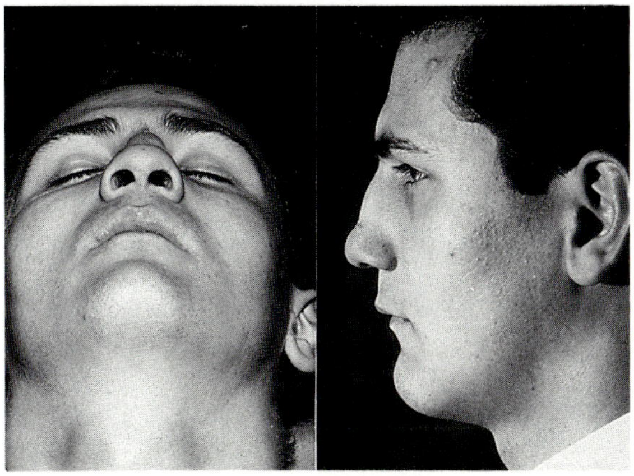

A

is missing, we sometimes use the mediocolumellar incision of Rethi or Sercer, to insert the cartilage strut (Fig. 163). This procedure also permits the additional correction of any scar retraction of the columella, and, if necessary, allows one to elongate the columella (Fig. 164). The disadvantage of Rethi's method lies in the aesthetic plane, because it rules out the creation of the double angle of the columella. Partial columellar retraction, without any loss of tip support, can be corrected using local septocolumellar skin advancement flaps, Converse's (1971) square flap (Fig. 165), or by using a horizontal V-Y advancement procedure (Figs. 166 and 167), as shown, in cases of excessive columellar retraction.

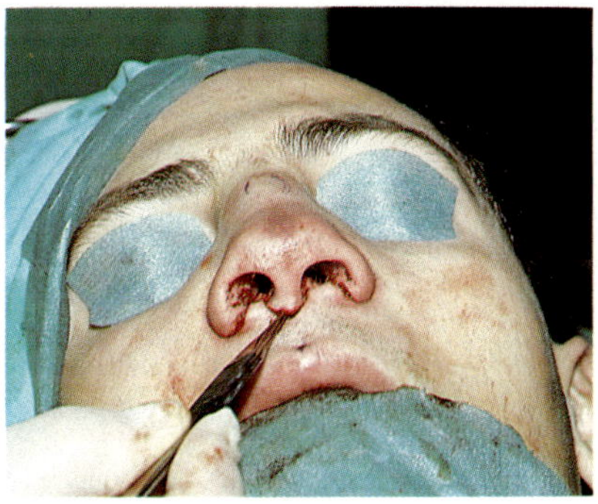

B

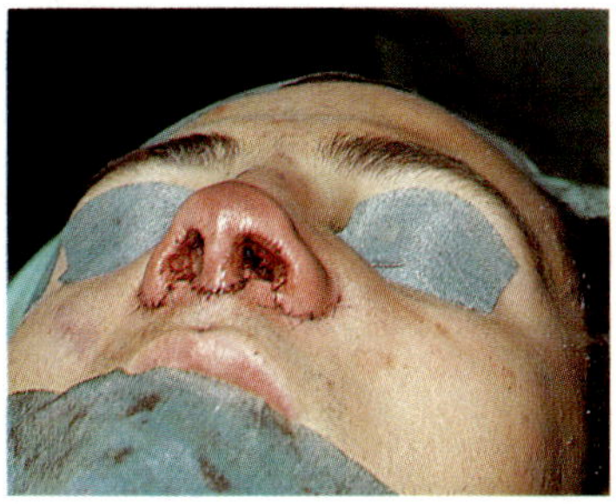

C

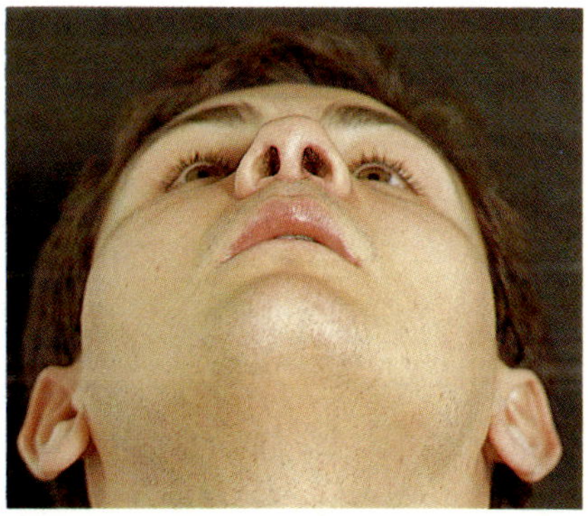

D

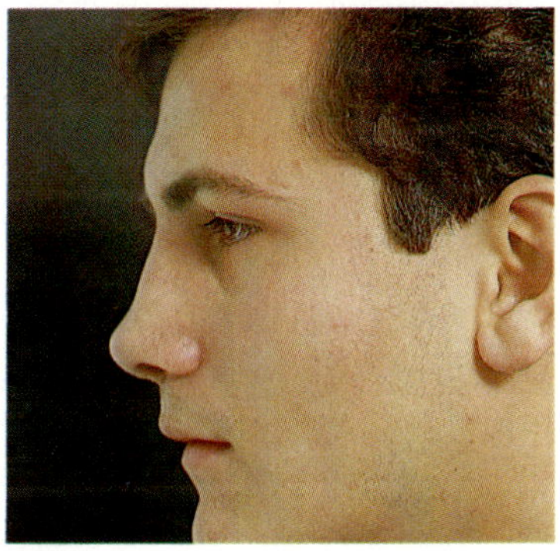

E

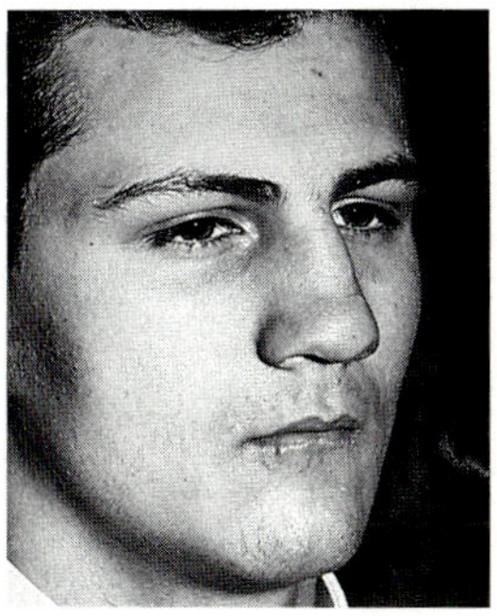

F

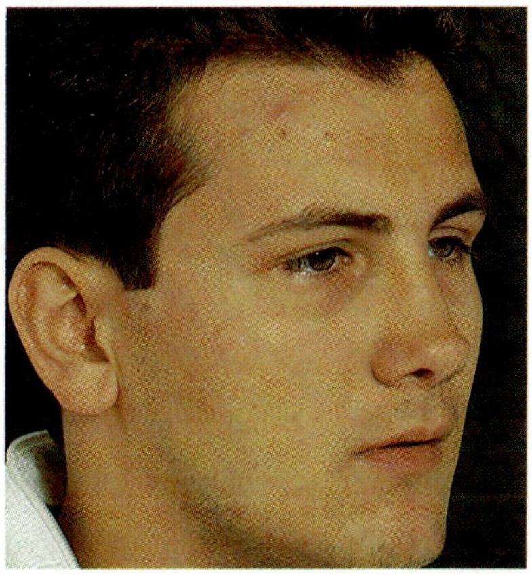

G

Fig. 162. Open procedure for elongation and support of the columella in a case of platyrhinia combined with closure of septal perforation (same patient as in Fig. 133. (A) Preoperative view. (B) Section of the columellar base continuing into the transfixion and bilateral alotomy. (C) Columella sutured after insertion of a strut of ear cartilage. (D and E) Result. (F and G) Pre- and postoperative half-profile view.

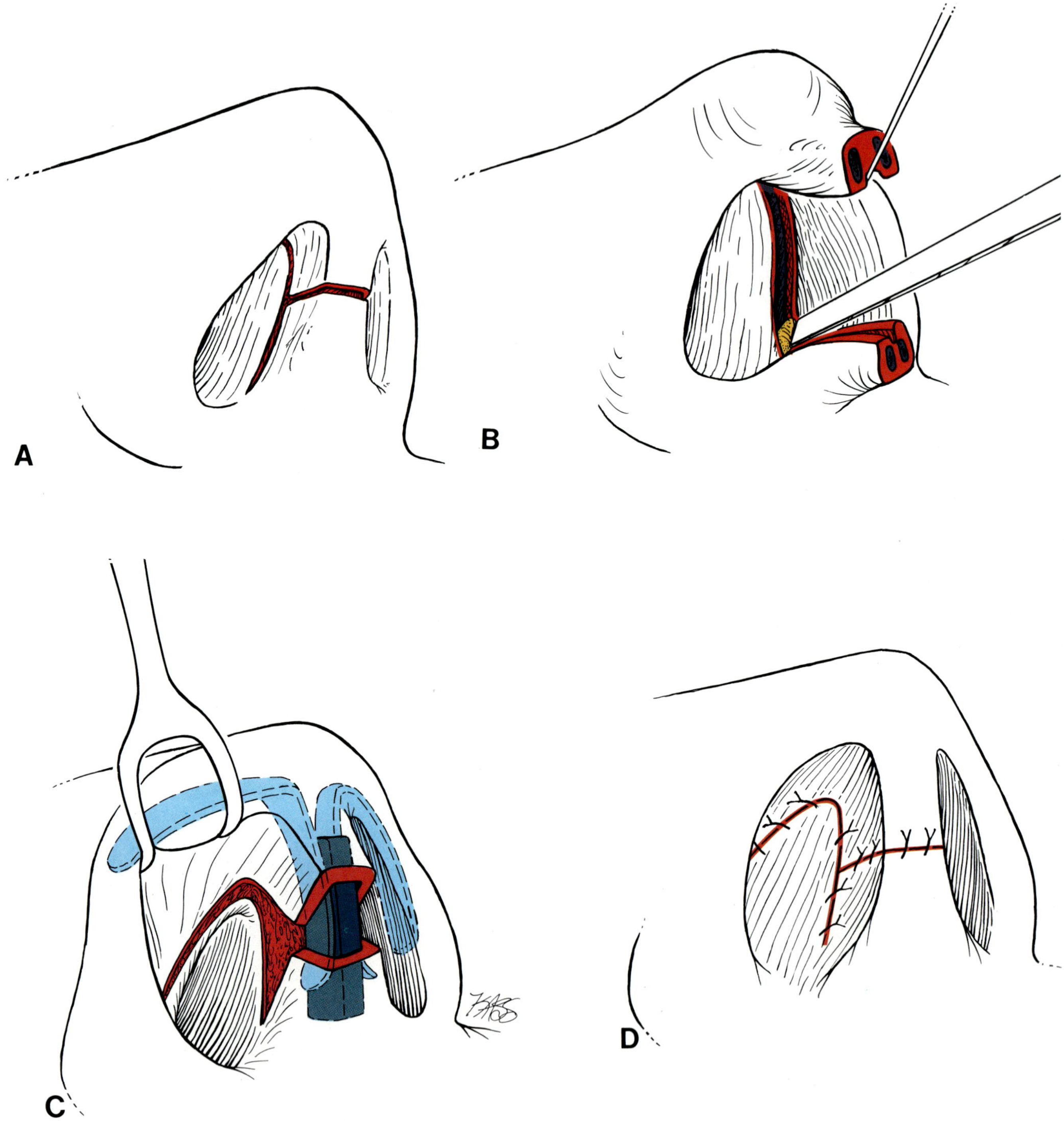

Fig. 163. Open access to septocolumellar area. (A) Transfixion incision and mediocolumellar transversal incision (Sercer). (B) Repositioning of nasal spine. A strut will be inserted into the columella through the open access. (C) Insertion of a cartilage strut from the septum into the columella through the open access. (D) Suture of the transversal incision.

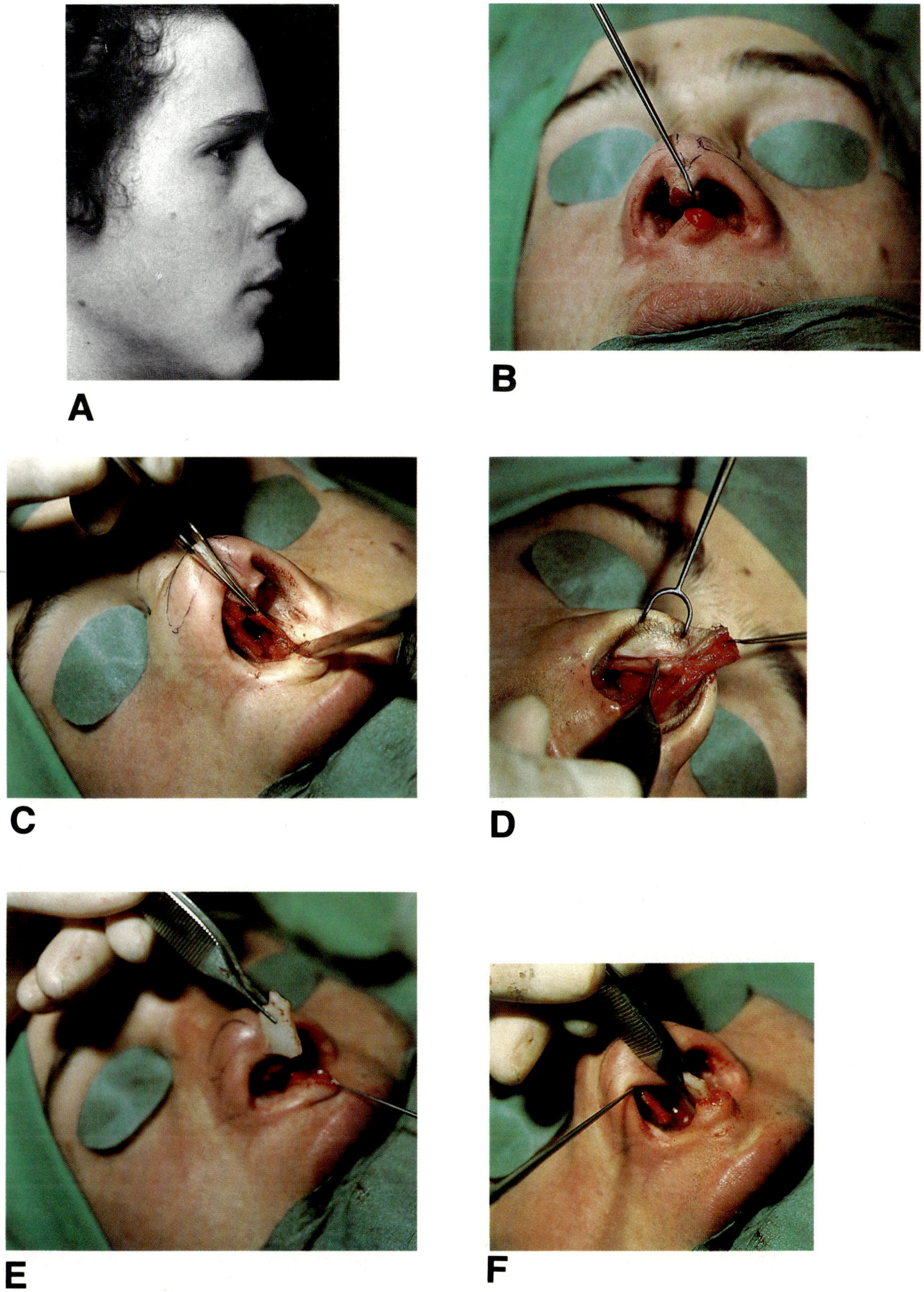

Fig. 164. continues.

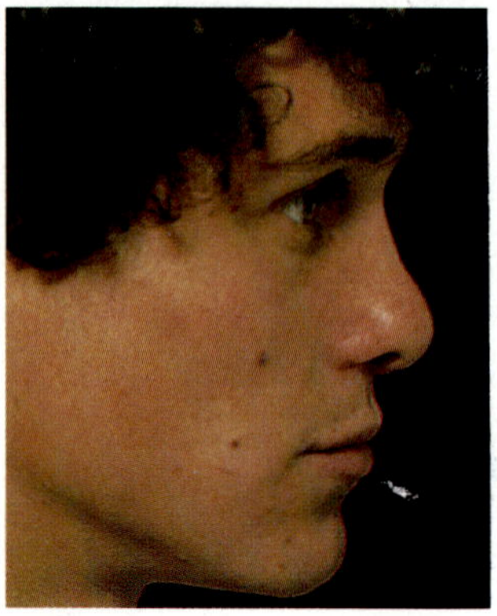

G

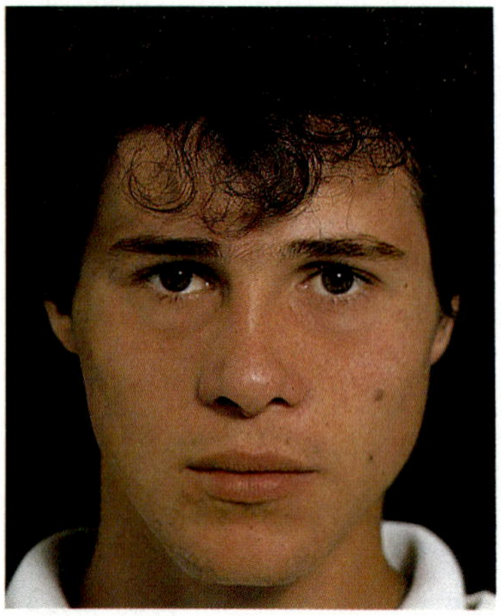

H

Fig. 164. Augmentation of the columella through external incision in a case of insufficient posttraumatic correction. (A) Preoperative profile. (B) Open access with transcolumellar incision. (C) Repositioning of the nasal spine with the chisel. (D) Trimming of the lower lateral cartilages with retrograde technique (evertion). (E and F) Insertion of a cartilaginous strut from the septum. (G and H) Late result.

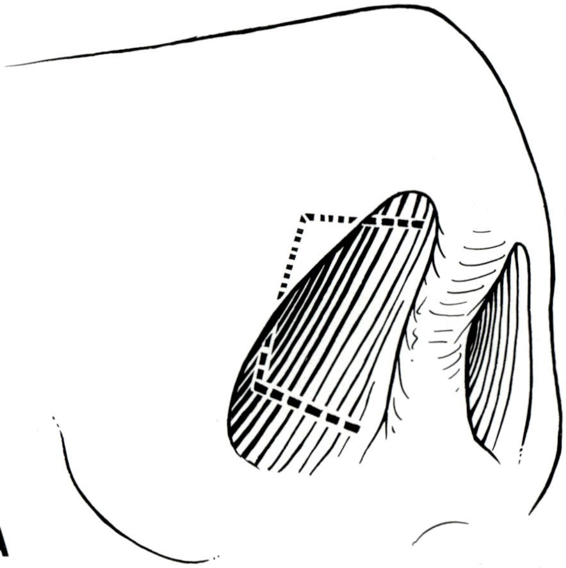

A

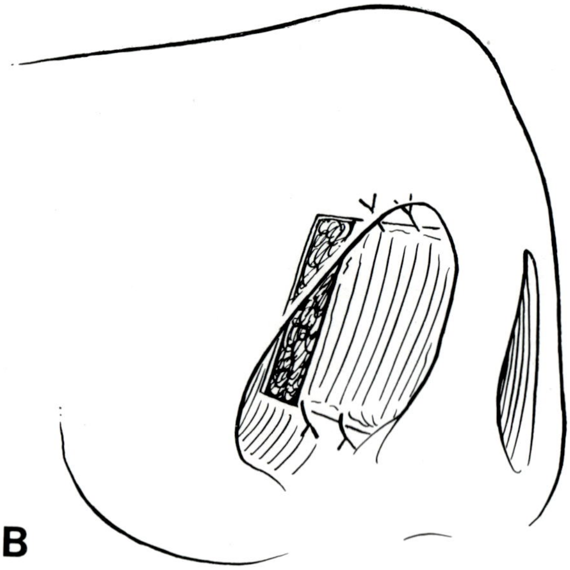

B

Fig. 165. Correction of retracted columella with skin advancement of Converse. (A) Retrograde advanced flap outlined. (B) Suture of the flap leaving a posterior raw surface which has to epithelize.

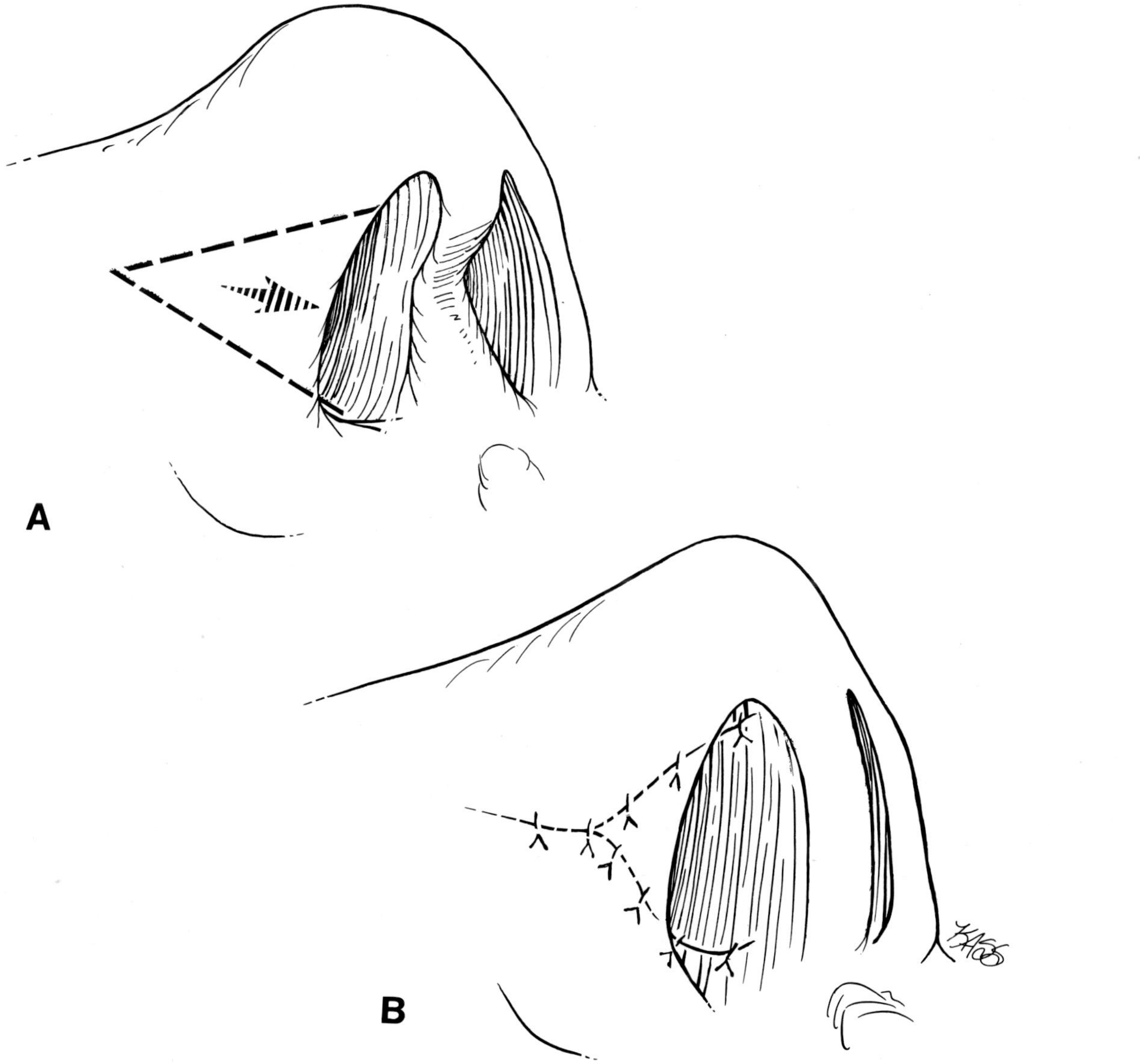

Fig. 166. Advancement of retracted columella with V-Y procedure (Meyer). (A) V- outlined in the septum reaching to the retracted columellar. (B) Y- sutured and columellar advanced.

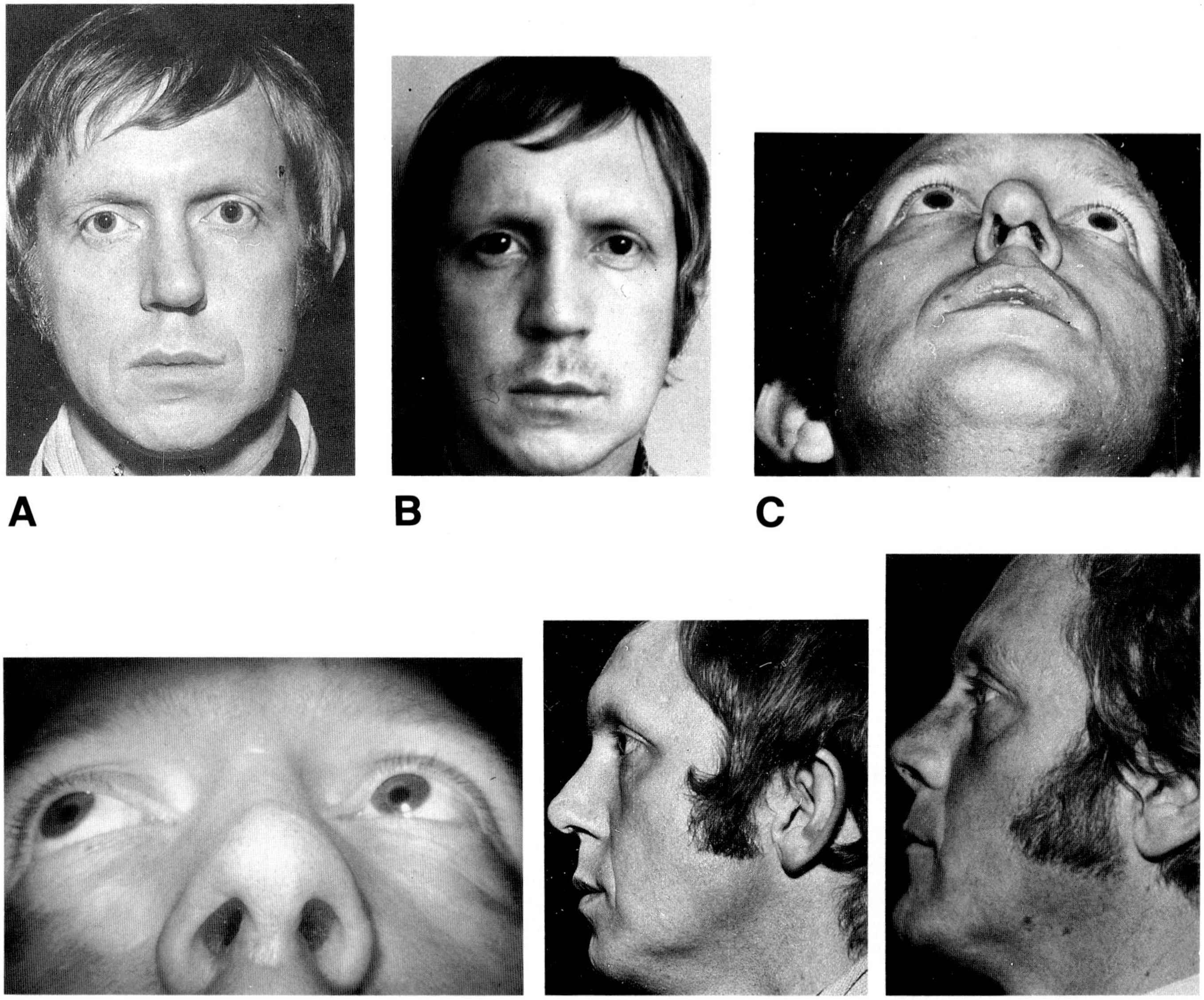

A B C D E F

Fig. 167. Correction of the traumatic retraction of the columella according to Fig. 166 Pre- and postoperative front views. (C and D) Pre- and posoperative axial views. (E and F) Pre- and postoperative profile views.

HANGING COLUMELLA

In the opposite way, the curved contour of a hanging columella is another unaesthetic detail of the nose, which can be secondary to a previous rhinoplasty. To correct it we like to resect a full-thickness part of the membranous septum. This resection is performed in a fusiform shape, at the level of the transfixion incision. A resection along the septocolumellar border is another way to correct a hanging columella (Fig. 168).

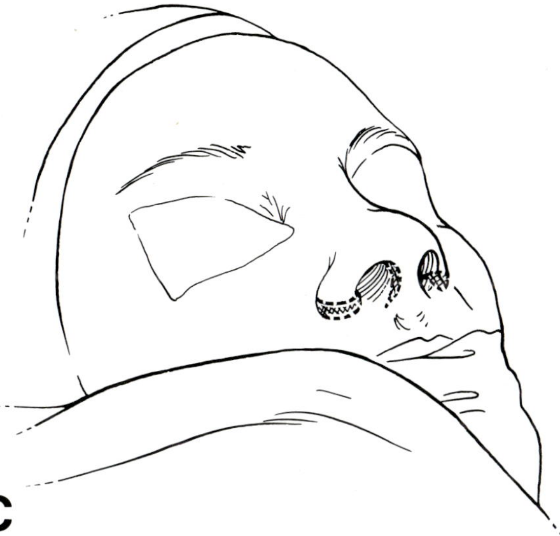

C

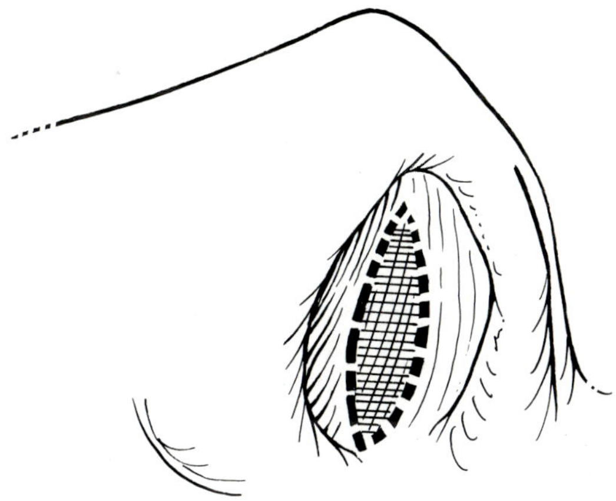

A

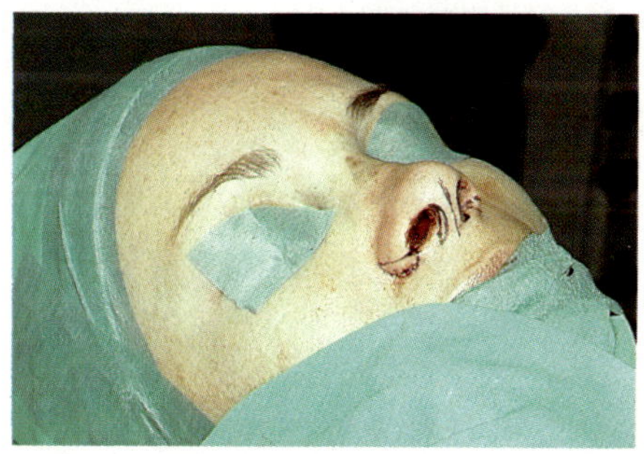

D

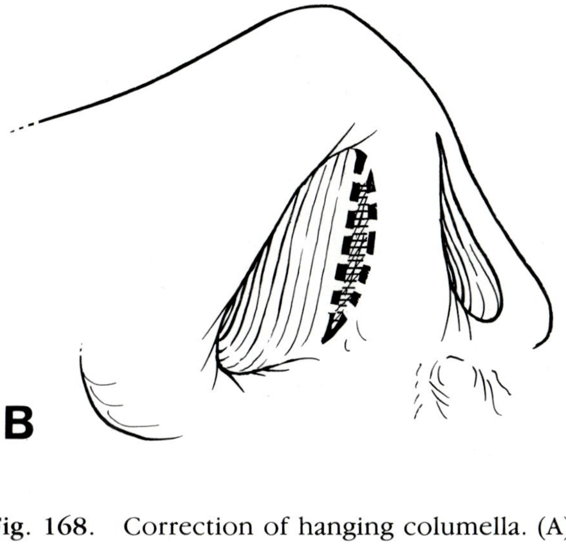

B

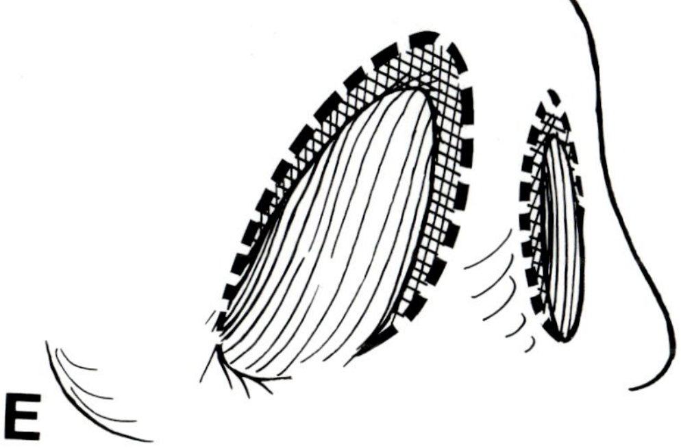

E

Fig. 168. Correction of hanging columella. (A) Full-thickness fusiform resection in the membranous septum. (B) Resection at the columellar border. (C and D) Strip resection at the columellar border combined with wedge resection at the alar base. (E) Simultaneous correction of hanging columella and broad columella.

BROAD COLUMELLA

We have already seen that the marginal commissure resection can be used in columellar lengthening. It can also be extended from the nostril to the columella for thinning down of both a broad columella and alae (Figs. 169 and 170). If a broad tip is associated with a short broad columella, we combine the tip and columella refinement with the lengthening of the columella, reinforced with a cartilage graft as described above (Fig. 171).

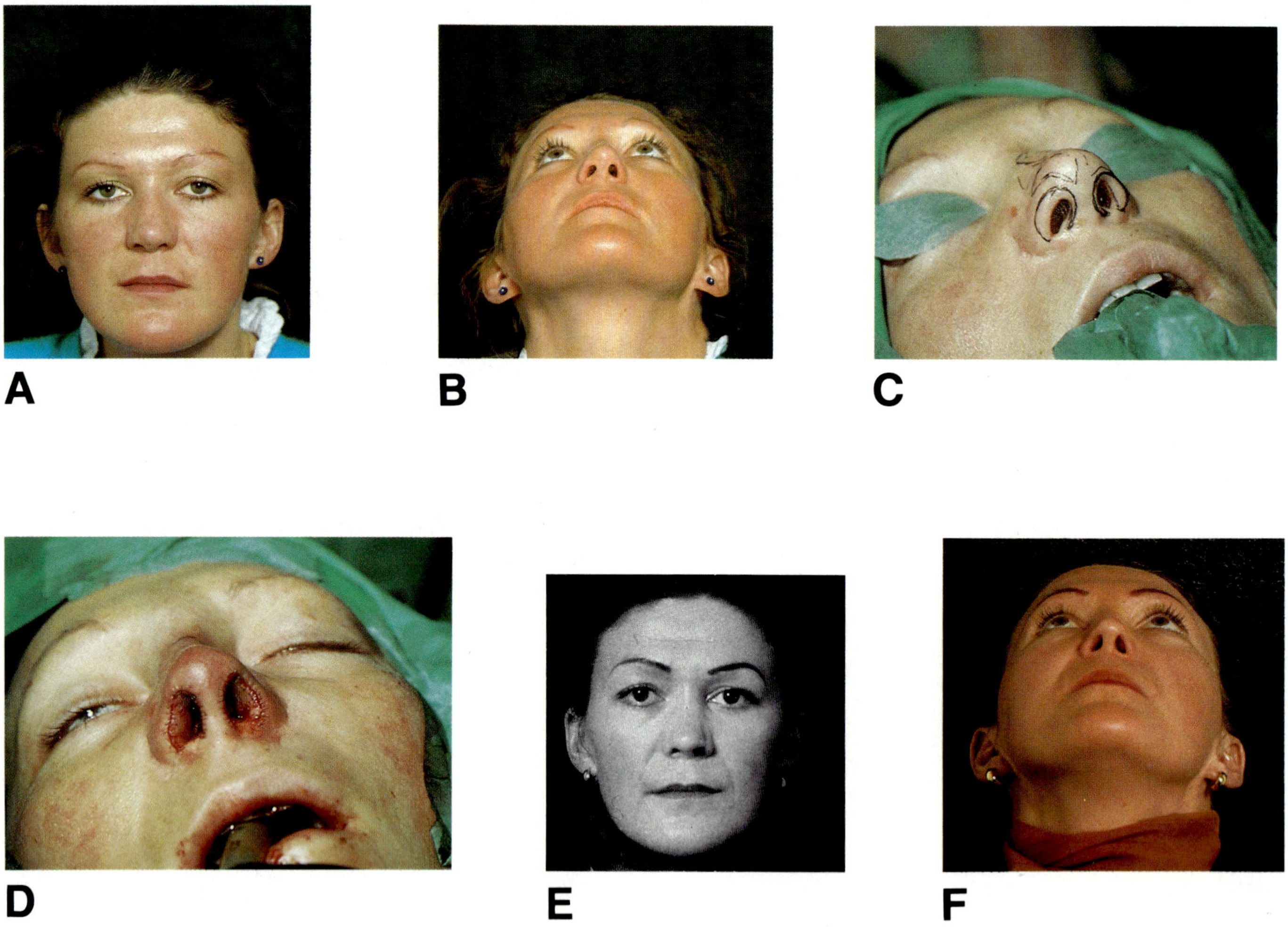

Fig. 169. Correction of broad columella and broad alar with marginal resections in a young woman after insufficient correction. (A and B) Preoperative views. (C) Outline of the resections according to Fig. 161E. (D) Alar and columellar rims sutured. (E and F) Result.

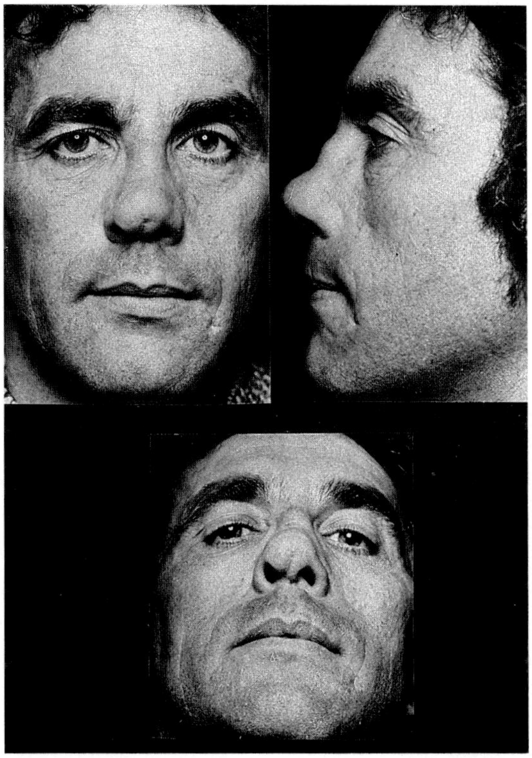

A

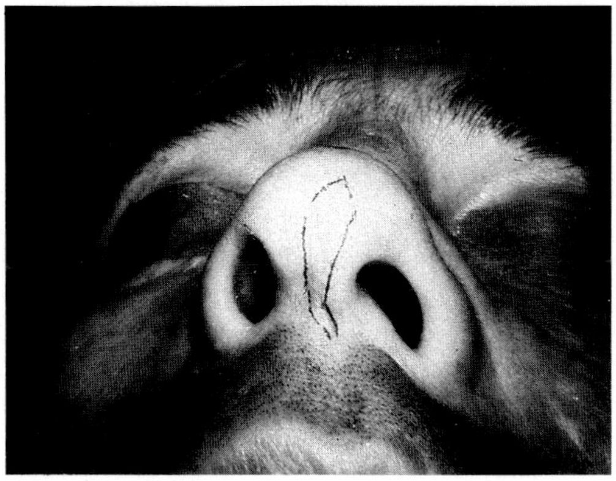

B

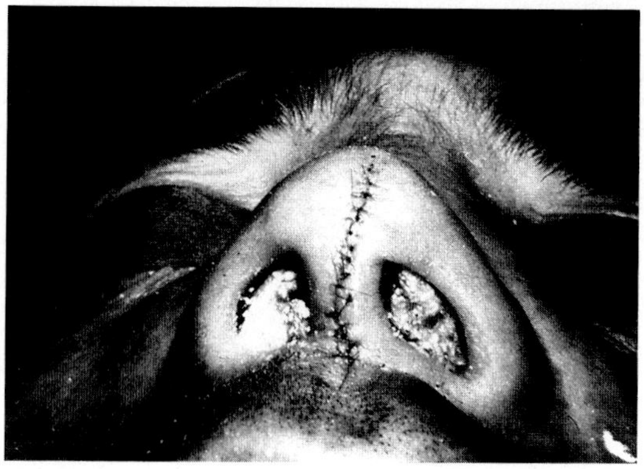

C

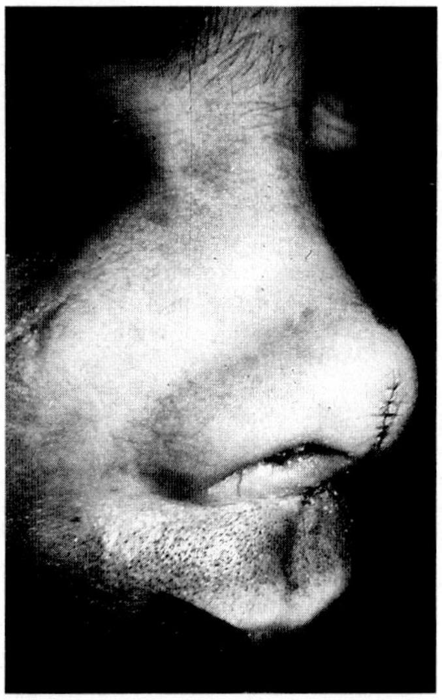

D

Fig. 170. Posttraumatic broad columella. (A) Preoperative views with thick and scarred tip and columella. (B) Midcolumella resection outlined. (C and D) End of the operation with sutured resection wound.

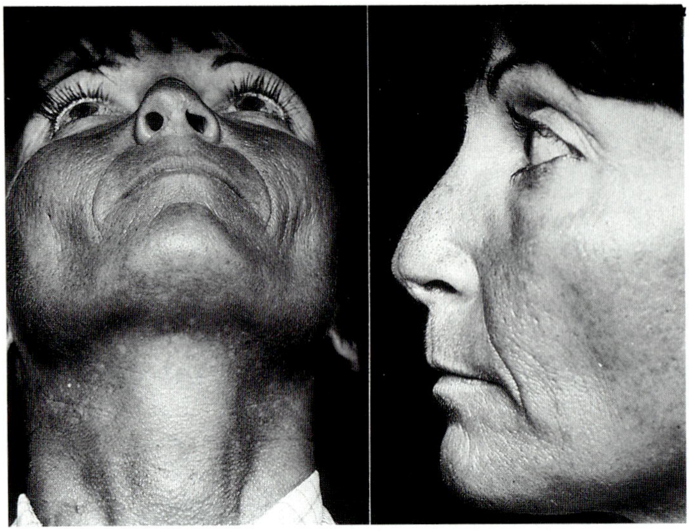

A

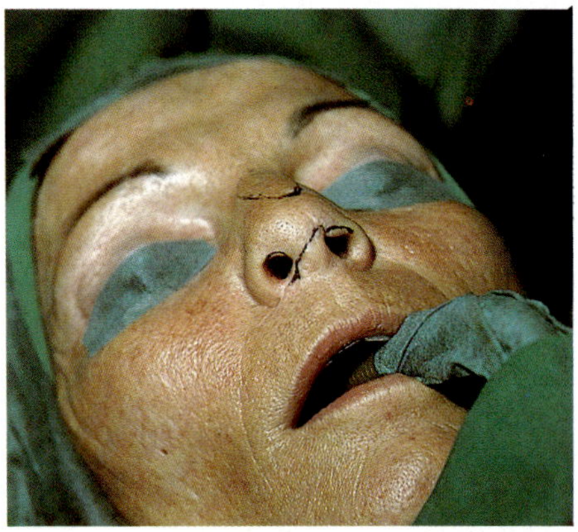

B

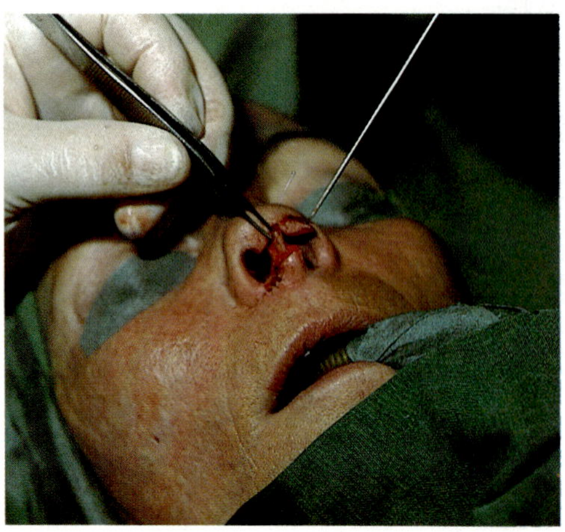

C

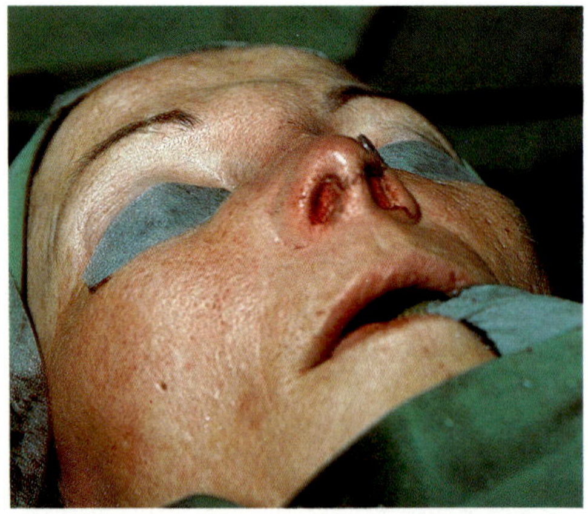

D

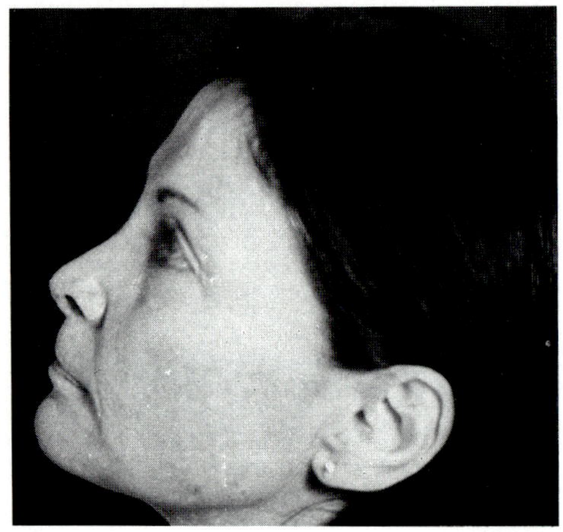

E

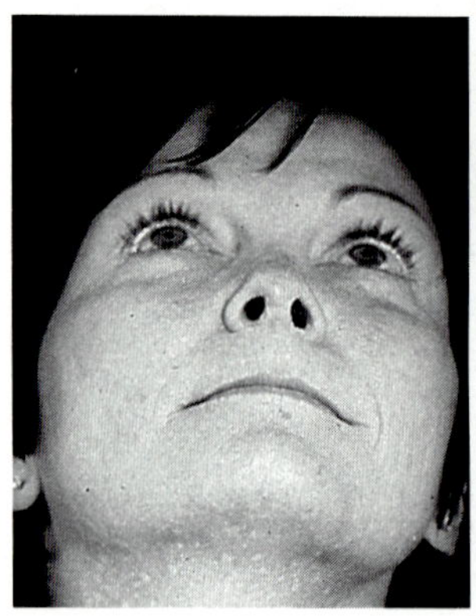

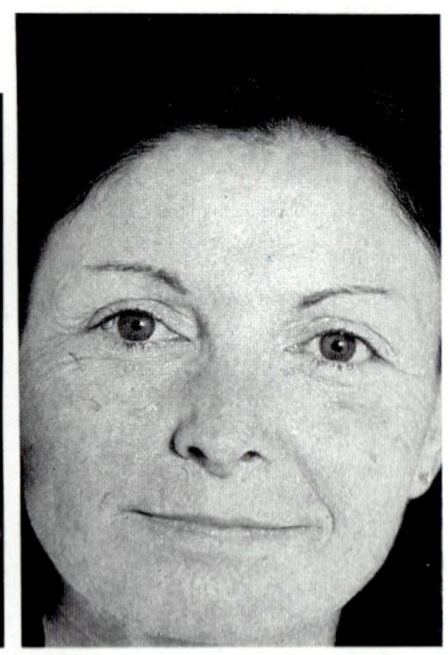

F G

Fig. 171. Posttraumatic broad and short columella with broad tip. (A) Preoperative views. (B) Oblique incision and marginal resection at the left nostril outlined. (C) Insertion of cartilage graft from the septum into the columella. (D) End of the operation with oblique advancement of the columella sutured. (E, F, and G) Late result.

OBLIQUE COLUMELLA AND OTHER PARTIAL DEFORMITIES OF THE COLUMELLA

The oblique columella is sometimes a sequela after a previous rhinoplasty and it spoils the balance of the nose. To reestablish a straight axis one has to modify at the same time the columella and the tip by sculpturing the lower lateral cartilage and performing both a marginal and a wedge resection of the columellar base (Figs. 172 and 173).

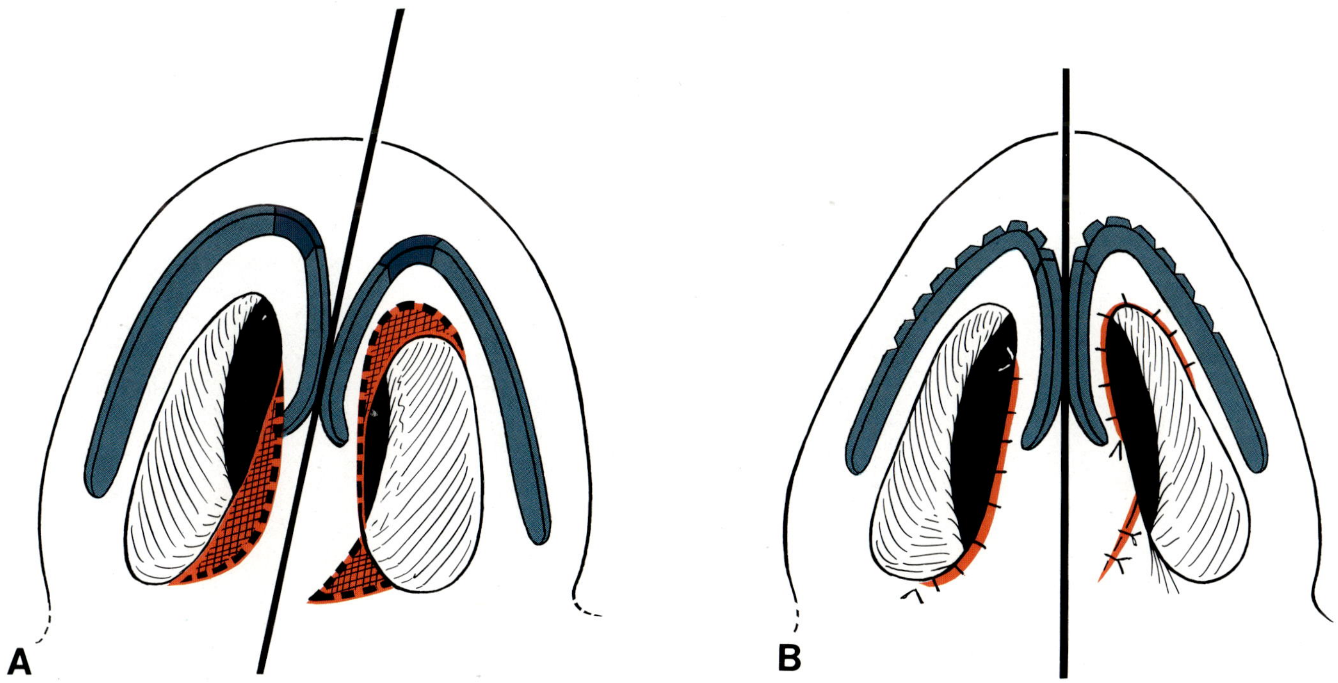

Fig. 172. Oblique columella. Correction with marginal and wedge resection at the columellar border and modeling of the lower lateral cartilages. (A) Resections outlined. (B) Equilibrated tip and columella.

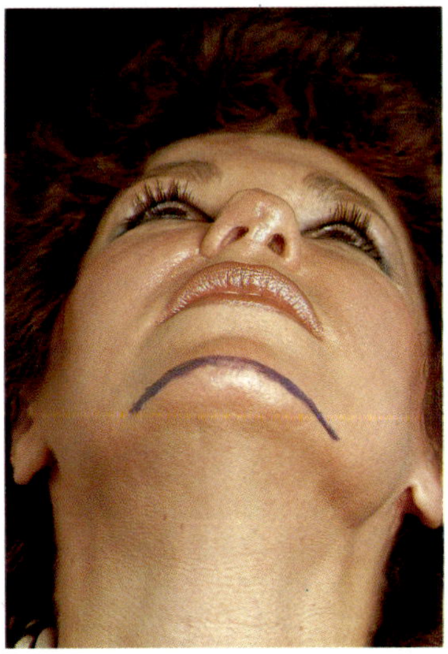

A

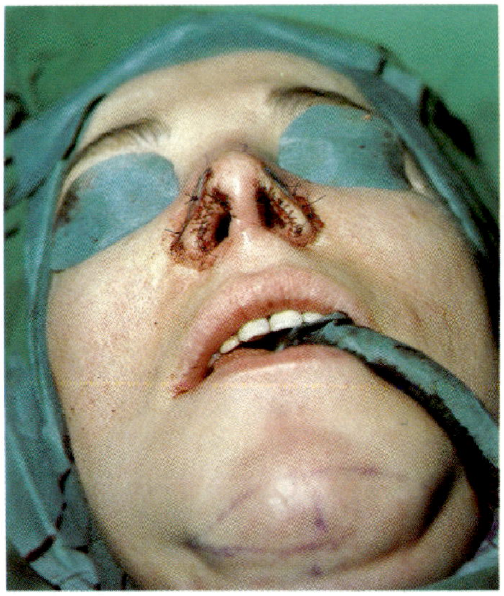

B

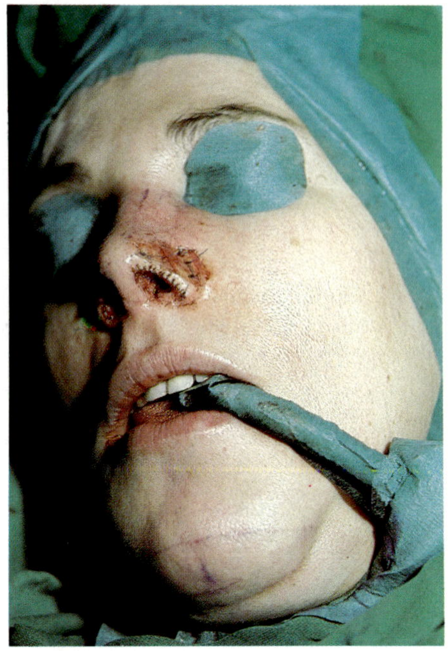

C

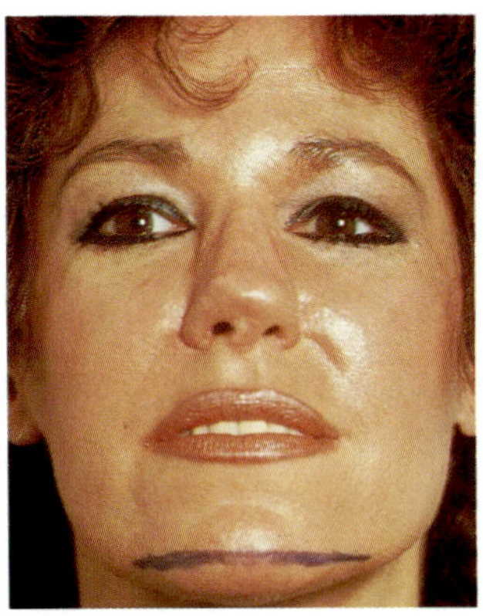

D

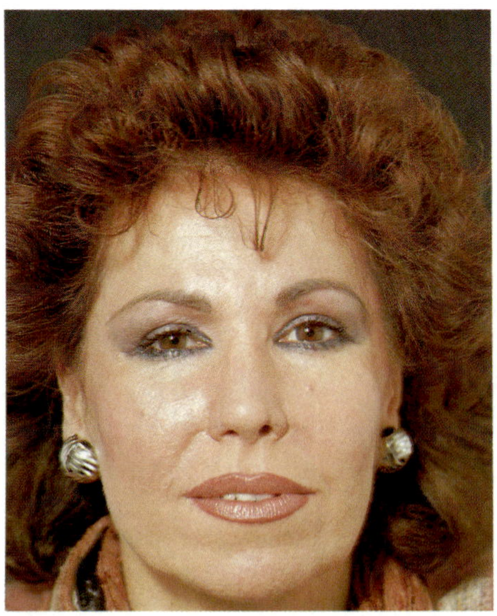

E

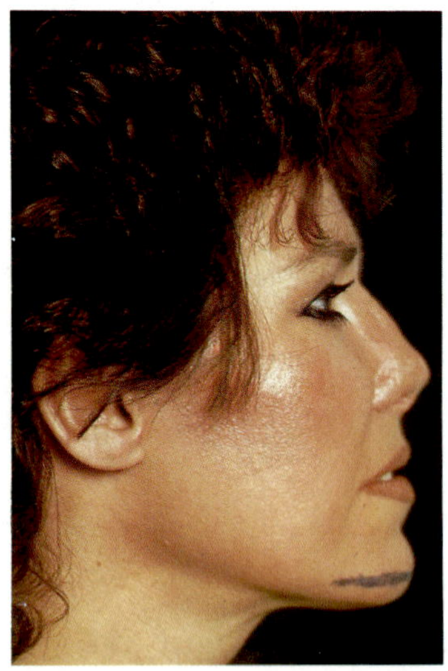

F

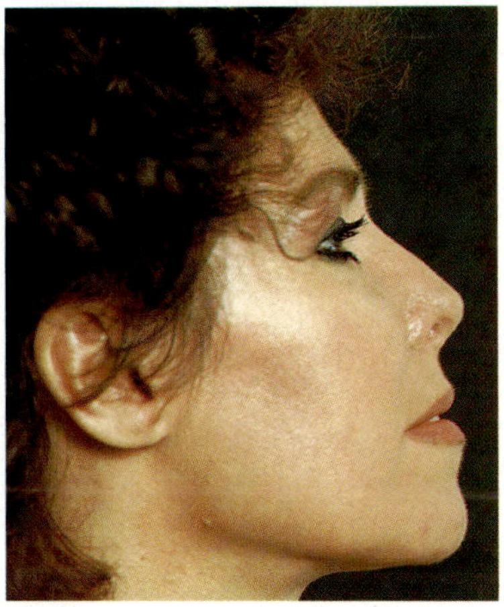

G

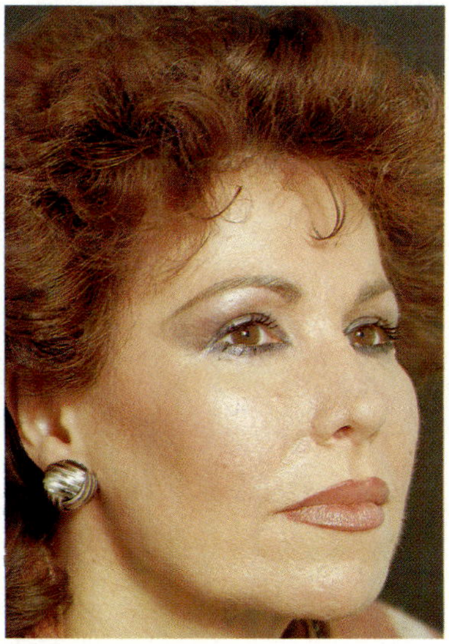

H

Fig. 173. Young lady with distorted nose, oblique columella, and impairment of nasal breathing after several corrective rhinoplasties. The columella was corrected with the technique shown in Fig. 172. (A) Preoperative axial view. (B and C) End of the operation. Cartilage from the septum grafted into the tip and columella and both alar. Right columellar border and both alar rims were trimmed and sutured. Transalar mattress sutures were tied over plastic sheets. A reduction of the mandibular contour and malar augmentation were performed. (D and E) Preoperative and postoperative front view. (F and G) Pre- and postoperative profile. (H) Postoperative half profile.

Other secondary, partial minor deformities of the columella have to be corrected by using the appropriate local procedures. A concave facet in the middle of the columella will be restored by introducing a cartilage graft in order to fill the depressed part (Fig. 174). Using a stronger and wider onlay we achieve, in addition, an increased accentuation of the double angle (Fig. 175).

A huge lobule associated with a depressed columella is thinned by wide lobulo-alar marginal resections as a complement to columellar onlay grafting (Fig. 176).

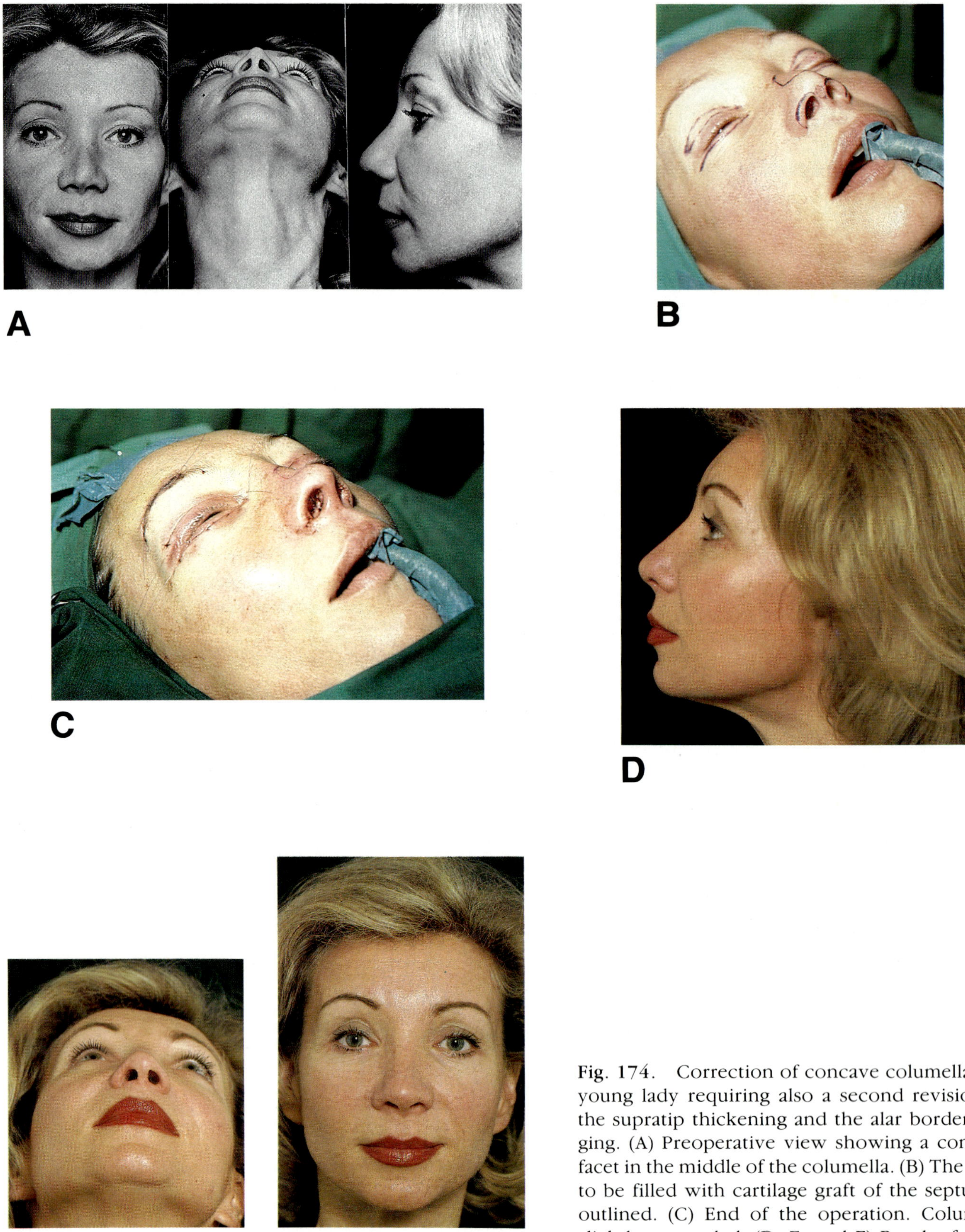

Fig. 174. Correction of concave columella in a young lady requiring also a second revision of the supratip thickening and the alar border sagging. (A) Preoperative view showing a concave facet in the middle of the columella. (B) The facet to be filled with cartilage graft of the septum is outlined. (C) End of the operation. Columella slightly protruded. (D, E, and F) Result after 14 months.

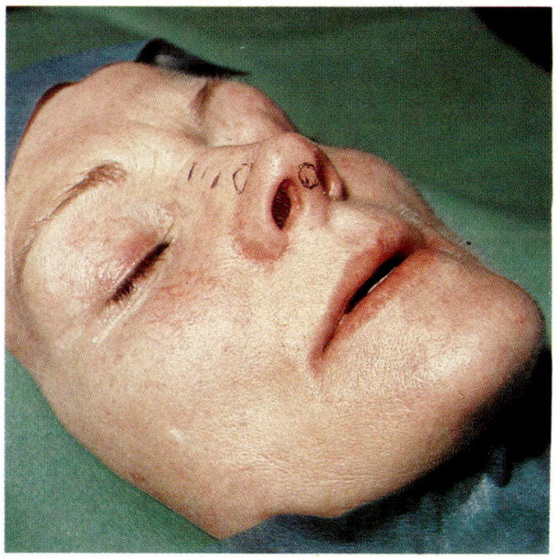

A

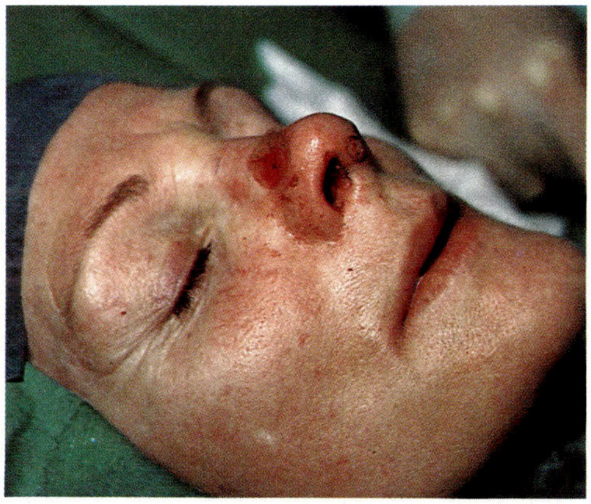

B

Fig. 175. Similar depressed facet at the columella requiring an onlay to augment and mark a double angle. (A) A too deep supraalar crease has to be corrected too, using cartilage graft as in the case of Fig. 279. (B) After insertion of an onlay the columella has a more natural shape.

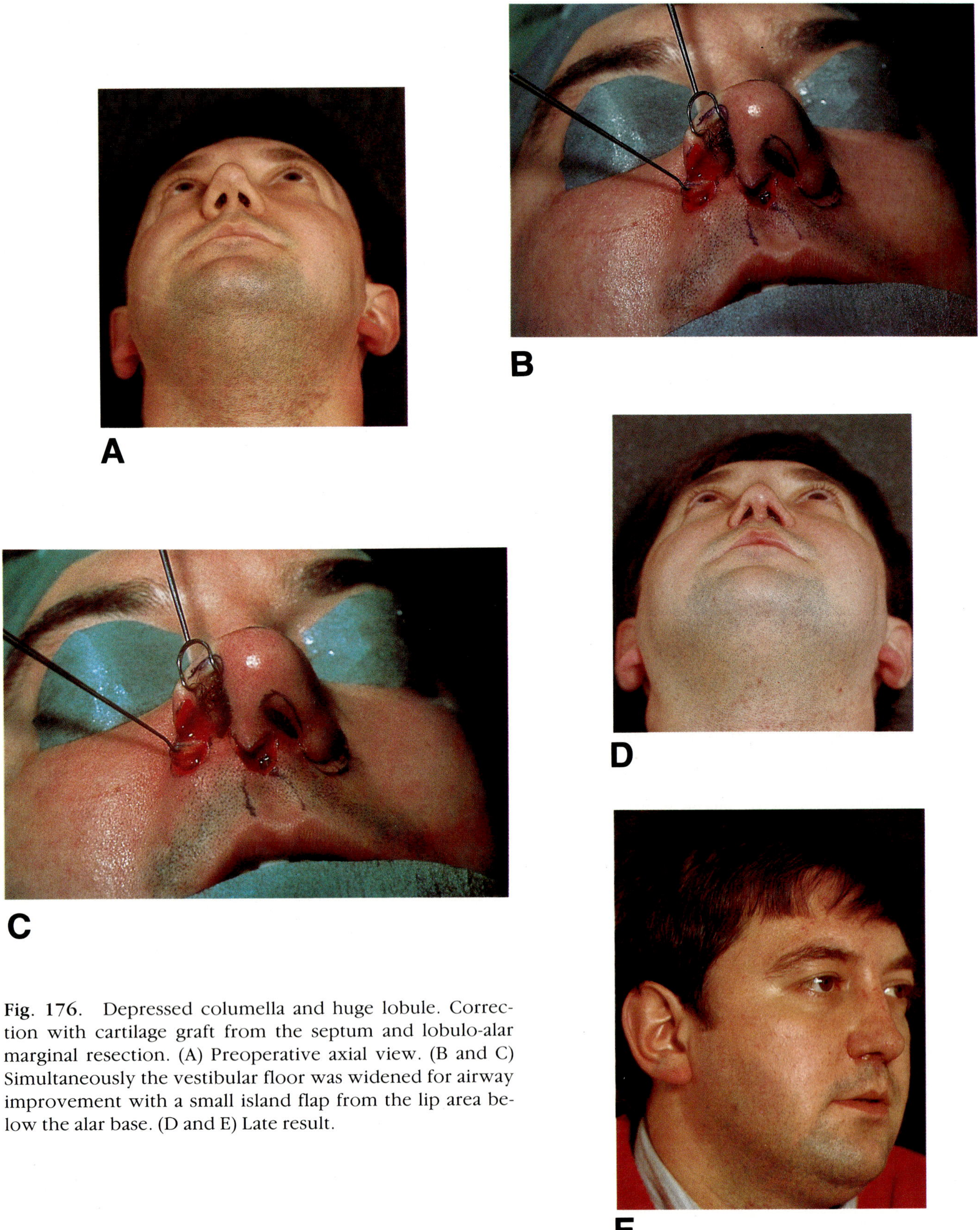

A

B

C

D

E

Fig. 176. Depressed columella and huge lobule. Correction with cartilage graft from the septum and lobulo-alar marginal resection. (A) Preoperative axial view. (B and C) Simultaneously the vestibular floor was widened for airway improvement with a small island flap from the lip area below the alar base. (D and E) Late result.

NASOLABIAL ANGLE

The transfixion incision is very helpful in effecting major changes needed in the tip-columella-lip complex. Through this incision we can vary the relationship between tip projection, the infratip region, columella angulation, the columello-labial junction, the central upper lip slope, the central upper lip prominence, and the position of the central lip-free border. The relationships and structures involved are what Webster (1975) calls the "tip-columella central upper lip aesthetic complex."

Janeke and Wright (1971) performed interesting anatomic demonstrations of alar cartilage variations and of the factors that provide nasal tip support, stressing the importance of inserting grafts into the columellar labial region in order to prevent tip drooping. Plumping the columellar-labial junction forward and downward makes the columello-labial angle more obtuse and raises the tip and anterior columella. This less acute angle is often desired, particularly in females, as it provides a younger-looking profile. The forward pull on the medial crura of the lower lateral cartilages gives the illusion of a tip rotation.

The modification of the nasolabial angle may be difficult to achieve in some cases of secondary rhinoplasty. While it is relatively easy to make a nasolabial angle and raise the upper lip, it is more difficult to lengthen a nose that has been previously overshortened. Thus, it is particularly difficult in revision surgery to place the nasolabial angle into the proper position in cases in which the nose is retruded and the lip too advanced. The resection of the spine and retropositioning of the angle by the use of mattress sutures that are passed through the periosteum of the nasal floor (Figs. 177A and B and Fig. 178) is therefore combined with an elongation of the septum, and of the nose, as described above.

The inverted suture of Daley (1944), termed a submerged suture by Aufricht (1969), has a similar effect (Fig. 177C). Instead of being passed twice transversely, the suture is introduced through the base of the columella to emerge in the middle of the columellar base where the philtrum begins. It is then introduced through the same puncture point in the skin and passed into the other vestibule from where it is passed transversely to the original vestibule and tied there. Using this triangular Daley-Aufricht suture one can bring an obtuse nasolabial angle to the normal 90 degrees, keeping the columellar base applied to the nasal spine.

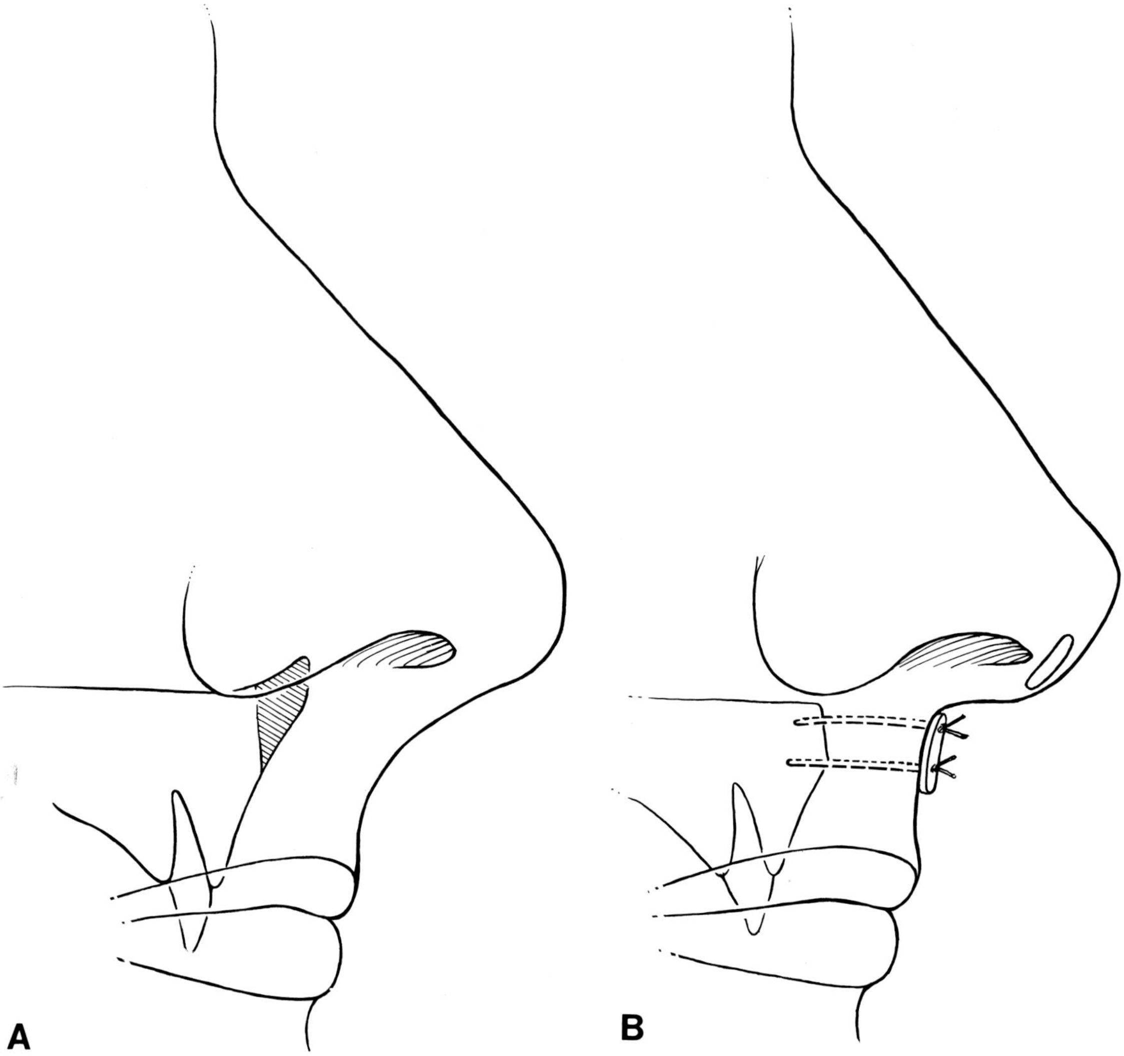

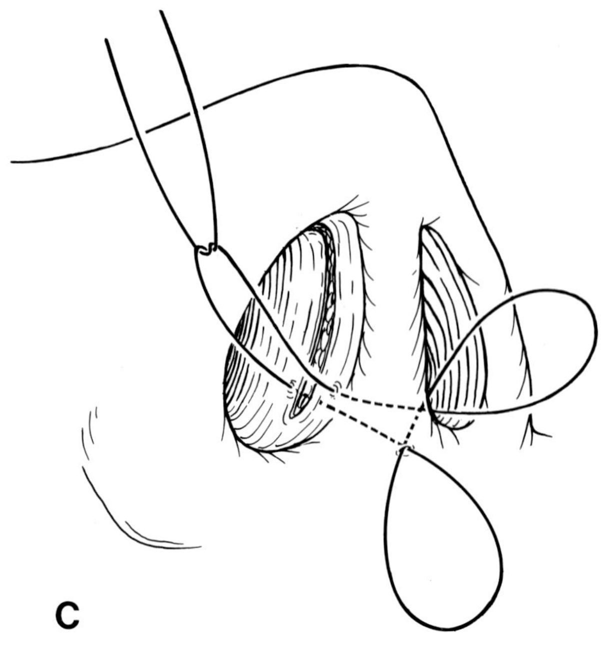

Fig. 177. Too obtuse nasolabial angle due to a too prominent spine. (A) The spine will be removed. (B) The philtrum is pulled backward with two mattress sutures anchored at the maxillary periosteum. (C) Inverted suture of Daley-Aufricht.

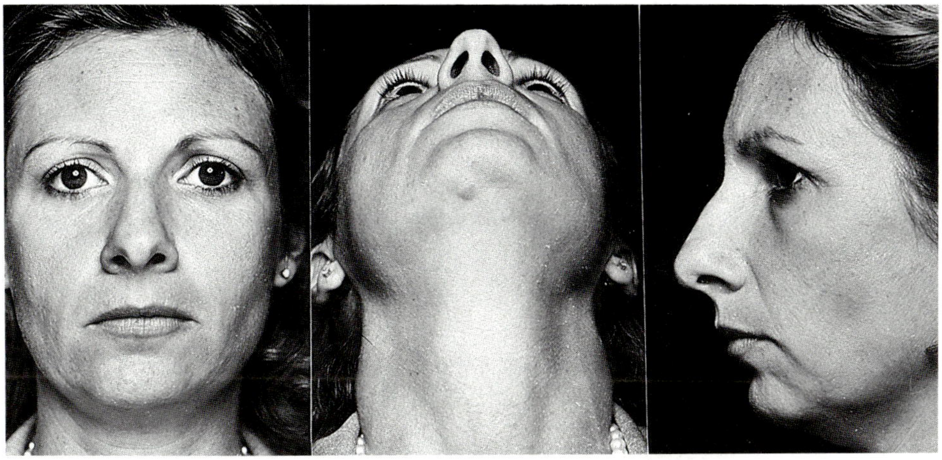

A

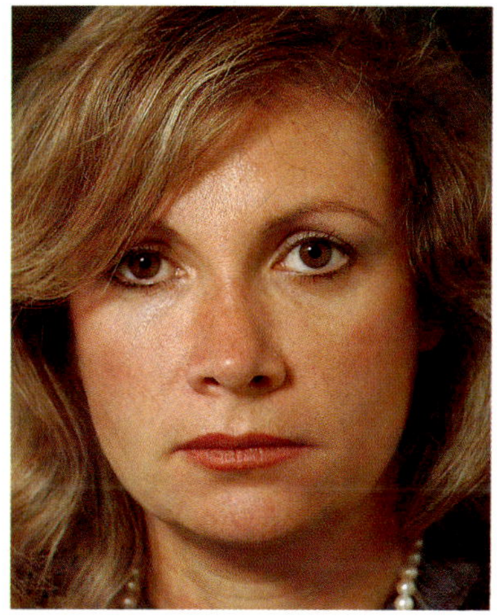

B

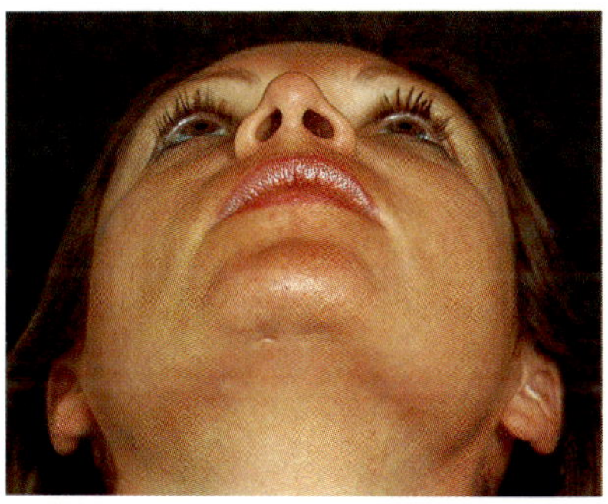

C

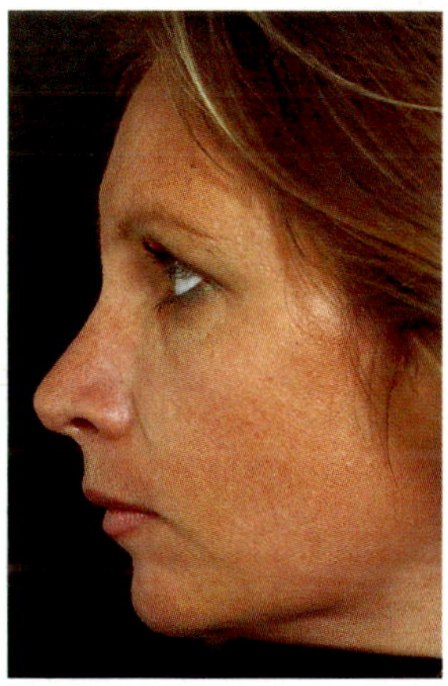

D

Fig. 178. Correction of a too short upper lip in a young woman after hump removal. The nasal spine has to be resected in order to allow the nasolabial angle to be shifted higher, giving the illusion of lengthening the lip. The prominence of the tip is also reduced. (A) Preoperative views. (B, C, and D) Postoperative views.

The procedure is the direct opposite if the nasolabial angle lies too far posteriorly and is too acute. The lengthening of the mucosa after an extramucosal dissection cannot be sufficiently obtained through the use of relaxing incisions or with the aid of small flaps. Instead, the addition of bone or cartilage or alloplastic material is necessary. For the correction of this deformity, a premaxillary onlay graft of Daley (1944) is applied. A cartilage graft from the septum or ear pavilion is introduced through the transfixion incision and is brought to lie in front of the spine and fixed with translabial mattress sutures as we described in 1964 (Denecke and Meyer) (Fig. 179).

Caronni (1972), Hinderer (1975), and Aiach (1982) proposed similar techniques with different materials. Hinderer (1975) uses a silicone implant.

In correcting the overshortened and "tight" nose, as well as the tethered lip, we also transsect the depressor septi nasi muscle through the transfixion incision by progressively dissecting forward using scissors until just under the skin of the columellar base and philtrum; this is the "lip-freeing" technique of Fred (1955). The cut is filled if necessary with cartilage, preventing the depressor fibers from reaching to themselves (see Chapter 3).

In the great majority of patients with hypoplasia of the middle third of the face, as well as with simple retrusion of the nasolabial angle, the surgical advancement or displacement of the maxilla and correction of the nasal base results in a subjective improvement in nasal air entry, which can also be verified objectively by rhinomanometric studies, as reported by Gottlieb and Masing (1984) and Rettinger and Masing (1986). This is due to an increase in the volume of the nasal skeleton and of the nasolabial angle, which improves nasal ventilation.

Through the same transfixion incision one

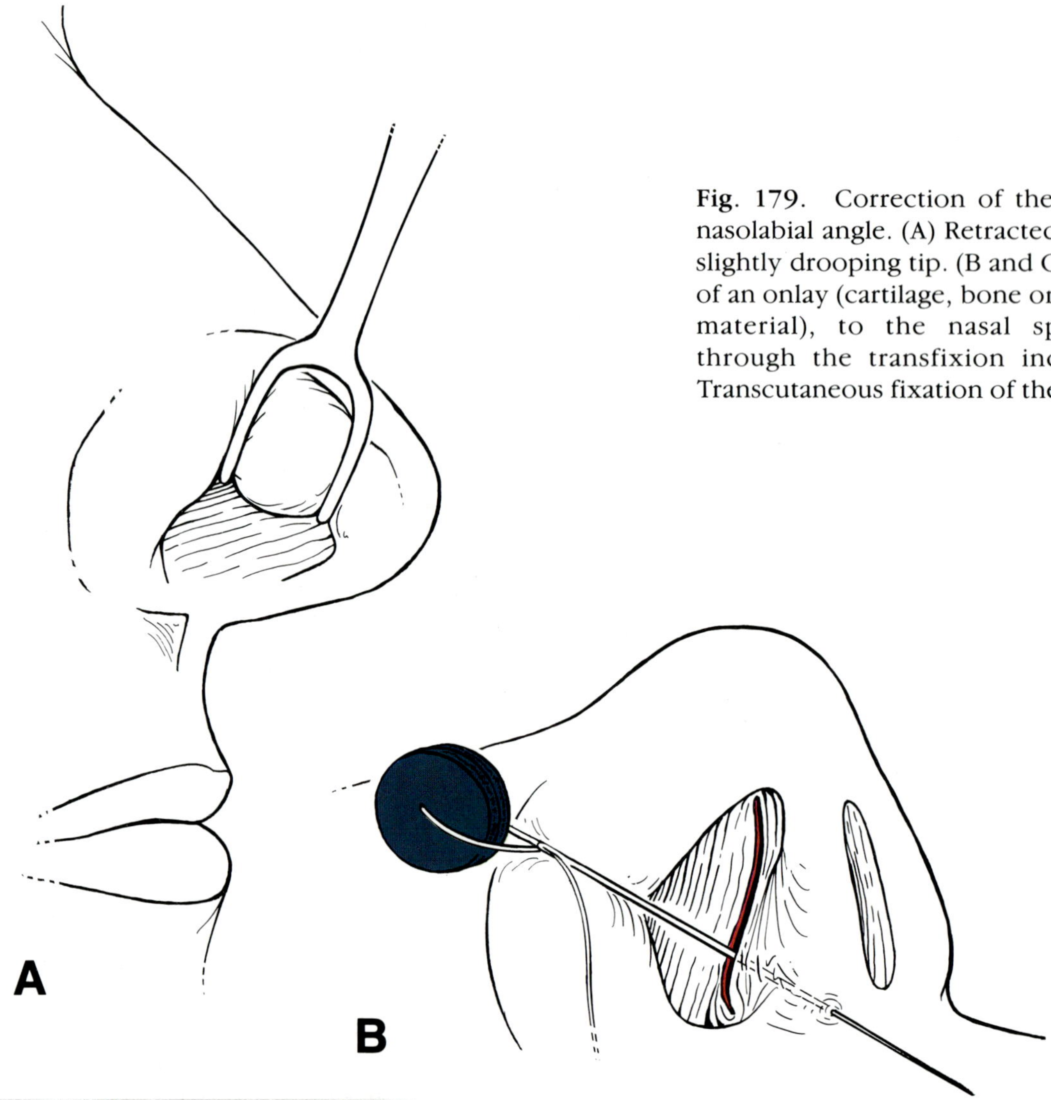

Fig. 179. Correction of the too acute nasolabial angle. (A) Retracted angle and slightly drooping tip. (B and C) Insertion of an onlay (cartilage, bone or alloplastic material), to the nasal spine level through the transfixion incision. (D) Transcutaneous fixation of the onlay.

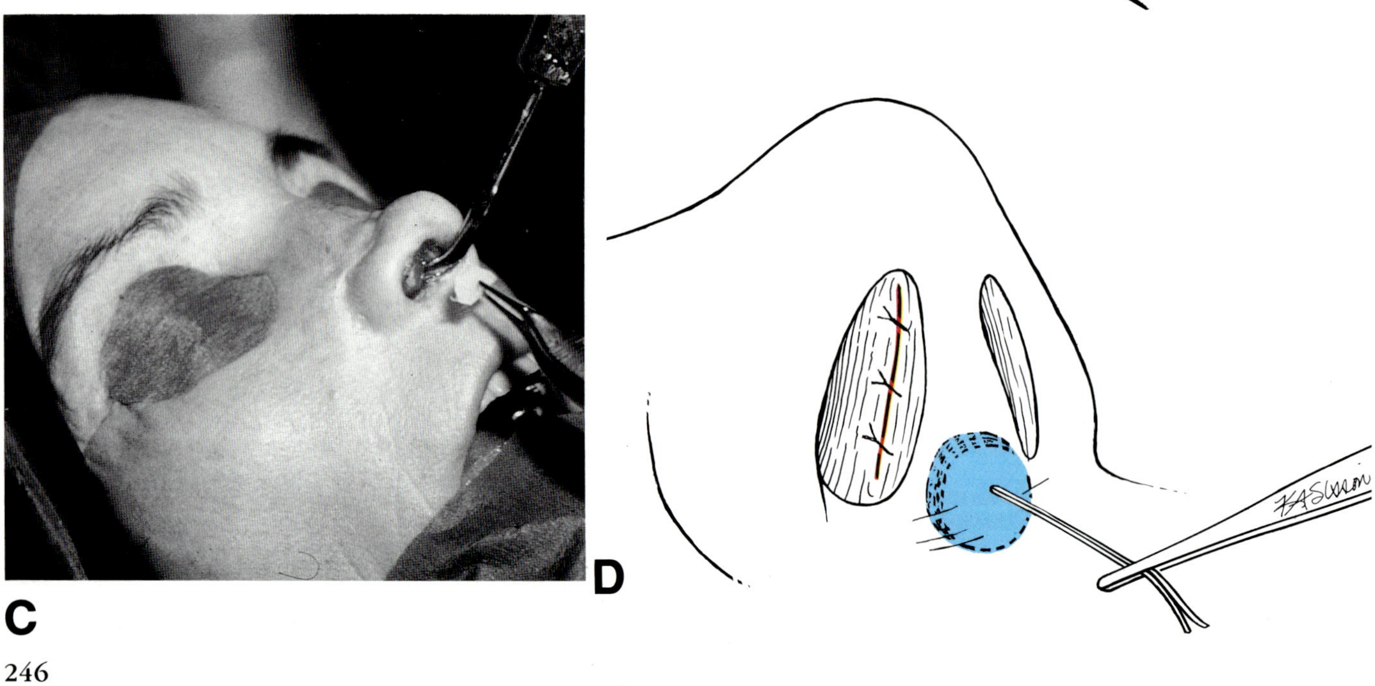

can reduce too prominent a sill of the vestibule by removing fat and subcutaneous tissue. In exceptional cases a fusiform horizontal skin resection is necessary on both sides to flatten an excessively high sill (Fig. 180). The defatting of the sill can also be done through an alar base incision (Figs. 181 and 182). Occasionally both the columella and the nostrils have to be shortened and placed more caudally. For this purpose, we simply perform the three basal resections (Fig. 183A). If at the same time the lip has to be shortened and the columellar base and alar bases displaced downwards into the upper lip, we combine the resections resulting in a buffalo-horn shaped skin excision (Figs. 183B, 184, 185, and 186). The lifting of the upper lip is usually sufficient to permit an additional augmentation cheiloplasty. In cases of very thin upper lips or in cases of sagging lips, correction can be obtained with a cutaneous strip resection at the cupids bows (Fig. 183). Instead of excising a buffalo-horn shaped strip of skin, the lifting of the upper lip can also be achieved by using bilateral S-shaped strip resections at the alar-lip junction, extending into the vestibular floor. By applying this technique, the columellar base is left at its original site (Fig. 187).

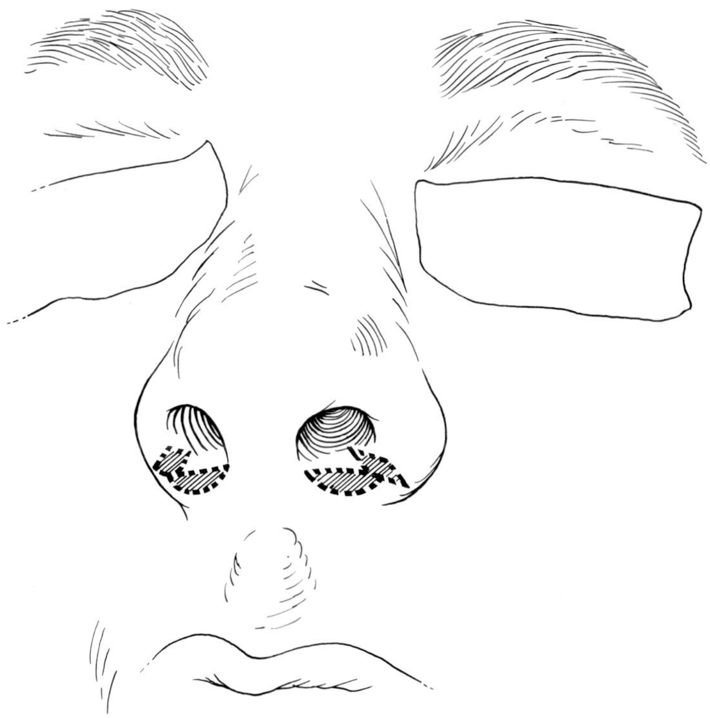

Fig. 180. Too prominent sill can be corrected by removing subcutaneous tissue through an incision or fusiform skin resection.

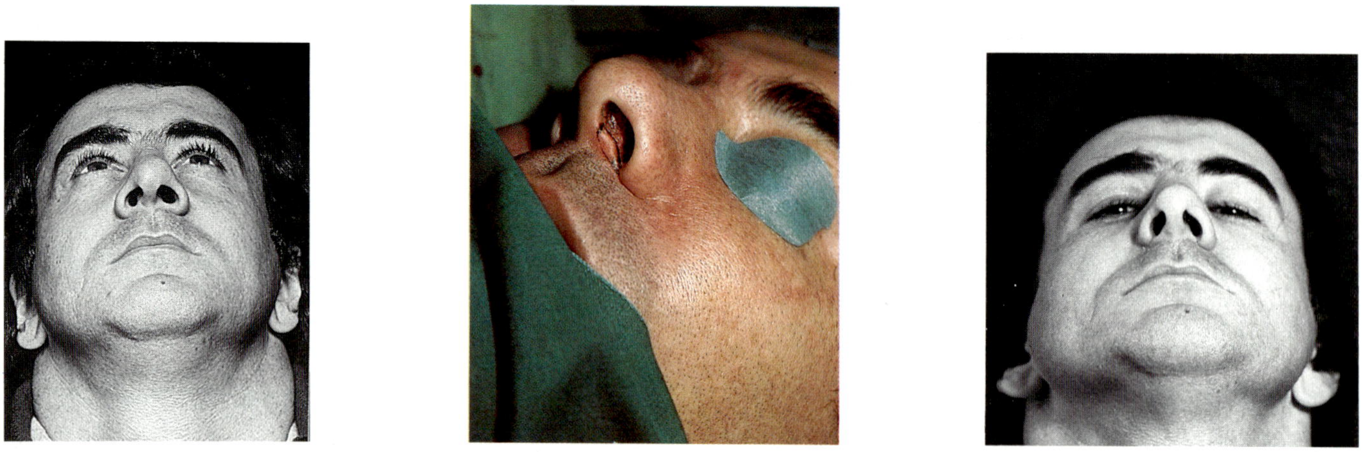

A **B** **C**

Fig. 181. Too prominent vestibular sill in a young man corrected by subcutaneous tissue resection through an alar base incision. (A) Axial view of the sills. (B) Outline of subcutaneous tissue to be removed. (C) Result after subcutaneous resection.

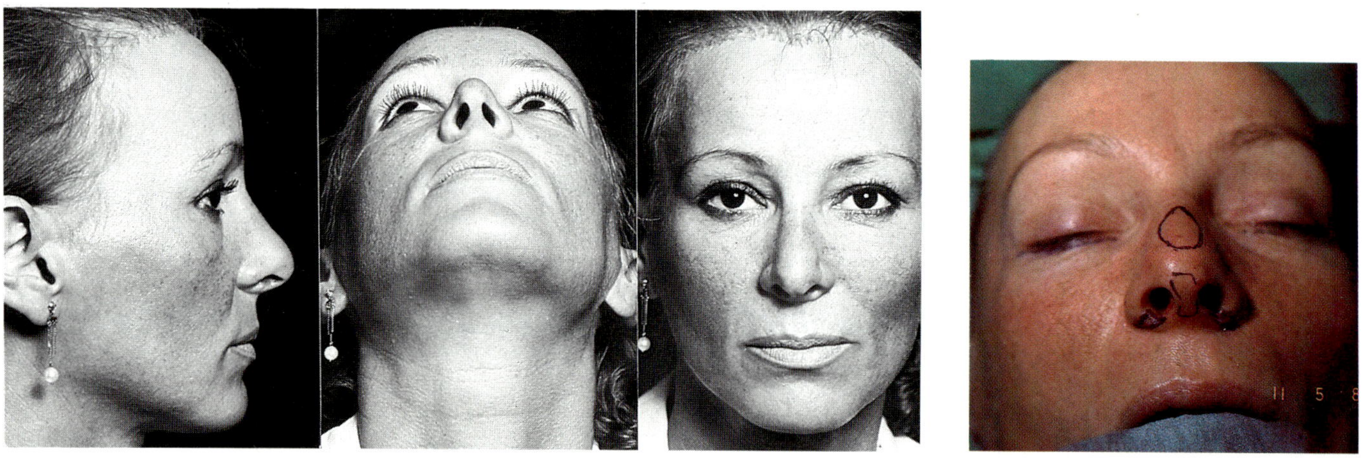

A **B**

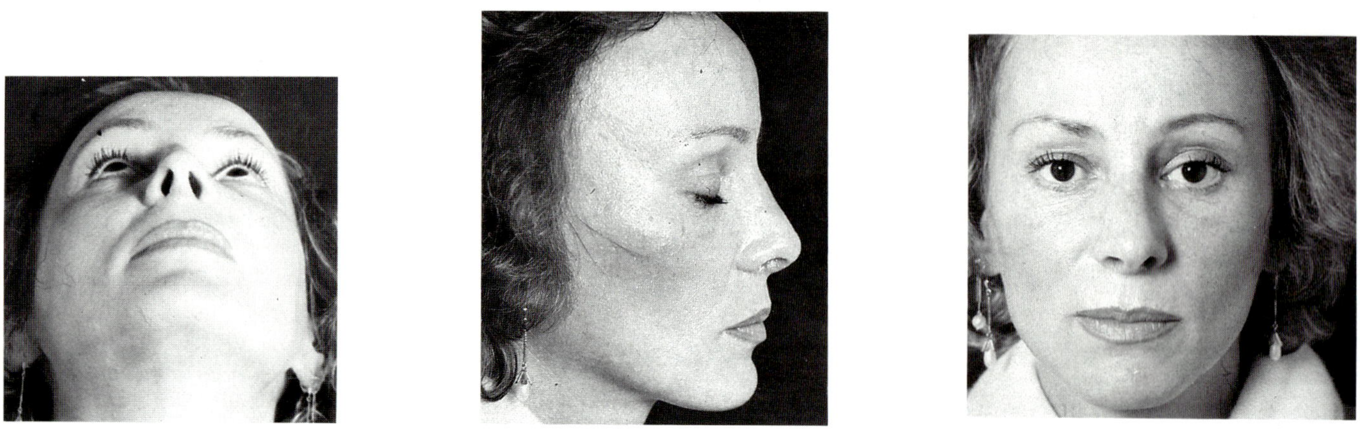

C **D** **E**

Fig. 182. Prominent sill giving an unattractive look to the nose of young female. It was reduced with the same resection combined with a supratip correction. (A) Preoperative views. Notice the high sill in profile view. (B) Resection of skin outlined. (C, D, and E) Result.

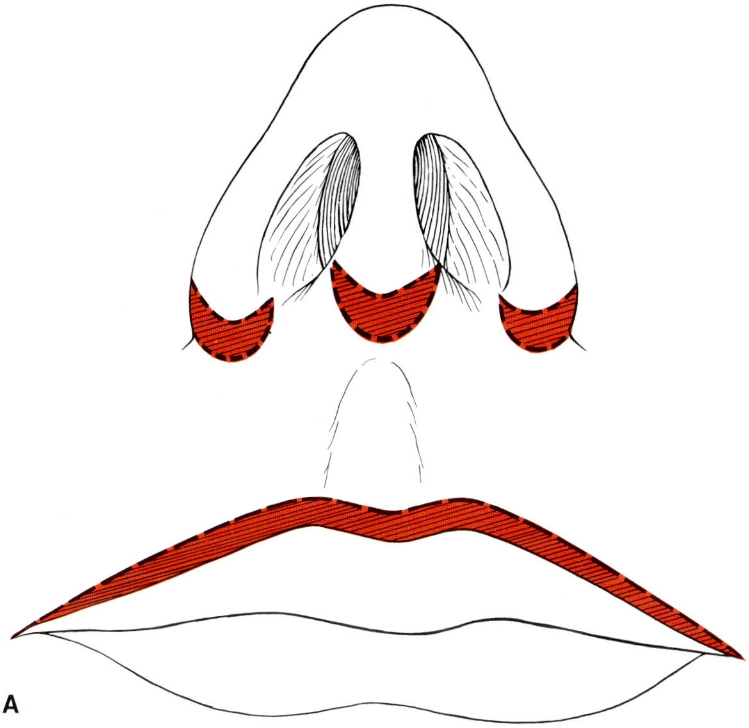

A

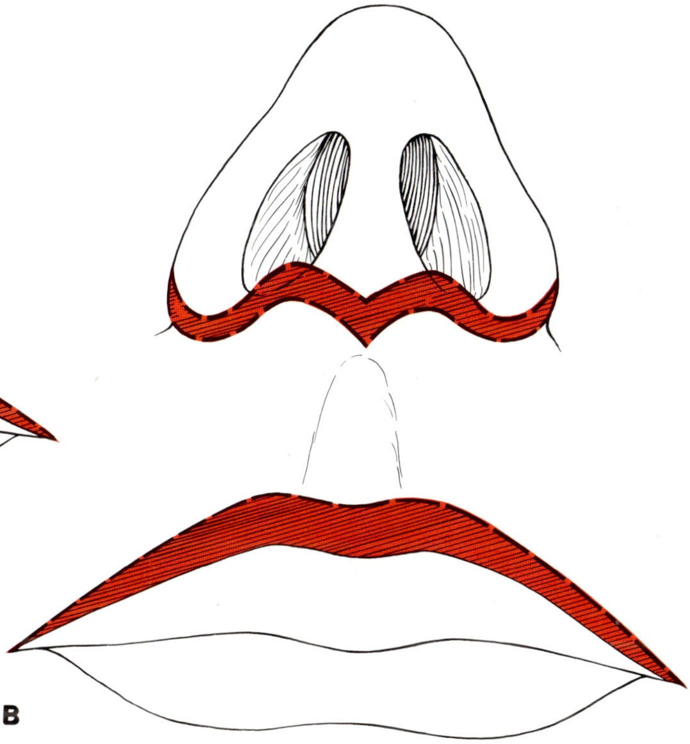

B

Fig. 183. (A) Shortening the upper lip by three isolated V-shaped resections at both alar and columellar base as well as by strip resection at the cupids bow, which is at the same time as an augmentation cheiloplasty. (B) Buffalo-horn-shaped excision along the nasolabial junction also shortens the too long lip and may be also combined with augmentation cheiloplasty.

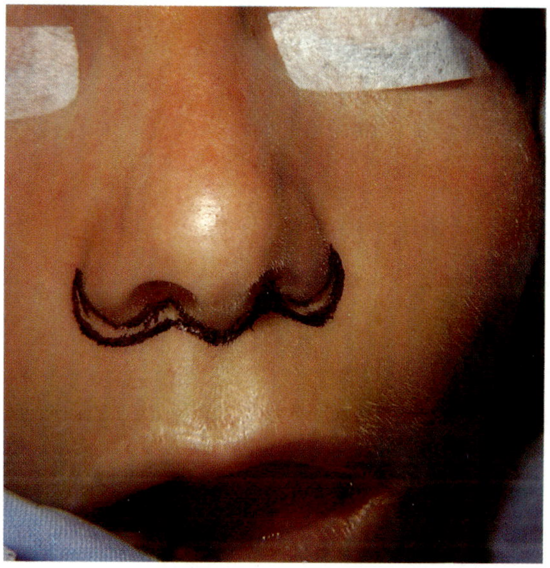

A

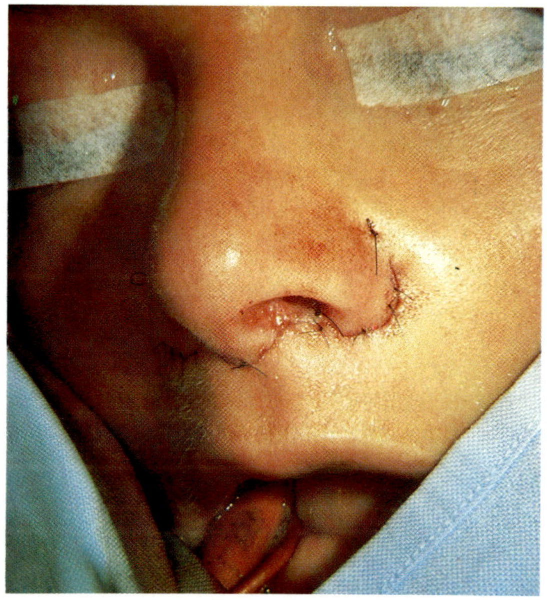

B

Fig. 184. Buffalo-horn-shaped excision along the nasolabial junction to shorten the upper lip. (A) Outline of the excision. (B) Subcuticlar and separated sutures.

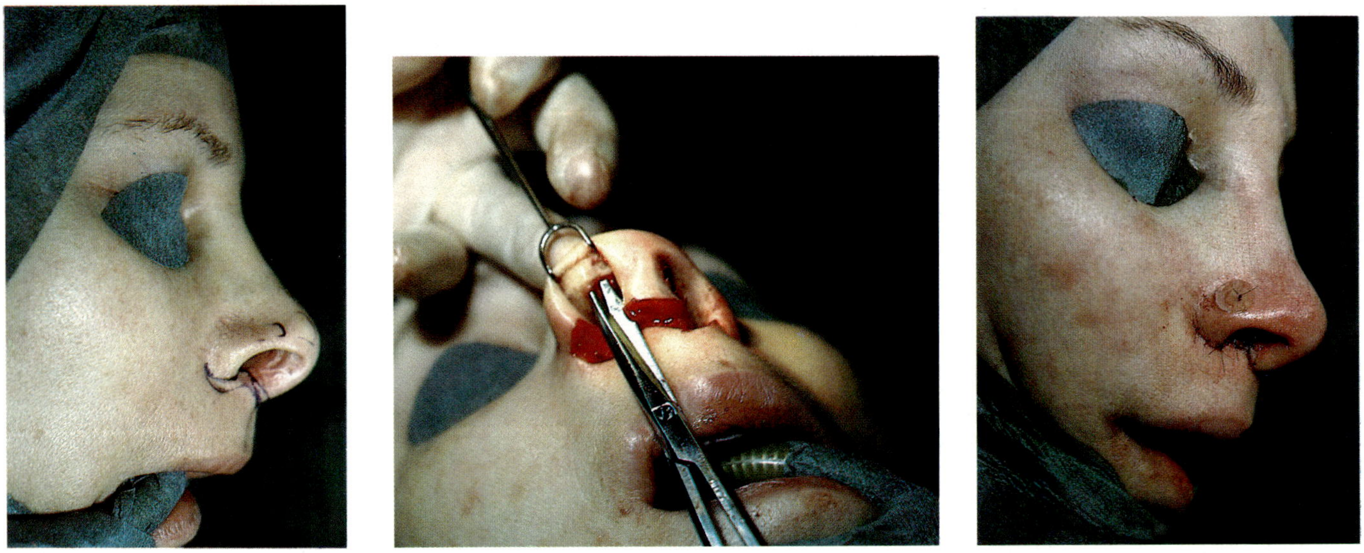

A **B** **C**

Fig. 185. Shortening the upper lip with buffalo-horn-shaped excision and correction of a sagging columella with full-thickness excision at the transfixion incision, as shown in Fig. 168 A. lowering the alar border and smoothening a supra-alar dimple, in a young female as a secondary procedure. (A) Outline of nasolabial excision and of the exaggerated supra-alar crease. (B) Correction of the alar retraction and of the supra-alar depression by insertion of a cartilage graft from the intercartilaginous incision by retrograde technique. (C) End of the operation with transalar mattress suture for fixation of the alar graft and suture of the buffalo-horn-shaped excision.

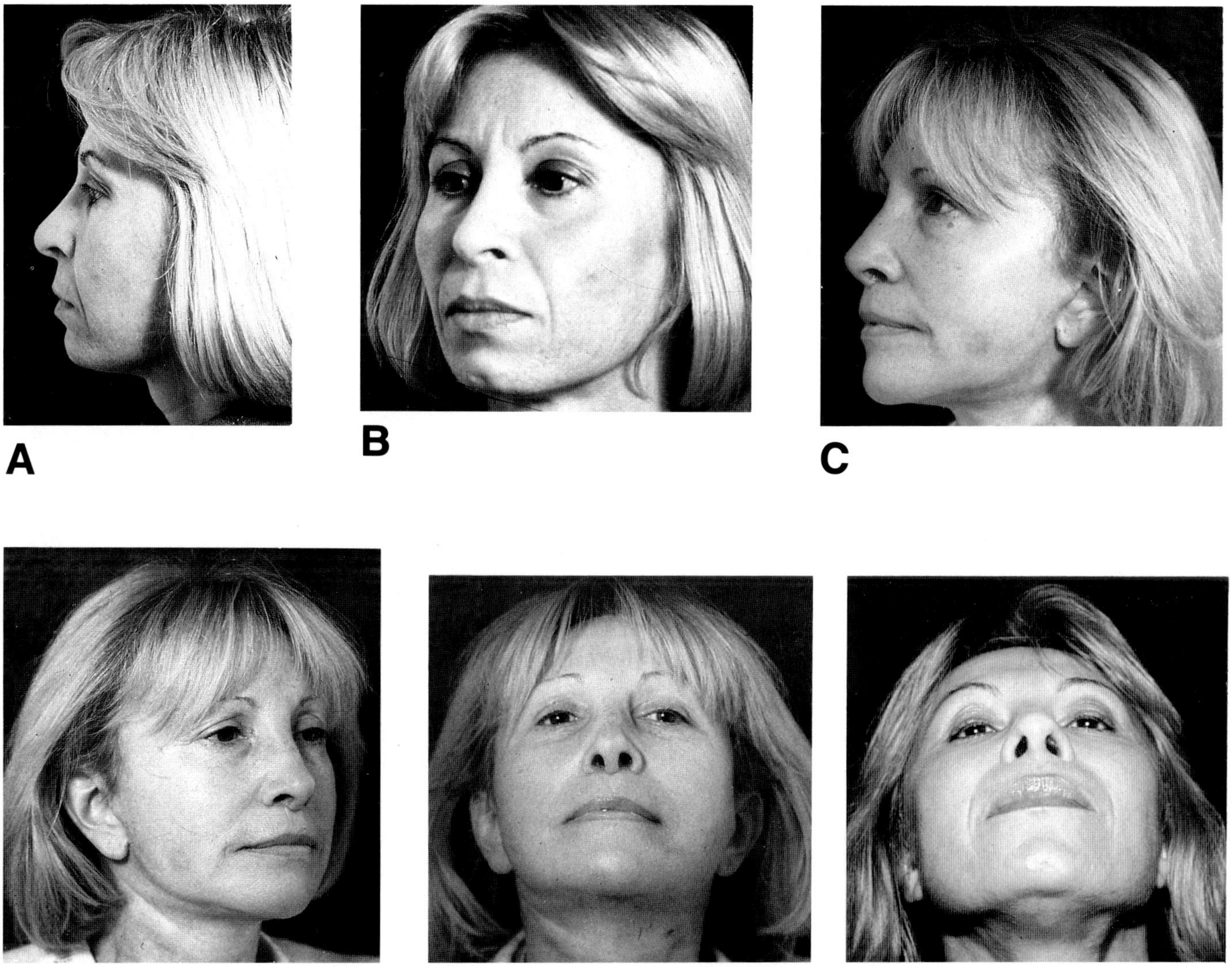

A B C D E F

Fig. 186. Young lady with too long upper lip, sagging of the tip, and supratip thickening after primary intervention. Shortening of the lip with buffalo-horn-shaped excision, supratip and tip correction in secondary procedure. (A and B) Preoperative views. (C, D, and E) Early result. (F) Late Result.

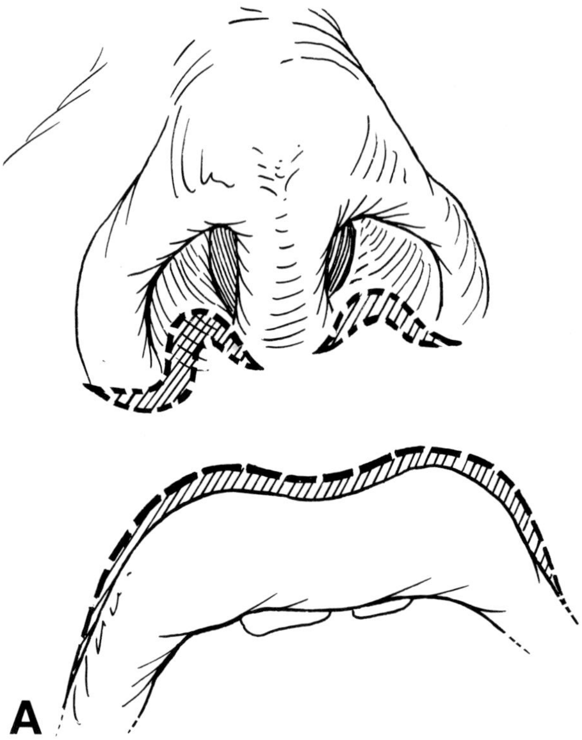

A

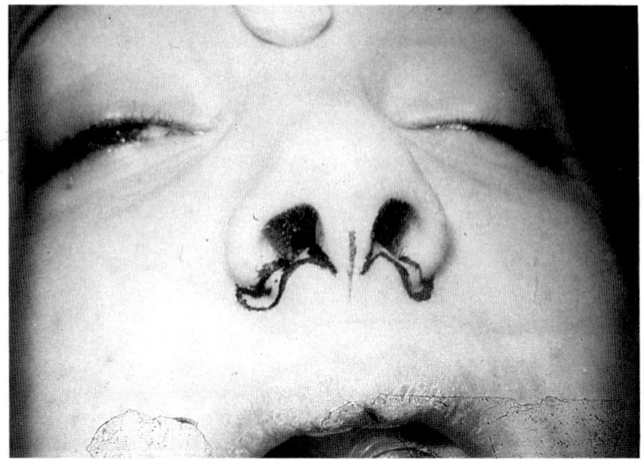

B

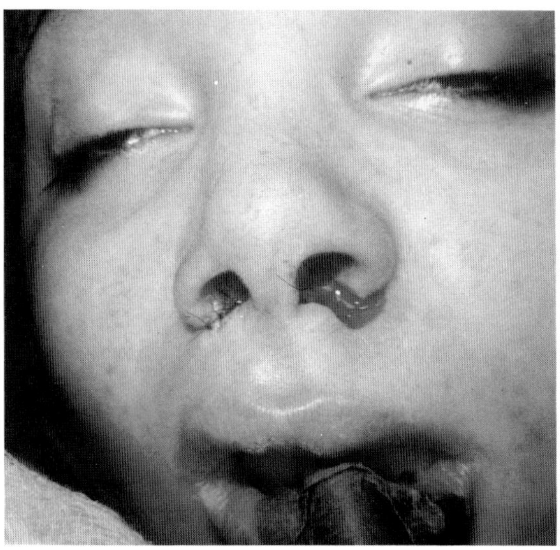

C

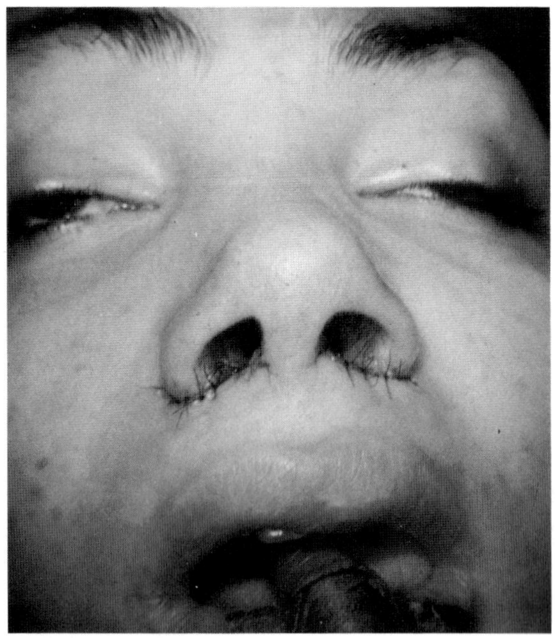

D

Fig. 187. Two separate excisions at the alar lip junction extending into the vestibular floor until the columellar base. (A and B) Outline of excisions. (C) Right side already lifted. Notice the upward shifting of the right lip side. (D) Suture on both sides.

TETHERED LIP

A tethered lip in which the gum is visible between the lip and the apex of the incisors is considered to be unaesthetic. Techniques utilized in the past to correct this have included shortening of the alveolar maxillary complex and closure of the labiogingival sulcus.

Our method decreases the elevation of the lip by means of the transsection of the depressor septi nasi muscle and levator labii inferiori, or myrtiform muscle, through the base of the transfixion incision, interposing the dorsal hump, if present, as a spacer, or, failing that, an ear cartilage or a bone graft from the iliac bone (Figs. 188–191). The gingiva is elevated from the anterior surface of the alveolus subperiosteally, allowing for relaxation and expansion of the gingivolabial fold and a downward shift of the lip. The levator labii superioris muscle is transsected laterally as far as the ala extends. The lip is then kept down with an interposed graft. The pocket is dissected as widely as necessary to fit the graft. In extreme cases of tethered lip we fix the graft with mattress sutures through the mucosa of the gingivolabial fold.

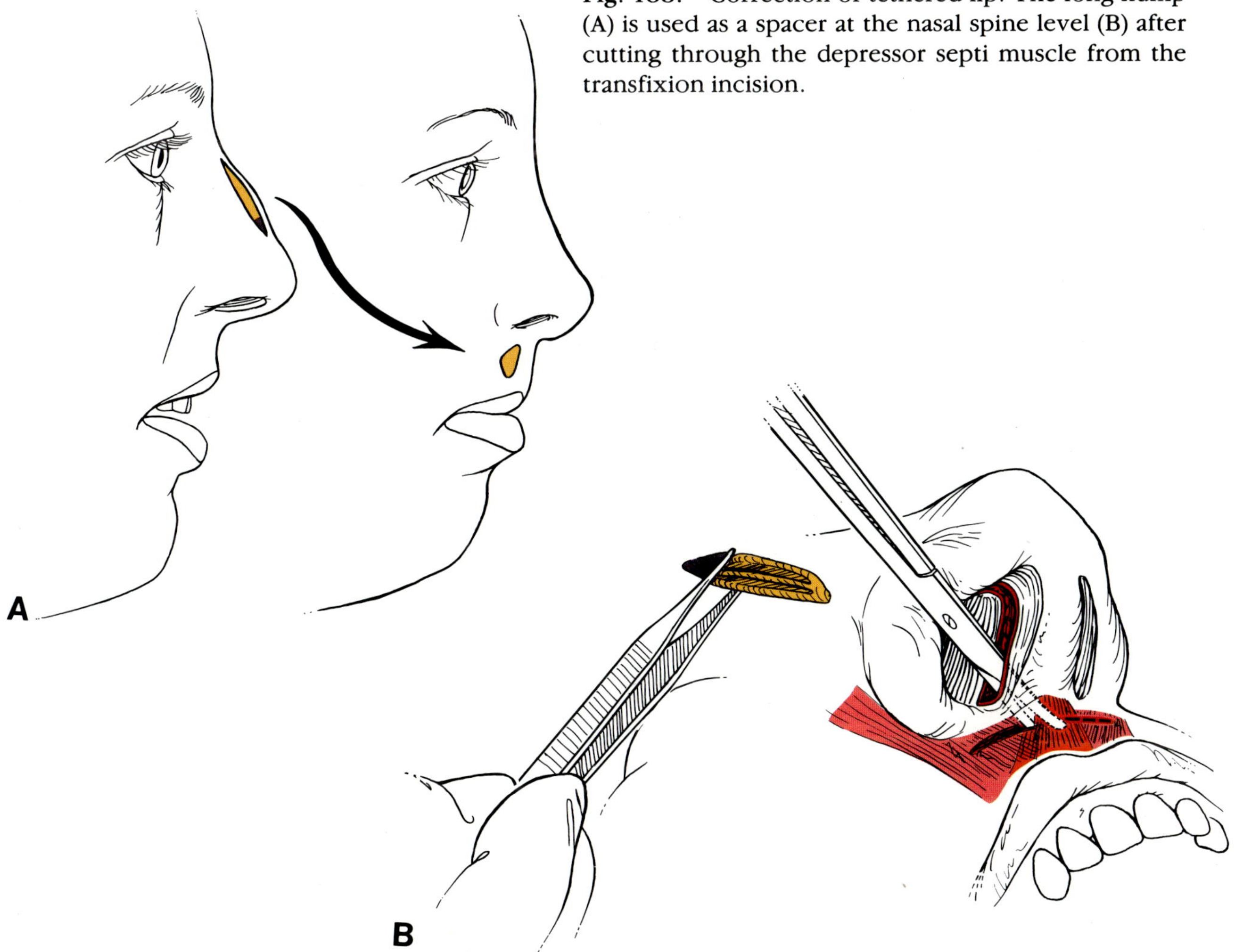

Fig. 188. Correction of tethered lip. The long hump (A) is used as a spacer at the nasal spine level (B) after cutting through the depressor septi muscle from the transfixion incision.

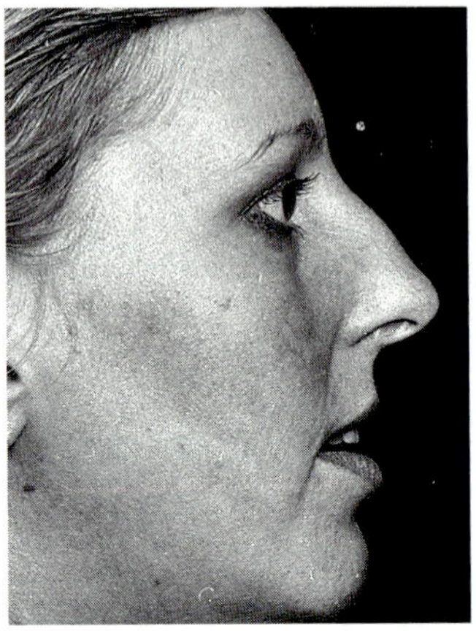

A

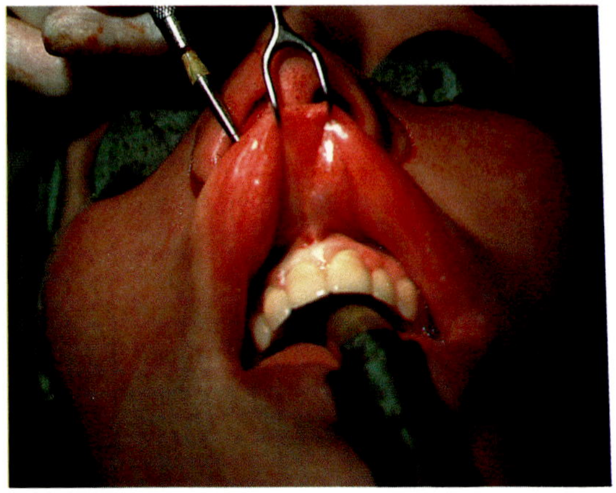

B

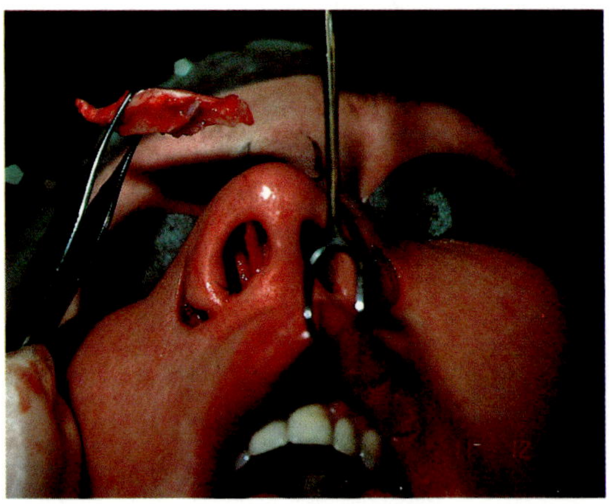

C

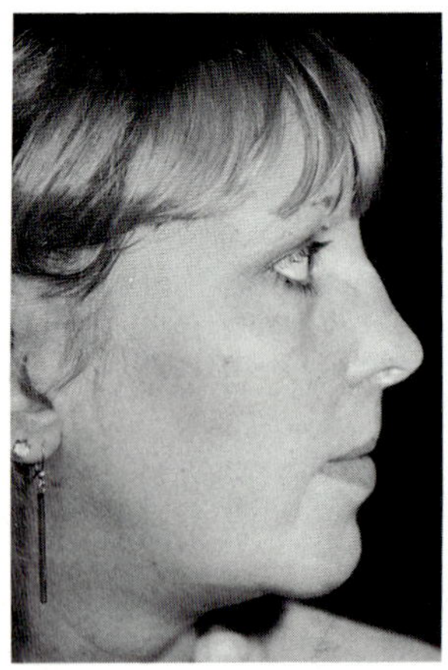

D

Fig. 189. Young woman with gummy smile operated according to Fig. 188, transferring the hump into a pocket at the nasal spine thus pushing downward the nasolabial and labial soft tissues. (A) Preoperative profile. (B) Dissection of the gingiva through the transfixion incision. (C) Hump of the nose will be reduced and inserted into the sublabial pocket. (D) New profile. The chin has been corrected too.

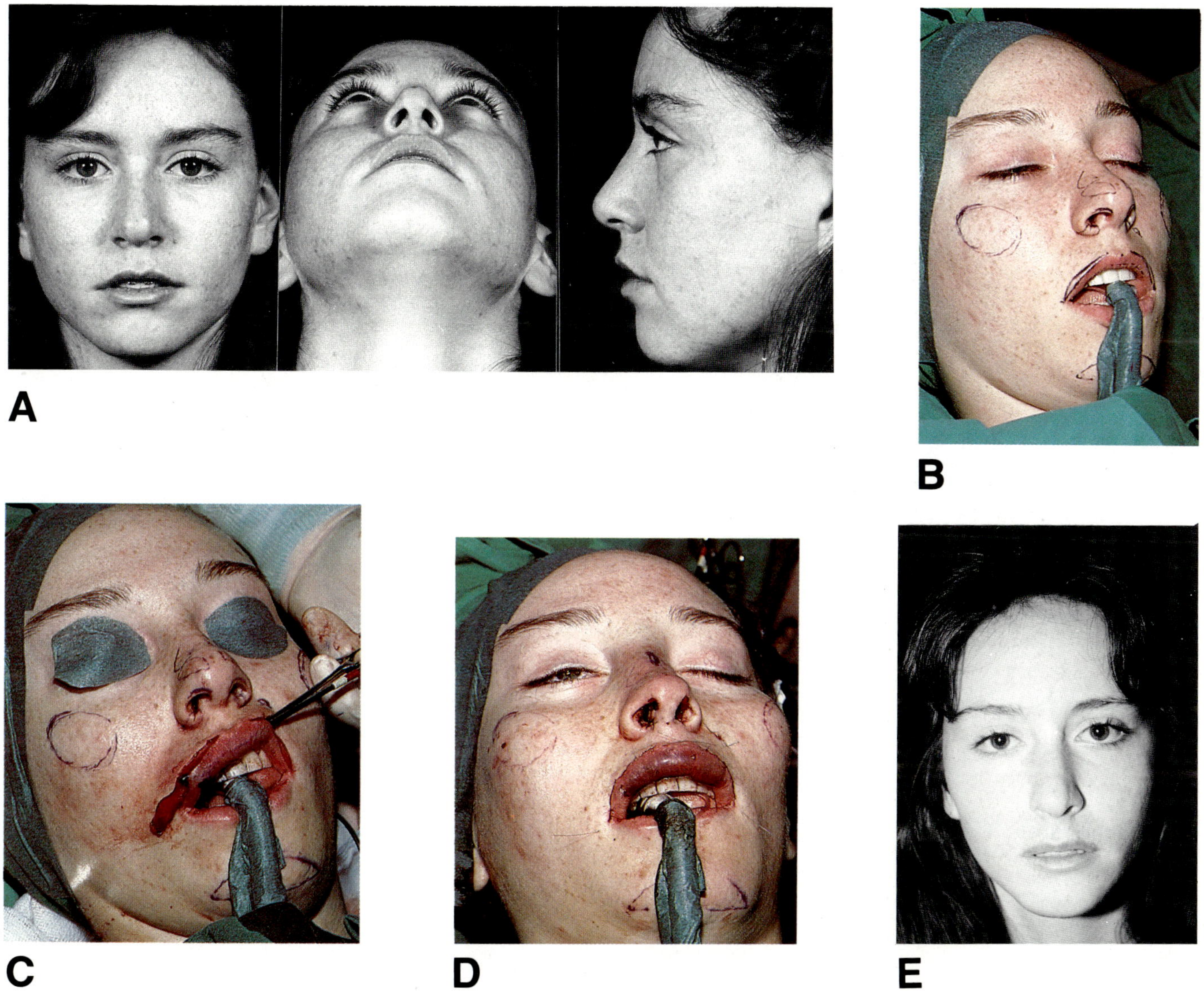

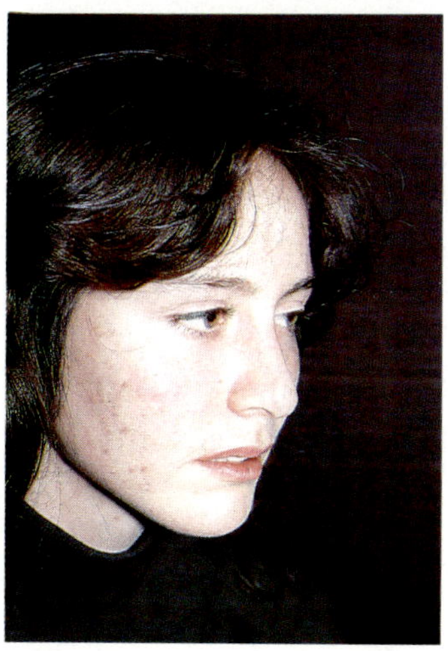

Fig. 190. Correction of the tethered lip combined with reduction of the vestibular sill, refinement of the nostril, and remodeling of the fascial contour in a young female. (A) Preoperative view. (B) Outline of the planned corrections. (C) Augmentation of the central part of the upper lip with temporal fascia. (D) End of the operation after malar and chin augmentation lip correction and nasal refinement. (E, F) Result.

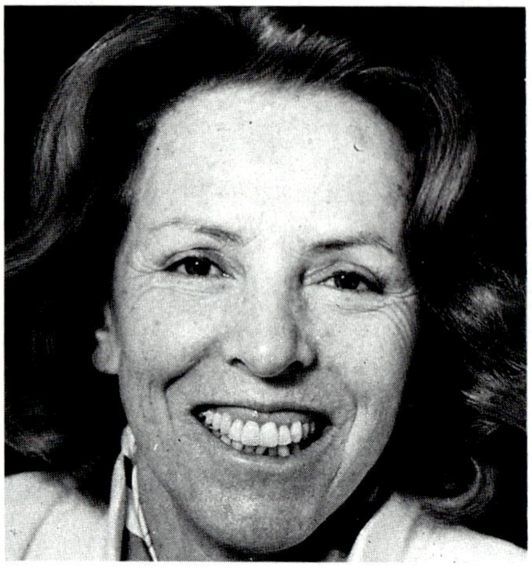

A

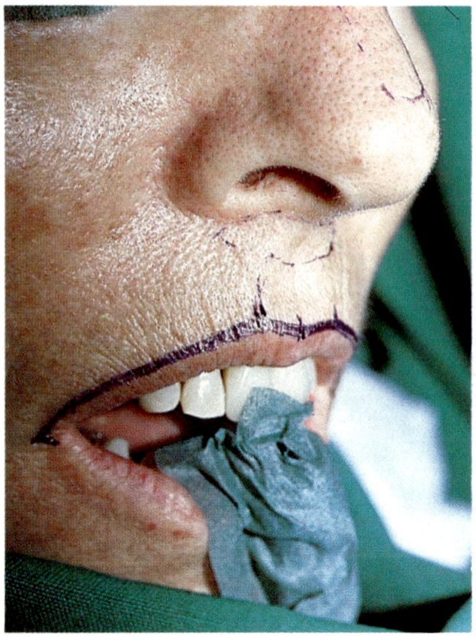

B

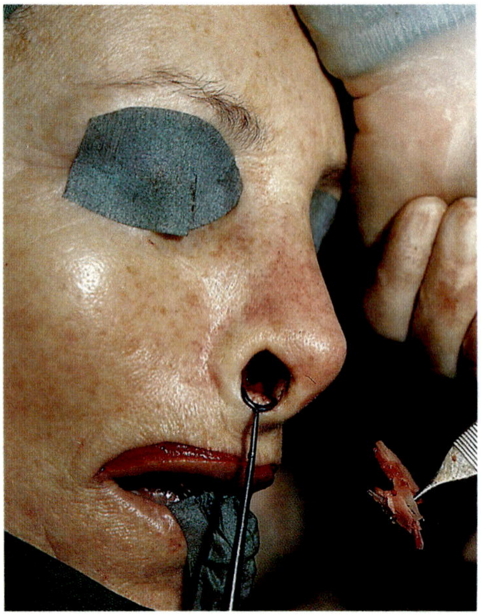

C

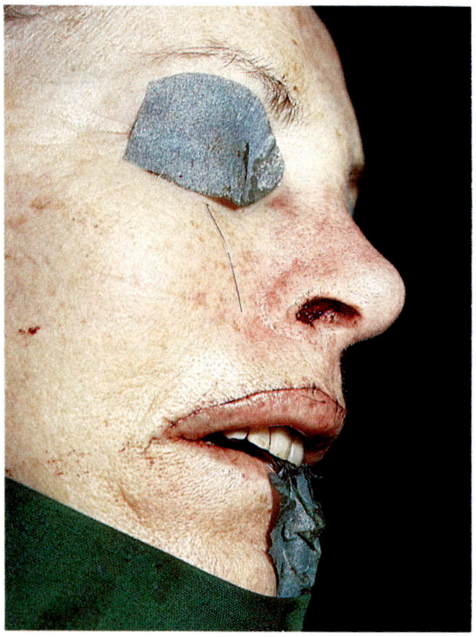

D

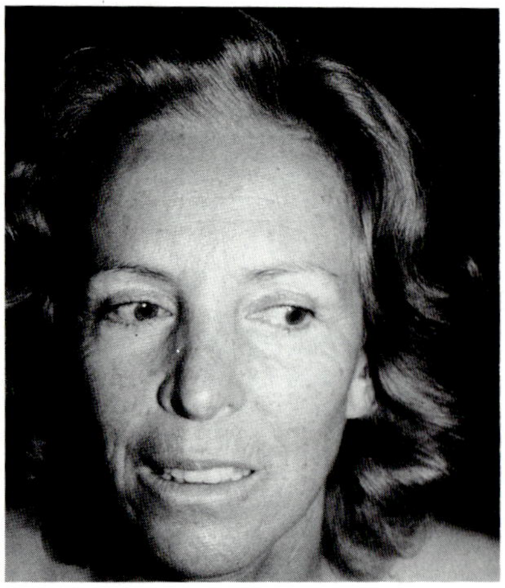

E

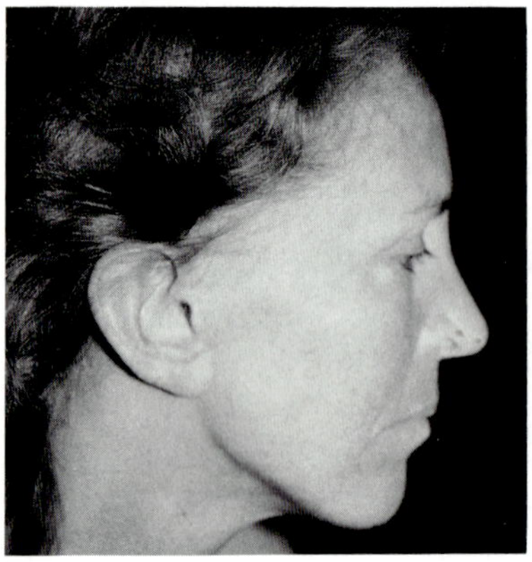

F

Fig. 191. Gummy smile in a middle-aged lady corrected in the same way. (A) Simultaneously the lip was shortened with a fine strip resection at the cupid's bow without interfering with its planned lowering. (B) Outline of hump, nasolabial onlay, and cupid's bow correction. (C) Insertion of hump into the lip. (D) End of the operation. (E and F) Result.

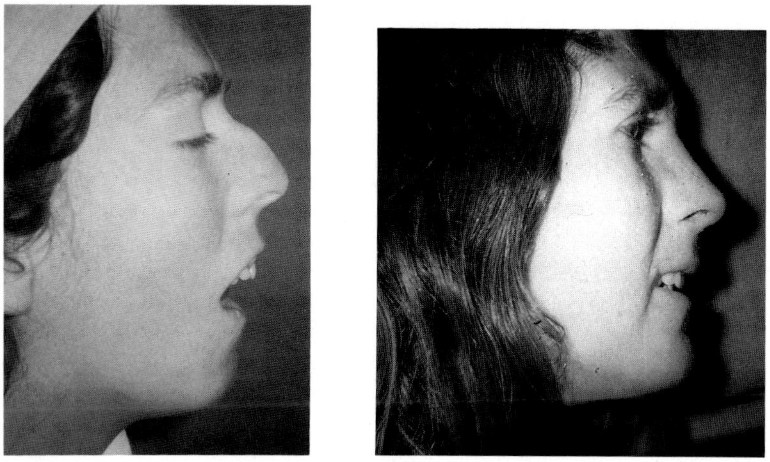

A B

Fig. 192. Another case of tethered lip operated in the same way. (A) Preoperative view. (B) Postoperative view after rhinoplasty and augmentation plasty.

The maxillary spine can be left intact, reduced, or enlarged by the same expanding graft according to the need of achieving a normal protrusion of the nasolabial fold. Ellenbogen and Swara (1984) proposed the same procedure using a custom carved spacer of silicone. They demonstrated how contraction of the elevator muscles (as seen with wrinkling of the nose) shows gum above the central incisors and how, by adding the action of the spreader-muscles, the gumminess is related to the excursion of the elevators.

Insertion of a spacer after partial transsection of the major elevators decreases the upward excursion of the elevators, thus eliminating the gumminess. When the spreader-muscles are brought into action, the gummy smile itself is corrected. In minor cases where only the hyperactivity of the levator muscles is the cause of the gummy smile the myectomy of the elevators suffices, without need to interpose autogenous or alloplastic material, as advocated by Miskinjar (1983).

In his book, Rees (1980) shows how resection of the nasal spine and of the caudal border of the cartilaginous septum, after freeing the lip with dissection of the alveolus and periosteum and with release of the low attachment of the frenulum, also corrects the tethered lip. In addition, the nasolabial angle has to be set at the proper level, the dorsum lowered, and the tip remodeled by resection of the outer portion of the lateral crus on each side. Furthermore, Rees performs a resection of the flared, widened columellar base by resecting the medial crura.

In extreme cases of a long maxilla with relation to the upper lip, causing the incisor to show and a gummy smile, the treatment should be a Lefort I impaction procedure as suggested by Kawamoto (1982). Therefore, such patients should be evaluated for vertical maxillary excess before deciding on a corrective procedure. In many cases the tethered lip is accompanied by a hump, thus producing a so-called tension nose.

THE TENSION NOSE

The tension nose is a condition in which the skin and mucosa of the nose have been stretched by disproportionate growth of the underlying bone and cartilage. Cottle (1960) stated that stretching of the mucosa thins out the blood vessels and nerves. This condition also occurs over sharp ridges and spurs in the nose and is connected to conditions of collapsed valves and alae as well as with narrow vestibules and a narrow cavity. The patient often complains of headache and difficulty in breathing. Chessen and Philpott (1955) pointed out that the tension nose typically has a long straight septum that seems to be trying to escape from the nose. The skin and mucosa are stretched thin. There is often a cartilaginous hump.

A slight septal deviation in the valve region can cause severe breathing problems. When the patient activates the depressor septi muscle for lowering the lip and the columellar base, the anteroinferior angle of the septal cartilage becomes visible through the skin in the weak triangle of Converse, and between the domes of the lower lateral cartilages.

According to Sputh (1985), repeated injury, inherited characteristics, or surgery may all produce a tension nose. Removal of the membranous septum can also cause tension. Inadequate removal of the anterior part of the septal cartilage during a rhinoplasty may produce a parrot beak effect, which is in fact really a cartilaginous hump creating tension.

Surgery of the tension nose relies on good surgery of the septum, upper lateral cartilages, and nasal bones. Parell et al (1982) pointed out that the thin skin leaves little error in surgical judgment or technique. The anomaly is treated with a complete septorhinoplasty and simultaneous correction of the excessively narrow and collapsing structures. The dorsum has to be lowered by reducing the bony and cartilaginous framework. The upper and lower lateral cartilages require the special treatment, described for the collapsing middle third of the nose in order to gain space at the level of the ballooning valve. In severe cases the valve angle is enlarged with a composite graft from the ear as described previously. In a few cases we have had to enlarge the vestibule and the nasal cavity as will be explained further on.

Both mucosal flaps in the caudal and anterior areas of the septum are elevated. All spurs and septal deviations should be corrected. The nasal dorsum is corrected through intercartilaginous incisions. The bony vault needs to be widened by outfractures. This surgery has the effect of lowering the nose and taking the stretch out of the mucosa and skin. Studies have shown that postoperatively, although the cross sectional area of the nasal valve is decreased, the angle of the valve is substantially increased. This, combined with the shortening of the upper lateral cartilages and their consequent increased rigidity, improves the aerodynamics of the narrow nose with relief of nasal obstruction (Arbour and Bilgen, 1986). Thus, the aesthetics and function of the nose are both improved (Fig. 192).

16

Residual Deformities of the Ala

HANGING (HOODING) ALA

The alar rim must have a harmonious line—not too low, not too high, not too straight, and not asymmetric. When the aesthetic relationship between the columella and the alar rim does not exist, or when the nose is significantly shortened by raising the columella, it may be necessary to raise the alar rim.

We see many operated noses, some presented at congresses, others in the literature, with a very beautiful profile, a perfect bony skeleton, and a good shape to the tip, where the only imperfection is a drooping lower lateral border, like the wings of a bird. This occurs because the operator did not have the courage to perform a marginal resection or other procedure for elevation.

We employ the following technique for accomplishing a rim elevation: (1) marginal resection, (2) trimming the caudal rim of the lateral crus of the alar cartilage and the caudal ventral border of the septal cartilage, (3) trimming the upper part of the lateral crus and the caudal ventral aspect of the septum, and (4) partial resection of the alar lining.

Marginal Resection

A wedge excised as a strip along the free border of each overlying side wall sculptures the nostril curve and regains the proper columella-ala relationship. In the book by Denecke and Meyer (1964/1967) we described the correction of a bilateral hare lip nose with marginal alar resections, and for the correction of the tip and lobule, a bilateral sickle-shaped excision on the anterior rim of the nostrils reaching the lobule. Millard (1967) published procedures with similar marginal resections.

Actually we perform marginal resections in about 10 percent of all primary and 20 percent of secondary rhinoplasties. As we (Meyer and Kesselring) explained in 1977 we mostly cut the edge of the nostril along its whole length (Figs. 193 D and 194) when the entire lower lateral rim is too low. On request we correct other anomalies, resecting the border only posteriorly (Figs. 193 B and 195) or anteriorly (Figs. 193 A and 196), or at either end (Fig. 193 C). The outline of

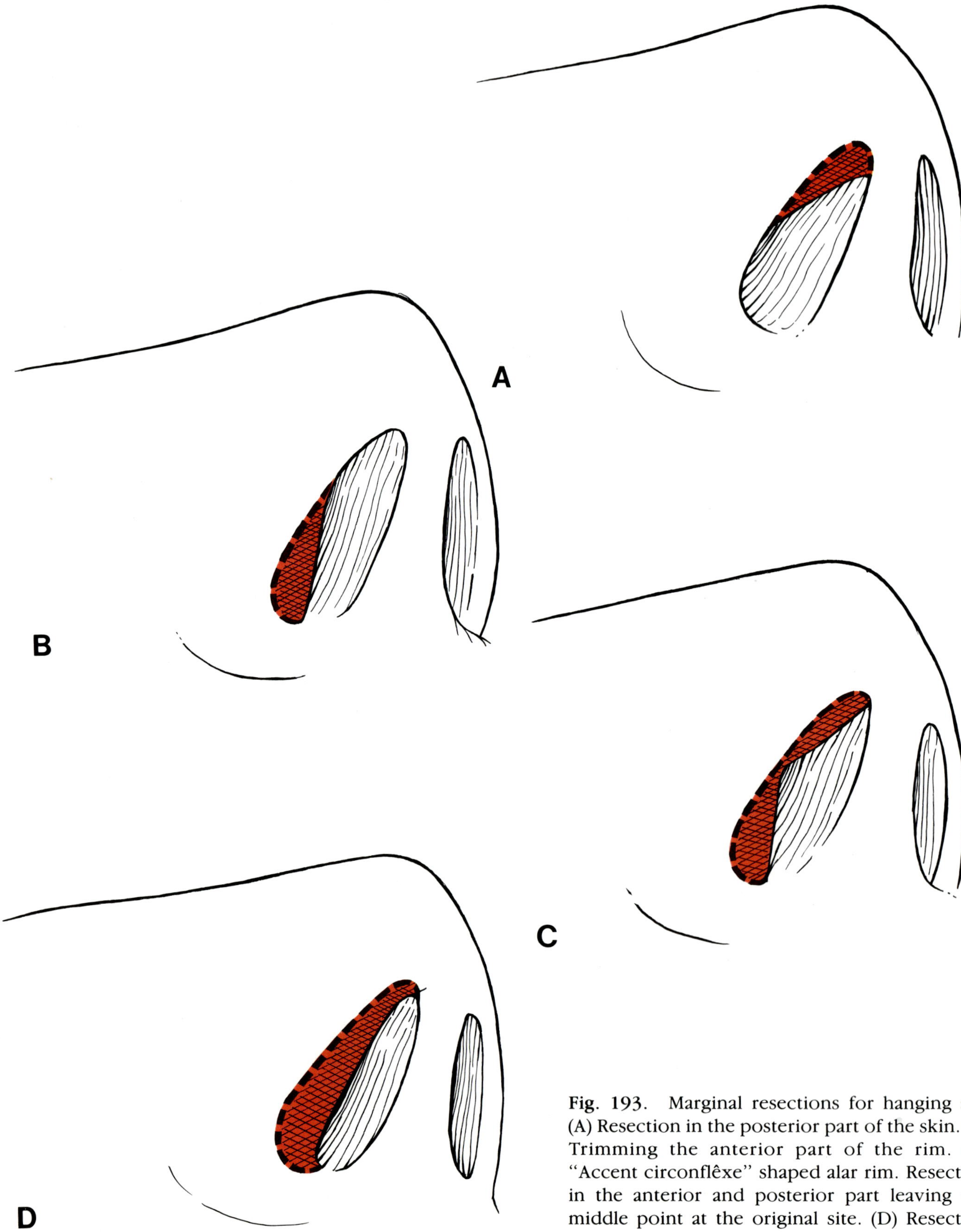

Fig. 193. Marginal resections for hanging ala. (A) Resection in the posterior part of the skin. (B) Trimming the anterior part of the rim. (C) "Accent circonflêxe" shaped alar rim. Resection in the anterior and posterior part leaving the middle point at the original site. (D) Resection along the entire rim.

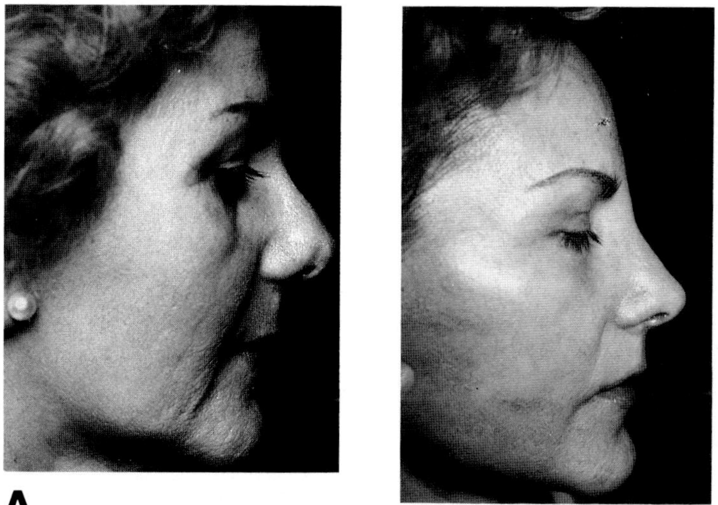

A B

Fig. 194. Alar border resection along the whole length in elderly lady operated three times before.

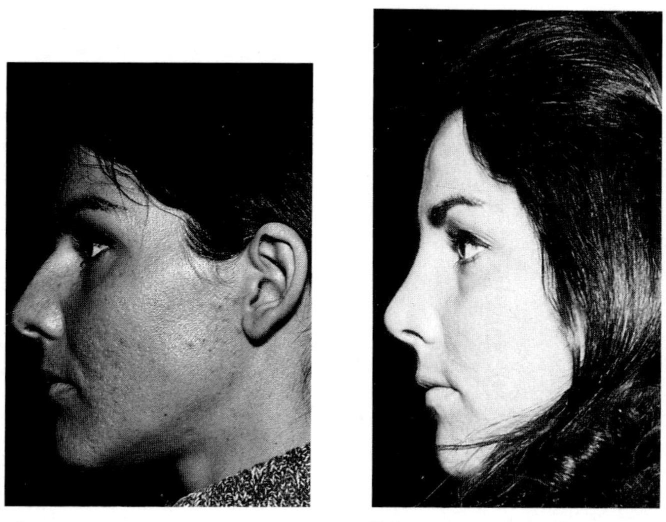

A B

Fig. 195. Sagging ala only in the posterior part. Correction with posterior resection.

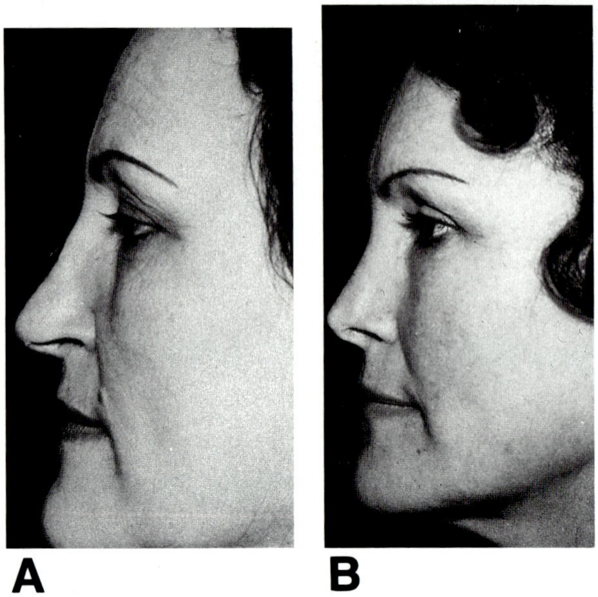

Fig. 196. Anterior marginal resection as secondary procedure.

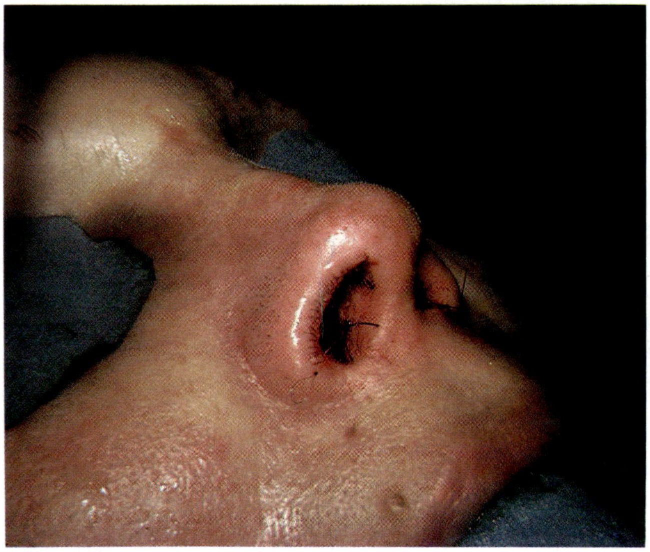

Fig. 197. "Over and over" or running suture of the trimmed alar rim in the whole length.

the wedge resection is marked carefully with a scalpel and the resection is carried out with a fine curved scissor. After cautious cauterization with a No. 15 blade the cut edges are approximated by over and over sutures of 6-0 nonabsorbable material (Fig. 197). These lower lateral rim resections are often combined with alar base resections according to Weir (1892), Seltzer (1949), Safian (1935), Converse (1964), and others. The rim resection can then fade into the alar base resection. These combinations have been described by Millard (1969), Meyer (1977), and Planas (1977) in caucasian flat and thick noses, by Boo-Chai (1986) in oriental noses, and by Spira (1966) and Avelar (1976) in negroid noses (Figs. 198 and 199). In 1983 Farina et al reported on the satisfactory results obtained in the correction of pseudo-crypto-columella by marginal resection of the hanging ala, something that they called S-shaped nasal wing.

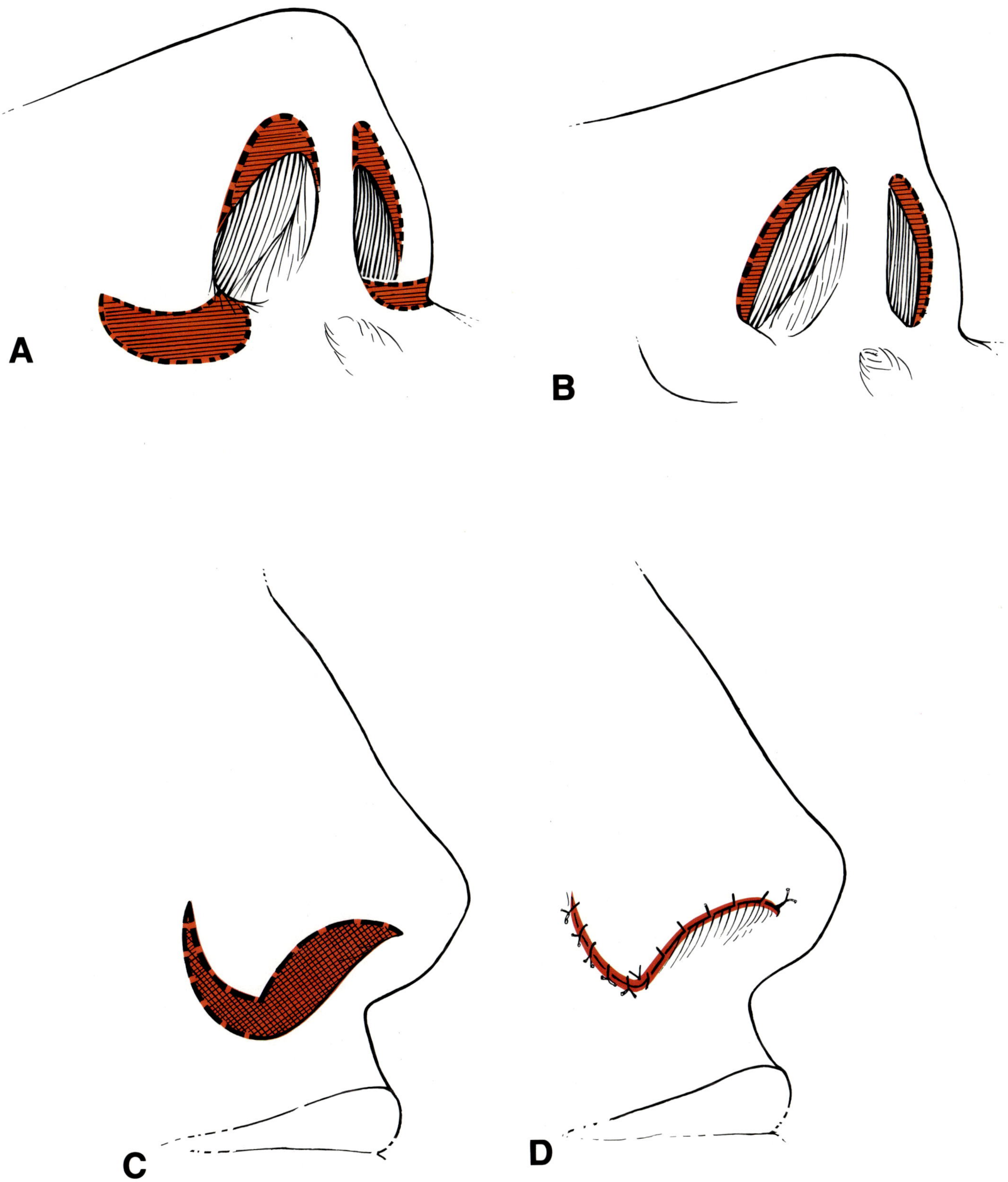

Fig. 198. continues.

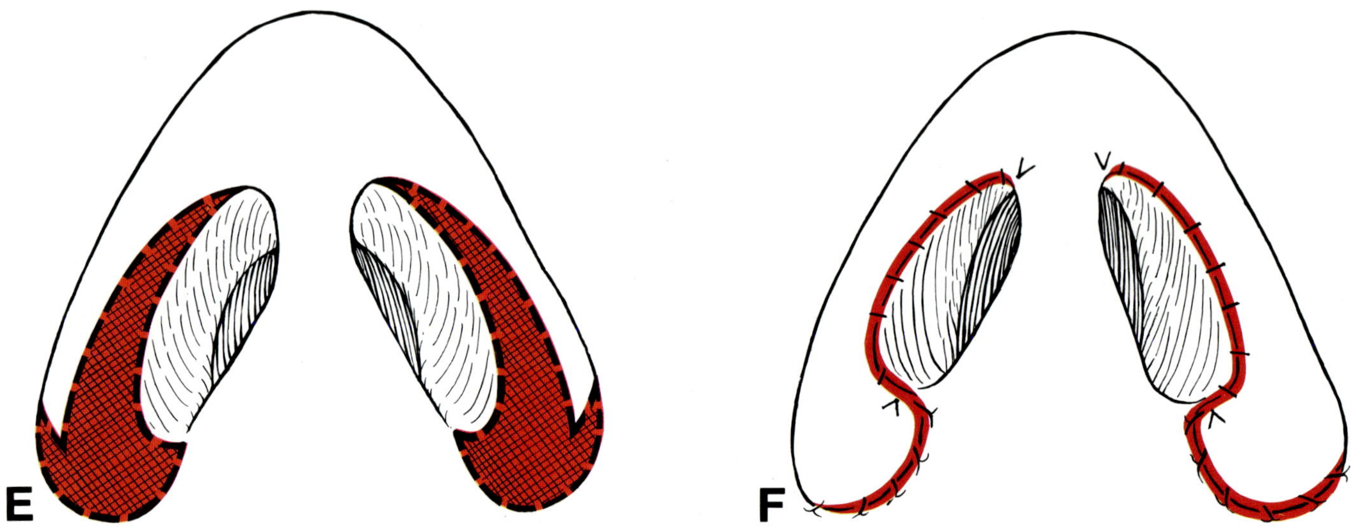

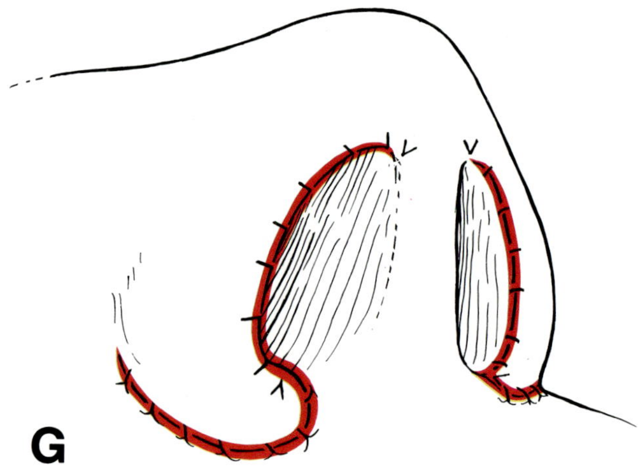

Fig. 198. (A) Wedge resection at the alar base combined with marginal alar resection in the anterior part. (B) Marginal resection along the entire alar rim. (C and D) Marginal resection following into the alar-wedge resection and suture. (E, F, and G) Same resection and suture in axial and half profile view.

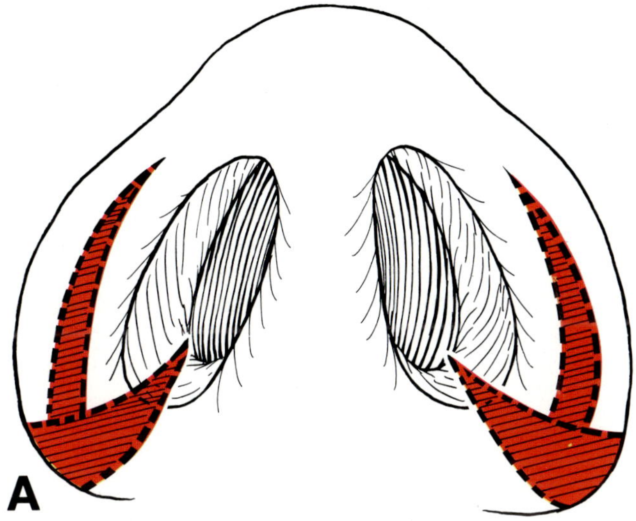

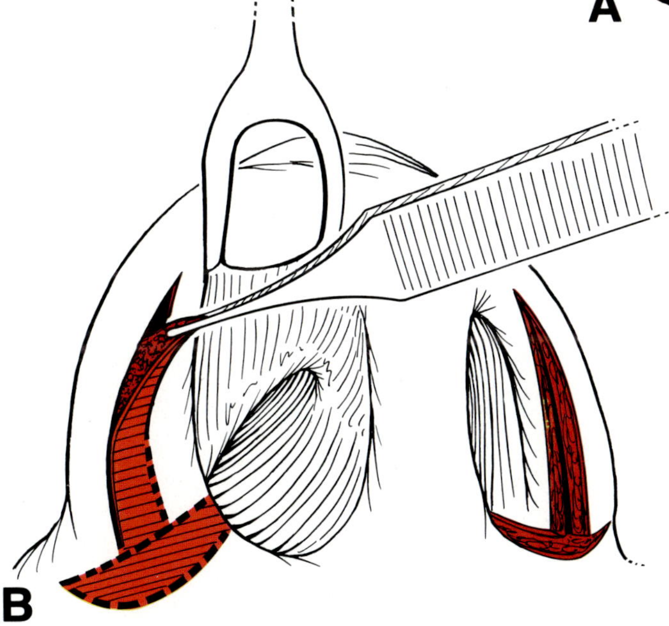

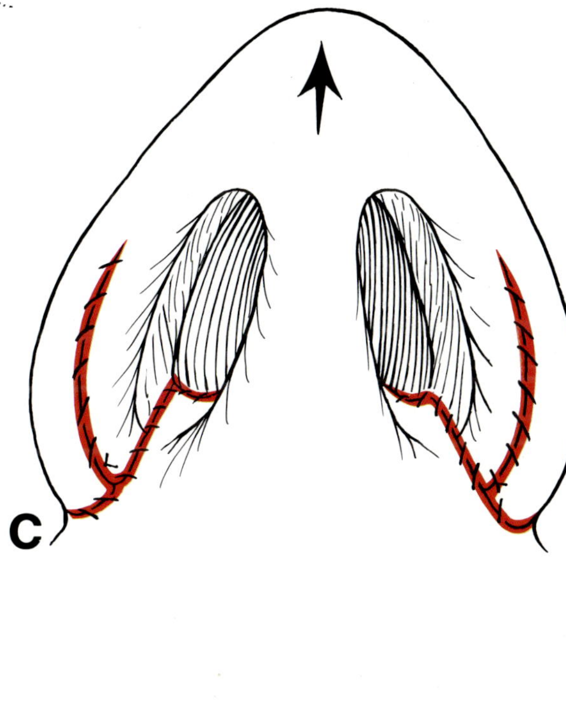

Fig. 199. Thinning the thick ala combined with alar base wedge resection. (A) Outline of excisions. (B) After the marginal resection a bevelled incision at the alar border permits a keel resection of cellulo-adipose tissue between the external and the internal skin layer of the ala. (C) "Over-and-over" suture at the alar rim and separate sutures at the base.

In many cases an important lowering of the bridge in highbridged noses with a hump has a flaring effect on the nostril, pushing the side wall and the alar border into a lower position. This sagging of the ala produces an unattractive shape in the profile view, especially when the columella is tilted backwards with septocolumellar mattress sutures, giving the impression of a pseudo-hidden columella. This can be corrected with inner wedge resections of vestibular skin, together with resection of the caudal border of the lateral crus of the lower lateral cartilage. Thus, at the end of the operation we always have to check if the width of the flaring nostril must still be reduced. In such cases a marginal resection then has to be added as a refining procedure.

In some patients the chief secondary deformity is not the thickness of the entire nasal tip but merely the thickness of the nostril margins. Reduction of such marginal thickness can be performed at the same time as the marginal resection by removing cellulo-adipose tissue between the two skin layers of the nostril, the external and the internal. This can be done with a blade, according to Fomon (1960) (Figs. 199 and 200) or by (blade) cauterization (Figs. 201 and 202). The marginal resection can be performed in a

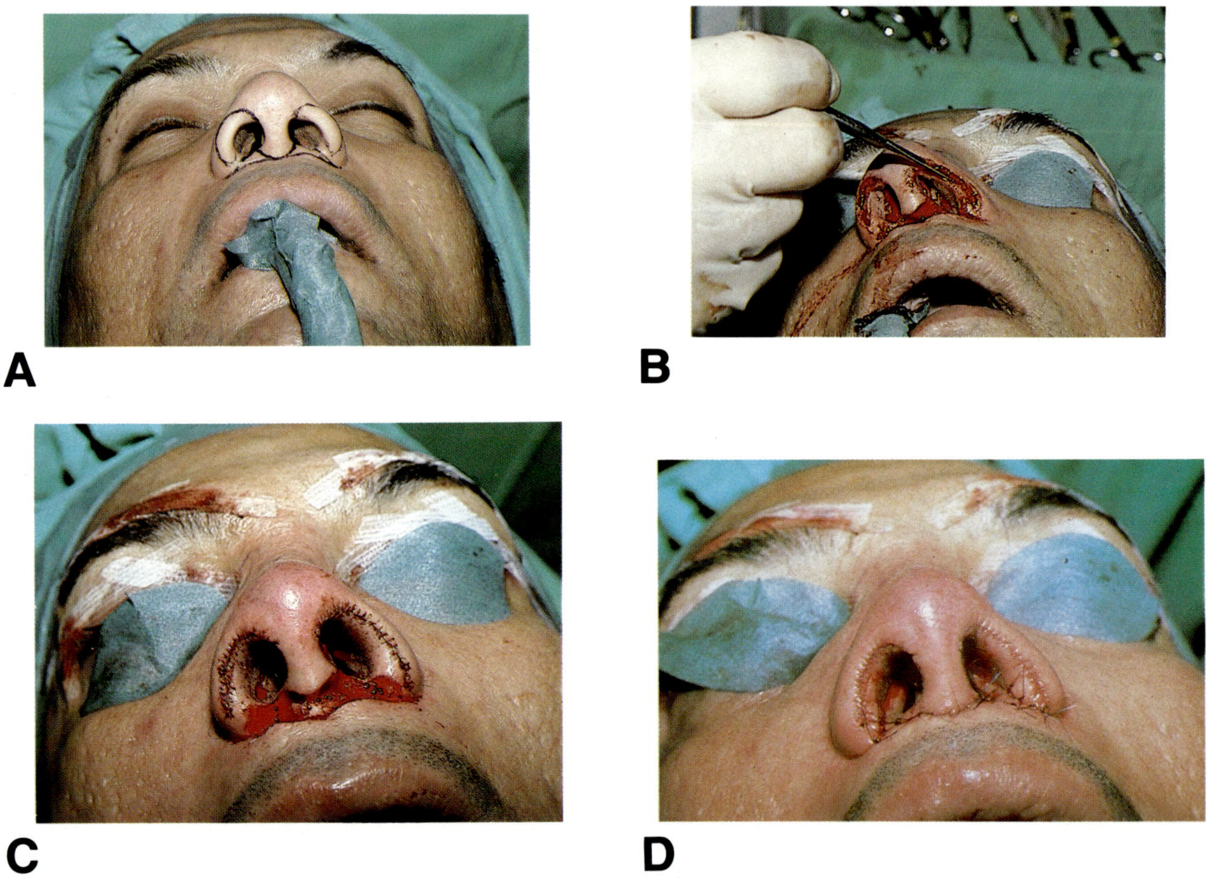

A B C D

Fig. 200. Resection of cellulo-adipose tissue in the ala. Width thinning was combined with buffalo-horn-shaped resection at the nasal base for shortening the lip and modeling the columellar-lip area with ear cartilage grafting. (A) Preoperative axial view. Outline of the skin excisions. (B) Thinning the ala with the knife. (C) Over-and-over running suture of the alar rim. (D) End of the operation.

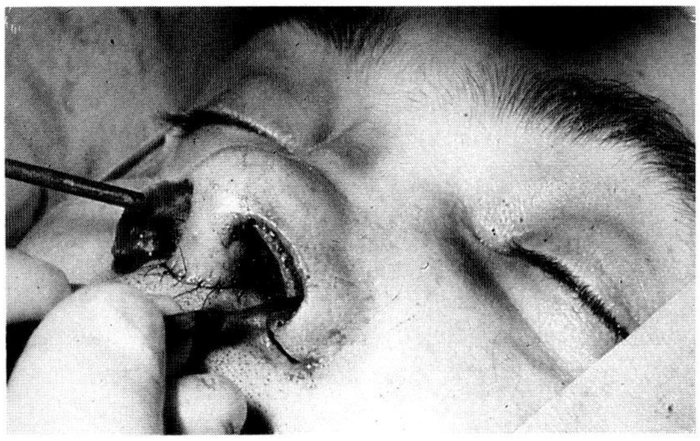

A

bevelled fashion by trimming more at the vestibular side, thus suturing the resection borders inside the vestibule, as Bernstein (1975) does. This has to be done very carefully to avoid thickening of the infolded border.

Trimming the Caudal Border of the Lateral Crus of the Alar Cartilage

Trimming the lateral crus of the alar cartilage at its caudal border combined with the trimming of the caudal ventral border of the quadrangular plate was recently described by McKinney and Stalnecker (1984). This is useful only in thin skinned noses because the rigid external skin of the ala does not allow the rim to conform to the new position of the cartilage. In our hands we have found this technique to be insufficient.

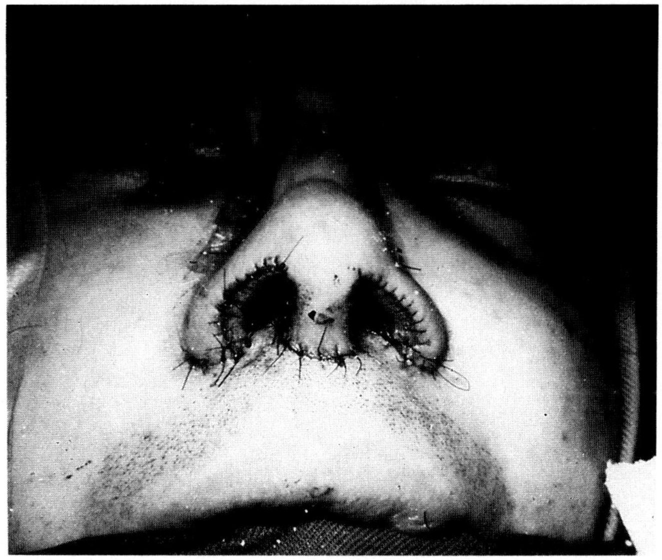

B

Fig. 201. (A) Thick ala can be thinned also by cautious cauterization. (B) Over-and-over running suture, a flat alar thinning.

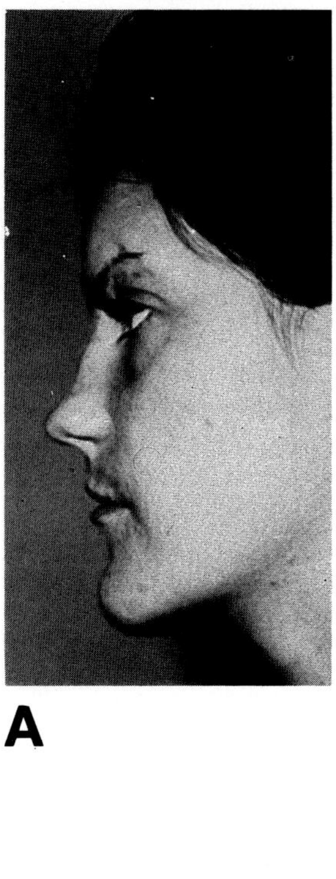

A

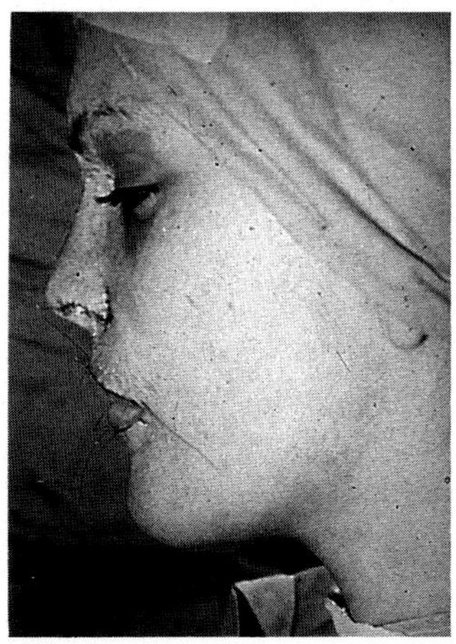

B

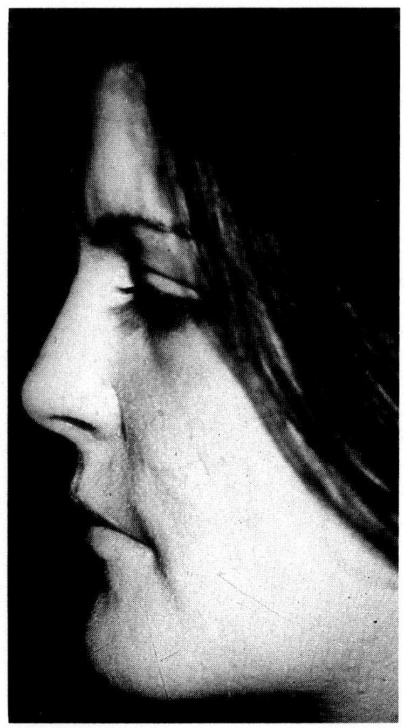

C

Fig. 202. Posttraumatic nose deformity with thick ala. Correction with thinning of the nostril as shown in Fig. 199. (A) Preoperative profile. (B) End of the operation. The cupid's bow lip is corrected simultaneously. (C) Result.

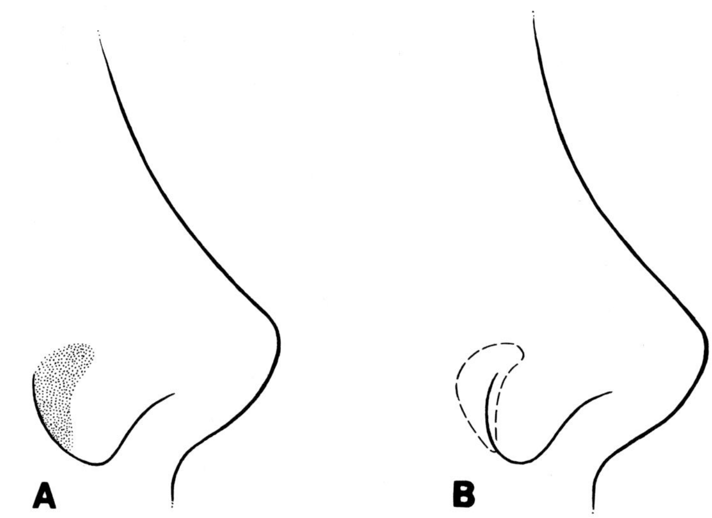

Fig. 203. Correction of a high supra-alar crease. From a lateral vestibular incision the upper alar area is defatted. (A) Area to be defatted. (B) Area defatted and ala-nasal crease lowered.

Trimming the Cephalic Portion of the Lateral Crus

Trimming the cephalic portion of the lateral crus, as in our standard tip modeling procedure, is also combined with shortening of the caudal ventral aspect of the septal cartilage, as done by McKinney and Stalnecker (1984). In most cases this does not adequately elevate the alar rim.

Excision of a Strip of Lining

By excising a strip of lining caudal to the internal valve underlying the region of the cephalic lateral crus, we can provide a better rim elevation. Eventually a cephalic part of the alar cartilage can be removed together with the piece of vestibular skin. This can be done at the level of the intercartilaginous incision. If one wants to perform this internal resection for pulling up the alar curtain at the valve as a retrograde resection then one has to suture the curtain in a proper elevated position to the upper border of the intercartilaginous incision and to the upper lateral cartilage. In certain cases we can avoid a marginal resection by utilizing this technique. When using this procedure there is the danger of a poor aesthetic result as the border of the nostril may become irregular or notched.

Lowering the Alar-Nasal Crease

Occasionally a patient presents with a high alar-nasal crease requiring its lowering with a reduction of the width of the ala. This can be done in a delicate manner by removing subcutaneous celluloadipose tissue from the nostril through a horizontal internal incision. The new lowered crease is then emphasized by a transcutaneous mattress suture knotted on a plastic sheet (Figs. 203 and 204).

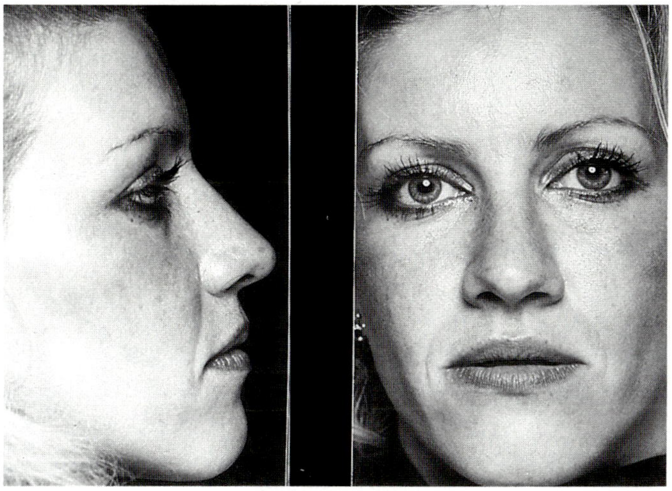

A

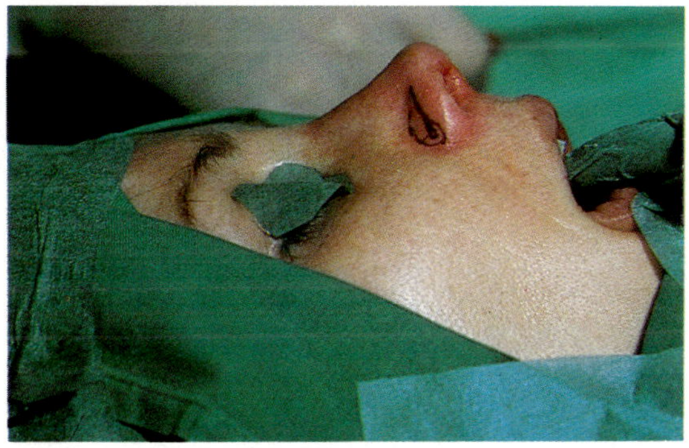

B

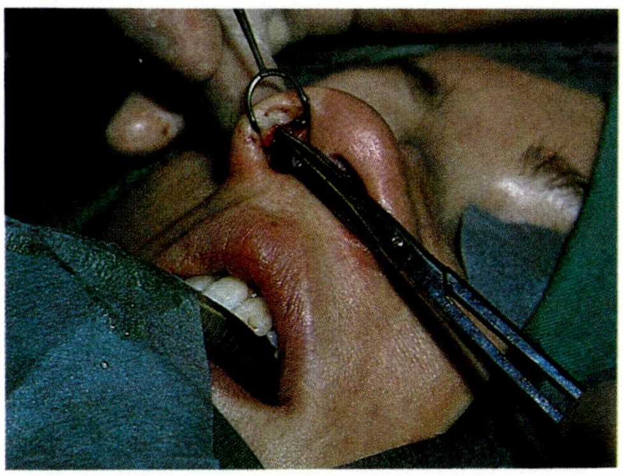

C

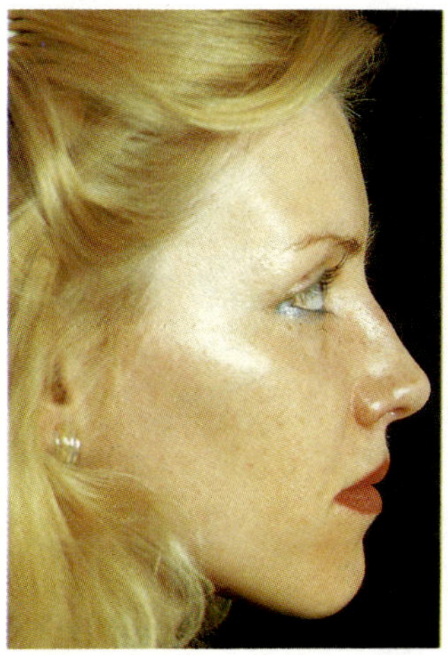

D

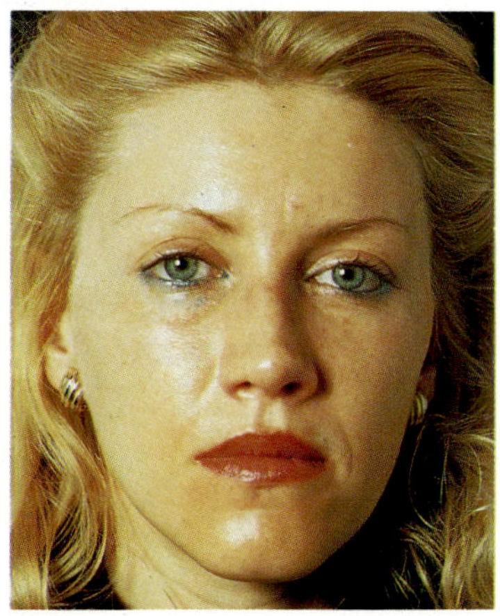

E

Fig. 204. Correction of high ala-nasal crease in a young woman. (A) Preoperative view. (B) Outline of the area to be defatted. (C) Defatting from a lateral vestibular incision. (D and E) Result with a finer alar base and lower supra-alar crease.

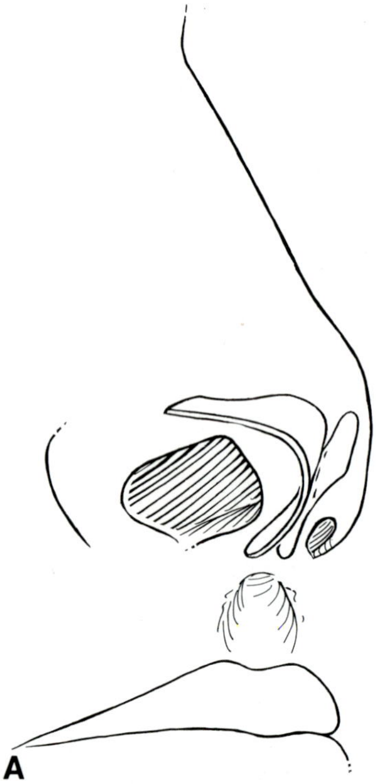

A

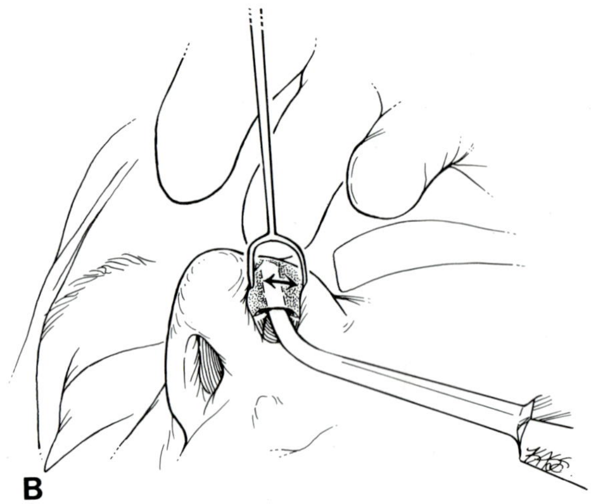

B

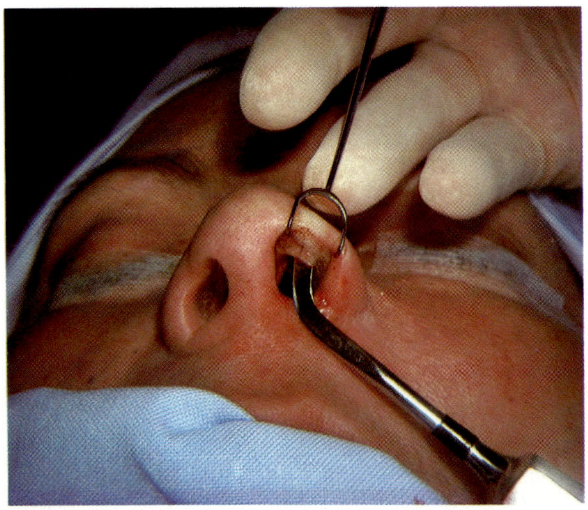

C

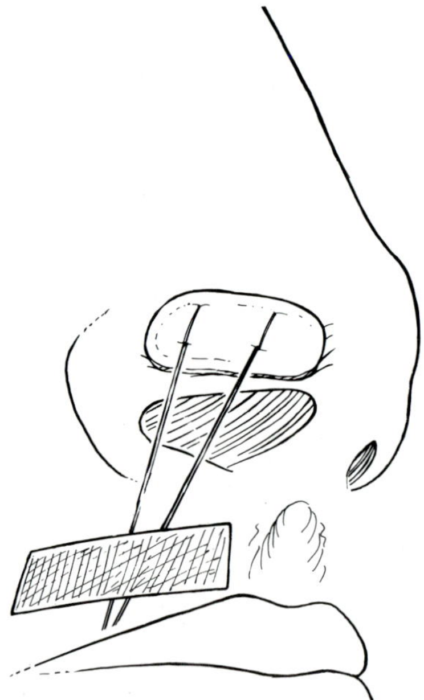

D

Fig. 205. Correction of high retracted ala (A) by lowering the border. (B and C) Elevation of a very marginal pocket in the ala from the intracartilaginous incision for reception of a cartilage graft from the septum. (D) Fixation of the cartilage graft with transalar mattress sutures that are pulled downward and taped to the upper lip.

LOWERING OF THE ALAR RIM

A slightly pronounced height to the alar ridge may have an attractive sensual look. But an excessive retraction of the alar border with a contour, like a French accent circonflexe (i.e., "ˆ"), becomes quite unattractive.

For lowering the alar rim in cases of excessive secondary retraction, Millard (1972) suggests swinging a transposition flap from the membranous septum to the ala, including a part of the medial crus. In most cases of too pronounced height to the alar edge, however, we prefer to use a technique that we advocated, consisting of an adequate dissection of the nostril and insertion of cartilage spacer (Meyer and Kesselring 1977).

If at the beginning of the operation such a correction is planned, the infracartilaginous vestibular incision of the luxation technique should be executed more within the vestibular wall, nearly at the level of a cartilage splitting incision. From this incision or from the intracutaneous or intercartilaginous incision an intracutaneous pocket between the external skin and vestibular skin can be created, approaching toward the margin with a fine blunt scissor in the region of the alar retraction. The pocket is enlarged with the curved Trelat elevator (Figs. 205 and 206) and pushed down with the marginal skin in order to make room for the reception of a rectangular or oval piece of cartilage harvested from the upper part of the lateral alar crus. One or two transalar mattress sutures tied over a plastic sheet with 5/0 unabsorbable thread will keep the cartilage transplant in situ and the whole alar rim in its new position (Figs. 205 and 206 F and G). A

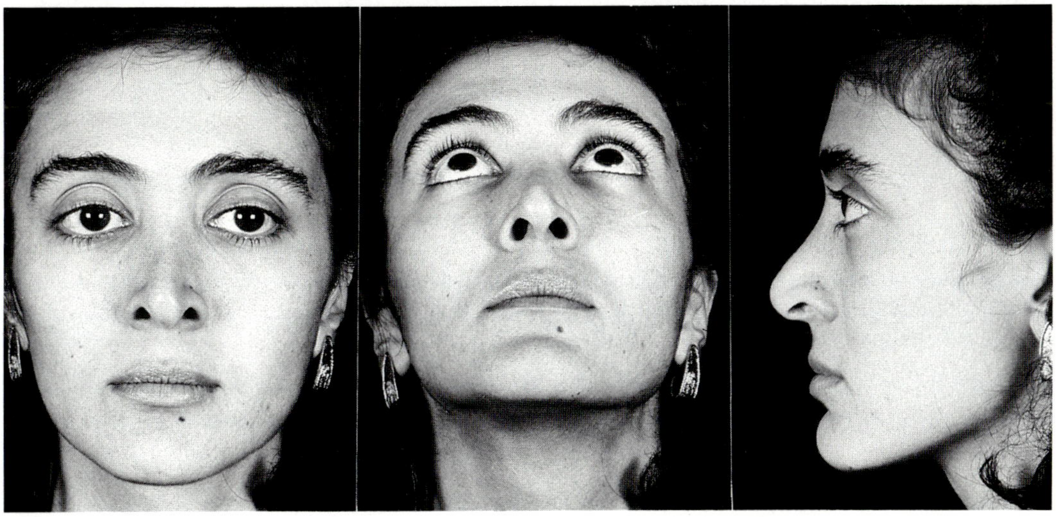

A

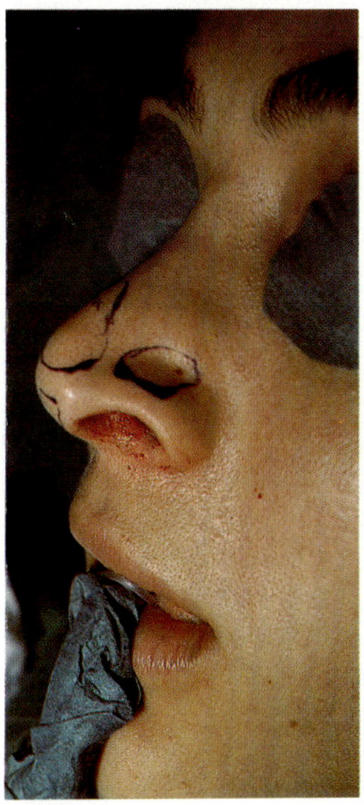

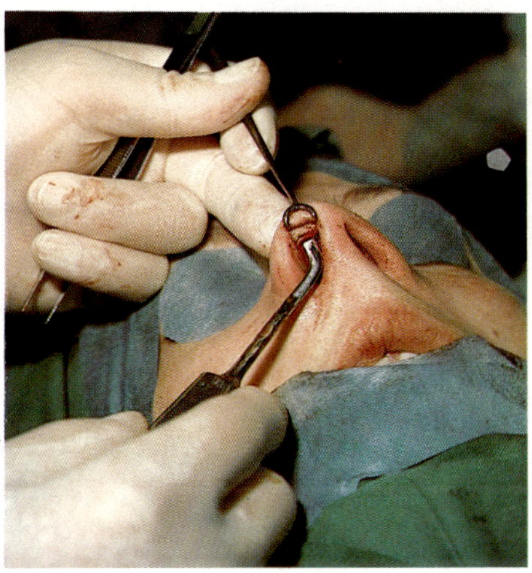

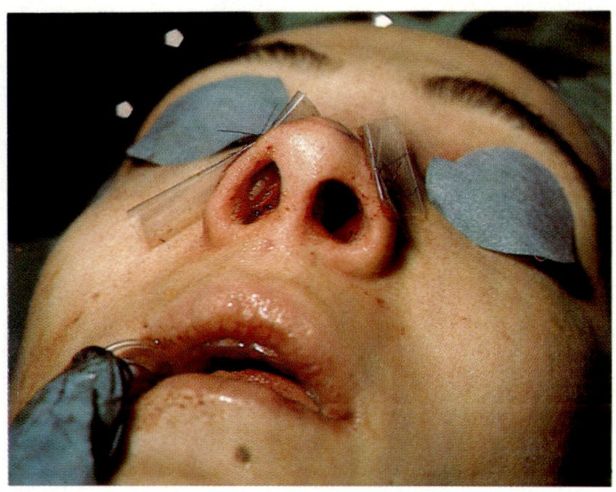

B **C** **D**

Fig. 206. continues.

Fig. 206. continued.

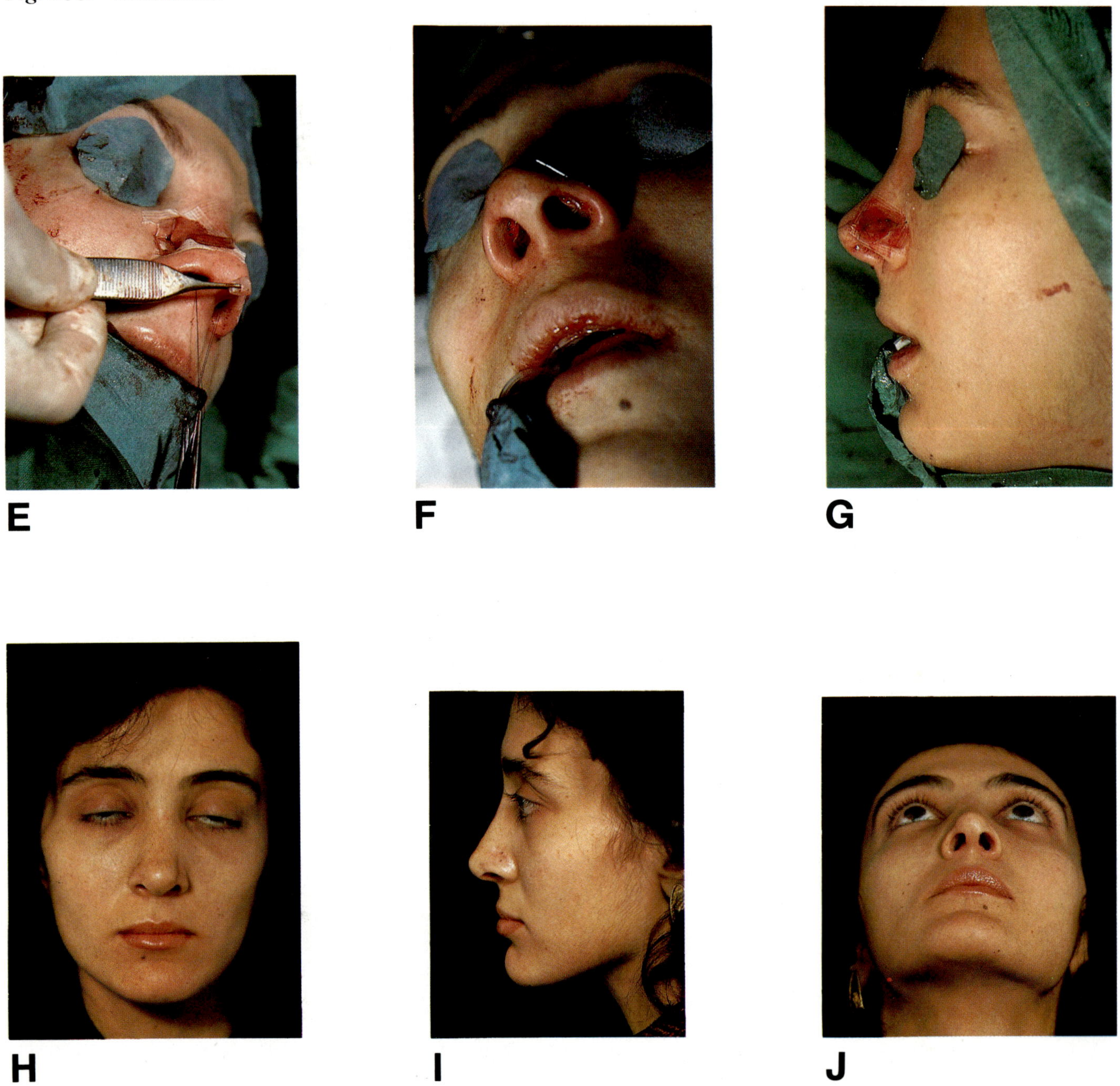

Fig. 206. Retracted ala, supratip thickening, and excessive depression at the supra-alar crease in a middle-aged lady. Combined correction of these secondary deformities. (A) Preoperative views. (B) Outline of the areas to be corrected: supratip tissue resection, tip definition with grafting, supra-alar depression to be filled, and retracted ala to be pulled downward. (C) Pocket formation in the right ala with the curved elevator of Trélat through the intracartilaginous incision. (D) Discorid cartilage graft from the septum is visible in the right pocket. (E) Lobular cartilaginous onlay about to be inserted for tip projection and definition. (F and G) Left transalar mattress sutures tied over a plastic sheet maintaining in place the spacer graft. (H, I, and J) Result.

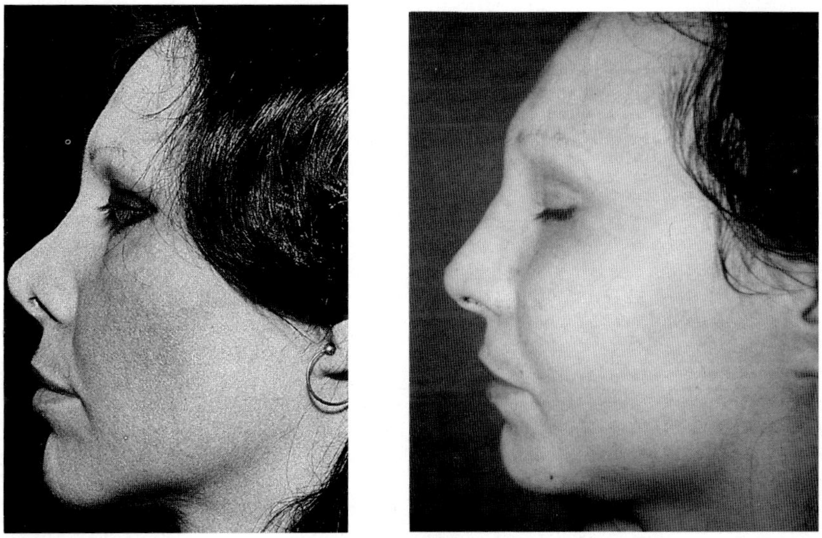

A B

Fig. 207. Middle-aged lady with retracted ala in the anterior part. In revision surgery the nose is lengthened and the alar rim lowered anteriorly with cartilage grafting and trimmed posteriorly. (A) Preoperative view. (B) Postoperative view.

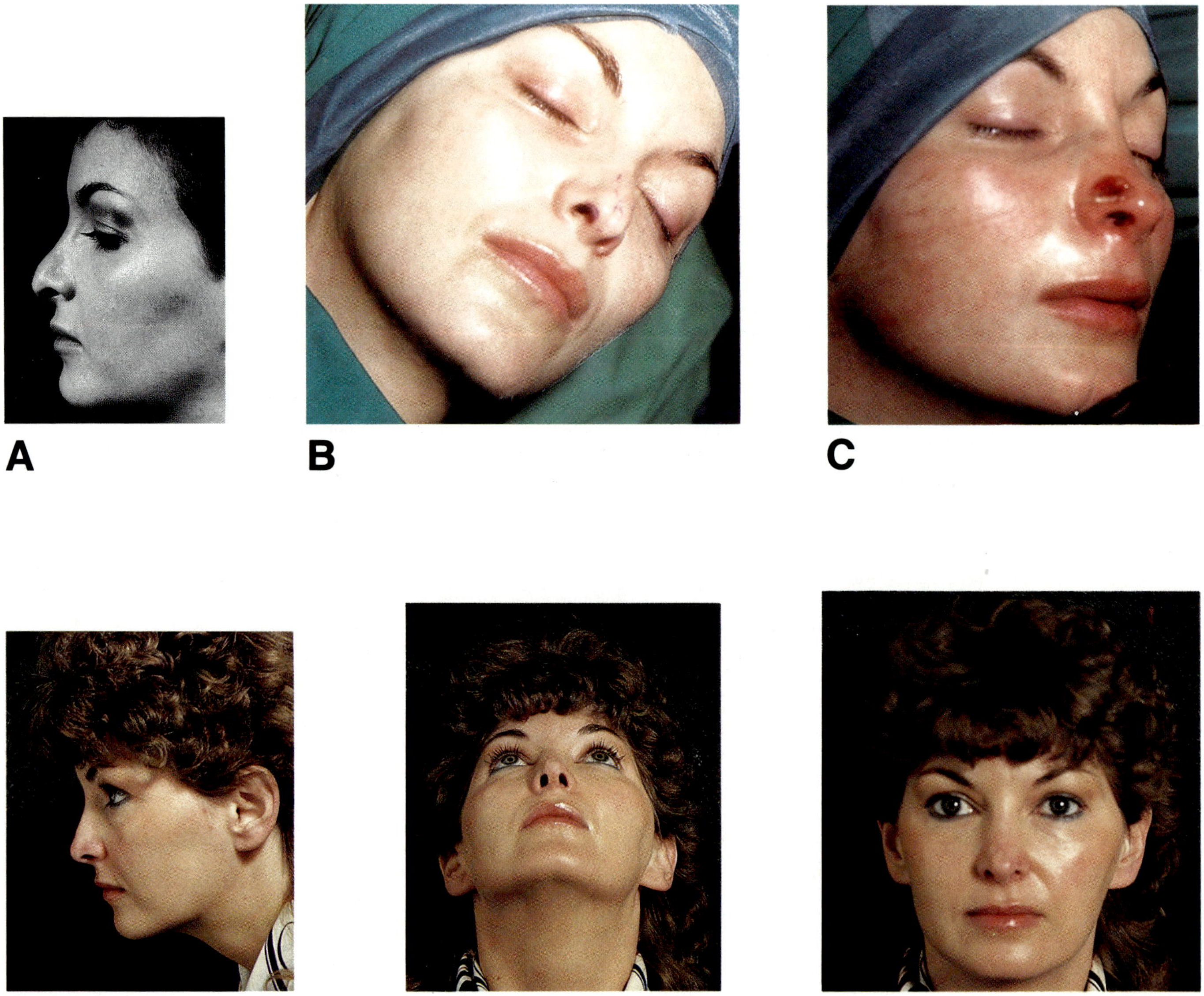

A B C D E F

Fig. 208. Young female with high alar border and polly beak. Alar correction using the method of Figure 205 and with marginal resection at the alar-columellar commissure. (A) Preoperative view. (B) Outline of dorsal reduction and commissural trimming. (C) End of the operation with transalar mattress sutures fixing inserted cartilage grafts. (D, E, and F) Result.

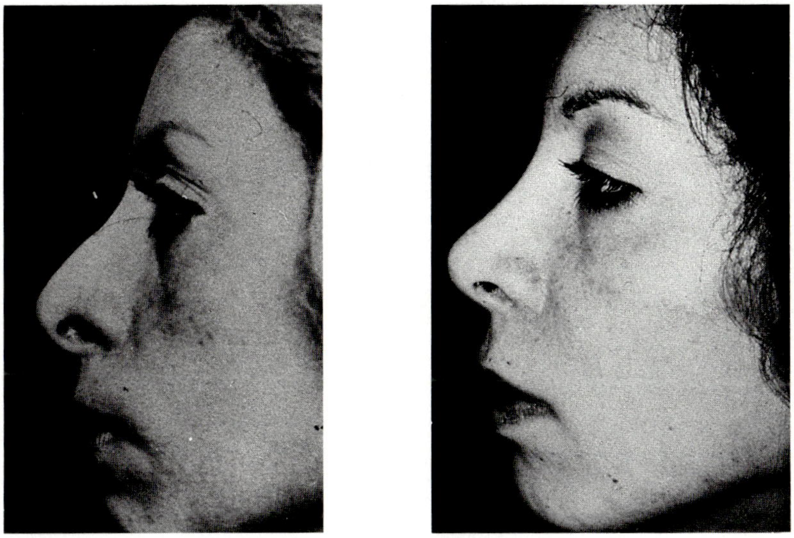

A B

Fig. 209. Alar retraction and supratip thickening in a young lady after two previous rhinoplasties. Lowering of the alar rim is combined with tip plasty and marginal resection at the lobulo-alar commissure. (A) Preoperative view. (B) Postoperative view.

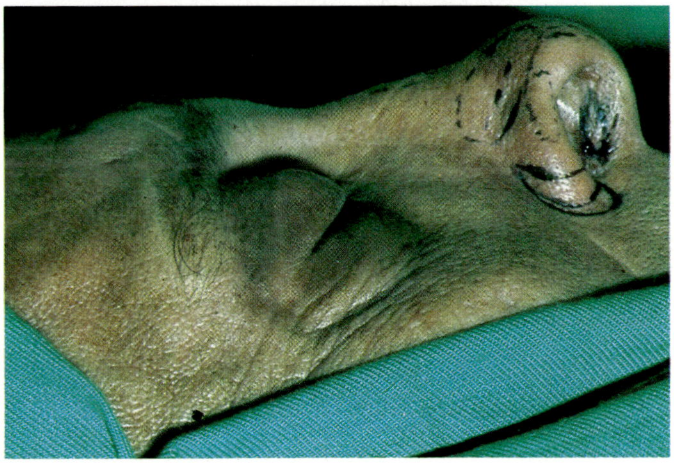

A

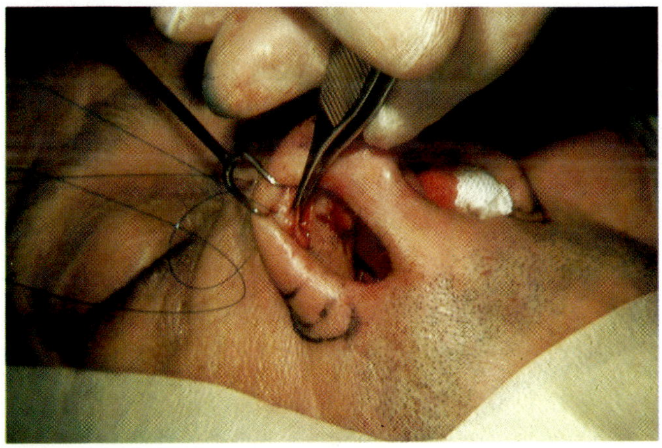

B

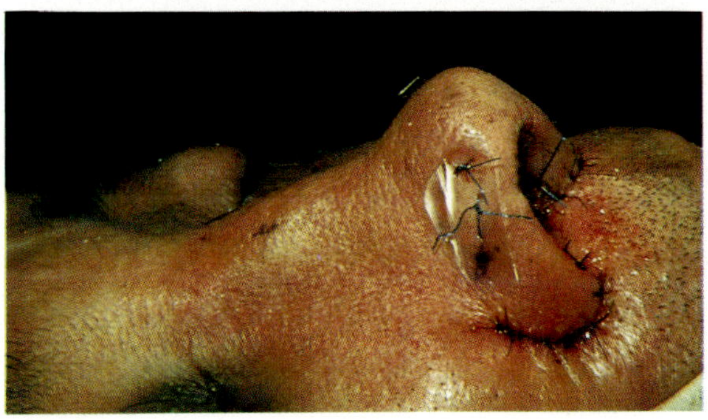

C

Fig. 210. Lowering of the ala combined with wedge resection at the alar base, which lowers the posterior part of the nostril. (A) Preoperative outline of the wedge resection. (B) Insertion of the cartilaginous spacer into the ala. (C) End of the operation.

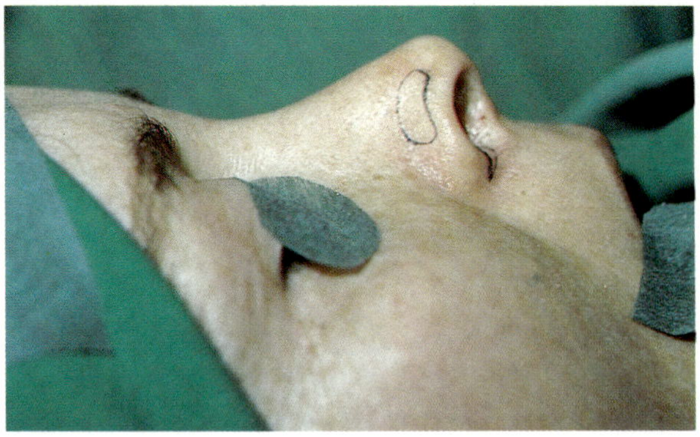

A

slight overcorrection at the end of the operation is of benefit to achieve a good permanent result. If necessary, in addition two small resections of the alar rim in front of and behind the point of the former retraction can improve the aesthetically appreciable rounded line of the rim (Figs. 207–209). In order to obtain a more marked lowering of the alar border, the base of the alar sweep can be cut and reinserted at a lower level towards the upper lip (Fig. 210). If an alotomy with alar base displacement or a basal Weir resection is necessary, the access for the alar pocket formation and for introducing the cartilaginous spacer can be obtained from the lateral side (Figs. 211). In traumatic cases, the alar rim can be lowered and refined at the commissure with marginal resection as well as partially reconstructed with skin graft transfer from the opposite alar base (Fig. 212).

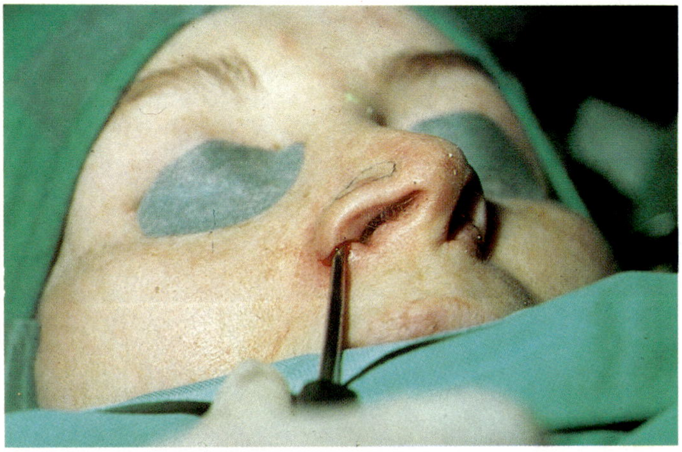

B

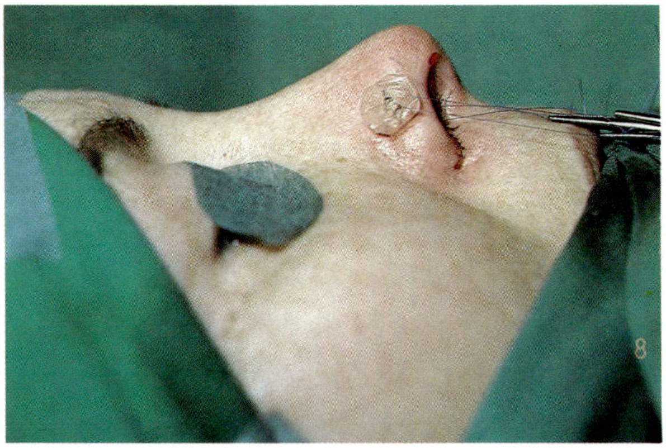

D

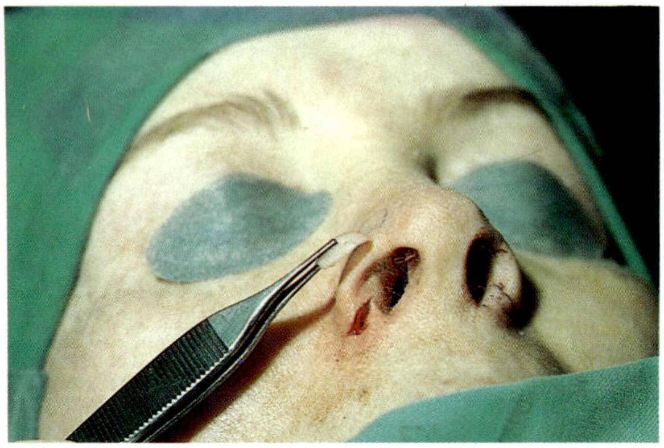

C

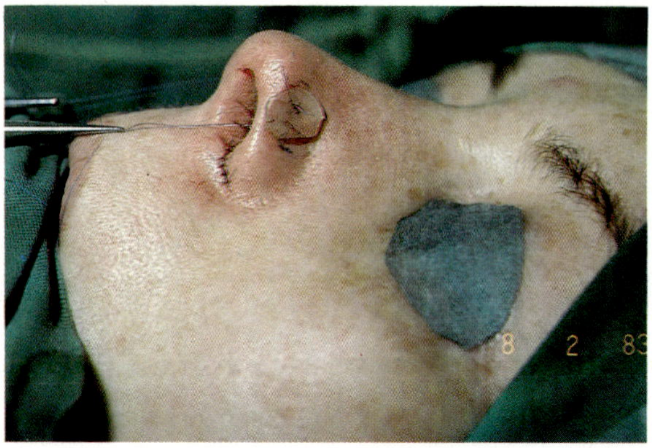

E

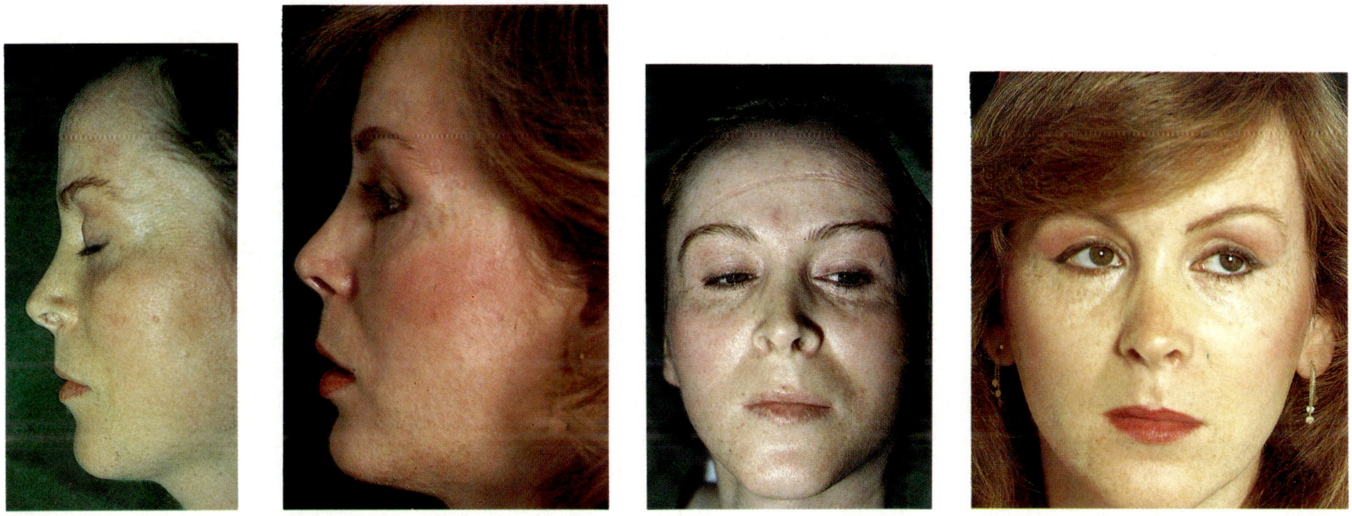

F G H I

Fig. 211. Correction of iatrogenic retracted alar base. (A) Outline of the site to place the cartilaginous graft. (B) From the alar base incision the alar pocket is elevated. (C) Discoid cartilage graft about to be inserted. (D and E) Transalar mattress sutures will be taped to the upper lip excercising a downward traction for one week. (F and G) Preoperative and postoperative profile. (H and I) Preoperative and postoperative front view.

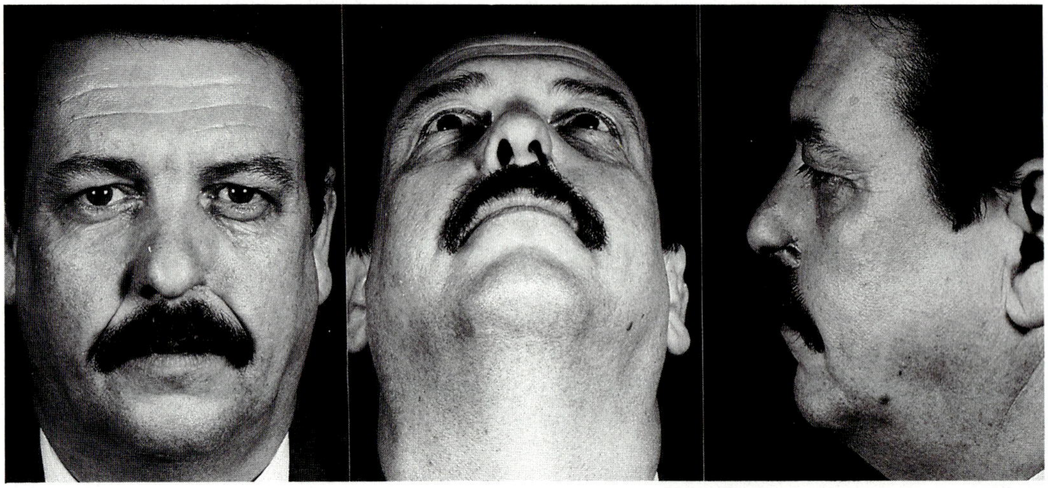

A

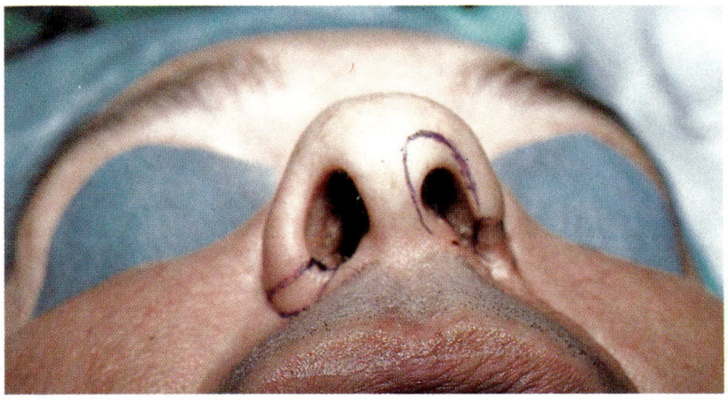

B

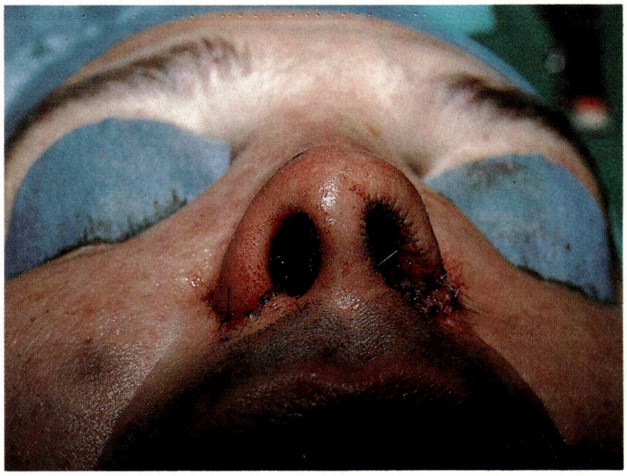

C

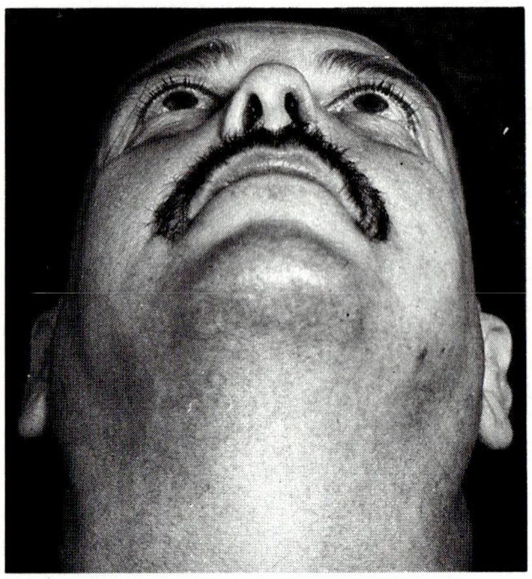

D

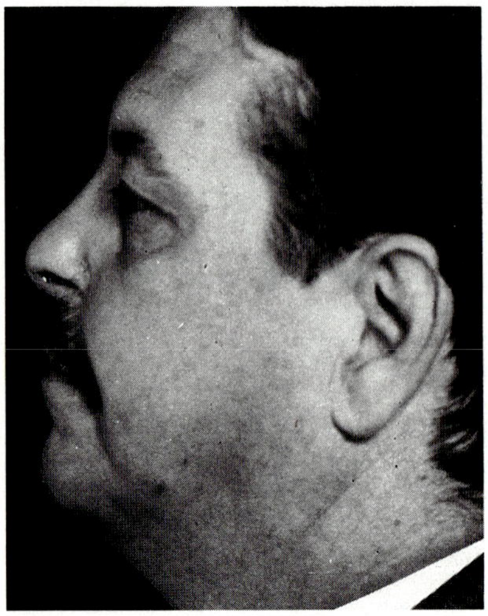

E

Fig. 212. Traumatic unilateral alar base defect in a middle-aged man. Correction with balanced resection of the opposite alar base and commissure resection on the defect side. The resected right alar skin is transferred to the left alar base to envelope the remnant fibrous wall. (A) Preoperative views. (B) Outline of the resections. (C) End of the operation with skin grafting from ala to ala and with suture of the resection at the alar-columellar commissure. (D and E) Result.

17

Stenosis and Atresia

The treatment of stenosis and atresia of the nose is an important task because the human being requires a free nasal airflow for the benefit of physical balance. The site of stenoses may be divided in three parts: (1) vestibule, (2) nasal cavity, and (3) choana. It may be unilateral or bilateral and range from slight to severe.

Anterior and/or posterior nasal stenosis may be congenital. They usually affect the lateral angle. Stenosis after trauma, infection, or surgery is more common. It may also result from ulceration of the nostril rim secondary to lupus, syphilis, burns, tumor excision, nasal intubation, and injudicious packing. In iatrogenic stenoses the most frequent surgical procedures preceding the deformity are rhinoplasty and cheiloplasty. On the other hand, it is also frequently seen after nasal reconstruction because the soft tissue brought into the defect tends to shrink. Skin grafts and composite grafts without rigid support also contract. Nasal stenosis in varying degrees is seen in patients with cleft lip after primary repair.

Fortunately, vestibular stenosis very seldom develops after aesthetic rhinoplasty even when marginal skin is excised for asymmetry. If the rim resection is more ambitious, as in cleft lip patients, the vestibular wall must be lined by free skin or composite graft to avoid postoperative stenosis.

We have had occasion to correct nasal stenosis following the use of packing with a lead string for a prolonged period. The string produces irritation at the lateral angle of the nostril, or multiple small lacerations, and this leads to a constricting scar.

For functional and aesthetic reasons, nasal stenosis demands correction. Early surgery is important particularly if the condition is encountered in children. In cases of total or subtotal reconstruction of the nostrils, the danger of shrinkage of the tissue is extremely high. In many such cases we have had to operate several times. A dilator formed by a PVC or silicone tube into a proper shape occasionally seems to be preferable and sufficient treatment.

STENOSES OF THE VESTIBULE

Basically scarring and retraction in the vestibule is due to the lack of nasal lining and sometimes to a loss of cartilage. Often an incision scar reaching the lateral angle of the vestibular floor or the alar border leads to such a deformity. In order to repair scarring stenosis of the nostril the lost skin or at least the cartilage has to be replaced. This can be done by using composite grafts taken from the auricle. In some cases of minimal scar contraction in the vestibule, grafting with preserved cartilage combined with a Z-plasty might be useful. After Z-plasty with or without full thickness skin grafting and with or without the application of a stent mold, the results are often acceptable.

Alar notches are usually unilateral, isolated defects that attract attention. Most result from trauma or from surgical extirpation of a neoplasm. Congenital notches also occur and range from isolated ones to severe defects associated with major craniofacial anomalies.

The surgical management of alar notches varies depending upon the severity of the defect. In the congenital cases, the width of the defect is usually obvious. Notches resulting from surgery or trauma, however, may be distorted by scar. One may have to recreate the defect before an appropriate technique for closure can be selected.

Rieger described in 1967 the use of a flap of dorsal nasal skin with the pedicle based on one side of the nose but comprising essentially all of the skin of the other side of the nose; the flap also included a triangular extension into the glabellar region. Rigg suggested in 1963 both lateral and medial bases for his dorsal skin flap, which also has a triangular extension into the glabellar region. Marchac (1985) reported the use of a Rieger flap that was modified somewhat. His diagram showed a flap taken much higher up in the glabellar region and forehead, which he rotated downward to repair a large defect of the middle of the nose. He reported on two cases and apparently used a vascular pedicle from just above and lateral to the inner canthus. Cronin diagrammed in 1983 a V-Y advancement from the glabella, combined with a rotation flap from the dorsum and side of the nose, also reaching the alar border.

If the scar of the notch is protruding into the lumen of the vestibule, producing a medial or lateral vestibular stenosis, we remove the subcutaneous fibrous tissue from the ala through an internal vestibular incision and replace the missing part of lower lateral cartilage with a shield-shaped graft from the septal quadrangular plate. The cartilaginous support is held in place with transalar mattress sutures (Fig. 213). The same procedure can be applied if the notch retraction is combined with external scarring necessitating, in addition, a Z-plasty of the alar skin (Figs. 214 and 215).

There are certain limitations to the use of *composite autografts* of skin and cartilage taken from the pinna, if minimal loss of the graft is to be achieved. It is very important for graft take that the first blood circulation to the graft be present some 3–6 hours post-transplantation. This is thought to occur through inoculation: that means end-to-end anastomosis of blood vessels within the skin and perichondrium of the graft and the recipient area vessels. Therefore, the size of the graft becomes the most important consideration. No part of the graft should be more than 1 cm away from the edge of the repaired defect. On the other hand, shrinkage of a composite graft may occur and has to be considered. Gentle handling of the graft is mandatory. Therefore, such a graft should only be held with skin hooks and sutures. For preparing the recipient area, excision of scar tissue is necessary.

The graft is sutured in place by atraumatic resorbable sutures of 5-0 and 6-0 size. To prevent impairment of inoculation, the minimum number of sutures should be used and subcutaneous sutures should be avoided. Gluing with fibrin tissue (see Chapter 10) helps to reduce the amount of sutures and to achieve complete hemostasis without using cautery.

As we stated in 1964 (Denecke and Meyer), the composite graft should be 1 mm thicker, longer, and broader than the defect. This is true even if the graft is taken as a preauricular graft, including the crus helicis as advocated by D. Baker (1987), who forms a very fine alar border repair that is especially important in female patients with alar loss. The skin of the lateral wall of the nose is then turned down for lining the nostril, according to F. Smith (1956). The external skin of this composite graft extends into the preauricular region as a triangular or rhomboid flap and will serve to cover the external nasal defect after moving down the Smith flap for lining (Figs. 216 and 217).

Avelar, Psillakis, and Viterbo (1984) are also

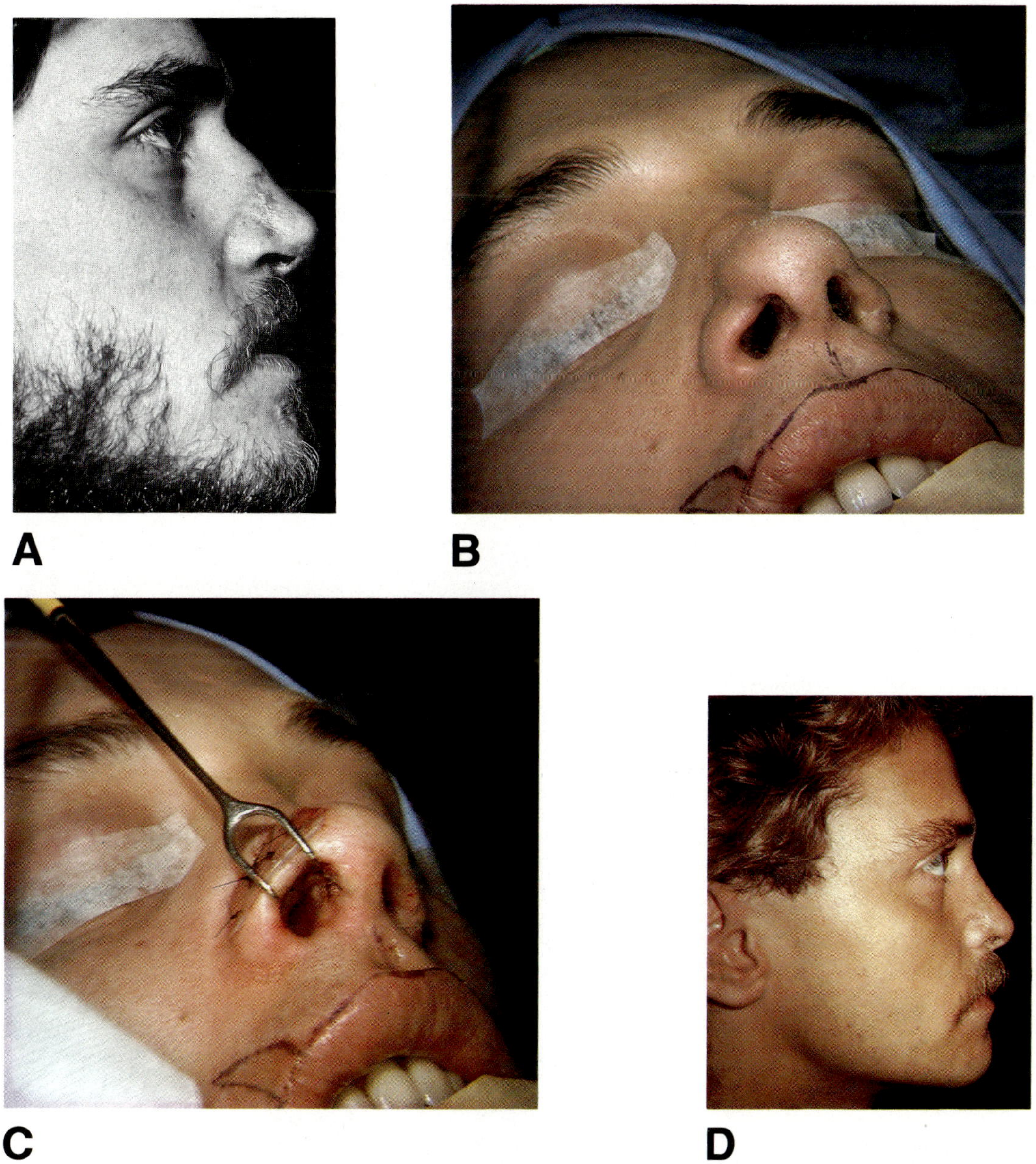

Fig. 213. Post-traumatic cicatricial retraction of the right ala obstructing the vestibule corrected with insertion of a slightly concave cartilage graft from the septum into a pocket at the scar level and fixation with transalar mattress sutures. (A) Preoperative profile. (B) Anterior stenosis visible. (C) End of the revision with intracartilaginous incision extended to the membranous septum and mattress sutures tied over a plastic sheet. (D) Postoperative profile.

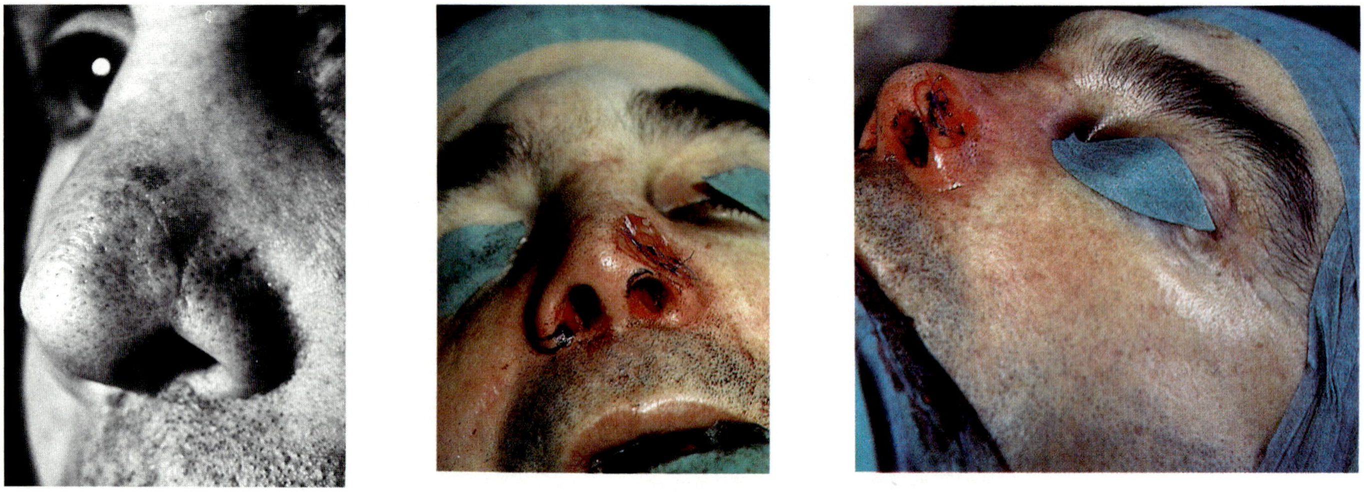

A B C

Fig. 214. Post-traumatic retraction of the left alar margin with impairment of the nasal airway corrected in the same way as Figure 214 and additional small external Z-plasty and anterior marginal resection. (A) Preoperative side view. (B) Mattress suture performed and marginal resection outlined. Reduction of the opposite nostril circumference at the nares by small wedge resection at the alar base. (C) End of the operation.

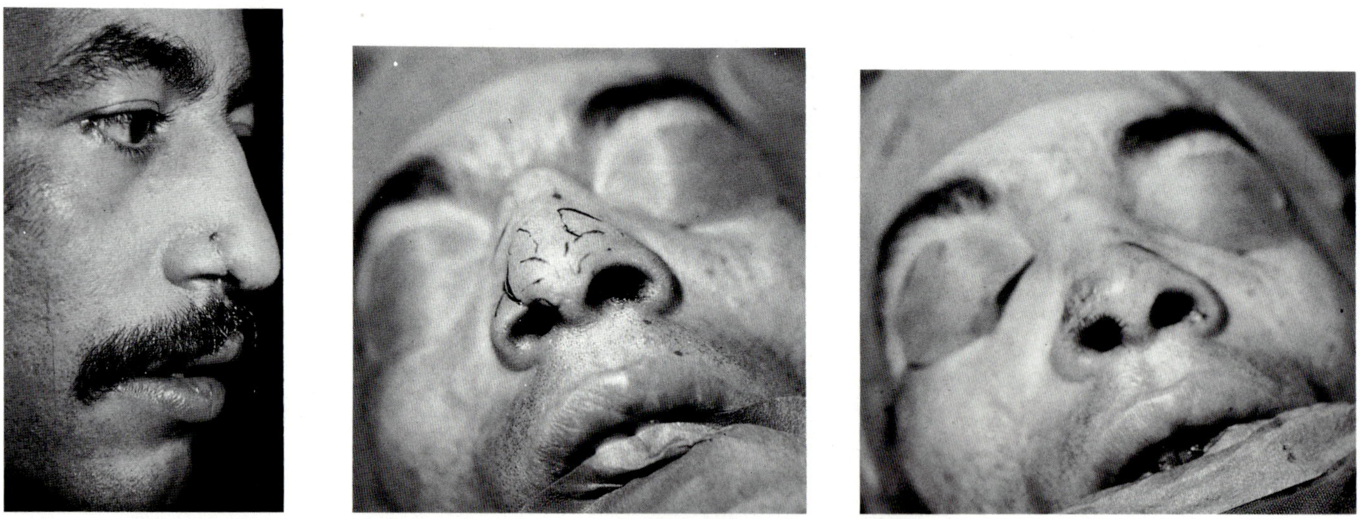

A B C

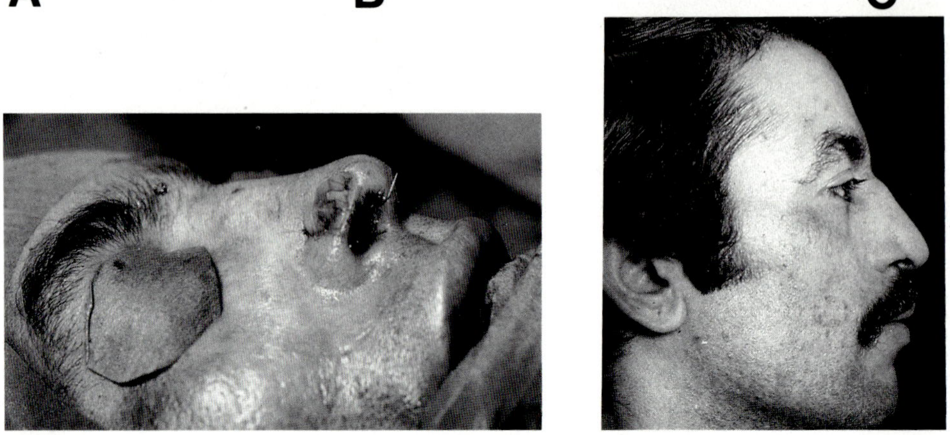

D E

Fig. 215. Similar post-traumatic case with retracted alar border corrected like case Figure 214 with Z-plasty and anterior rim resection. (A) Preoperative view. (B) Outline of the Z-plasty and alar border trimming. (C and D) End of the operation. (E) Result.

using large composite grafts up to 30 cm^2 from the retroauricular region in the reconstruction of the nasal deformities, applying a similar technique as suggested by Converse (reported in Denecke and Meyer, 1964).

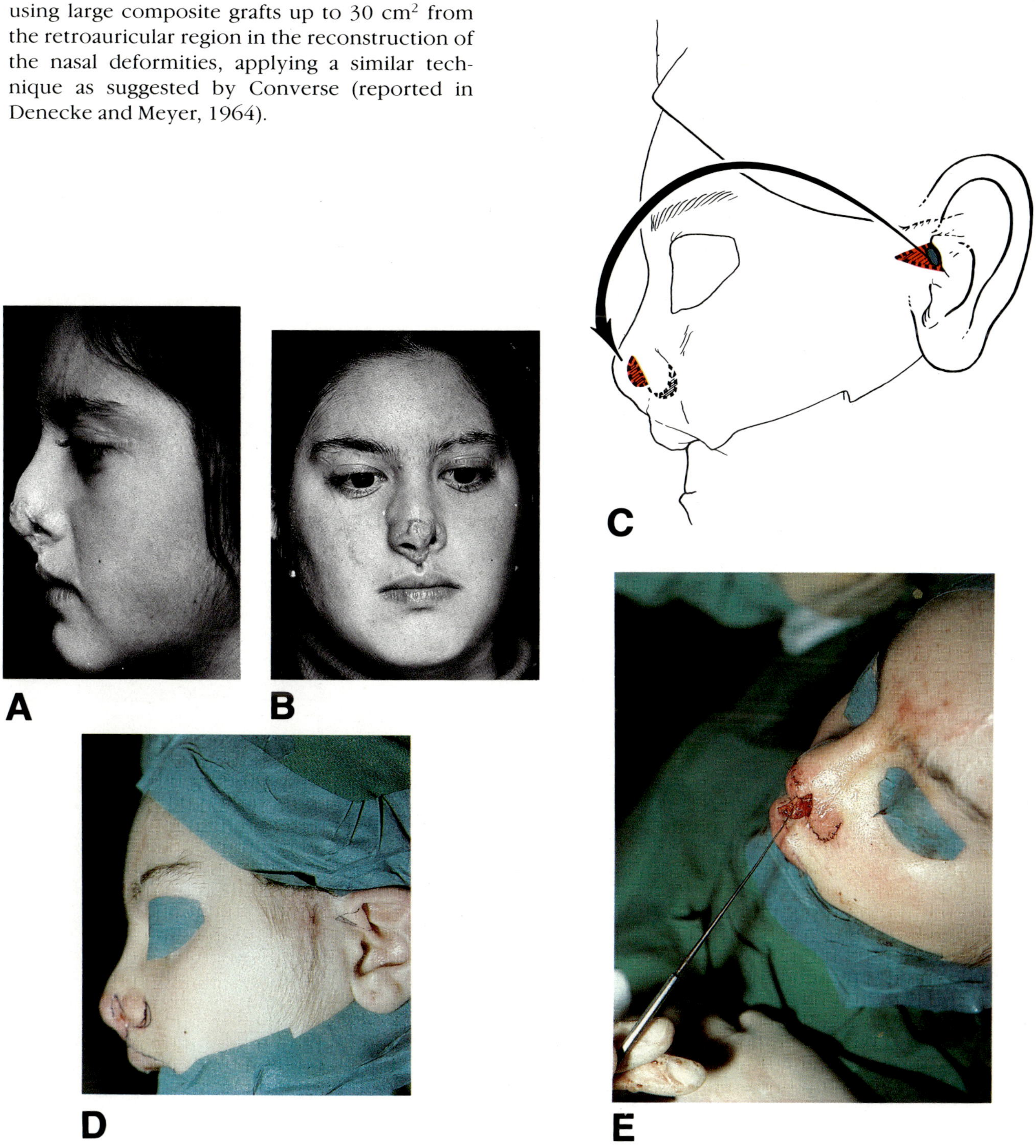

Fig. 216. Young girl after car accident with scar stenosis of the left nostril corrected with composite graft from the ear. (A and B) Preoperative view. (C and D) Outline of scar incisions at the ala and of the preauricular composite graft including a part of the cartilage of the crus helicis. (E) Composite graft transferred and sutured at the alar border, will cover the alar defect.

Fig. 216. continues.

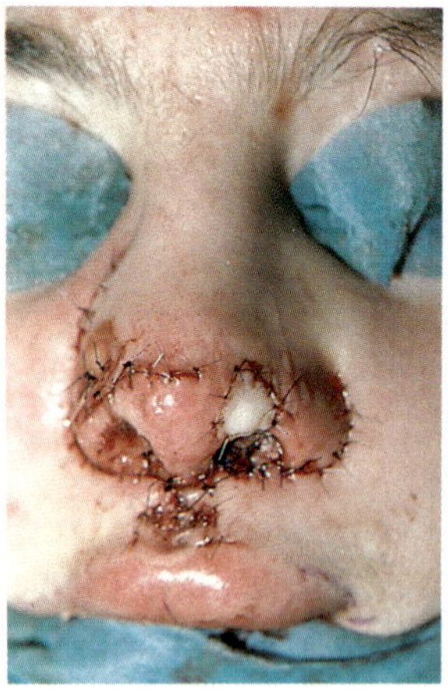

F

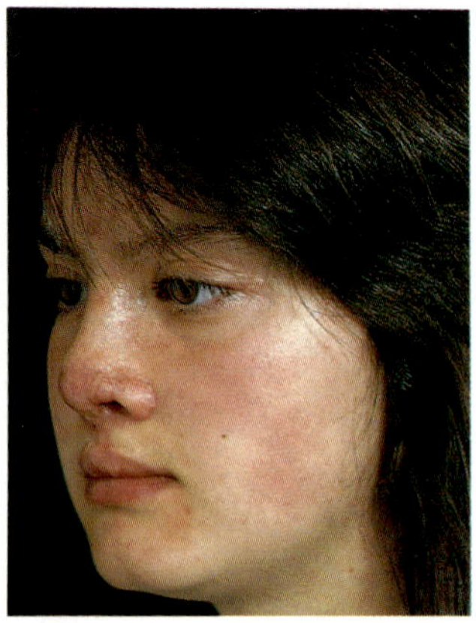

G

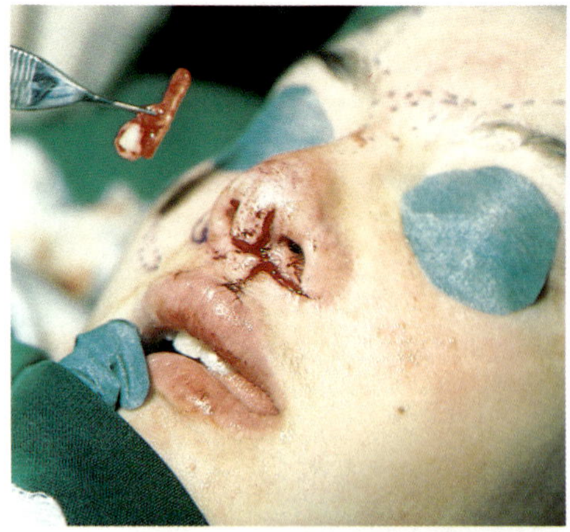

K

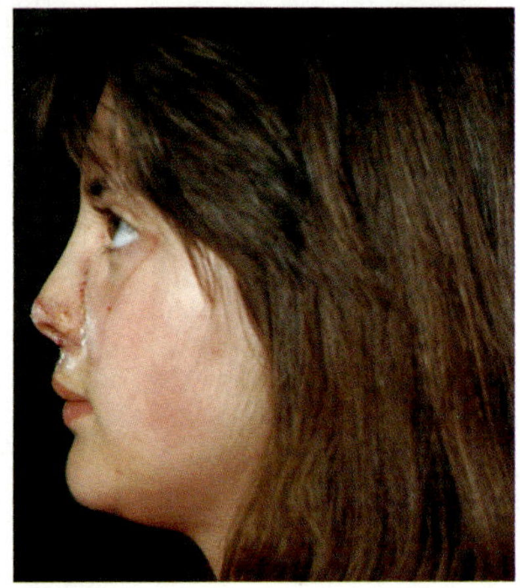

L

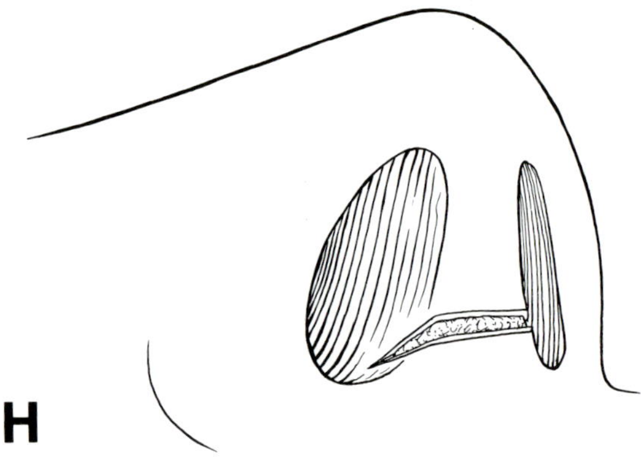

H

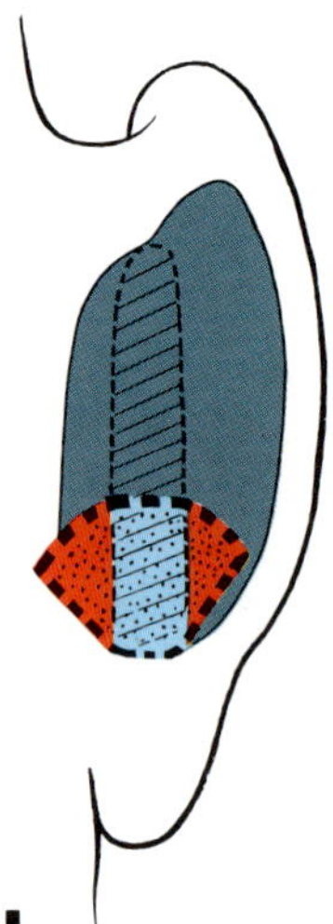

I

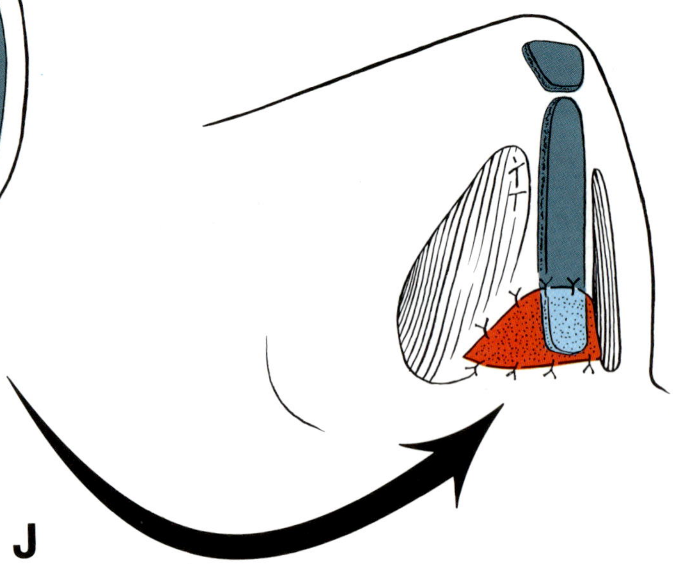

J

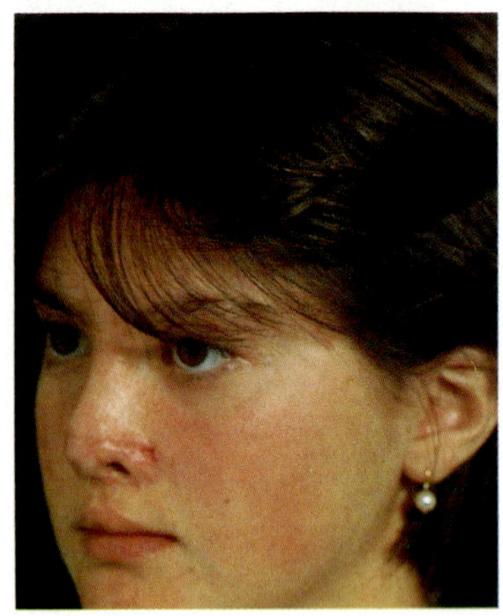

M

Fig. 217. *(continues)* (F) Graft sutured. (G) Graft in site after 2 months. (H, I, J, and K) Later lengthening of the columella with a straight composite graft from the ear concha. A skin rectangle will be sutured to the columellar base, and the cartilage batten will produce protrusion of the tip. (L) Second composite graft in site after two weeks. (M) Early result.

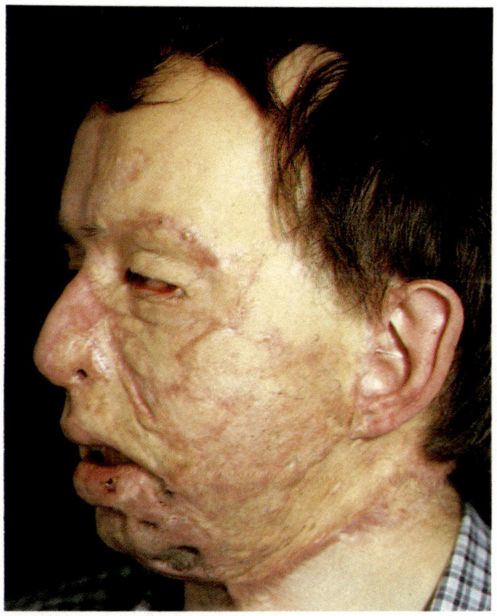

A

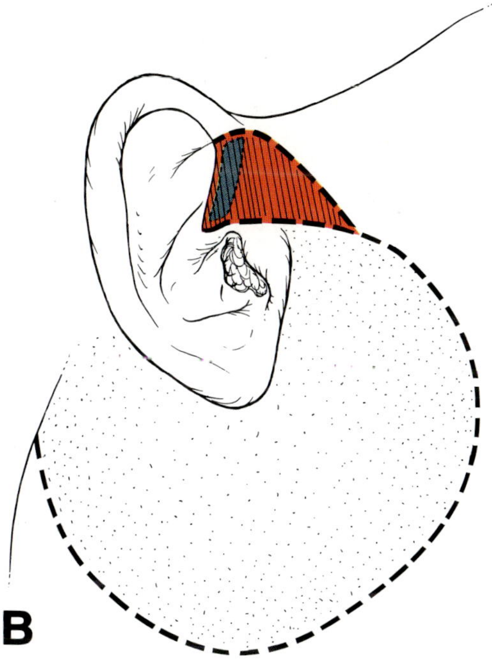

B

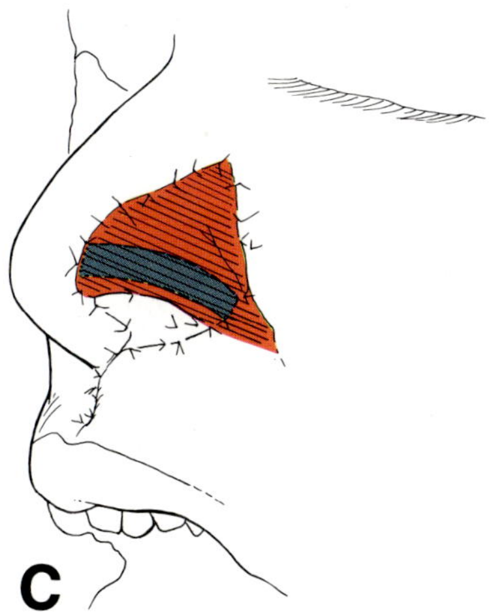

C

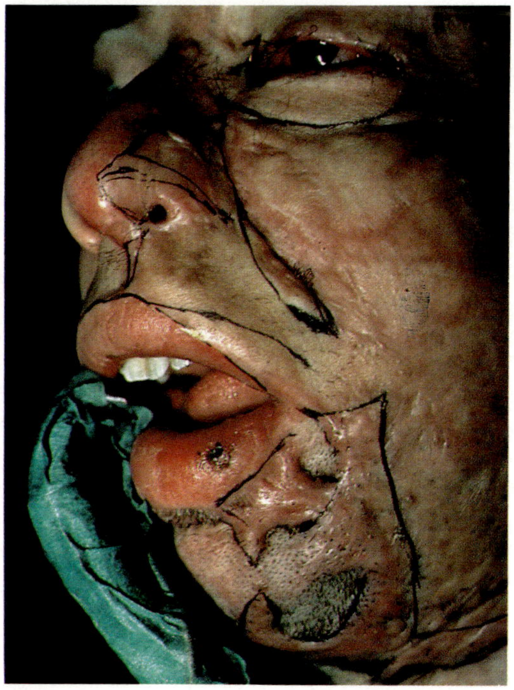

D

Fig. 217. continues.

Fig. 217. continued.

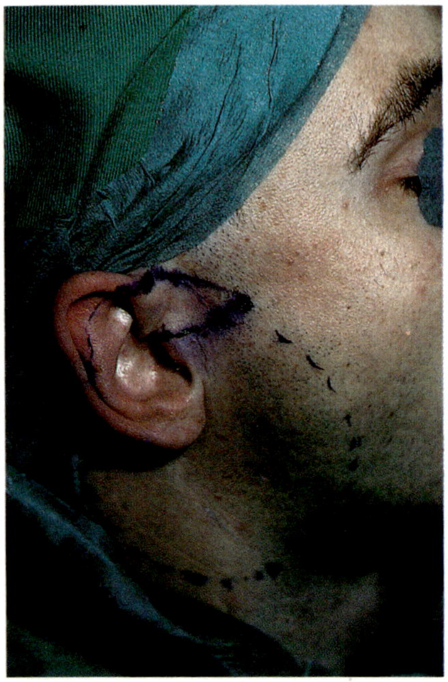

E

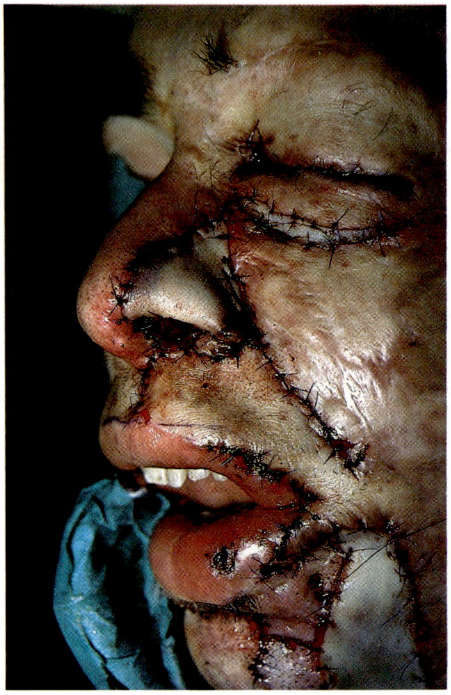

F

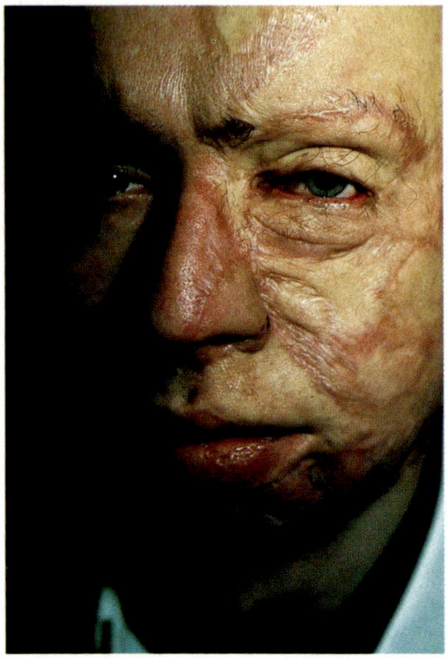

G

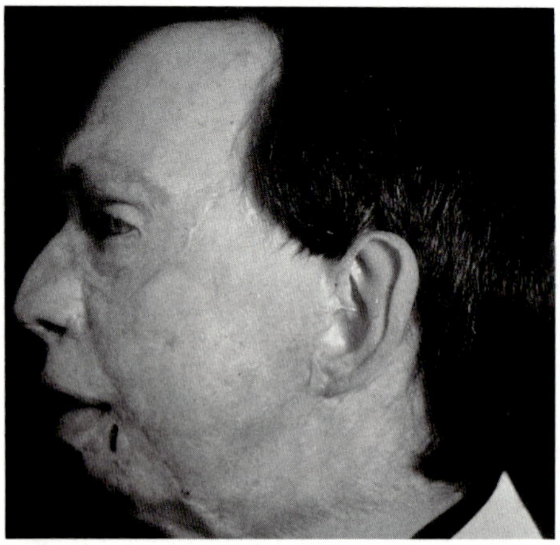

H

Fig. 217. More severe stenosis of the left nare after burn trauma in a young man, repaired with the same, but larger preauricular composite graft. (A) Preoperative aspect. (B and C) Transfer of the composite graft to the nasal defect in a drawing. A periauricular rotation flap in the donor area is illustrated. A first scar revision is combined with the nasal repair. (D) The nostril stenosis will be excised. (E) Preauricular donor area outlined. (F) Graft transferred. (G) Early result. (H) Late result.

For vestibular stenosis secondary to total and partial reconstruction of the nose we use the same preauricular composite graft, including the cartilage of the crus helicis, to substitute for the lateral lining of the vestibule. After removal of scar tissue from the lateral wall and the anterior commissure of the vestibule, we insert the composite graft in a reverse fashion to cover the resulting raw area, suturing the auricular border to the nostril and columellar border (Fig. 218). A rim reconstruction in cases of partial nasal repair can be performed with a smaller auricular composite graft that includes only the inner aspect of the crus helicis (Figs. 219 and 220).

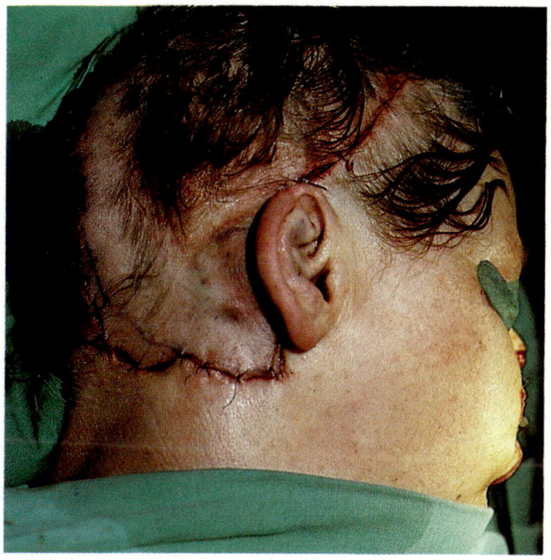

B

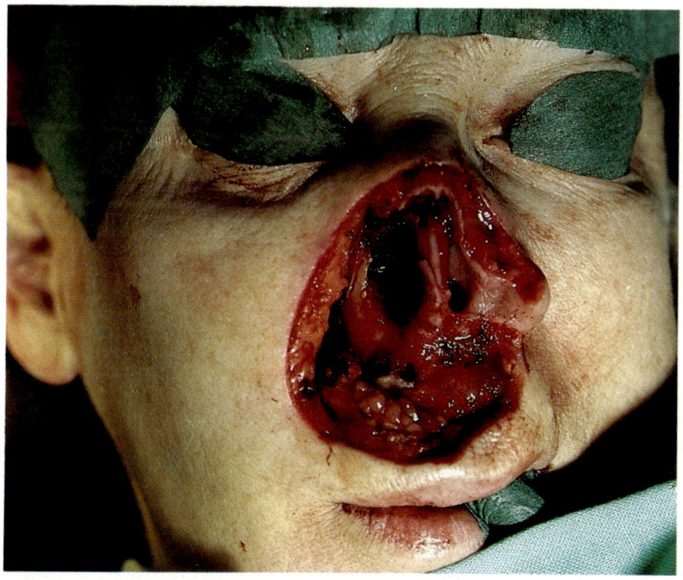

A

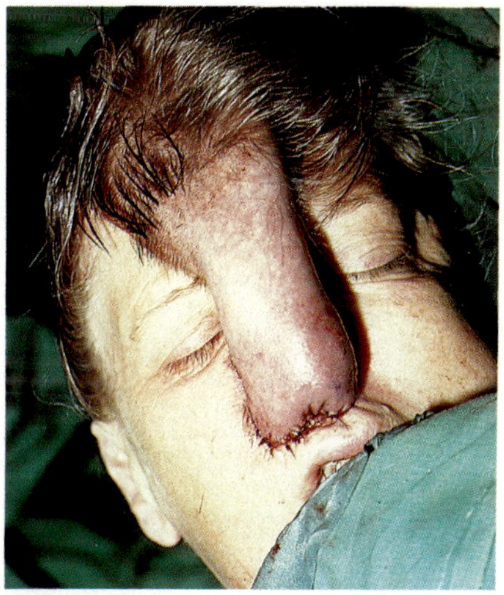

C

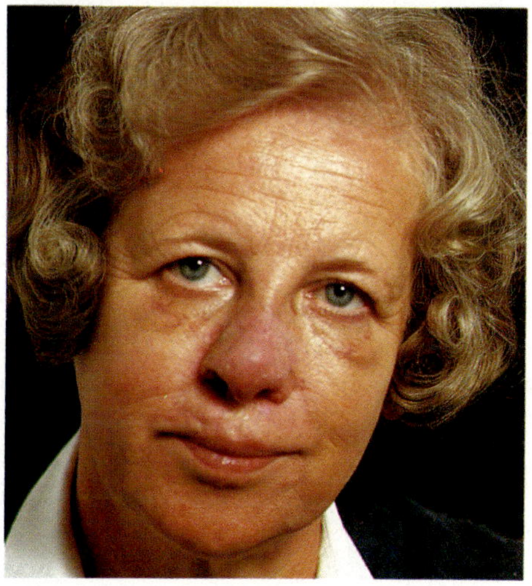

D

Fig. 218. continues.

Fig. 218. continued.

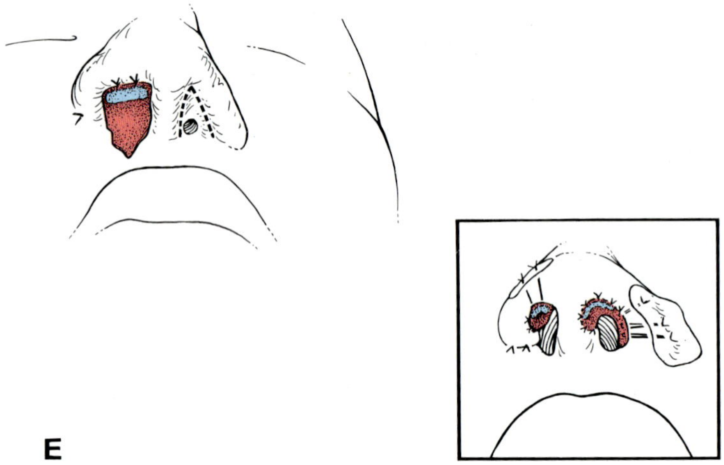

E

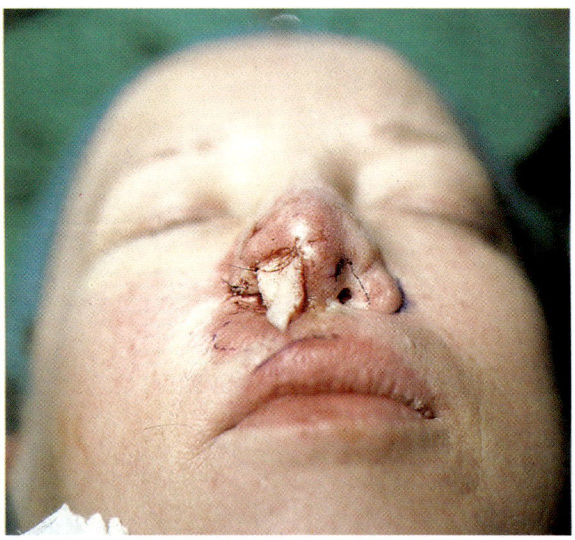

F

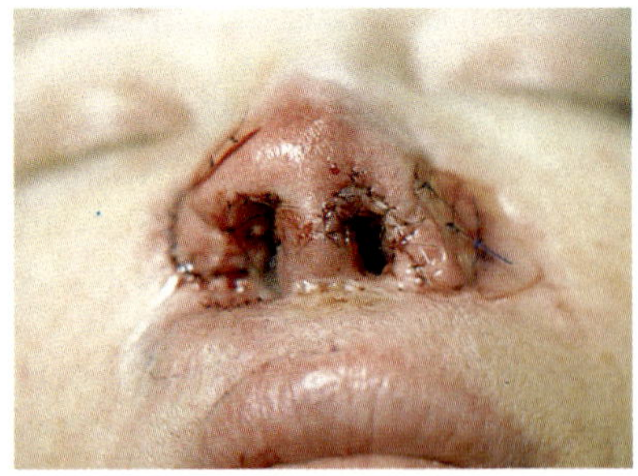

G

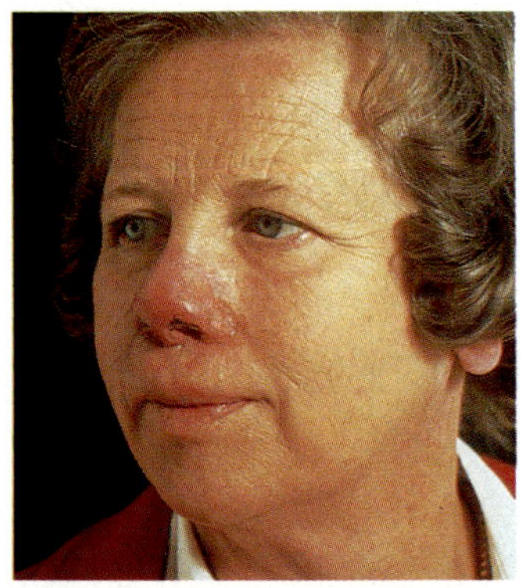

H

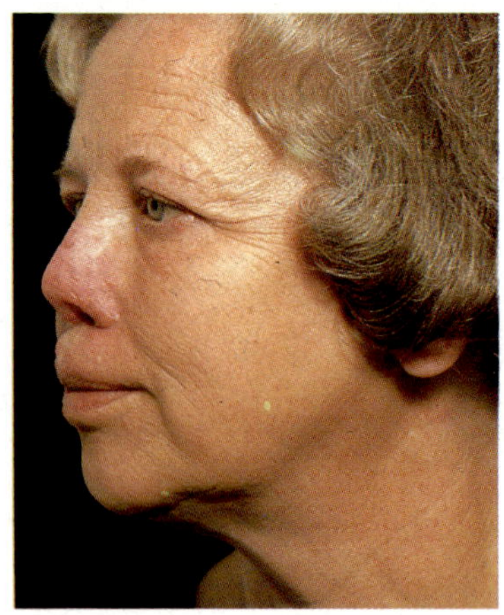

I

Fig. 218. (A) Middle-aged woman with large nasolabial defect after tumor removal. The defect is repaired with a fronto-parieto-occipital flap of Galvao (1981) leaving a scar free forehead. The secondary nostril stenosis was managed with a composite graft from the crus helicis of the ear. (B) Delay of Galvao flap. (C) Transfer of the flap. (D) Provisional good result, but with nostril stenosis. (E, F, and G) Preauricular composite graft from the right ear is sutured to the border of the right ala and will be folded inside to line the lateral vestibular wall. The same graft from the left ear is inserted in the left tissue defect to provide the alar border and lining for the vestibule. (H and I) Late result.

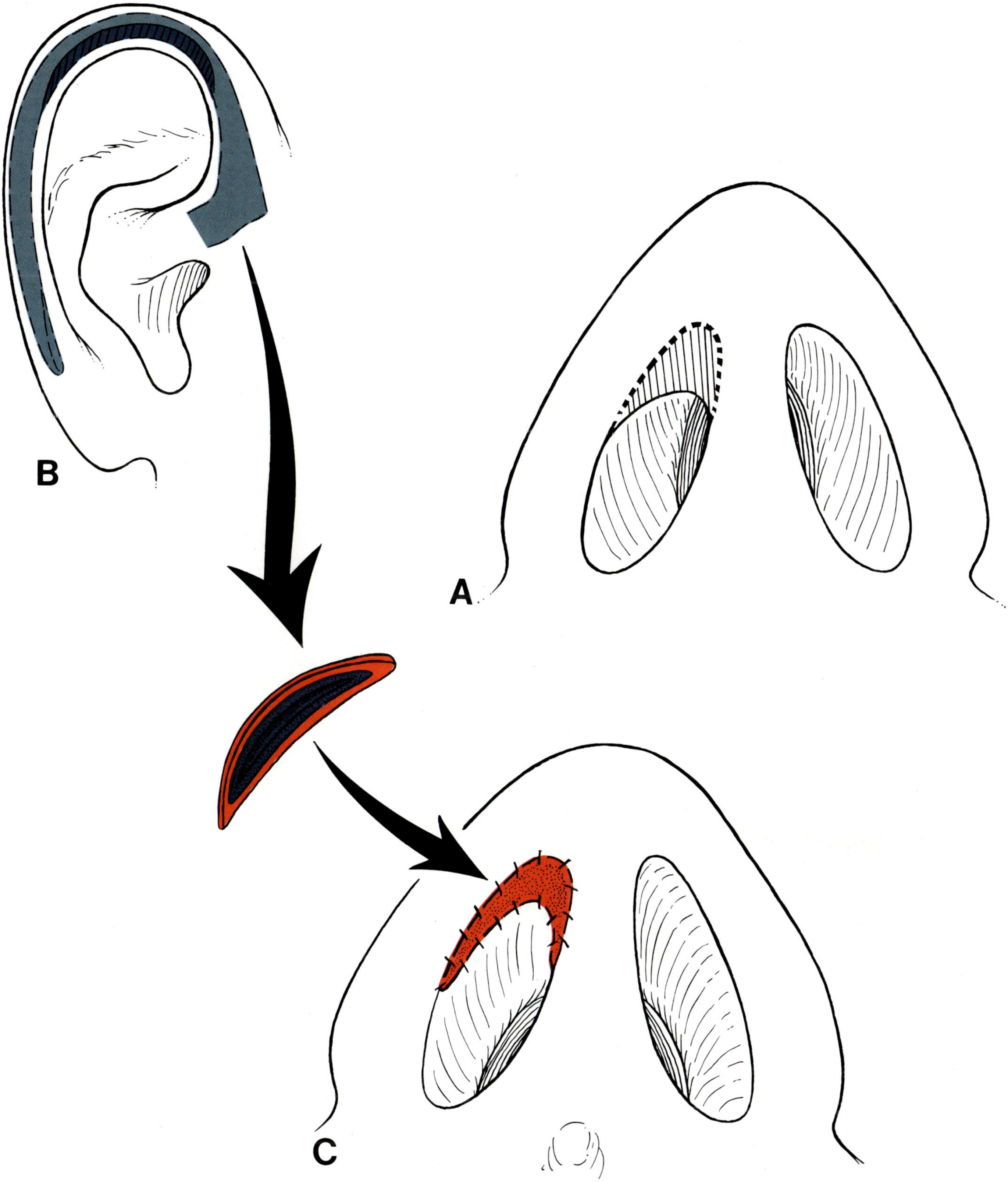

Fig. 219. (A) Composite graft from the ear for correction of anterior web stenosis of the vestibule. (B) Chondrocutaneous graft from the inner posterior aspect of the helix. (C) Graft sutured to the lobular-alar commissure.

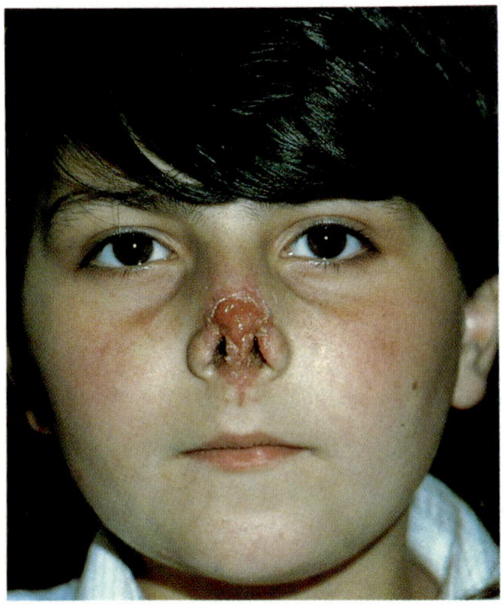

A

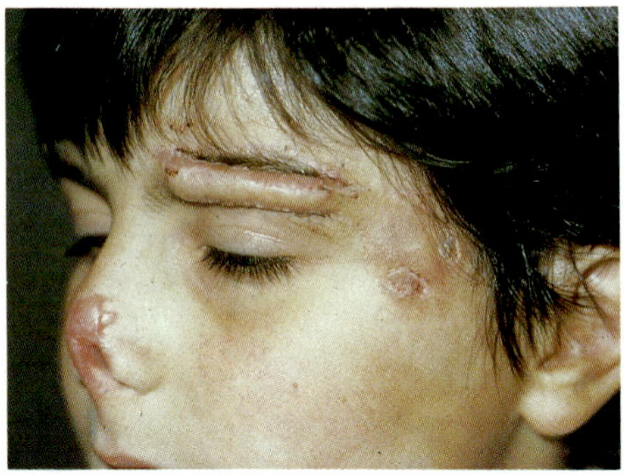

B

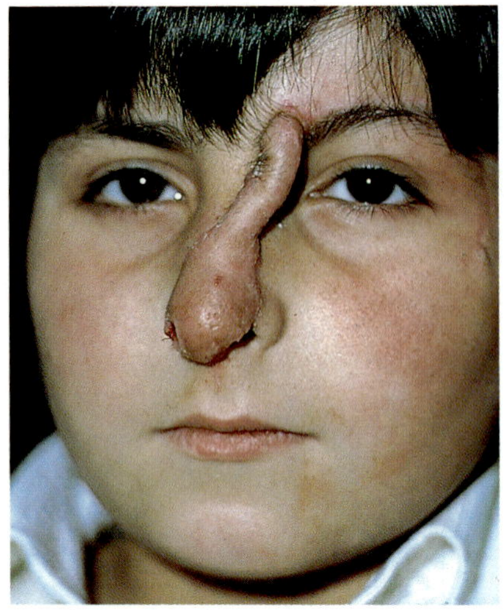

C

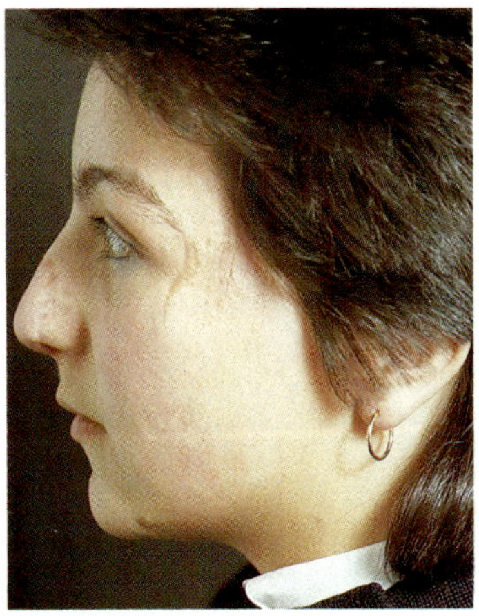

D

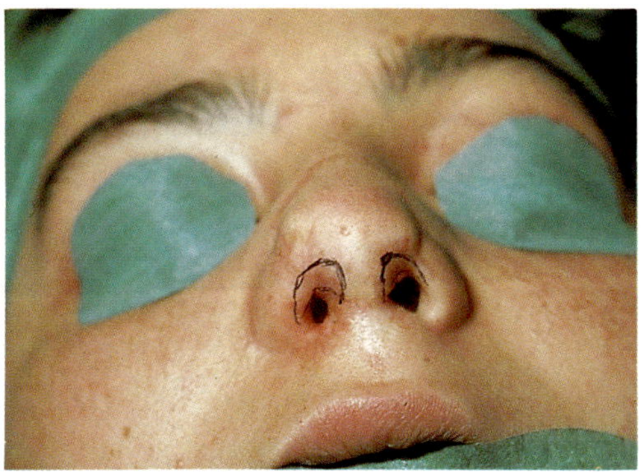

E

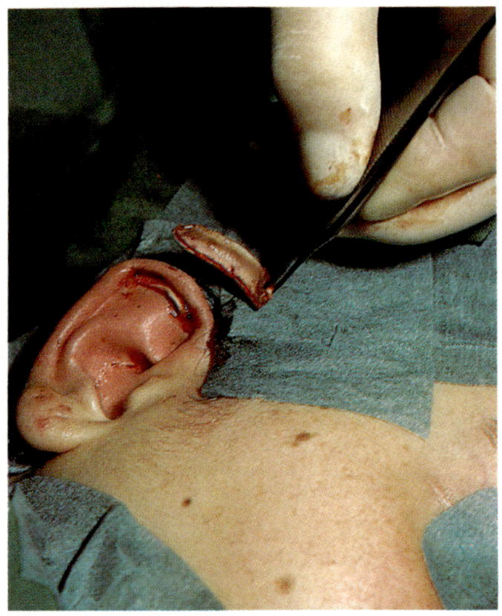

F

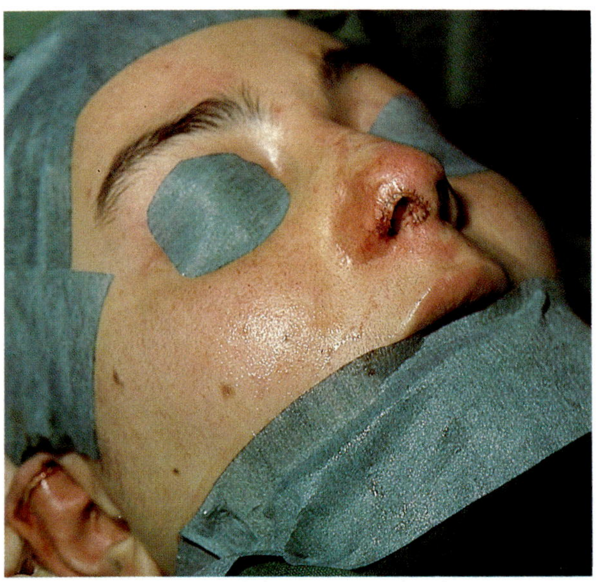

G

Fig. 220. This 10-year-old girl underwent a three stage procedure with frontotemporal flap (Schmid, 1952; Meyer, 1960) for partial reconstruction of the nose, after dog bite lesion. The aesthetic result was very satisfactory. But as in many other reconstructed noses an anterior stenosis of the vestibule developed necessitating a further intervention to improve nasal function. From the right pinna a helical composite graft was sutured to the lobular-alar commissure after removal of a cicatricial stenosing web. (A) Patient before partial reconstruction. (B) Frontotemporal flap prepared after first stage. (C) Flap transferred. (D) Result after three interventions. (E) Bilateral anterior web stenosis of the vestibule before correction. (F) Composite graft from the helix. (G) Graft sutured to the lobular-alar commissure. *Fig. 220. continues.*

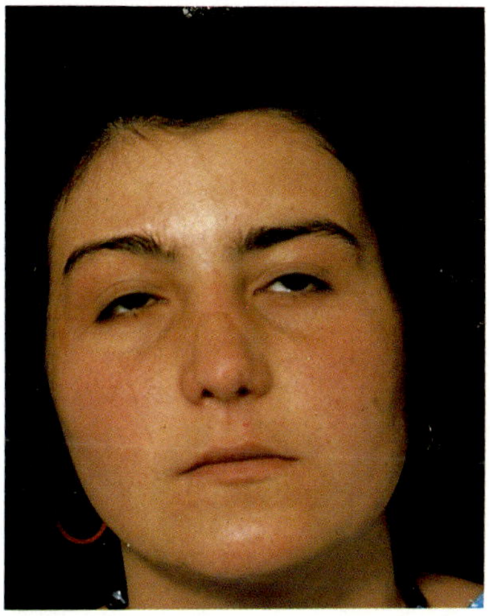

H

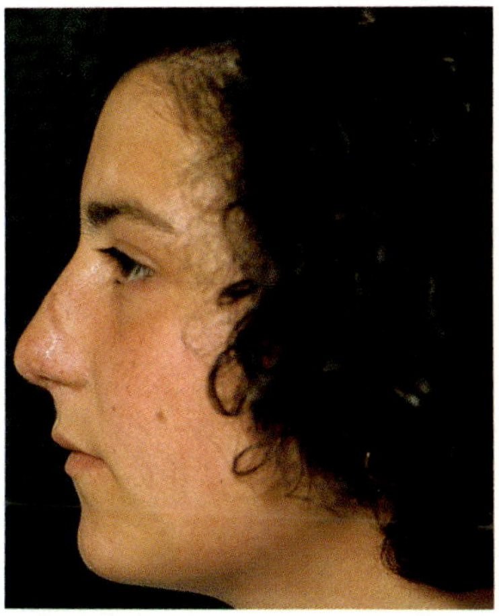

I

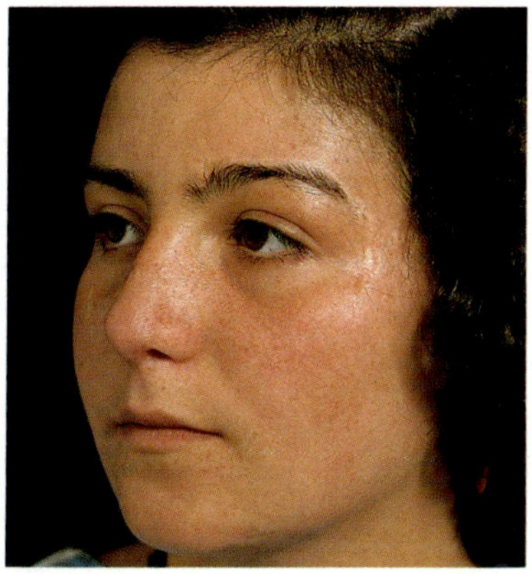

J

Fig. 220. continued. (H, I, and J) Final result.

For vestibular stenosis we form a *three dimensional Z-plasty* with two skin flaps that are dissected in the frontal anterior wall of the web. Both flaps are elevated. The raw surface of the posterior wall of the web is visible and can be thinned by removing scar tissue. Two flaps are cut also in this posterior wall. The two anterior flaps are turned onto the septum and to the lateral wall. The two posterior flaps are transposed forward to the vestibular floor. Transalar and transcolumellar mattress sutures maintain the flaps in position (Figs. 221 and 222).

For many years, particularly in cases of cleft nose, we used a technique that consisted of elevating a laterally based septal flap forward and grafting the donor septal area with a full thickness skin graft. In the same period we developed another similar technique for the treatment of acquired stenosis in adults. A laterally based paranasal flap is transposed into the vestibular floor, lining also the lateral aspect of the vestibule (Fig. 223). The septocolumellar defect is lined by a free skin graft. It seems that skin grafting of a rather rigid septum would help to maintain the circumference of the nasal vestibule.

The surgical procedure chosen depends on the location of the vestibular stenosis, the thickness of the obstructing wall, and the status of the alae. Excision of an obstructing membrane is generally insufficient. The ring-like occluding scar will recur. Such a scar should be opened by introducing a laterally and inferiorly based flap into the nasal floor and lateral vestibular wall. This is then anchored at its alar attachment by mattress sutures, as advocated by Lemoine (1931).

Dufourmentel (1973) combined this method with a full-thickness postauricular skin graft to the inner surface of the ala. We use composite ear grafts because the nostril needs cartilaginous support. Composite grafts are ideal for vestibular reconstruction and lining because of their tightly adherent skin covering and thin pliable cartilage. The length of the graft is not as critical for its take as is the width.

Only minimal stenosis of the lateral angle or the anterior dome can be simply incised, as proposed by Fomon (1948). After excision of the scar, the posterior membrane is removed and the anterior membrane is sutured against the wall. Sometimes, for a minor stenosis corrected by Z-plasty with or without full-thickness or composite grafting, a stent mold is helpful.

In cases of stenosis at the anterior commissure, Joseph's (1932) method can be used advantageously. A triangular flap based on the septum and including the superficial layers of the area of stenosis is elevated to remove the underlying connective and fatty tissue. Another triangular flap, based laterally, is formed along the inner and posterior wall of the stenosis. We prefer to use composite grafts from the ear to substitute for the first flap in these cases. The nasal vestibule is enlarged and deepened along its floor by means of a transposition flap from the cheek lateral to the base of the alae. As an extension of this technique, we use a free skin graft to complete the lining of the vestibule on the columellar septal wall.

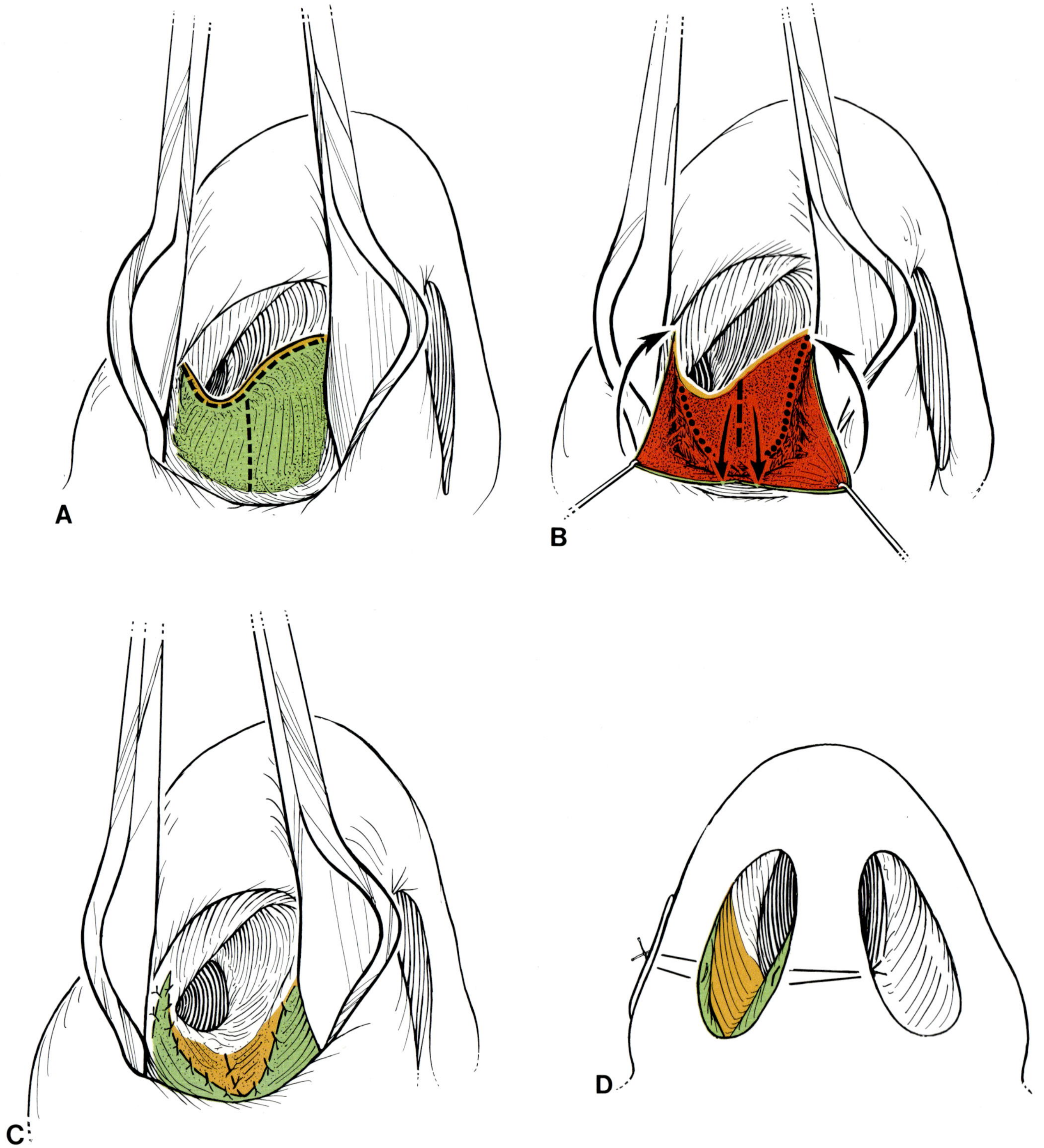

Fig. 221. Correction of vestibular web stenosis by three dimensional Z-plasty. (A) Two skin flaps are dissected in the frontal anterior wall of the web. (B) Both flaps are elevated. The raw surface of the posterior wall of the web is visible and can be thinned by removing scar tissue. Two flaps are cut also in this posterior wall. (C) The two anterior flaps are turned one to the septal wall, the other to the lateral vestibular wall. The two posterior flaps are transposed forward to the vestibular floor. (D) Transalar and transcolumellar mattress sutures holding the flaps in place.

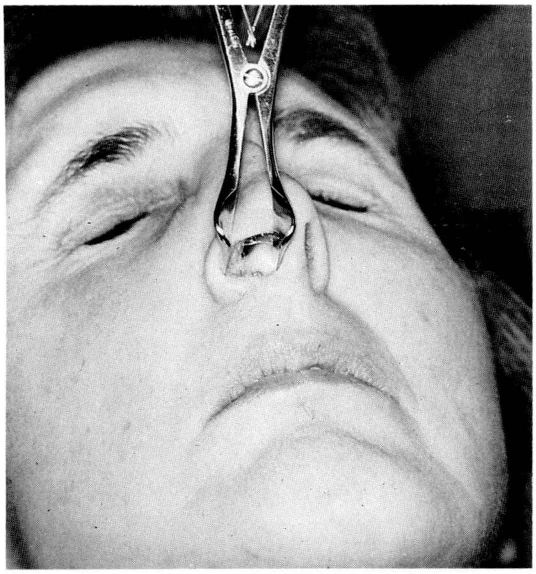

A

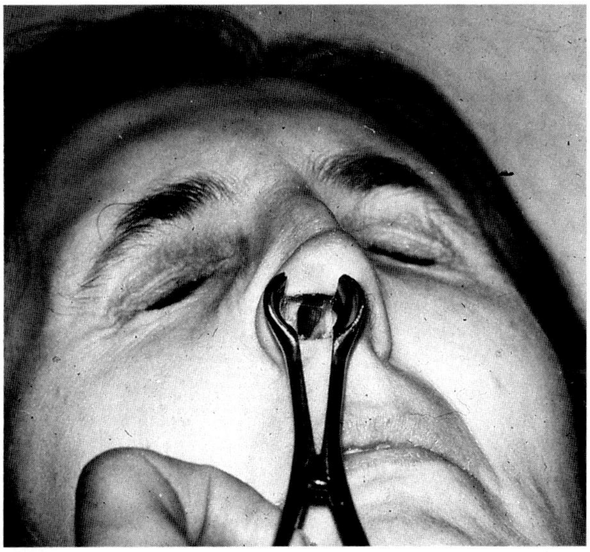

B

Fig. 222. Middle-aged woman with web stenosis of the left vestibule corrected using the method of three dimensional Z-plasties. (A) Preoperative view with stenosis. (B) Stenosis eliminated.

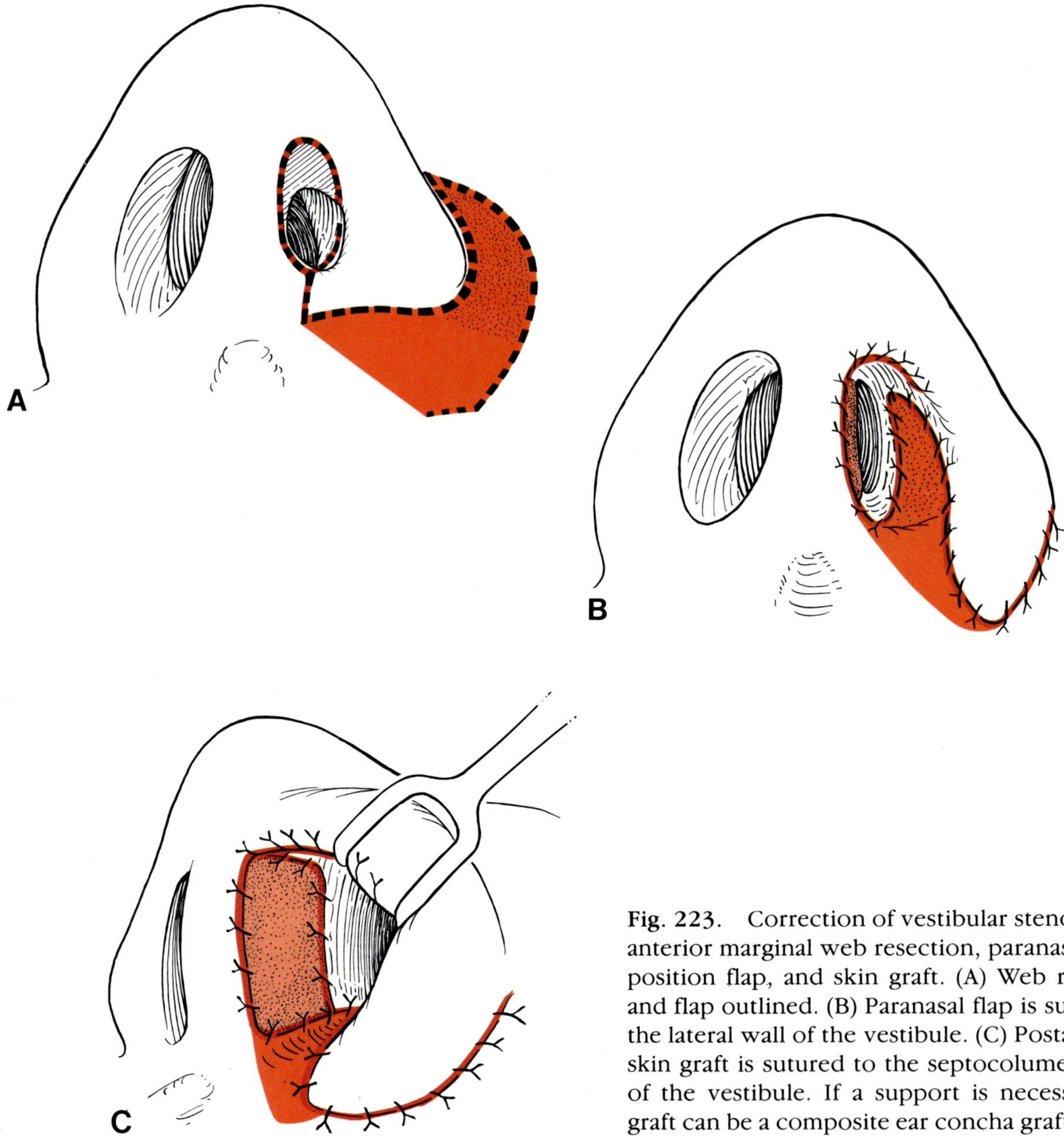

Fig. 223. Correction of vestibular stenosis with anterior marginal web resection, paranasal transposition flap, and skin graft. (A) Web resection and flap outlined. (B) Paranasal flap is sutured to the lateral wall of the vestibule. (C) Postauricular skin graft is sutured to the septocolumellar wall of the vestibule. If a support is necessary this graft can be a composite ear concha graft.

To prevent recurrent scar contraction in the lateral vestibular angle we use a personal technique, described in 1972 in the book *Unfavorable Results in Plastic Surgery* by Goldwyn. An inferiorly based flap is outlined on the external surface of the stenosing web, the base being at the inferior part of the columella and extending laterally along the future inferior nasal rim.

This flap is then transposed to line the nasal floor after excision of the inner surface of the web. The flap is not always necessary. After the excision of a fibrocicatricial block, producing stenosing of the vestibular floor, a paranasal island flap is carried into the vestibule to rebuild the skin lining, covering both the floor and the lateral wall of the vestibule (*see* Fig. 230). When the scarring process affects only the vestibular floor we can enlarge this lower stenosis by using only the paranasal flap (Fig. 224). This flap was first described by us (Meyer and Kesselring, 1977) and subsequently by Conley, Sachs, and Donovan (1982), who renamed it the mini alar base myocutaneous flap. We transfer this flap to the vestibular floor, either through a tunnel under the alar base (Fig. 225) or with the help of a complementary alotomy (Figs. 226–229). The

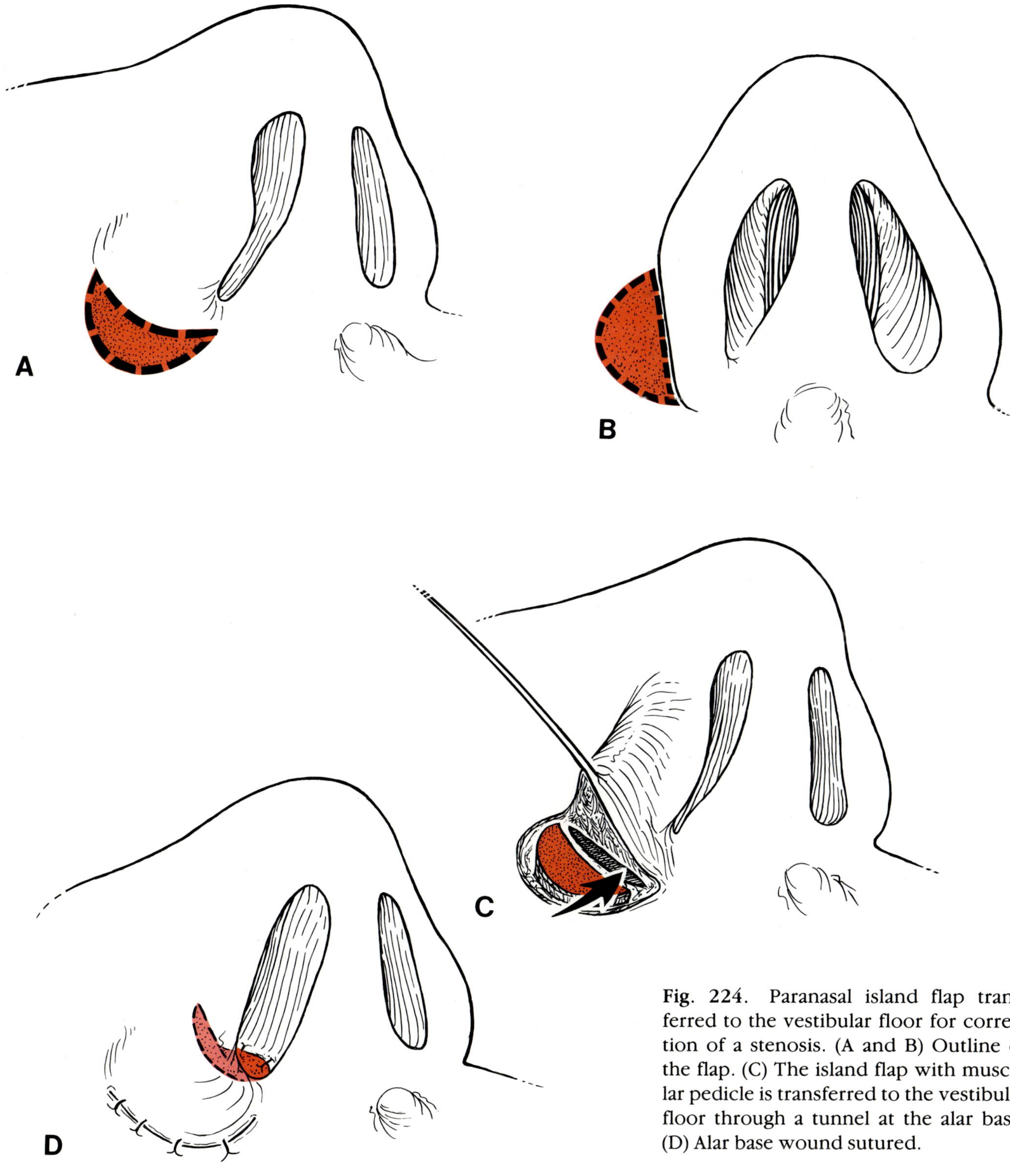

Fig. 224. Paranasal island flap transferred to the vestibular floor for correction of a stenosis. (A and B) Outline of the flap. (C) The island flap with muscular pedicle is transferred to the vestibular floor through a tunnel at the alar base. (D) Alar base wound sutured.

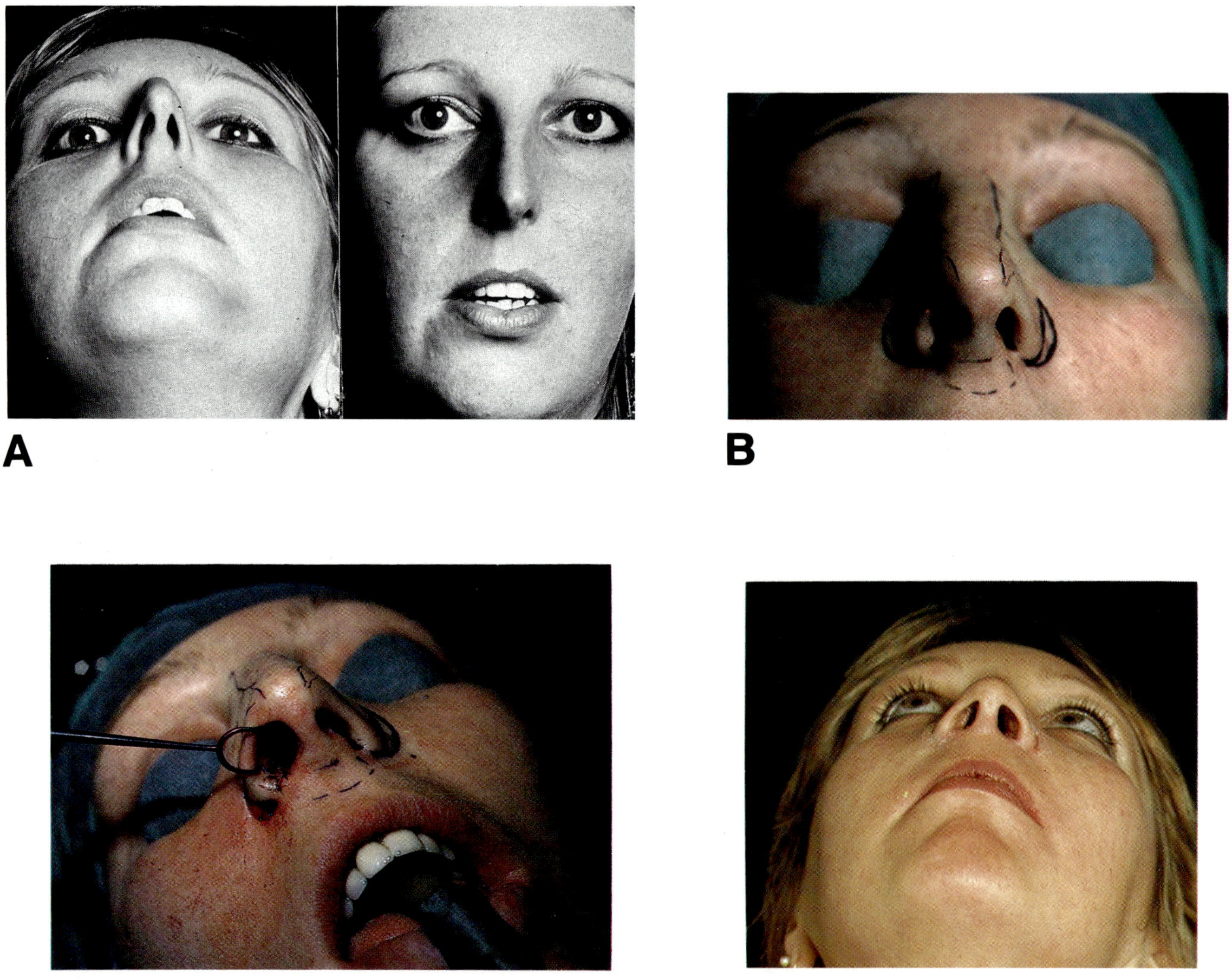

Fig. 225. Young lady with narrow nasal pyramid and especially narrow vestibule on both sides. For enlarging the vestibule bilateral paranasal myocutaneous island flaps were used. This is the same patient in Fig. 189, operated concomitantly for tethered lip. (A) Preoperative axial view. (B) Both island flaps outlined. (C) Right flap transferred and sutured to the vestibular floor. (D) Axial view of the enlarged vestibules one year later. In the same intervention osteotomies are also performed with lateral displacement of the nasal bones and nasal cavity (see Fig. 237).

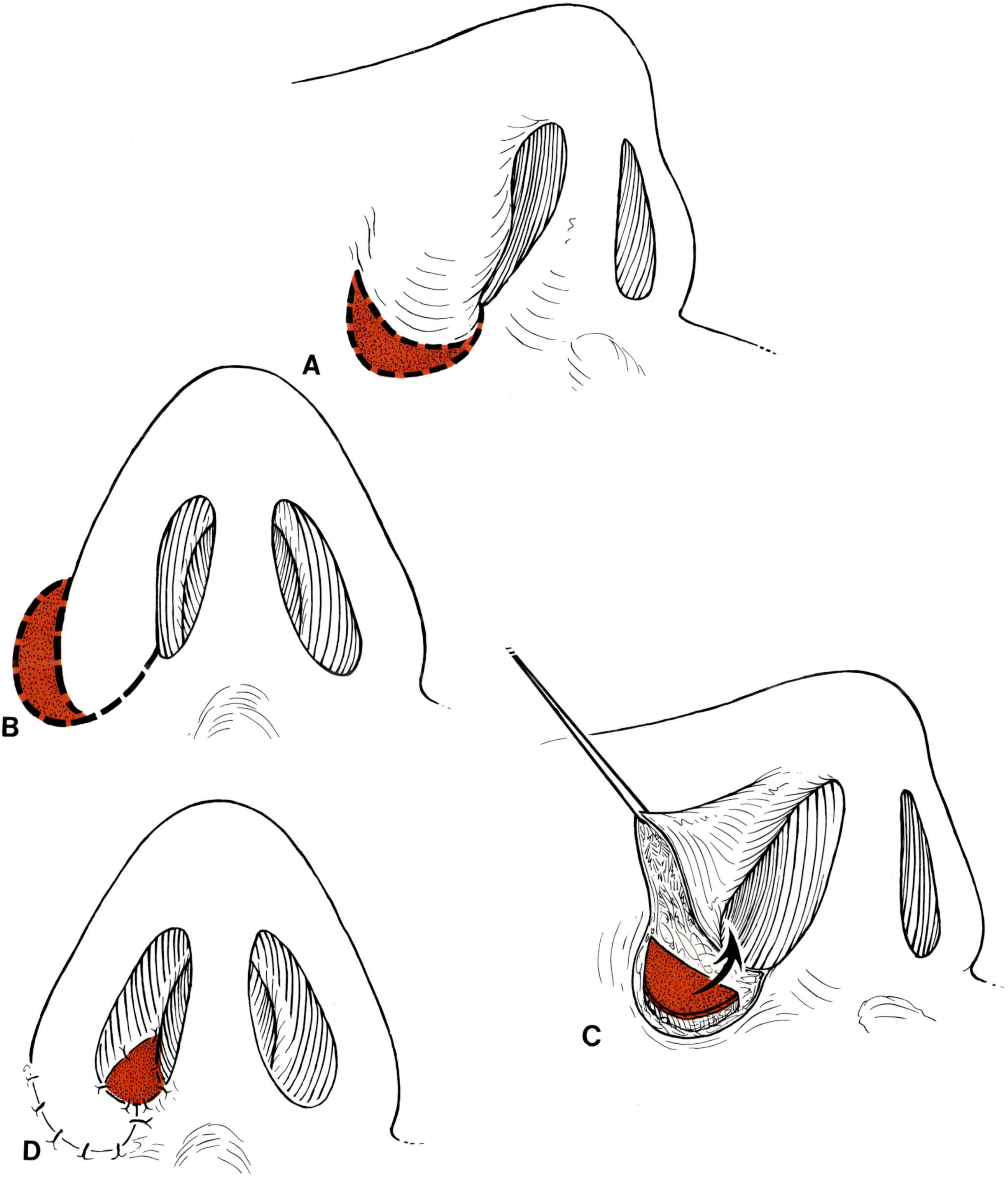

Fig. 226. The same myocutaneous island flap is transferred to the vestibular floor with the help of an alotomy. (A and B) Flap and alar base section outlined. (C) Transfer of the flap. (D) Flap and donor site sutured.

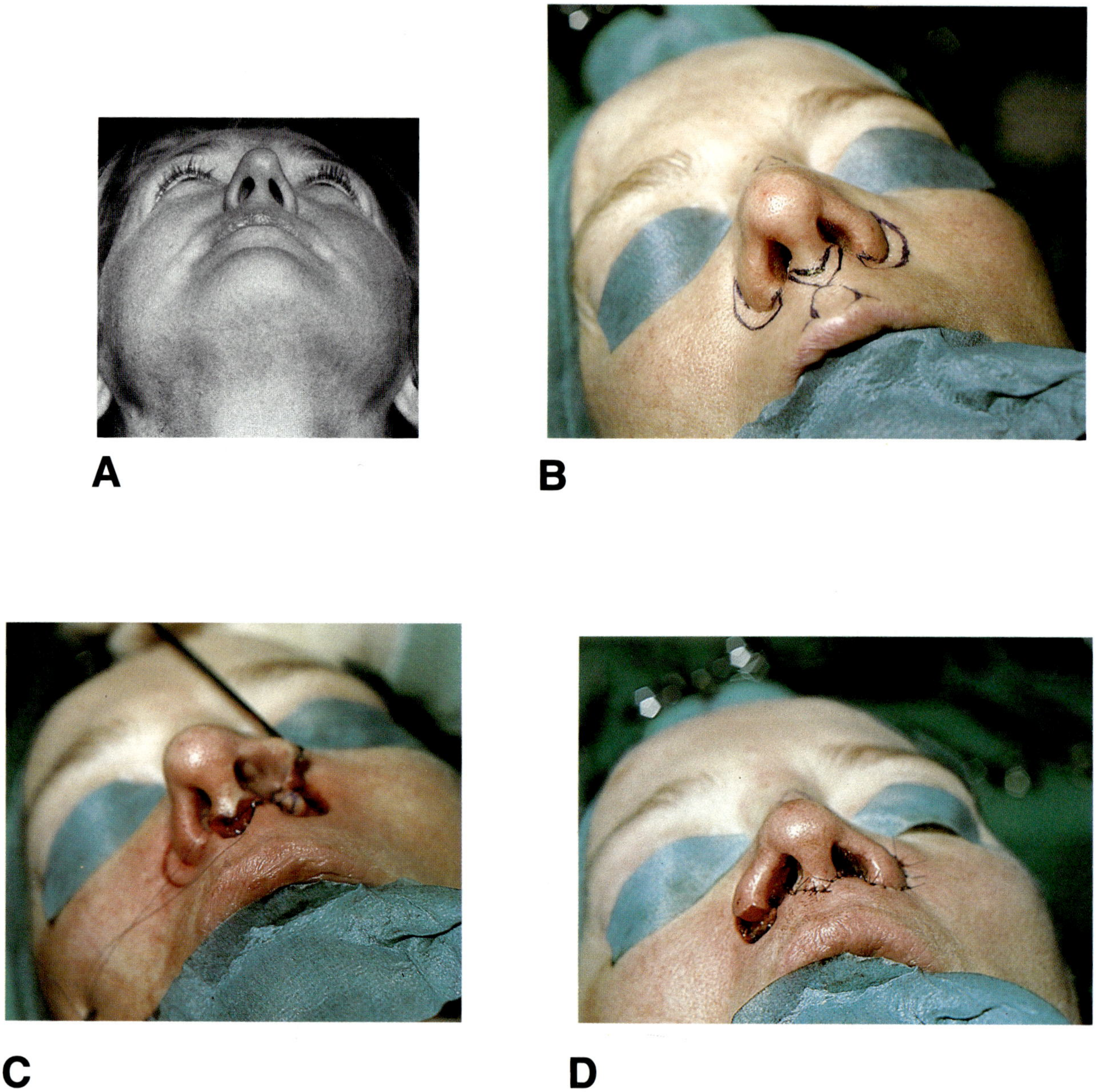

Fig. 227. Middle-aged female with narrow vestibule and airway impairment treated with bilateral paranasal island flaps shortening at the same time the upper lip with alar base displacement. (A) Preoperative view. (B) Outline of the island flaps and columellar base excision. (C) Left island flap moving to the vestibular floor right flap incised and V-shaped strip of skin excised at the columellar base. (D) Left alar base and columellar base displaced more caudally. On the right side the flap is sutured but not yet the alar base.

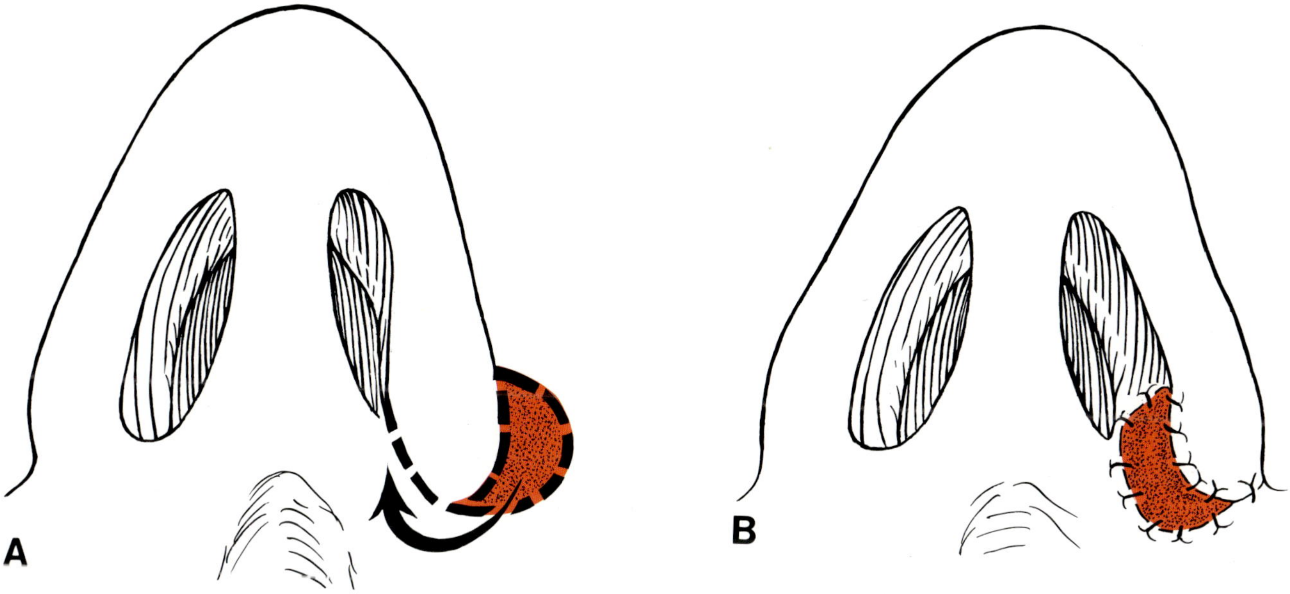

Fig. 228. (A and B) The same island flap can also form a new sill of the vestibule producing a most symmetrical aspect of the nasal base.

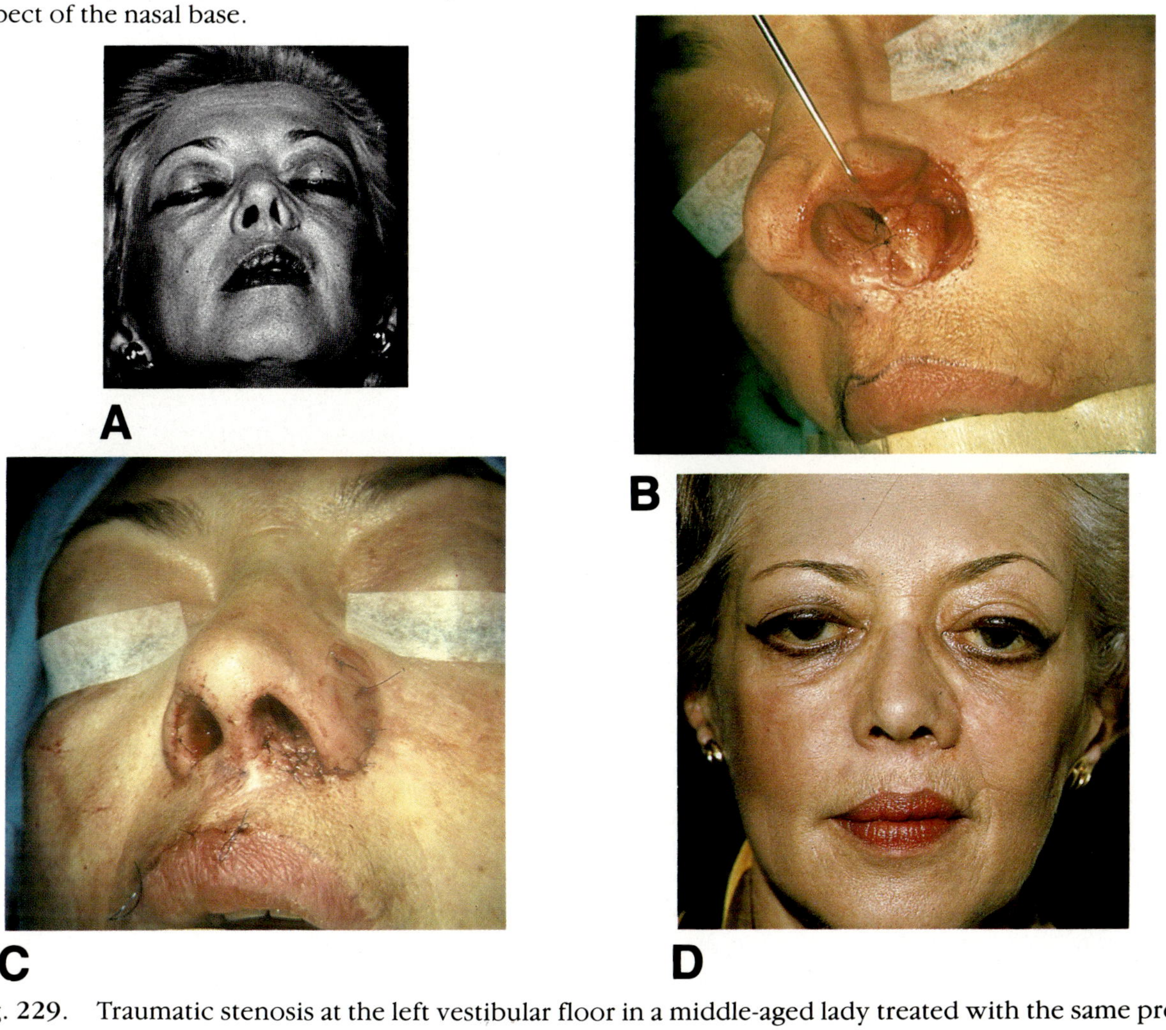

Fig. 229. Traumatic stenosis at the left vestibular floor in a middle-aged lady treated with the same procedure. (A) Preoperative axial view. (B) Transfer of the flaps. (C) The flap covers the lateral portion of the vestibular floor and provides a part of the sill and lateral lining. (D) Result.

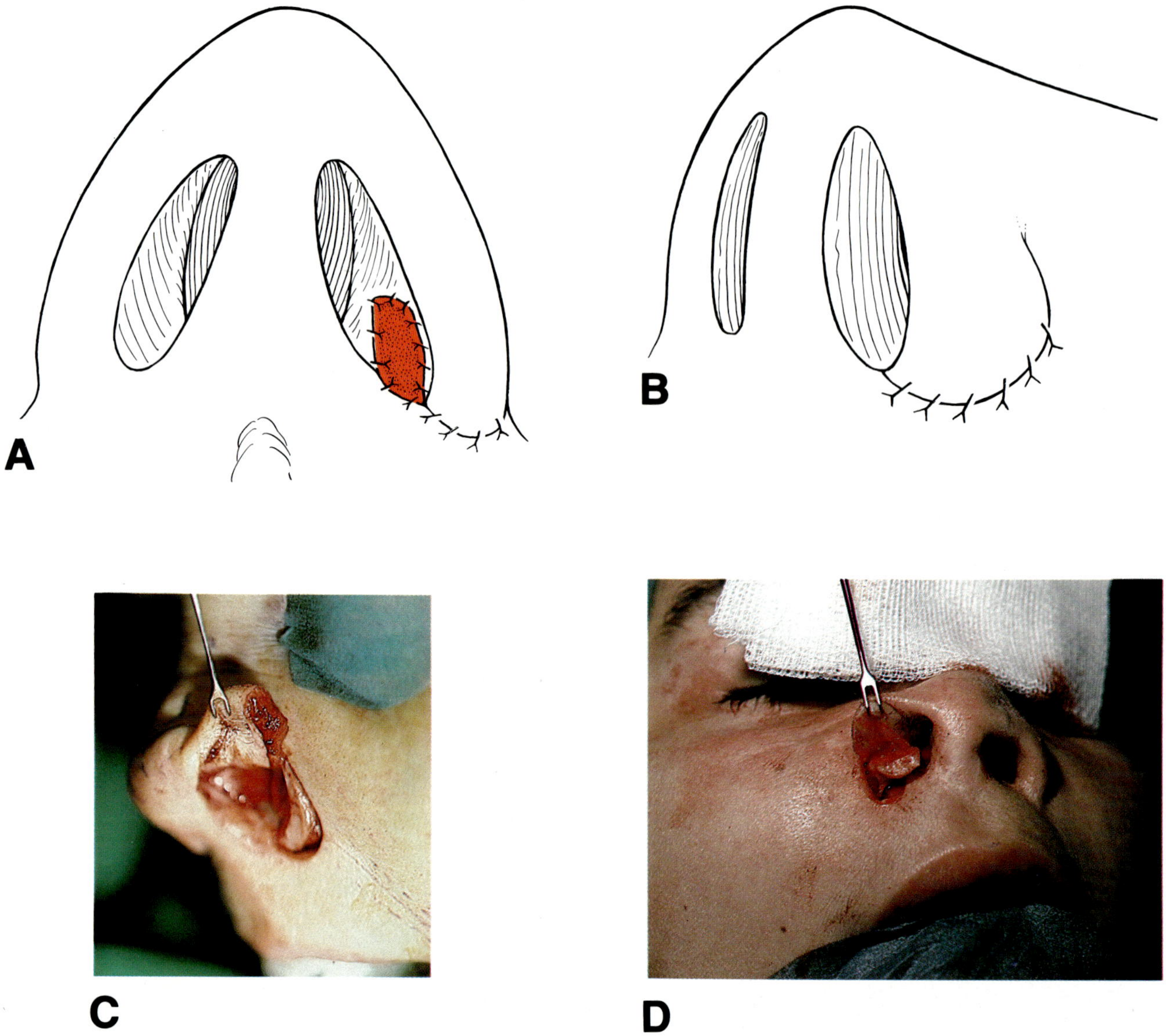

Fig. 230. In these two cases the same island flap could be inverted inside the vestibule to enlarge the lateral wall. (A and B) Design showing the transferred flap and the alar base suture. (C and D) Two cases showing such a flap transfer.

use of the paranasal island flap can be extended to the treatment of stenosis located at the lower part of the ala. In such conditions, this myocutaneous island flap is inverted inside the vestibule to enlarge and rebuild its lateral wall (Fig. 230). By transferring this flap to the basal portion of the ala, we can, in addition, elongate the ala on its stenosed side.

The alar base wedge, as outlined for use as a Weir resection, can also be utilized as an island flap to enlarge the vestibule by rotating it into the lateral vestibular wall as shown in Figure 231. As a supplementary measure to increase the height of the alae, a composite auricular graft is used, taken from the inner aspect of the crus helicis. In this region, the skin is extremely adherent to the cartilage, an important advantage for the eventual take of the graft (Fig. 232). The subcutaneous pedicle of this flap exerts a lateral traction on the vestibular angle, keeping the floor sufficiently wide. To replace the loss of tissue following excision of scars from the vault of the nasal vestibule, the nostril may also be lined by means of a composite auricular graft from the crus helicis.

In some cases, the scarring process also retracts the columella, which needs to be lengthened by one of the procedures we have already

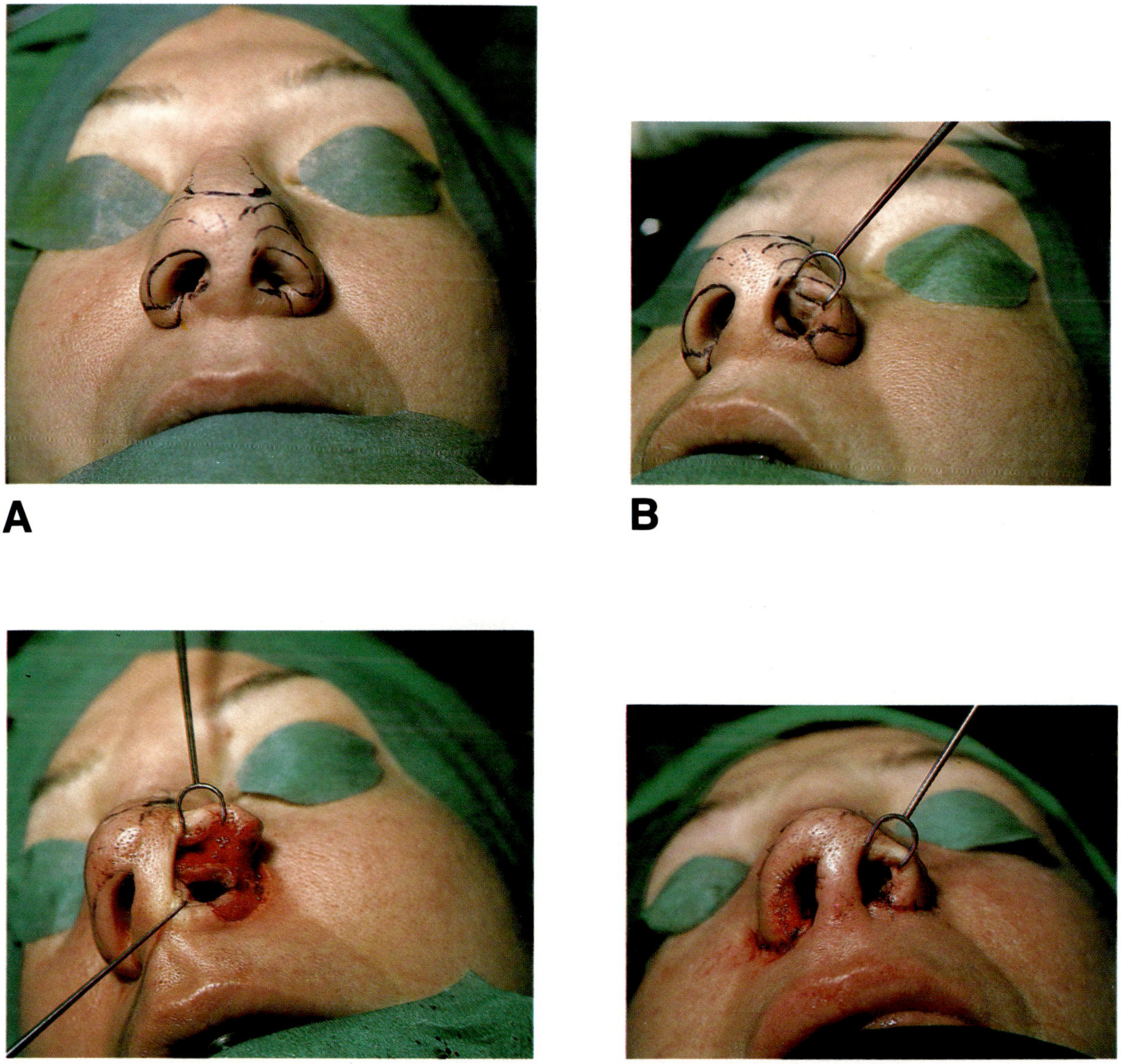

A B C D

Fig. 231. The island flap is in this case of traumatic shortness of the left ala completely inverted in order to form the basal part of the lateral vestibular wall, thus elongating the ala on the stenosed side. (A) Weir edge to be resected at the right alar base and a similar wedge outlined at the left side. The latter will not be resected but turned inside to provide additional lining of the lateral vestibular wall. (B) Vestibular stenosis visible. (C) Rotation of the flap. (D) Suture of the flap for widening the alar lining. The basal border of the alar wedge has been sutured to the vestibular alar base and the antero-superior border of the wedge has become the inner attachment of the ala to the vestibular floor.

described. In a 2-year-old child we needed two nasal flaps and two buccal mucosal flaps for building up a nonexistent wall and floor of the vestibule (Fig. 233).

After excessive removal of vestibular skin a partial stenosis of the nasal airway resulted in the region of the domes. Stenosis may extend both medially and laterally to create a circular con-

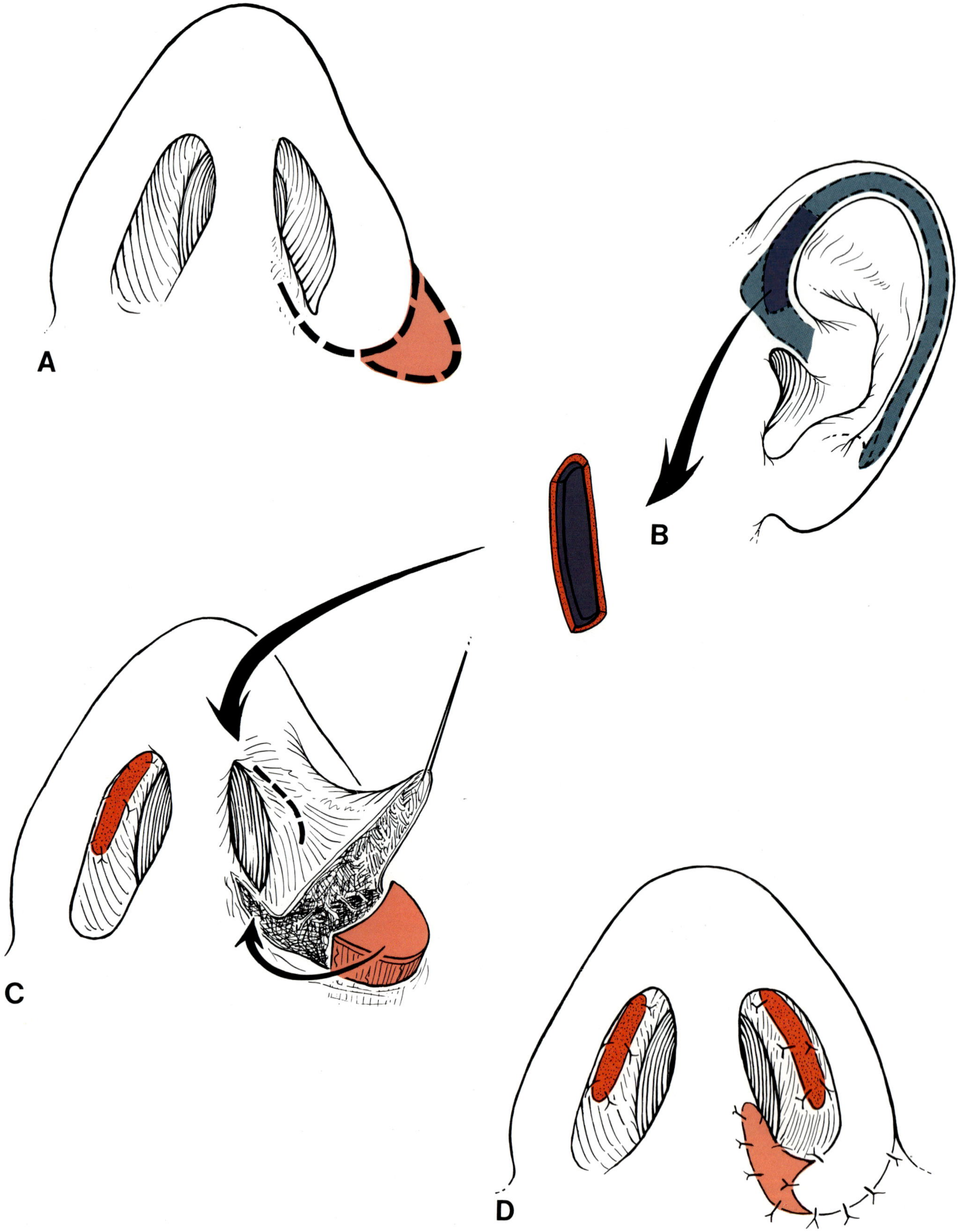

Fig. 232. (A, B, C, D) Correction of severe vestibular stenosis with a paranasal island flap (like Fig. 226) and auricular composite graft (like Fig. 86).

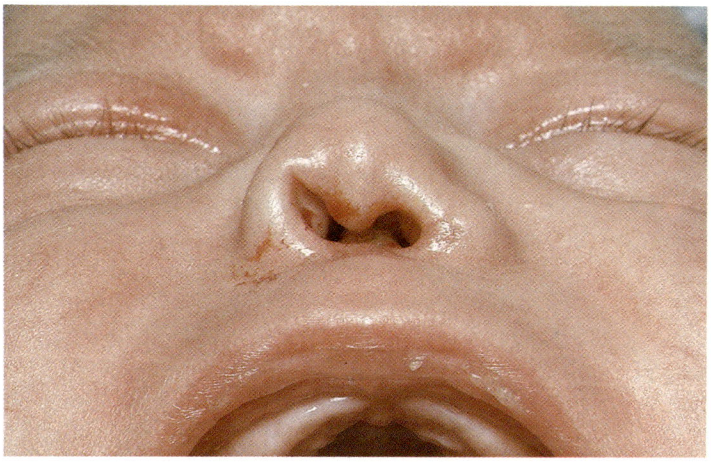

A

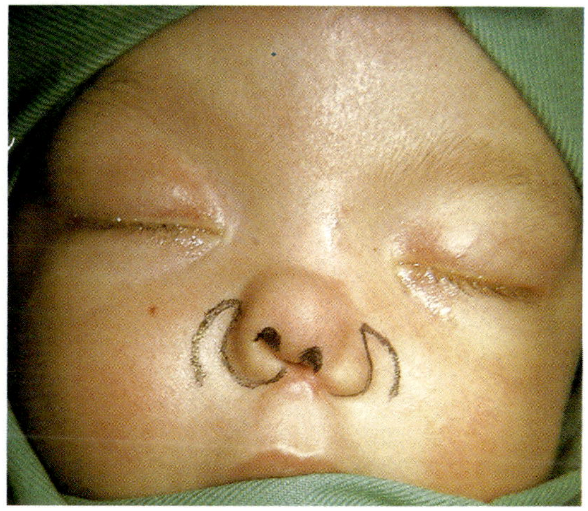

B

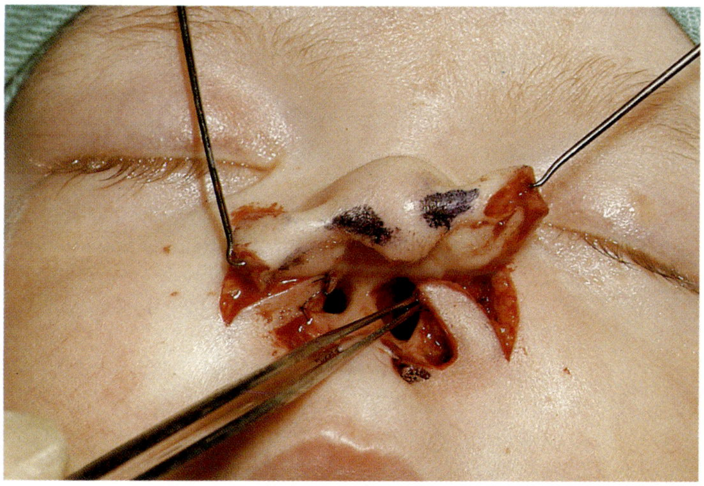

C

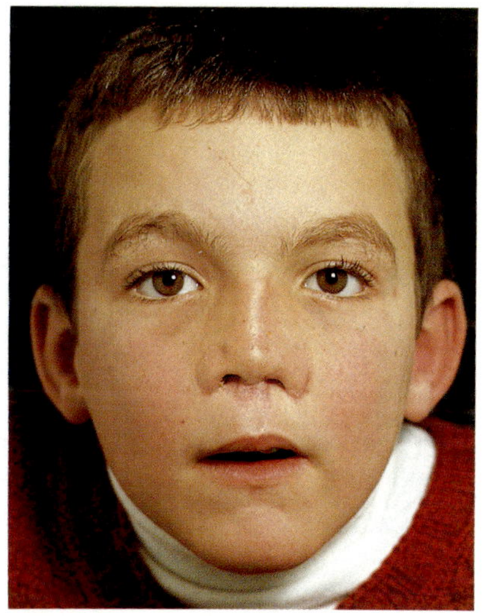

E

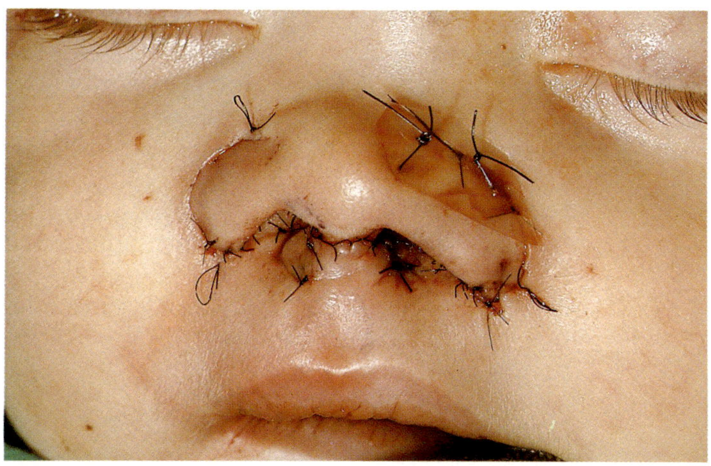

D

Fig. 233. Treatment of severe bilateral stenosis in a 2-year-old child with stenosis due to iatrogenic septocolumellar necrosis. (A) Preoperative view. (B and C) Bilateral paranasal flaps are transposed into the vestibule to build a part of the lateral wall. The columella is lengthened by skin resection at the ala-columellar commissure. (D) Overcorrected situation at the end of the operation. (E) Late result with sufficient nasal breathing but requiring aesthetic improvement, which is planned. *(Fig. 233 continues.)*

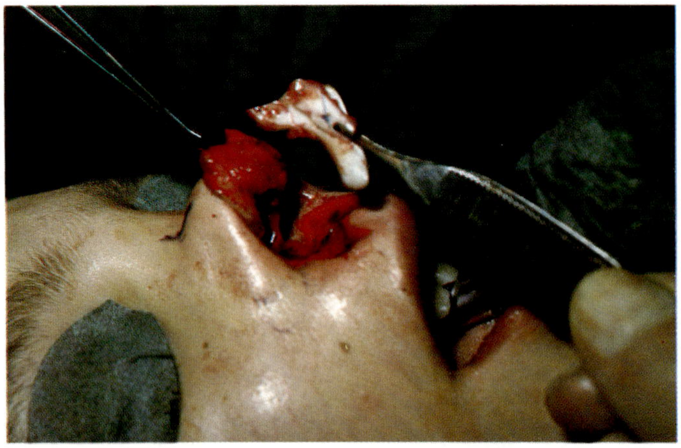

F

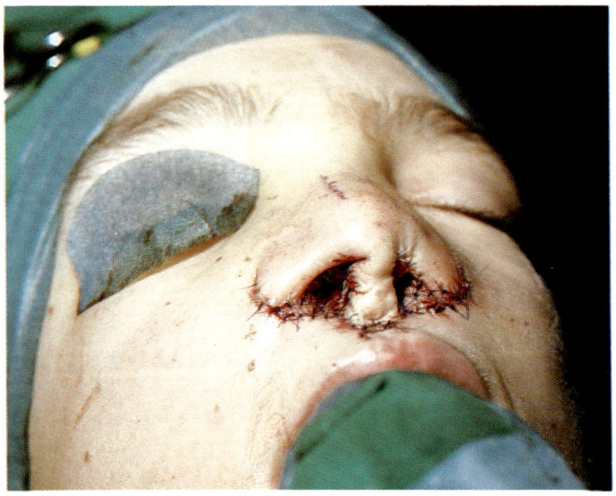

G

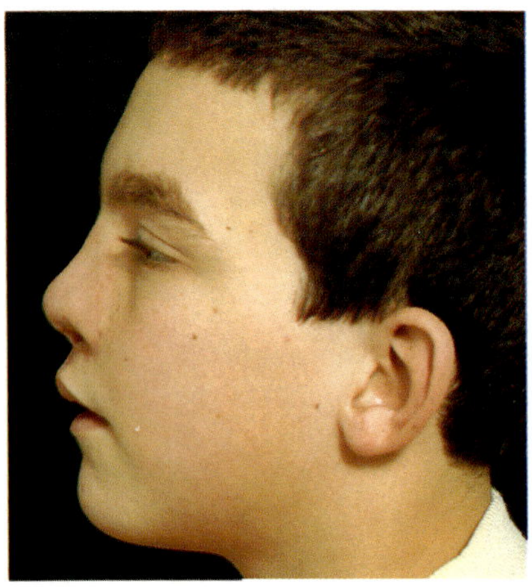

H

Fig. 233 *(continued.)* (F and G) Tip-columella augmentation with L-shaped graft at the age of 11 years. (H) Final result.

traction. An inward pull of the external nasal structures ensues because both the overlying skin and the cartilage components have been weakened. The treatment of this deformity requires removal of the intranasal scar tissue and cicatricial bands by a combination of internal or external Z-plasty procedures and the use of full-thickness skin grafts to cover the raw areas.

To correct hare lip noses and extremely large lobules or broad alo-columellar commissure, we have developed the *infolding method,* derived from the plication of the forehead flap used in nasal reconstruction. It consists basically of thinning the skin at the commissure of the nostril and in the anterior part of the excessively broad columella and then folding it inwards after partial excision of the alar cartilage. The margin of the ala is lifted to the same level as that of the opposite side. Together with the excess alar cartilage we remove the fibrous tissue, filling the broad commissure and leaving the skin intact (Figs. 234–236).

The newly shaped nostril is held in place with three or more mattress sutures slung over a plastic sheet. This of course jeopardizes the blood supply of the infolded skin, but not enough to produce necrosis. There is less danger of secondary narrowing and stenosing of the vestibule with this technique than in other procedures experienced by us.

In cases of marked asymmetry as in a harelip nose, we complete the vestibular lining with an additional composite graft from the ear (see Chapter 20).

The use of skin to fill large mucosal defects in the nose should be avoided if possible because it may lead to formation of ozena-like dryness with crusts, since the skin has no mucous glands. For us, free or pedicled oral mucosa has proved to be the best grafting material for the inner lining of the nose. The long mucosal flap, whose base is in the region of the gingivobuccal fold, is passed to the nasal defect through a tunnel between the oral vestibule and the nasal spine, as described by Jeschek (1960) in his ozena operation and by us for the closure of large septal perforations.

We have also used the buccal flap in children with extensive stenoses of the vestibule and the nasal cavity, as we did in the case of Figure 233.

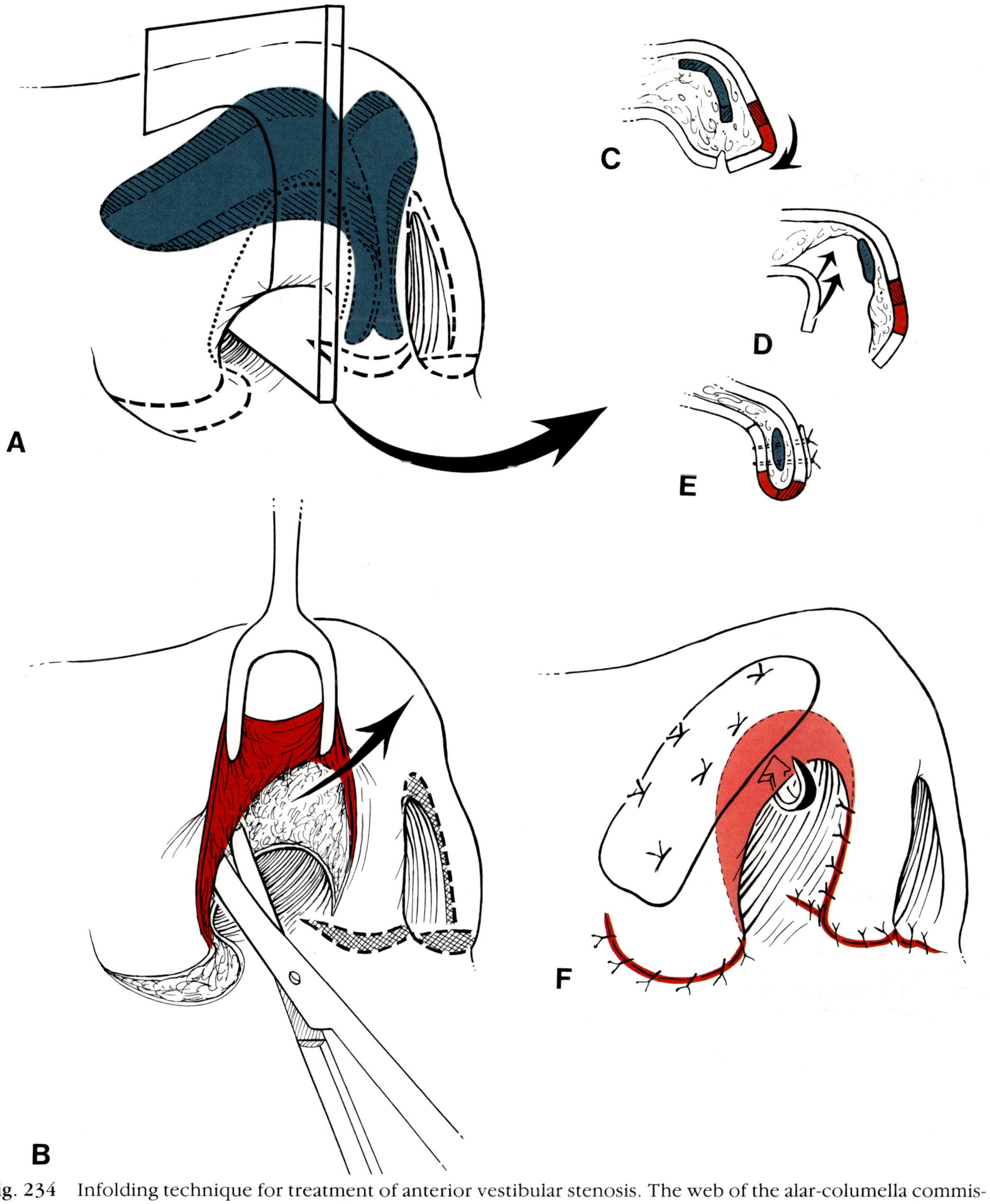

Fig. 234 Infolding technique for treatment of anterior vestibular stenosis. The web of the alar-columella commissure is not resected but subcutaneously defatted from a vestibular incision and folded into the vestibule to form a new dome. (A) The lower lateral cartilage is trimmed caudally and cranially. At the same stage the alae and the columella are reduced by basal resections. (B, C, D, E, and F) Defatting the web (infolding the skin of the web) which is fixed in the new position by transalar mattress sutures. (D and E) Cross section through the ala shows the rotation movement of the skin of the web to reduce external surface and augment internal lining surface.

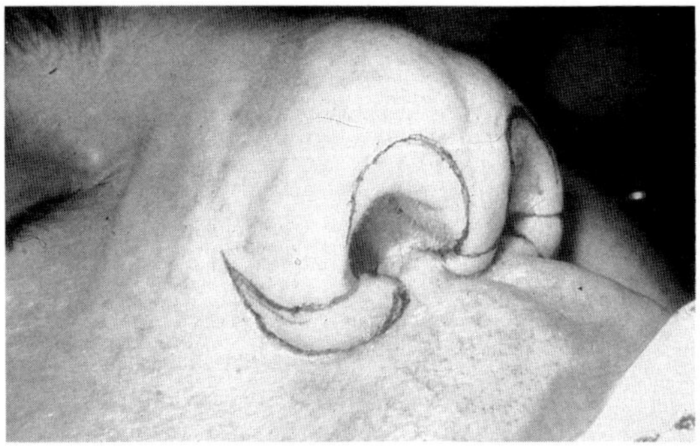

A

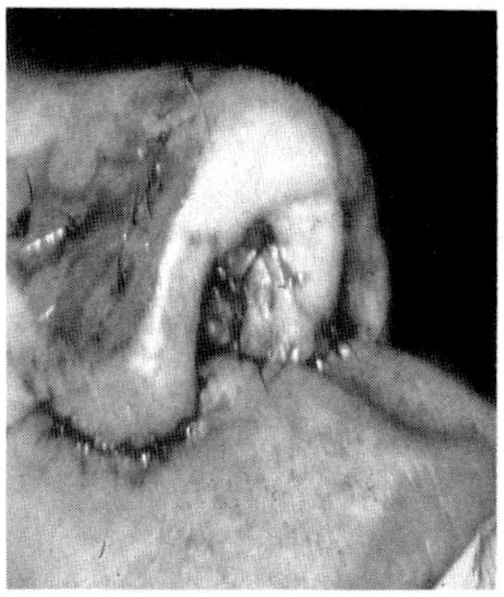

B

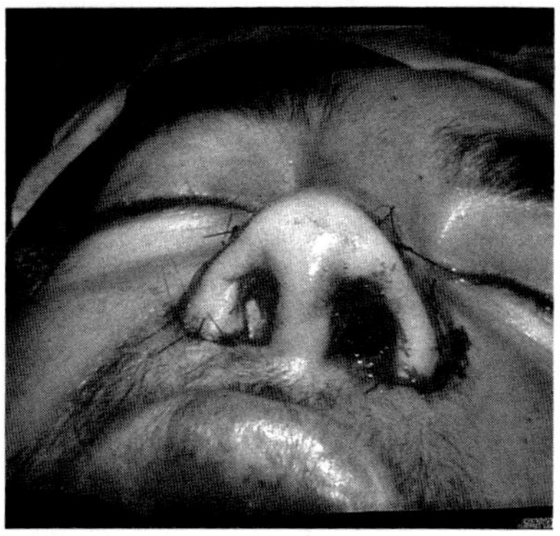

C

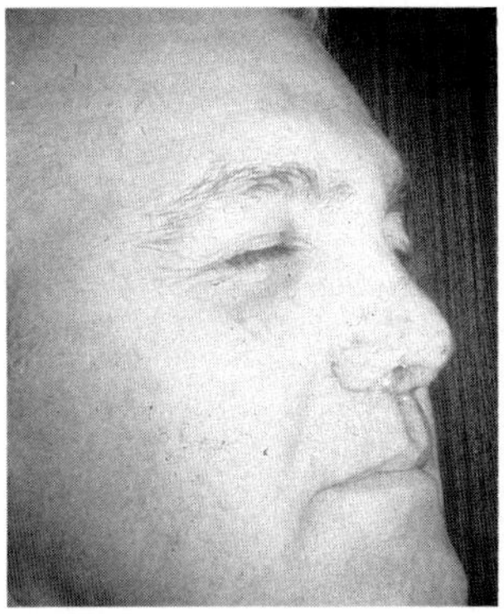

D

Fig. 235. Anterior web stenosis in a middle-aged man corrected with the infolding method. (A) Preoperative outline of the columellar-alar area to be defatted and infolded and of the basal alar and columellar excisions. (B and C) End of the operation. Infolded external skin of the stenosing web that has become internal vestibular lining. Transalar fixation with mattress sutures visible. (D) Late result.

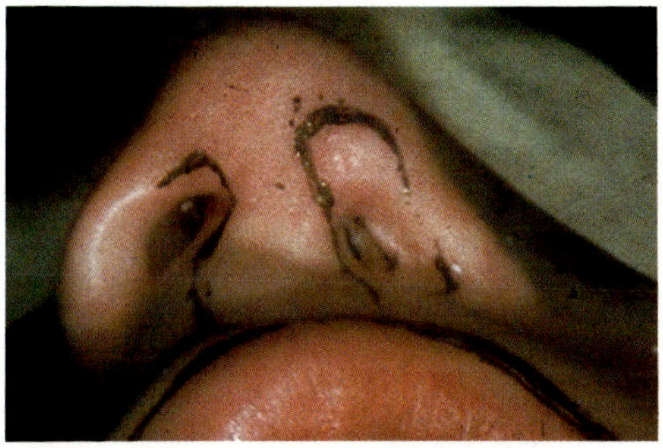

A

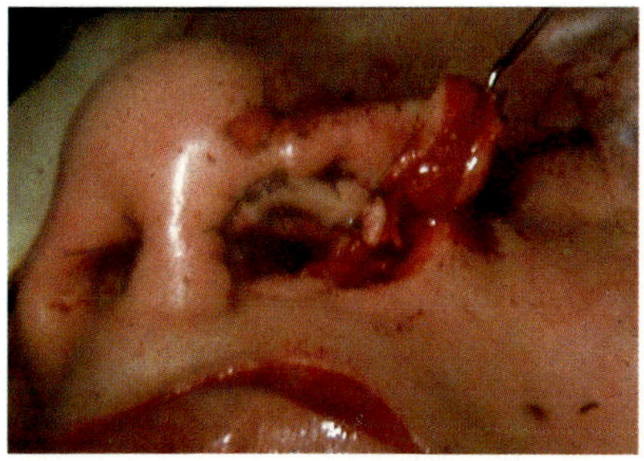

B

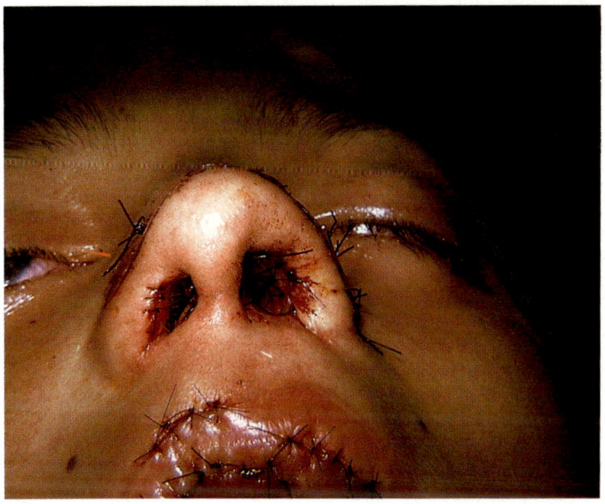

C

Fig. 236. For treatment of a severe stenosis the infolding techinque can be combined with a skin graft or composite graft completing the vestibular lining. (A) Stenosing web to be infolded is outlined. (B) Composite graft sutured to the lateral wall of the vestibule as a complement to the anterior web infolding. (C) In a child the enlargement of the vestibule always has to be an overcorrection taking into account the subsequent retraction. Transalar mattress sutures are holding the infolded skin and the graft in place after a supplementary refinement.

NARROW NASAL CAVITIES

Extremely narrow nasal cavities are quite rare. Usually these are found in hump noses and tension noses combined with tethered lips. The narrowness is found in the bony structures of the nasal cavity, the external bony pyramid, or in the vestibule. The etiology of both deformities is usually congenital. Occasionally we encounter excessively narrow cavities caused by iatrogenic injuries or trauma.

Following septoplasty and turbinate operations, the lumen of the nasal cavity can then be reduced by maximal synechia formation. The best operative procedure in such cases of extensive synechia is to remove the adherent fibrous tissue from the septum and from the turbinates. The septal mucosa should be preserved as much as possible, at least on one side. If a concomitant septal deviation is present we dissect the mucoperichondrium and mucoperiosteum on both sides, usually before removal of the synechial tissue. The resection of adherent scars essentially deprives the lateral wall of the cavity of mucosa. Thus, the denuded area will be principally situated over the surface of the turbinates and agger nasi, which is best grafted with buccal mucosa.

If the synechia extends to the choana pulling the turbinates medially, producing a complete stenosis leaving only a minimal airway passage below the inferior turbinate, we repair the surface of the denuded lateral wall and in addition, we increase the size of the cavity by lateral displacement of the nasal-antral wall. This can be accomplished by circular osteotomy of the nasal cavity and lateral displacement of the wall, as illustrated in Figure 237, or through the maxillary sinus with the Caldwell luc approach. Stents

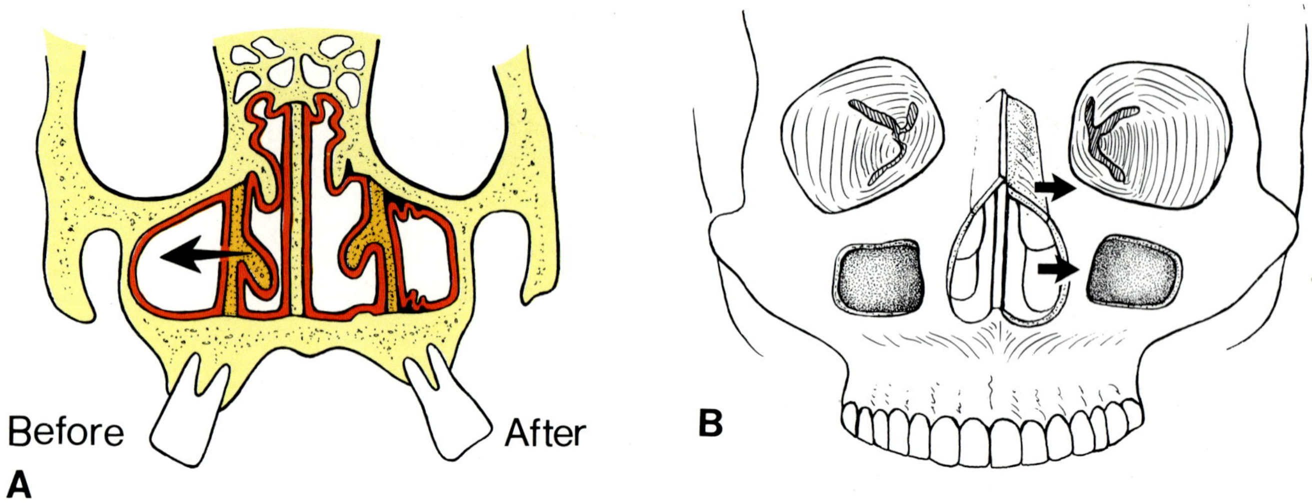

Fig. 237. In cases of too narrow nasal cavity we widen it, displacing laterally the antronasal wall through the maxillary sinus dissecting the mucoperiosteum all around the wall and mobilizing the bone with a fine chisel (A). (B) The reverse techinque is used for treatment of ozena (see Fig. 240).

must be placed for at least 2 weeks. A very effective airway splint that we use sometimes is the custom-made Doyle silicone splint, which consists of two wings with an air passage on each side.

For widening the nasal cavity we still use the procedure described by us in 1964/1967 by Denecke and Meyer, combining a submucosal lateral displacement of the internal antronasal wall, with the lateralization of the nasal bones. We proceed through the maxillary sinus with subcutaneous and submucosal mobilization of the antronasal wall and perform lateral osteotomy through the gingivobuccal incision. Through the same access port we can perform the lateral displacement of the walls of the external bony pyramid after the paramedian and transverse osteotomies through the intercartilaginous incision. This is the reverse of the surgical treatment of the excessively large cavity of the ozena nose. From the oral vestibule we fashion a large opening into the maxillary sinus and mobilize its medial wall circumferentially with a chisel or a burr. The thin mucosa of the sinus may be removed from the medial wall but the nasal mucosa should be preserved as much as possible. The bony wall, including the turbinates, is dislocated laterally.

Also, through the sublabial approach, the piriform crest may be removed if necessary using a chisel from the nasomaxillary suture line to the floor of the nose. The lower section and the bony wall is displaced laterally into the sinus by finger pressure exerted through the nostril or with an elevator. The result is a considerable enlargement of the piriform aperture in the lower part of the nose and the nasal cavity itself.

The external nasal walls are also laterally displaced after completing the usual osteotomies. The bony plates can now be lifted over the lateral edge of the lateral osteotomy with an elevator or with the Walsham forceps and placed in the subperiosteal pocket at the side of the lateral osteotomy.

The lateral edge of the lateral osteotomy can also be trimmed away with a forceps, saw, drill, or chisel, taking care not to injure the periosteum, permitting the medial edge of lateral osteotomy to be repositioned more laterally. This double lateral displacement of internal and external nasal walls provides a maximal widening of the nasal cavities. The walls have to be kept in their new position with copious packing of the cavities, or by utilizing luminal splints that have to be maintained in place for 1–2 weeks and to be changed if necessary (Figs. 237–239).

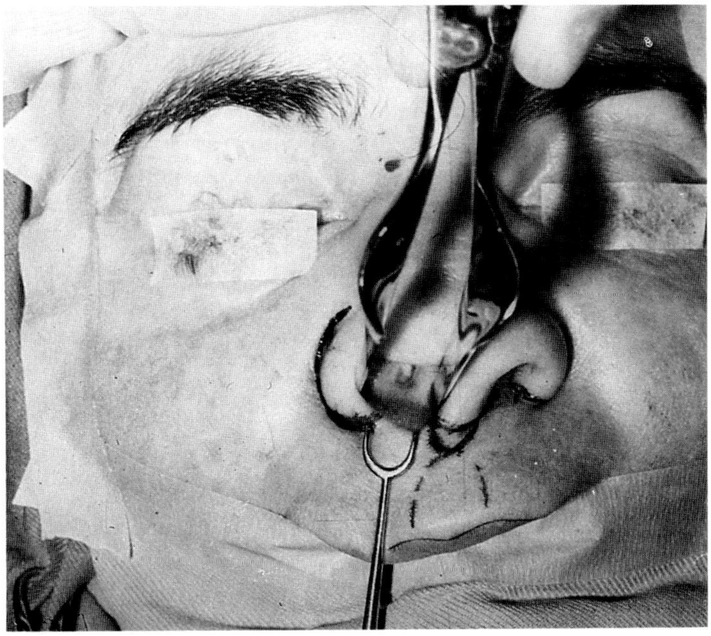

A

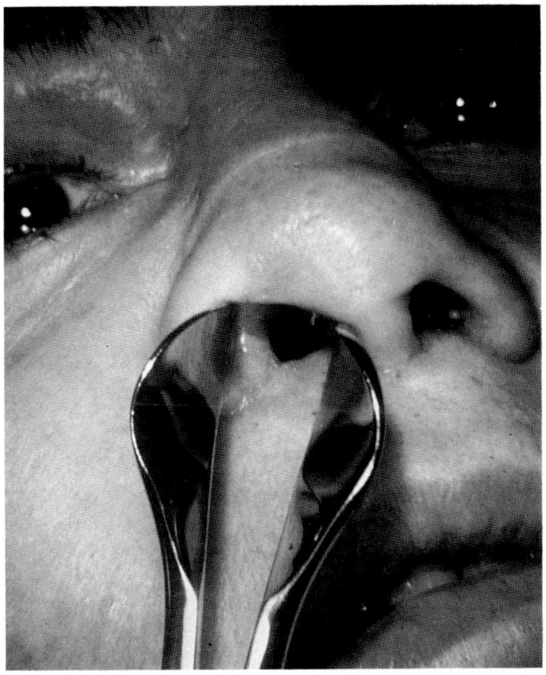

B

Fig. 238. Iatrogenic stenosis of the left vestibule and nasal cavity in a middle-aged woman treated with the method shown in Fig. 237, displacing laterally the antronasal wall. (A) Stenosis visible. (B) Vestibule and cavity widened—1 year after surgery.

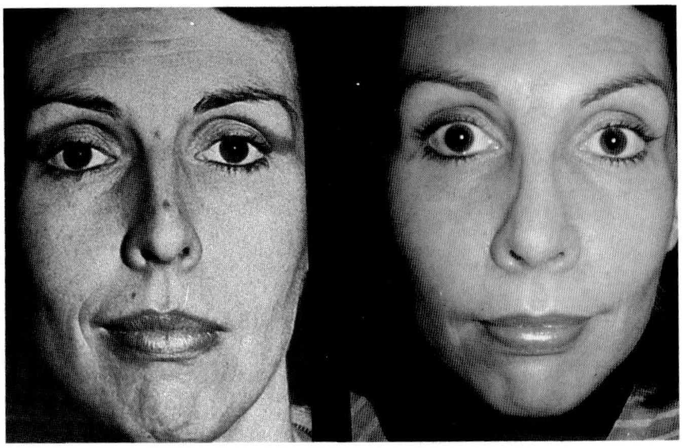

A

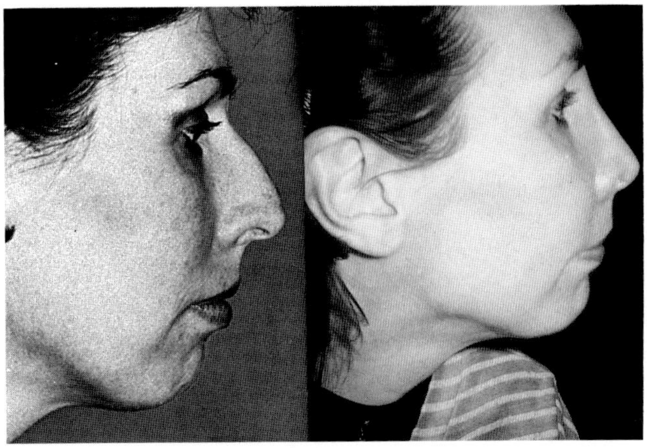

B

Fig. 239. Middle-aged female with narrow nasal pyramid and narrow cavity corrected with usual osteotomies and lateral displacement of the nasal bones and with lateral displacement of the antronasal wall of the cavity. (A) Preoperative and postoperative front view. (B) Preoperative and postoperative profile.

CORRECTION OF THE OZENA NOSE

The pathognomonic nasal shape of the ozena nose was described by the terms "Zaufal's nose" in Germany and "Tarnaud's platyrrhinia" in France. Platyrrhinia combined with cacosmia differentiates the ozena from simple chronic atrophic rhinitis. The pathogenesis of ozena is still unknown today. Thus, lacking in etiology, the surgeon can only obtain a result that provides only a partial chemical improvement while attempting to control the local symptoms. Most of today's methods of surgical treatment are directed toward the reduction of the width of the nasal cavities and hold the only possibility of influencing the symptomatology of ozena. The best known methods are relatively obsolete. Those are the procedures of Lautenschläeger (1934, 1952), Hinsberg (1921), Seiffert (1922, 1955), Halle (1924), Eckert-Moebius (1923, 1965), Ramadier and Eyries (1948), and Rethi (1960). Jeschek's technique (1969) is still applied by Ey (1984), as mentioned above.

In 1961 we advocated the combination of an external narrowing rhinoplasty with reduction of the nasal cavity size. The external rhinoplasty completes the narrowing of the nasal cavities and makes it more effective. We proceed in a manner opposite to that used in widening the nasal cavities as described above.

Through an incision in the oral vestibule the anterior wall of the maxillary sinus is exposed. The periosteum is pushed medially as far as the piriform aperture. The mucoperichondrium of the inferior nasal meatus is dissected with an elevator from the exposed piriform crest superiorly, toward the agger nasi and the middle meatus. The maxillary sinus is opened in a Caldwell-Luc fashion. If the sinus mucosa is thin and not inflamed, we leave it in place. If it appears thickened we remove it. The antronasal wall is now cut circumferentially with a chisel or a drill. The partially elevated mucoperiosteum of the nasal cavity is preserved and the mobilized bony wall is pushed medially. In this way one is able to displace the wall to the extent that it possible for it to lie against the septum without tearing the mucosa.

In order to hold the displaced antronasal wall in its new position and to narrow the lumen in the transition zone from the vestibule to the nasal cavity even more we insert a wedged costal cartilage graft, autologous or homologous, next to the piriform crest. It is held in place without any fixation suture. Our homologous grafts are stored at $-4°C$. Packing of the considerably narrowed nasal cavities is not necessary and neither is packing of the maxillary sinus.

The cavity narrowing procedure is followed by the external correction of the nose (of the platyrrhinia). We perform the usual osteotomies with medial repositioning of the nasal bones and the frontal process of the maxilla. The narrowing of the external nasal pyramid begins at the point where the internal narrowing of the cavities stops. If we compare the nose to a house, we can say that not only are the walls pushed inward, but that also the gabled roof adapts itself to the new spatial relationship and participates in the narrowing (Fig. 240–242).

CHOANAL ATRESIA

Congenital choanal atresia is a rare malformation that is more frequently unilateral than bilateral. There is a less frequent membranous form mostly located posteriorly by the edge of the soft palate. The more usual form is completely or partially bony and occurs more anteriorly at the transition of the bony to the soft palate. In babies a unilateral choanal atresia can be suspected when unusual breathing difficulty during feeding or unilateral rhinorrhea is present. The diagnosis is made by nasal endoscopy, conventional x-ray with contrast instilled into the nares, or by CT.

Recurrent cyanosis and dysphagia with asphyxia-like symptoms while feeding indicate the possible existence of bilateral atresia. As an emergency procedure the early establishment of a satisfactory oral airway by inserting an oropharyngeal tube is mandatory. Tracheotomy should be avoided because of the decannulation problems. According to Fearon et al (1968), and Dehaen and Clement (1985), neonates with bilateral choanal atresia and severe breathing difficulties should have an opening in both choanae made as soon as possible under general anesthesia. With visual control via the nose, the surgeon makes a small hole in the center of the bony choanal plate. The small opening is enlarged with a diamond burr. The other side is opened in the same way and an aspiration tube is inserted bilaterally and attached to one another in front of the nares.

Most authors prefer the transnasal approach in neonates and infants below 2 years of age in spite of some disadvantages of this method, such

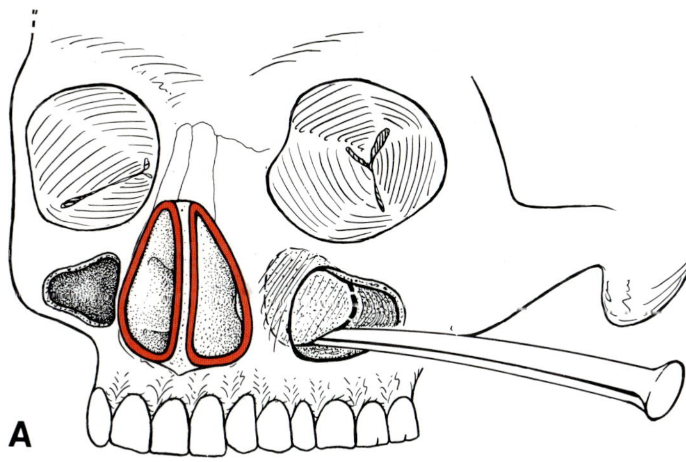

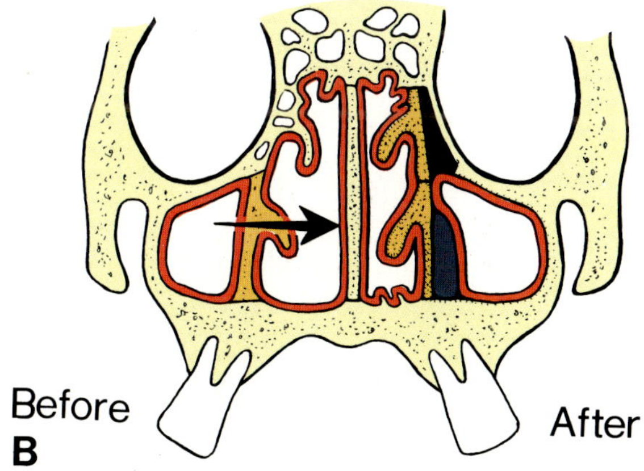

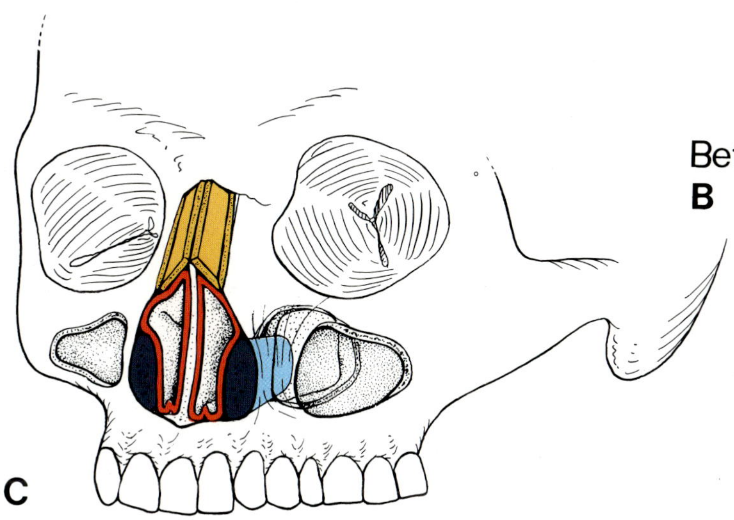

Fig. 240. The reverse technique of that shown in Fig. 237. A is used for treatment of the ozena as narrowing procedure moving medially the antronasal wall. (A) Mobilization of the medial wall of the maxillary sinus. (B) Displacement of the wall. (C) Bilateral fixation with rib cartilage wedge.

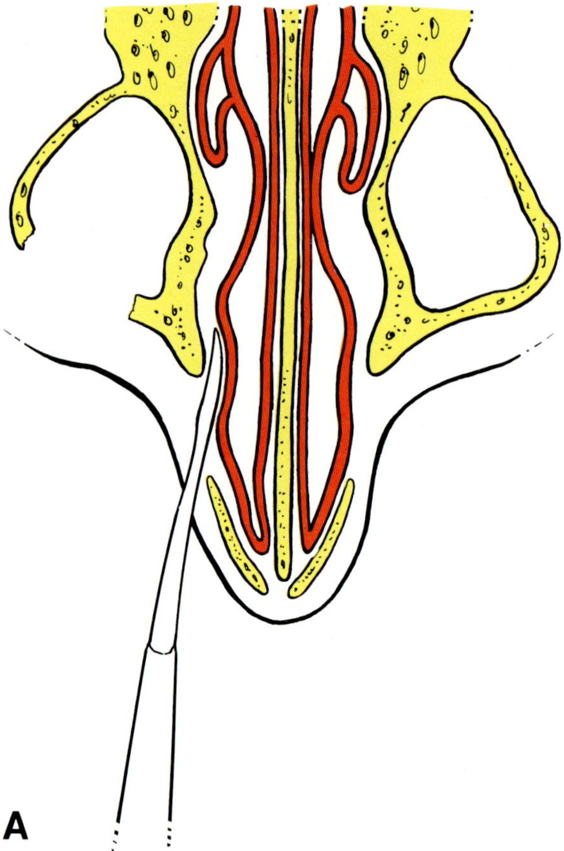

A

Fig. 241. Narrowing of the nasal cavities for treatment of ozena. The antral-nasal wall is medially displaced after mucoperiosteal dissection and mobilization of the base by circumferential osteotomy through the maxillary sinus. (A) Bilateral mucoperichondral dissection from a lateral vestibular incision (axial view). (B) Displacement of the wall and wedging with a costal cartilage graft (axial view). (C) Displacement and wedging in front view.

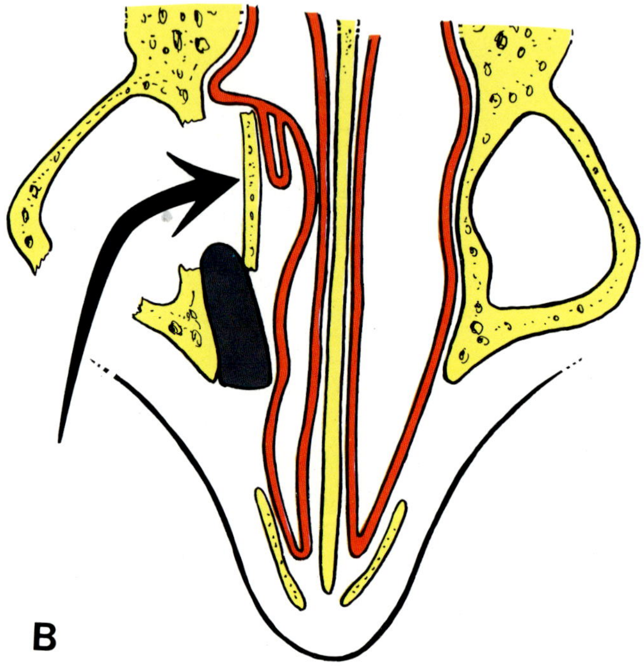

B

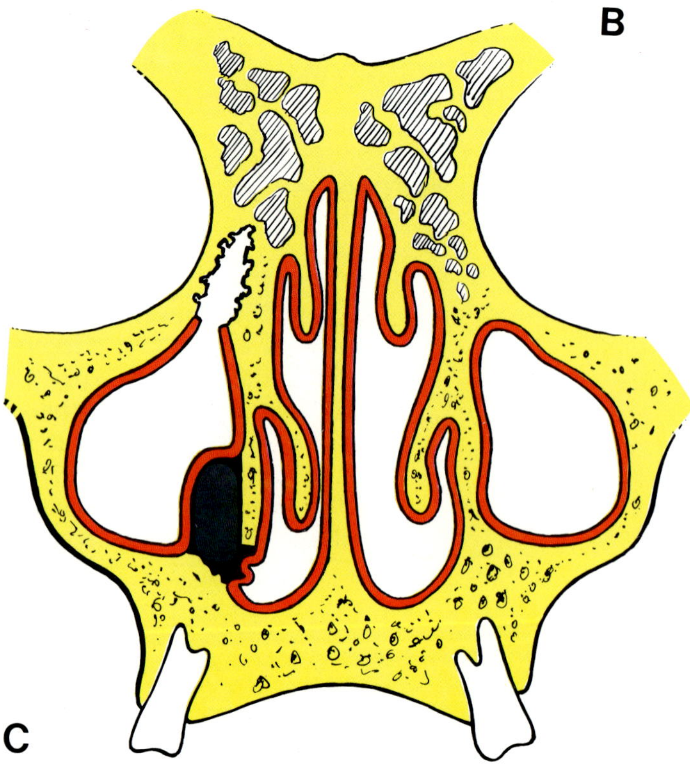

C

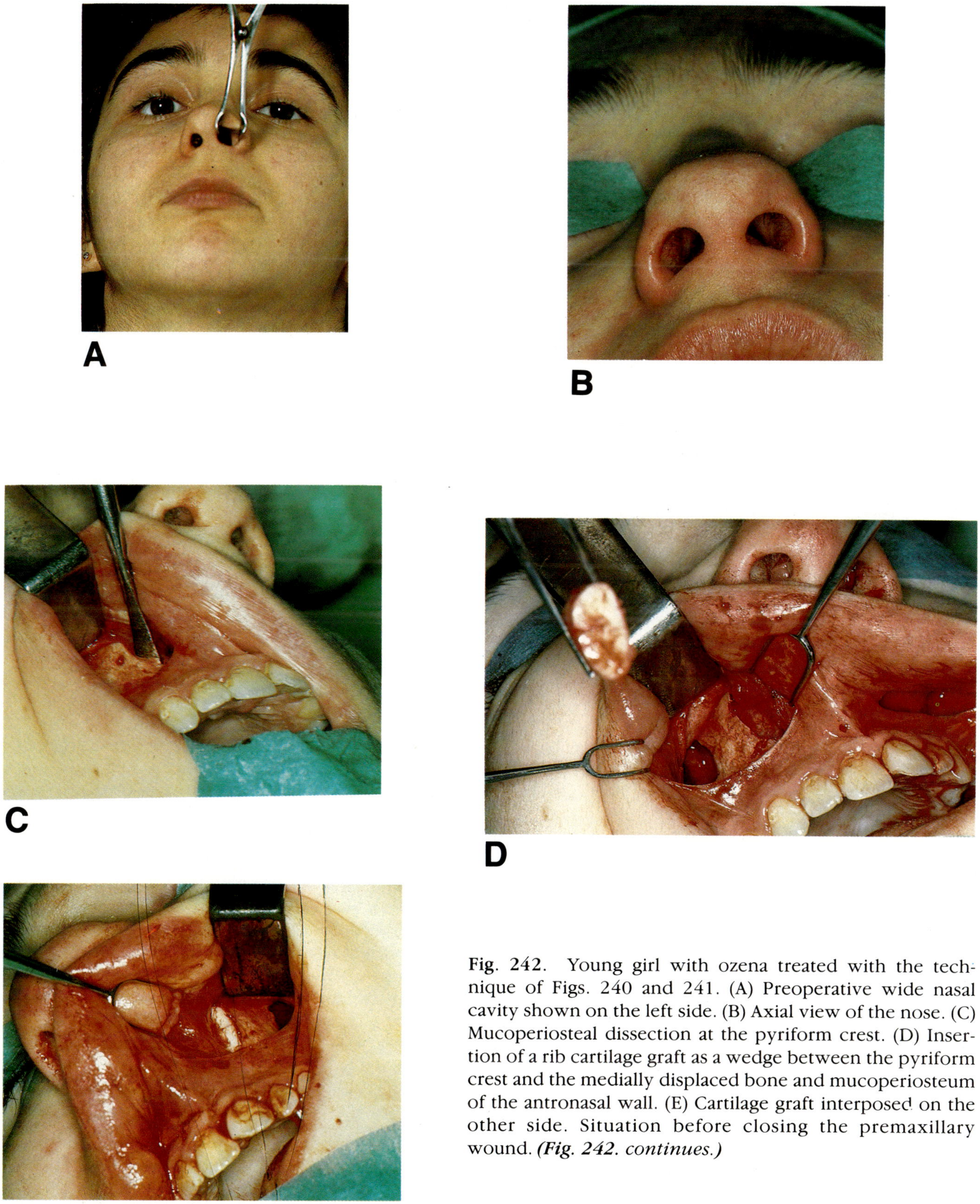

A

B

C

D

E

Fig. 242. Young girl with ozena treated with the technique of Figs. 240 and 241. (A) Preoperative wide nasal cavity shown on the left side. (B) Axial view of the nose. (C) Mucoperiosteal dissection at the pyriform crest. (D) Insertion of a rib cartilage graft as a wedge between the pyriform crest and the medially displaced bone and mucoperiosteum of the antronasal wall. (E) Cartilage graft interposed on the other side. Situation before closing the premaxillary wound. ***(Fig. 242. continues.)***

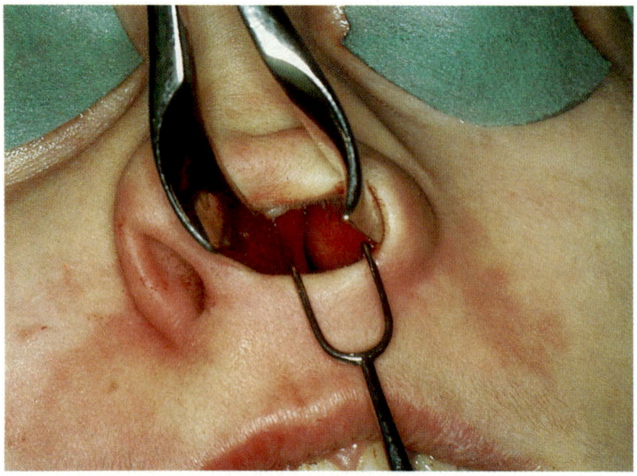

F

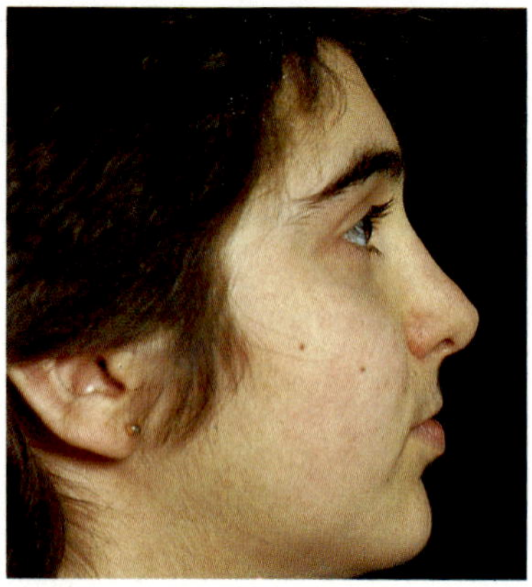

G

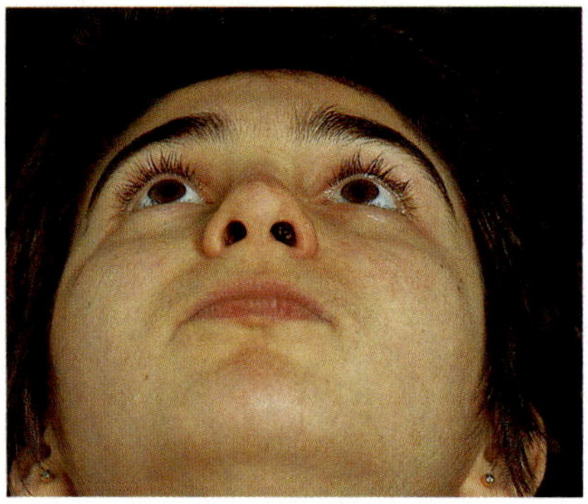

H

Fig. 242. *(continued).* (F) Resulting narrowed nasal cavity. (G and H) Postoperative view of the patient.

as the risk of producing a false passage and lesions at the site of the posterior nasopharyngeal wall. To prevent these complications, Dehaen and Clement (1985) use a diamond burr instead of a chisel or trocar, and operate under control from the front as well as from the rear.

For treatment of the bony atresia we use the burr and the chisel. Still other authors work with a sharp curette, a CO_2 laser, or a microrongeur. The definitive surgery for unilateral atresia can be performed at the age of 5 months, or at 2 years, or at 16 years, according to different authors (Cinelli, 1966; Beinfield, 1959; Uffenorde, 1909; and others).

Among the four approaches now commonly recognized as most useful, the transpalatine approach is actually the most often used in children more than 2 years old. It was recommended by Brunk (1909), Steinzeug (1933), Schweckendiek (1937), and later also by Sheehan (1949), Blair (1931), Ruddy (1941), Aboulker (1951), Owens (1965), Wilson (1957), and McGowern (1961). We consider this open access the most secure and employ it in infants, children, and adults. Various incisions in the palatal mucosa have been published, such as the median incision of Ruddy (1945), the double basement door incision of Schweckendiek (1937), the M-shaped incision by Steinzeng (1933), the tongue-shaped incision posteriorly based flap of Owens (1965) (Fig. 243 A, B, and C), and the T-shaped incision of Meyer (Fig. 243 D and 244), which is described in the book by Denecke and Meyer (1964/1967). With our procedure the superior portion of the T-incision lies in the soft palate near the border of the bony palate where the atresia is to be found. The two palatal mucoperiosteal flaps are folded laterally, exposing the hard palate that is opened in the area of the atresia. The nasal and pharyngeal mucosa are dissected from off the atresia plate. The completely freed bony atresia wall can now be removed with a chisel, burr, or Craig forceps. In the two dissected mucous membranes we cut an oval window the size of the normal choana and let the mucosal borders approximate each other at the remaining sill of the atresia, pressing them against the surrounding walls. If necessary, we suture them with absorbable material or glue them down with fibrin adhesive. Wilson (1957) cuts three mucosa flaps to cover the new raw surface of the bone.

For bilateral atresia we proceed on both sides in the same way and introduce a round luminal splint or a commercial splint of special shape and with air passage to fit the nasal cavity. Before suturing the T-incision we place 2–6 mattress sutures of 4-0 absorbable thread through the mucosal borders at the atresia site, passing them through the mucoperiosteal flaps and tying them over the palatal mucosa after closing the palate incision (Figs. 243 and 244). The after care is also of utmost importance.

To retain the size of the lumen obtained by this surgical intervention the patient has to use rubber or silicone catheters. In the postoperative period, if a stenosis is observed by endoscopy, the stenosing borders have to be controlled by laser trimming.

Other approaches for the correction of choanal atresia are the transseptal, transantral, and transnasal ones. The transseptal approach was proposed by Uffenorde (1909) and von Eicken (1911), Herrmann (1974), and others. The transantral repair was recommended by Wright and Shambaugh (1967), and the transnasal access by Rethi (1960), Beinfield (1959), Tschopp and Morrow (1966), Masing (1974), Ey (1984), and others. The descriptions of all these techniques can be found in the book by Denecke and Meyer (1965/1967).

Like Flake et al. (1964), Owens (1965), Hall et al. (1982), Bobin et al. (1983), and Theogarai et al. (1983), we also recommend the transpalatine access for children under 12 months of age and even in infants at 1 to 2 months of age, while other authors like Herrmann (1974), Fearon et al (1968), Dahen and Clement (1985), Piquet et al (1984), as well as Prescott (1986), prefer actually the transnasal approach in these cases.

For membranous atresia, which occurs only in 10 percent of all choana atresias according to Healy (year), we proceed in the same way using the transpalatal approach or a transnasal one, also using a CO_2 laser, as advocated by this same author. He stresses that a thin bony plate can only be removed partially by this method because a plate more than 1 mm thick must be resected with a microrongeur. If we proceed by the transpalatal approach we can also split the soft palate back to the level of the atresia, which is usually situated more posteriorly than a bony atretic plate. In this fashion, or through the T-shaped incision (Meyer, 1964), it is possible to apply the double cruciate technique of Straith (1939) for auricular atresia, which is illustrated in Denecke and Meyer's (1965/1967) book. A vertical cross incision is made in the anterior membrane, and an oblique cross incision in the posterior one, forming four flaps on each side. The anterior four flaps are rotated posteriorly and the posterior ones are folded anteriorly. The eight flaps come into an approximately congruent position and are pressed against the wall. If necessary they can be sutured with absorbable thread or glued with fibrin adhesive and held tightly with packing.

Complete cicatricial closure of the posterior part of the nasal cavity and of the choana can occur after septal and turbinate surgery or too aggressive a correction of an ozena nose. Also, it can be the result of lues or other specific infections. The removal of the cicatricial web is performed as described for treating bony atresia. After removal of the fibrous scar tissue new mucous membrane tissue must occasionally be provided for complete epithelialization of the resulting defect. In these cases we use a transseptal approach and apply free mucosal grafts from the cheek, which are sutured and glued with fibrin adhesive.

NASOPHARYNGEAL OR PALATOPHARYNGEAL ATRESIA AND STENOSES

Another very rare affliction of the nasal airway is the cicatricial connection of the soft palate to the posterior wall of the pharynx. Nasopharyngeal atresia and stenoses can still actually be caused by infectious diseases such as diphtheria, rhinoscleroma, smallpox, leprosy, pemphigus, and coryza. The more frequent causes are iatrogenic, post tonsillectomies and adenoidectomies, or after tumor surgery. Very rarely they are present as congenital malformation. We have never encountered such a case.

The symptoms are the same in velopharyngeal atresia and stenoses as they are in unilateral choanal atresia. Speech disturbance (rhinolalia clausa) is minor, consisting of the loss of reso-

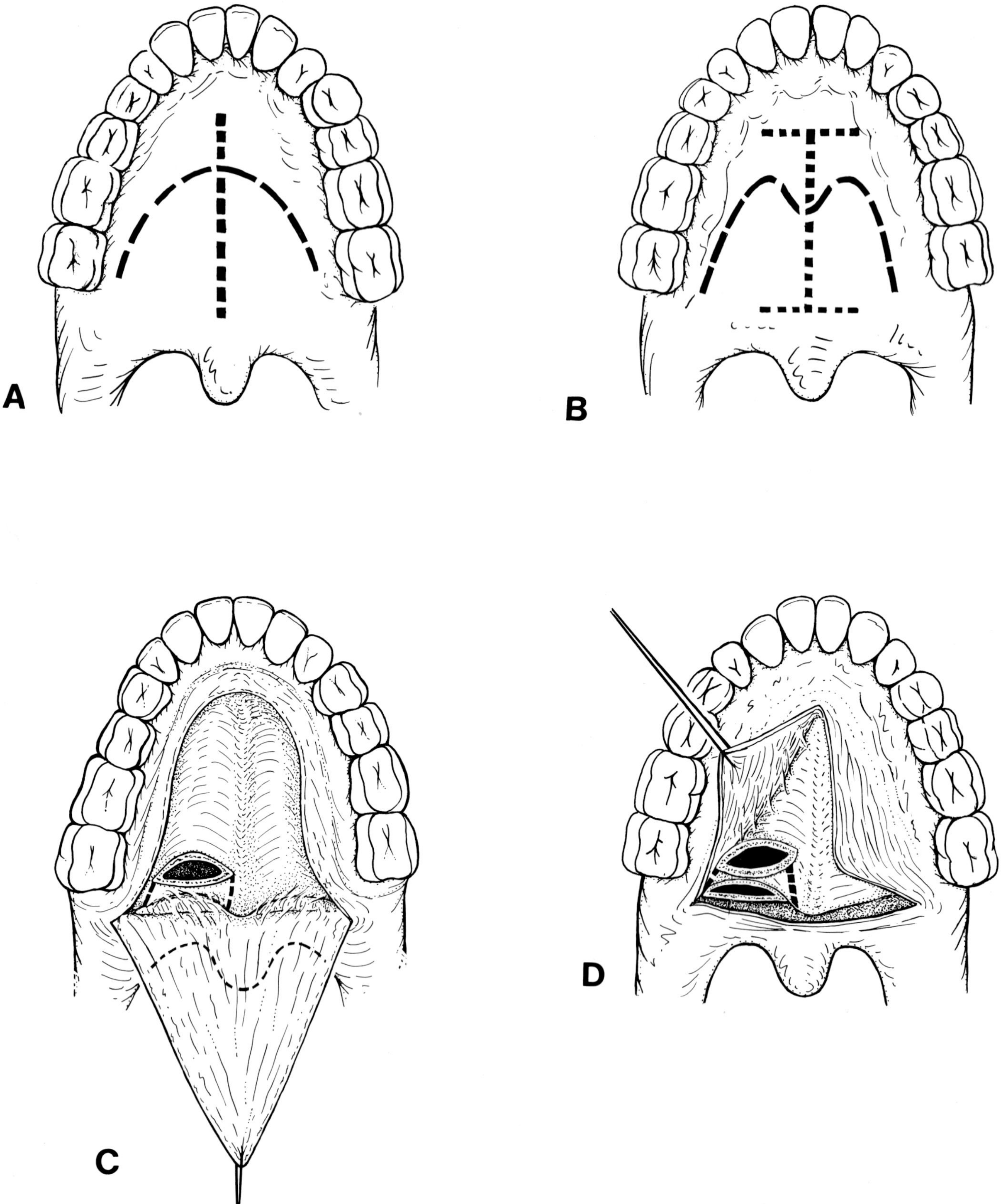

Fig. 243. Transpalatal approach for removal of choanal atresia. (A) Blair's median incision and Ruddy's curved incision. (B) Door like incision of Schweckendieck and Steinzeug's M-shaped incision. (C) Tongue-shaped incision (Owens) and flap folded back. (D) T-shaped incision (Meyer). The mucoperiosteal flap of the palate is folded back after T-shaped incision (Meyer). The soft palate is pushed backward and the nasal cavity is opened in front of the atresia while the nasal mucosa is preserved.

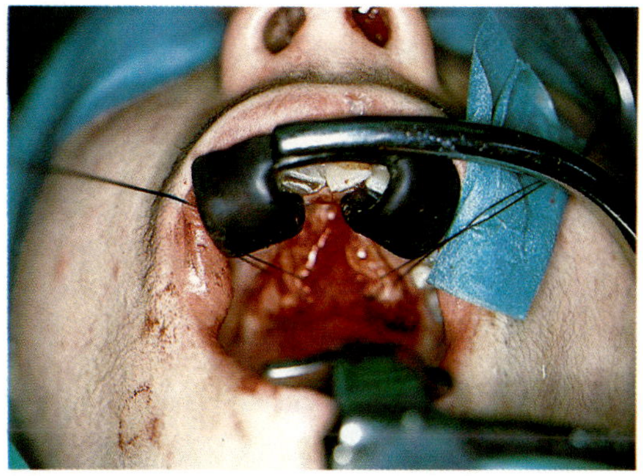

B

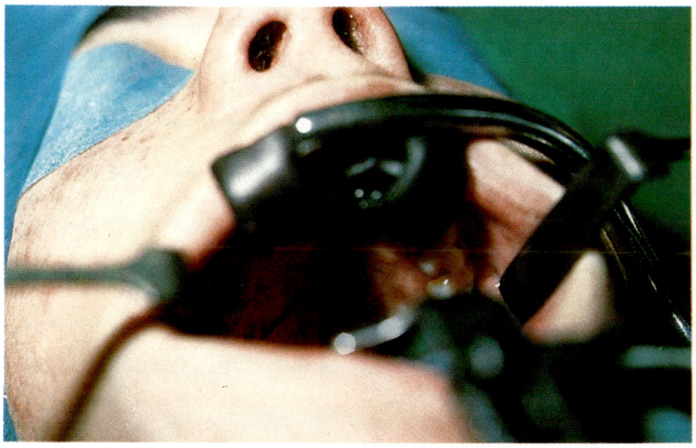

A

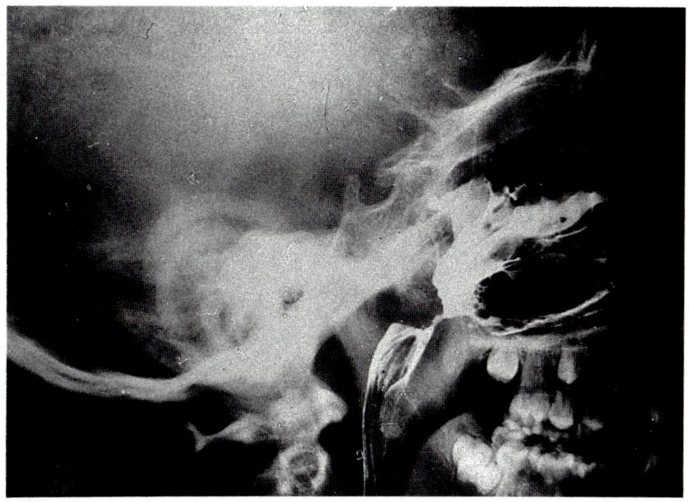

D

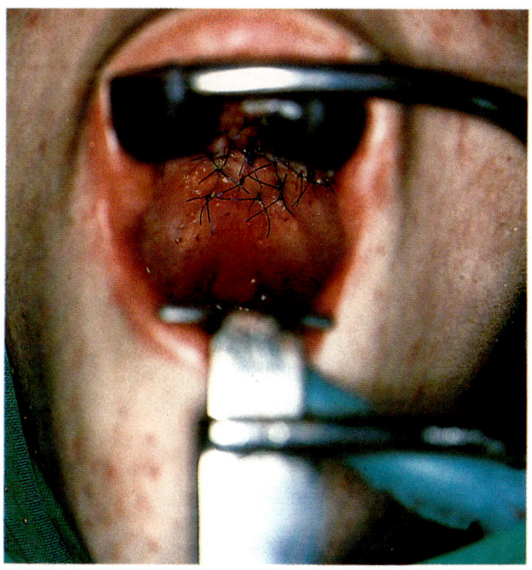

C

Fig. 244. Transpalatal approach for removal of choanal atresia in a young boy. (A) T-shaped incision (Meyer) outlined. (B) Open access to the bony palate. (C) View of the palatal suture. (D and E) X-ray with contrast before and after the operation.

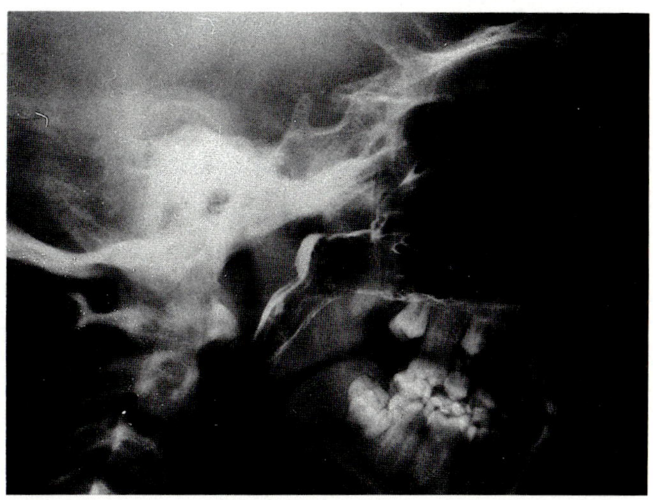

E

nance. Various methods have been described for sectioning the cicatricial wall—removal of the fibrous scar tissue separating the wound surfaces and obtaining epithelial cover by grafting.

Rethi (1948) recommended splitting of the entire soft palate while protecting the uvula and suturing the borders of the resulting defect. In the old literature we find descriptions of obturators and dilators that are now obsolete.

Immediate coverage of the resulting wound after resection of the obstructing wall with skin grafts is advocated by Liebermann (1932), McLaughlin (1950), and Denny and Wilson (1957). Free skin grafts are better tolerated in the pharynx and in the oral cavity than in the nose.

We use mucosal grafts from the cheek to cover the defects in the nasopharyngeal ring. For covering extensive defects of the pharyngeal wall, we transfer a flap from the cheek mucosa through a tunnel at the buccinator crest and the retromolar trigone. The tunneled segment of the flap must be deepithelialized (Fig. 245). The buccal flap is horizontally oriented, sparing the parotid duct and its orifice. The base of the elongated diamond shaped flap is located superiorly in the retromolar area. The submucosal deepithelialized base of the pedicle must be kept sufficiently wide to maintain the vascular supply to the island. Behind the submucosal tunnel the flap is rotated into the rhinopharyngeal defect. A similar flap was used by Culf, Chong, and Cramer in 1974 for lengthening the palate in cases of velopharyngeal incompetence. An intraoral mucosal flap can also be transferred as a myocutaneous flap based on the buccinator muscle, as it has been shown by Bozola (1985) for closure of palatal defects. We question whether the width of the pedicle would interfere with normal mandibular movement with the increased tissue mass found at the buccinator crest.

All the types of local mucosal flaps should be sutured circumferentially with nonabsorbable material and glued with fibrin adhesive very meticulously because packing is not indicated in this region. We consider a stent, a sponge rubber plug, or a hard obturator anchored to a palatal plate unnecessary. Absolute immobilization of a graft on the posterior wall of the pharynx and on the velum is difficult since the oro-pharyngo-palatal muscles move with every act of swallowing, which could conceivably also cause displacement of a packing. We proceed without using a nasopharyngeal obturator. We use flaps because they are less affected by the movement of the pharyngeal and palatal muscles than are free grafts. Rethi (1959) described pharyngeal flaps rotated into the posterior surface of the soft palate and held in place with mattress sutures.

Other procedures using local flaps for the elimination of nasopharyngeal atresia have been described by Vaughan (1946) and Kazanjian (1946) and reproduced in the book by Denecke and Meyer (1964/1967). Kazanjian's method is the only one among these with which we have some experience. It consists of placing two local mucosal flaps on each side of the atresia. The velopharyngeal flap is outlined on the oral side of the atresia, inferiorly based, and extends as far as the midline of the soft palate. It has to cover the raw surface of the epipharyngeal wall. The oval wound is resurfaced with a cheek mucosal transposition flap that is outlined below the Stenson's duct. We have performed this procedure bilaterally, but it can also be used unilaterally. In all these procedures it is important to not produce an abnormally large nasopharyngeal opening, which could be complicated by rhinolalia aperta and nasopharyngeal reflux (Fig. 246).

VELOPHARYNGOPLASTY

The most common etiologies of velopharyngeal incompetence are cleft palate (repaired, fibrotic, hypodynamic), submucous cleft palate, palatal paresis or paralysis, congenitally short palate, a large nasopharynx, and acquired palatal defects.

Adequate functioning of the valve is necessary for the development of sufficient oral air pressure necessary for the correct production of various sounds. When velopharyngeal valving is incomplete, the resulting speech is deficient in oral air pressure and is characterized by nasal air escape and hypernasality.

Twenty to thirty percent of children who were born with palatal defects experience velopharyngeal incompetence after primary repair. Furthermore, it may present as a congenital defect such as in individuals with a large nasopharynx.

Velopharyngeal incompetence with nasal escape in the absence of overt cleft palate has been reported in patients with a congenitally large pharynx and short palate (Randall et al, 1960; Birrell, 1966; Owsley et al, 1967; Jackson et al, 1980), in postadenoidectomy cases (Gibb, 1956; Calnan, 1971), and cases of neurologic disorders of the glossopharyngeal nerve.

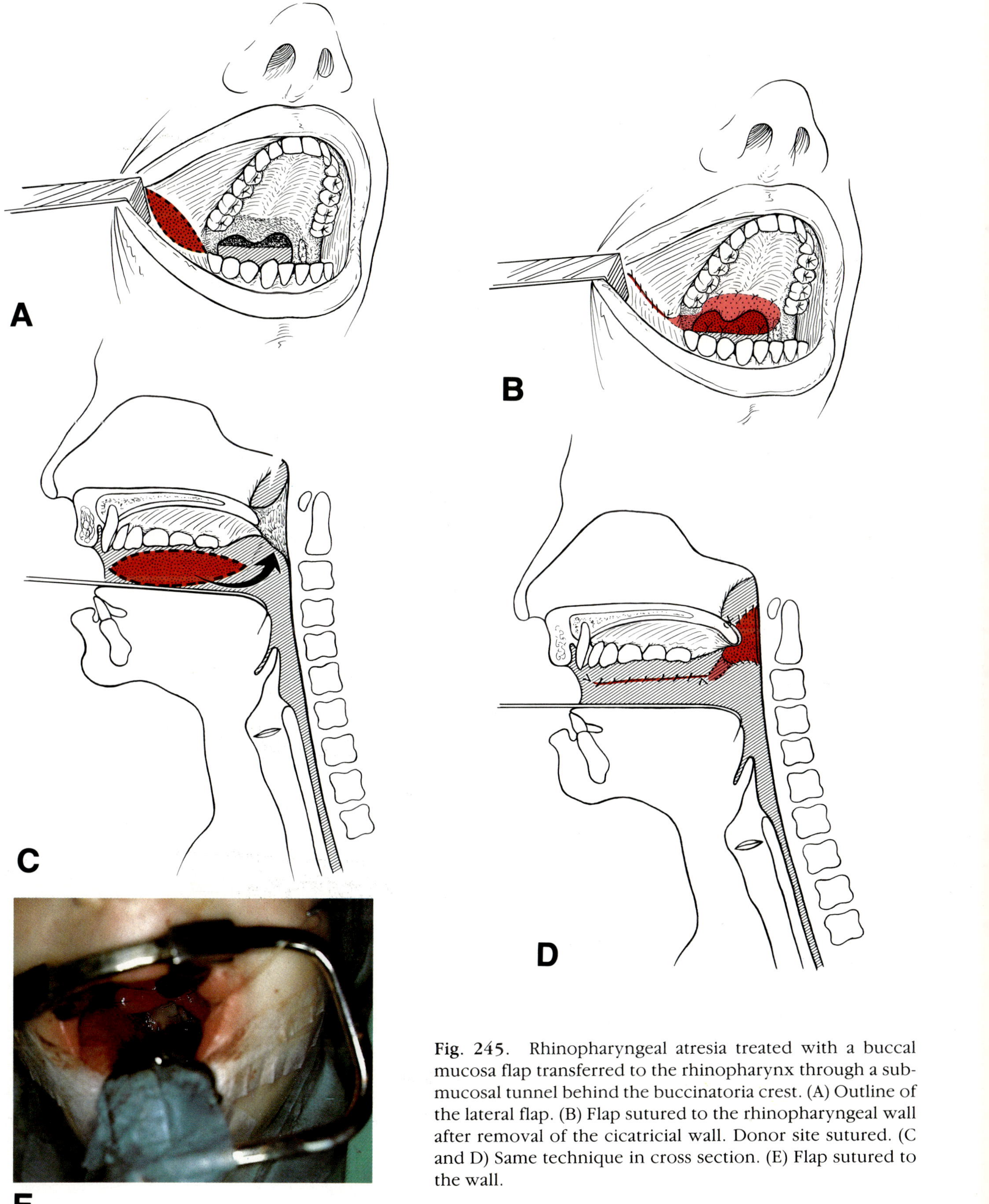

Fig. 245. Rhinopharyngeal atresia treated with a buccal mucosa flap transferred to the rhinopharynx through a submucosal tunnel behind the buccinatoria crest. (A) Outline of the lateral flap. (B) Flap sutured to the rhinopharyngeal wall after removal of the cicatricial wall. Donor site sutured. (C and D) Same technique in cross section. (E) Flap sutured to the wall.

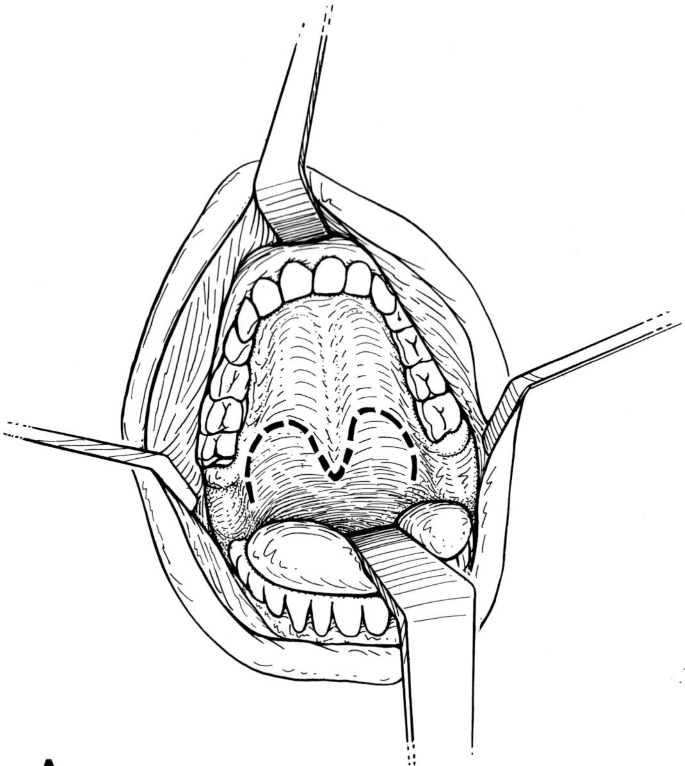

A

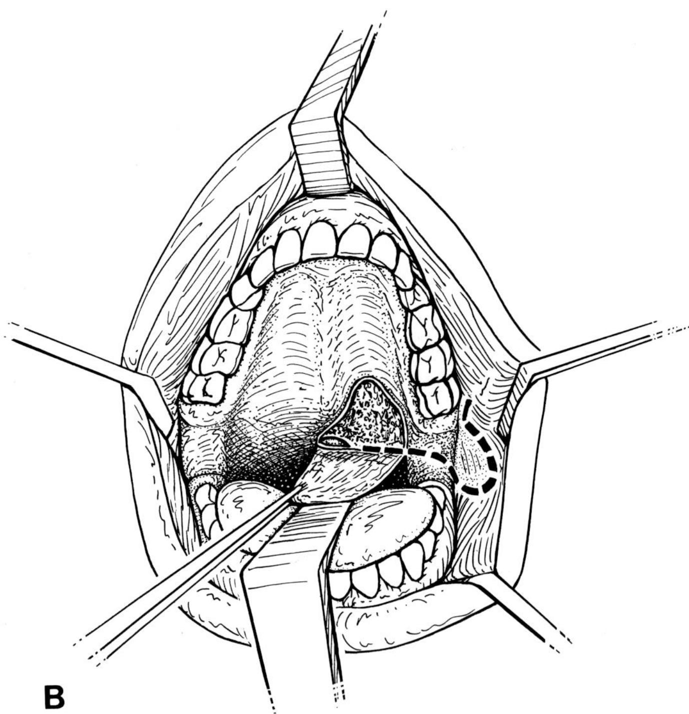

B

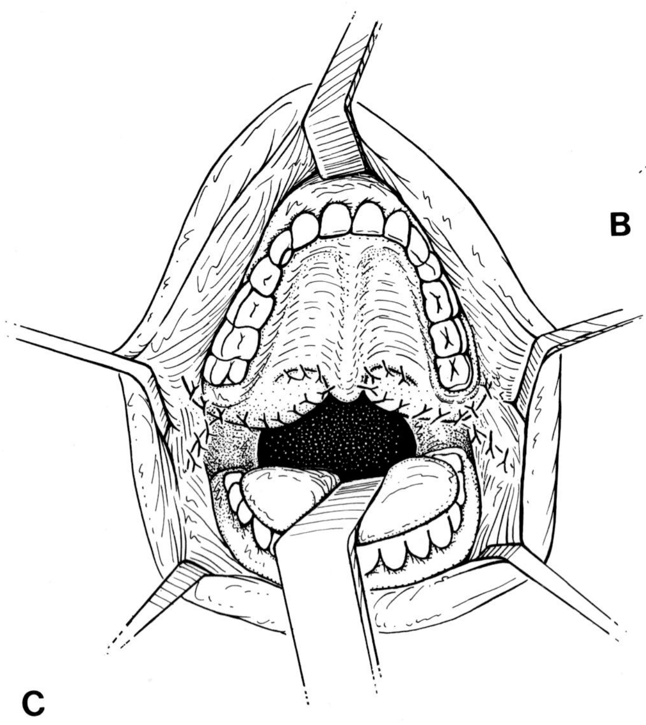

C

Fig. 246. Treatment of nasopharyngeal atresia with Kazanjian method. (A) Incision for formation of an inferiorly based velar mucosa flap. (B) Velar mucosal flap is elevated. Scar tissue is removed. Dotted line indicates the donor site of a mucosa flap from the cheek for covering the raw surface on the anterior wall of the soft palate. (C) End of the operation with bilateral elimination of the atresia. Cheek mucosa has been swung into the donor areas on the anterior surface of the soft palate bilaterally.

The evaluation of the patient with velopharyngeal incompetence includes a history and physical, as well as fiberoptic examination which may prove helpful, audiometry because of the high incidence of associated middle ear disease, cephalometry radiology of the palate, and speech analysis. Future diagnostic tools may include the ultrasonic measurement of oral and nasal airflow, air pressure measurements, and acoustic spectrographic analysis.

Surgical approaches for treatment may be broadly grouped into four basic types, with additional combinations of each that will be considered later: (1) pharyngeal flap procedure, (2) anterior displacement of the posterior nasopharynx (augmentation), (3) medial displacement of the lateral walls of the nasopharynx, and (4) retrodisplacement of the velum. Up to a decade ago the most common treatment for velopharyngeal incompetence was the medium pharyngeal flap, inferiorly based (Schoenborn, 1954; Rosenthal, 1951) or superiorly based (Bardenheuer, 1892; Sanvenero-Rosselli, 1935; Conway, 1955; Owsley et al, 1966).

Another possibility is to reduce the width of the nasopharyngeal aperture in the anteroposterior dimension. Wardill described in 1928 a method that produced a permanent ridge of fibrous tissue on the posterior pharyngeal wall. The elevated velum then contacts the ridge to achieve velopharyngeal closure. The ridge was created by making a transverse incision through the superior constrictor at the level of Passavant's ridge and suturing the tissue vertically. A similar "push forward" of the epipharyngeal wall by inserting autogenous rib cartilage into a submucous pocket, through a transverse incision was advocated by Vinas and Jager in 1971.

Hynes described in 1956 the construction of a permanent ridge on the posterior pharyngeal wall with two flaps elevated bilaterally, containing the salpingopharyngeal muscle, and rotated one against the other. The author did not recommend the use of this procedure in children under 10 years because of the associated technical difficulty.

In 1968 Orticochea advocated a dynamic sphincter velopharyngoplasty in which two lateral pharyngeal flaps and an inferiorly based third flap converge in the middle of the pharyngeal wall. The two lateral flaps are joined end-to-end in the midline, with the medial edges sutured to the median pharyngeal flap and the lateral edges rolled and sutured to one another raw surface to raw surface.

Reichert (1974) and Jackson (1983) also described a pharyngoplasty resulting in a narrowing of the nasopharynx and creating a dynamic muscular sphincter. The base of the pharyngopalatine arch is rotated horizontally into a raw triangular area made by a high transverse incision in the posterior pharyngeal wall. A lower lateral triangle of mucosa is elevated for the closure of the lateral resulting defect.

We developed a similar, but simpler, procedure. The dynamic muscle sphincter is made up of two velopharyngeal Z-plasties. Two musculomucosal walls join in the midline, leaving a heart-shaped rhinopharyngeal lumen. The lateral walls of the new rhinopharynx are formed by converging the posterior velopharyngeal pillars that contain the palatopharyngeus muscle. The posterior pillars of the lateral pharyngeal wall are detached at their lower half and transposed to the medial pharyngeal wall, reaching the midline. They remain joined to the lateral pharyngeal wall. In the lower lateral part of the pharynx, we cut a mucosal triangle by dissecting from off the prevertebral ligament, and transpose it laterally, thus covering the raw surface left after the transposition of the first triangular pillar flap, thereby realizing a velopharyngeal Z-plasty. The mobility of the palatopharyngeus muscle is at least partially maintained. We suture the four flaps. The two converging extremities of the lateral flaps are sutured together in the midline (Fig. 247–249). Occasionally a bifid uvula is connected concurrently with median sutures.

In a discussion on failures, in follow-up to Orticochea (1983), Jackson (1983), in reviewing the late results of his procedure, observes that when an inferior flap is used, the sphincter is often placed too low and cannot contribute enough to the integrated closure of the velopharyngeal area. Jackson stated that by inserting the lateral flaps higher on the posterior pharyngeal wall, the composite function of the sphincter, lateral pharyngeal walls, and soft palate is more satisfactory, and better closure is obtained. We do not share this opinion because in our method of extended double Z-plasties we incise a little lower than Jackson and Reichert and have obtained the same good speech results with postoperative speech therapy. We believe, however, that an important factor to achieve a

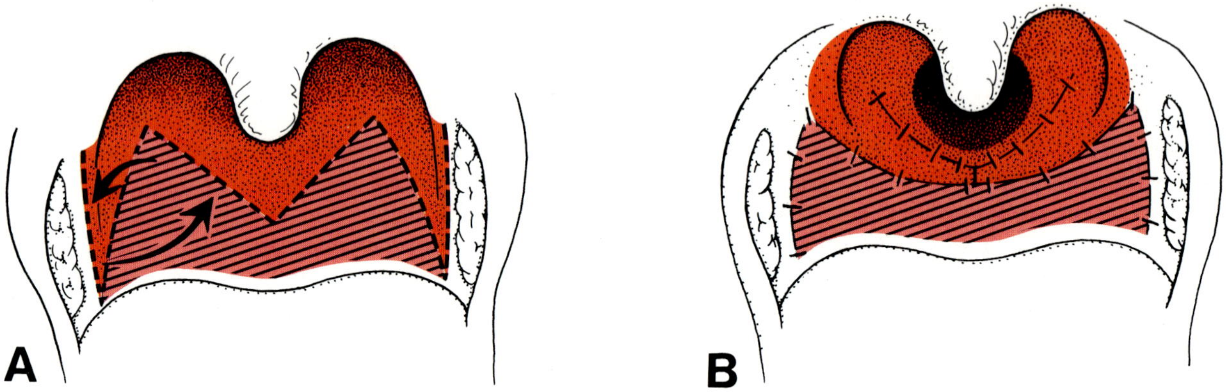

Fig. 247. Velopharyngoplasty of Meyer. Bilateral Z-plasty of posterior tonsillar pillar and posterior pharyngeal wall forming a small heart shaped rhinopharyngeal lumen. (A) Outline of the incisions. (B) Sutures after Z-plasty with transposition of superiorly based posterior tonsillar pillar flap to the midline of the posterior pharyngeal wall.

good functional result is that the flap attachment on the wall should be as broad as possible. In any case, we note that with the median velopharyngeal flap used up to 10 years ago we were not getting the same good results as with the sphincter velopharyngoplasty, which is partially dynamic, the mobility dependent on wound healing. Thus, we join Jackson in hoping that in the future the more common static methods will decline in popularity, and more surgeons will choose to use the more sophisticated philosophy to speech improvement found in the sphincter reconstruction.

In many cases of severe velopharyngeal incompetence due to a shortening of the soft palate, the lateral velopharyngoplasty is not sufficient to compensate for the loss of velar ascension and posterior displacement. In such cases we combine our method with a push back procedure. Such palate elongating techniques are known as the retrodisplacement procedures of Ganzer (1917), Veau (1922), Kilner (1932, 1958), and Wardill (1928) using an M-shaped incision, Dorrance (1925) with the inverted U-incision as well as elongation achieved with transposition flaps such as Millard's small mucoperiosteal flap (1966), and the sandwich flap of Moore and Chong (1967), which are larger island flaps. Other lengthening procedures include Edgerton's (1977) island flap, and Cochran's

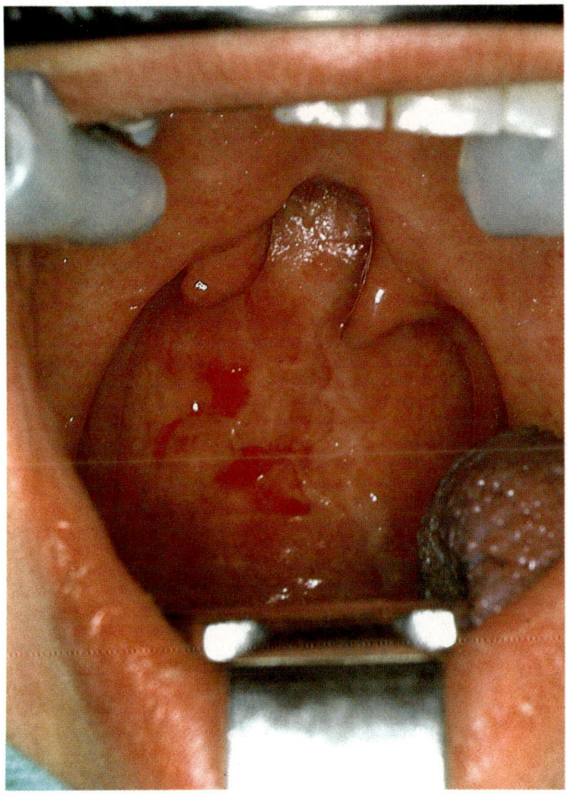

A

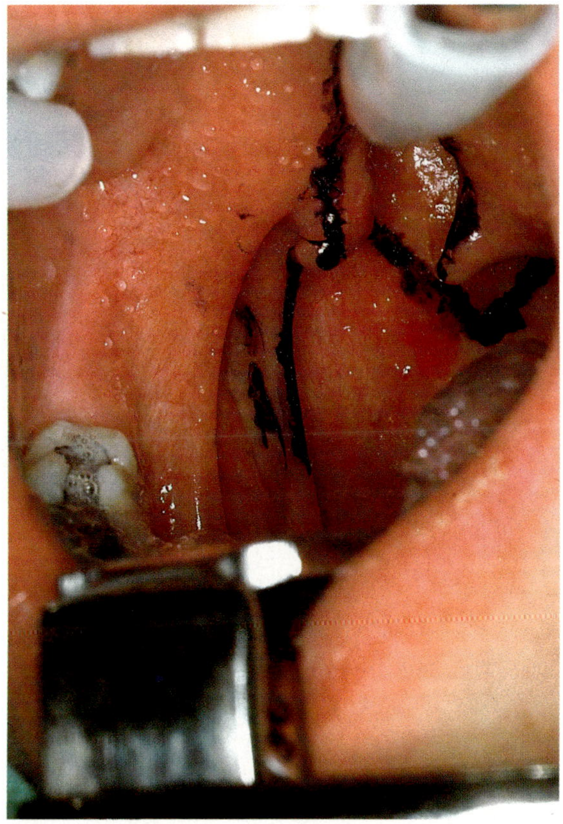

B

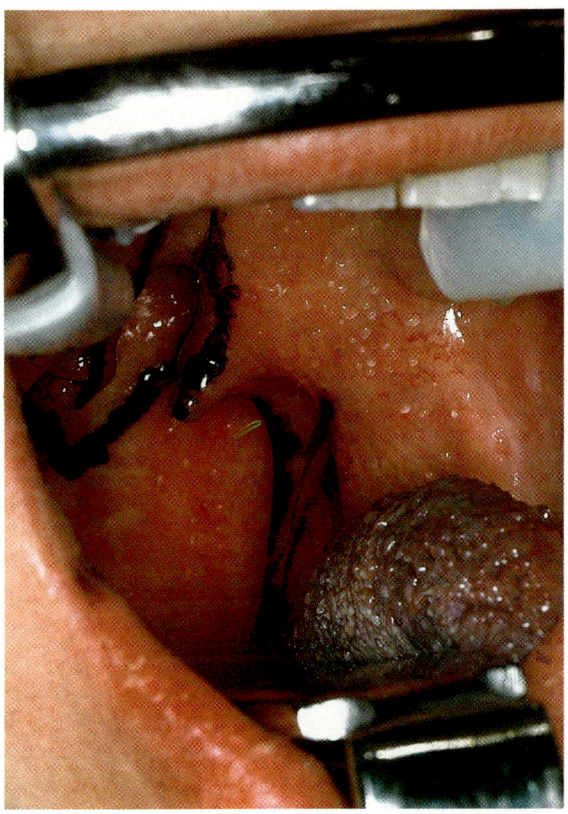

C

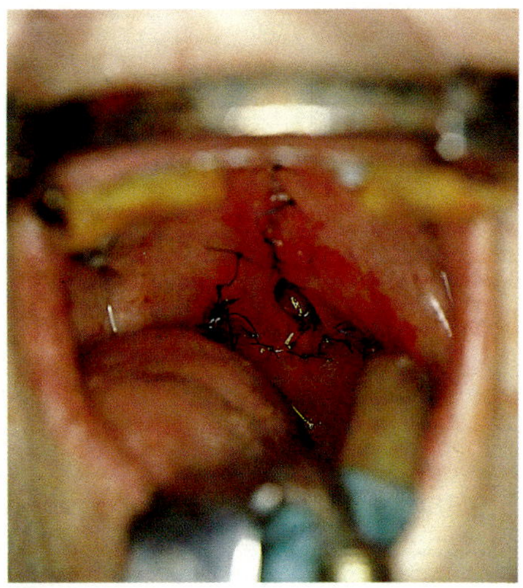

D

Fig. 248. Same velopharyngoplasty. Wide rhinopharyngeal area with cleft of the soft palate and bifid uvula. Correction with method of Fig. 247 and with closure of the soft palate. (A) Preoperative situation. (B and C) Outline of the incisions. (D) Flaps sutured and cleft closed at the end of the operation. The rhinopharyngeal passage is considerably narrowed.

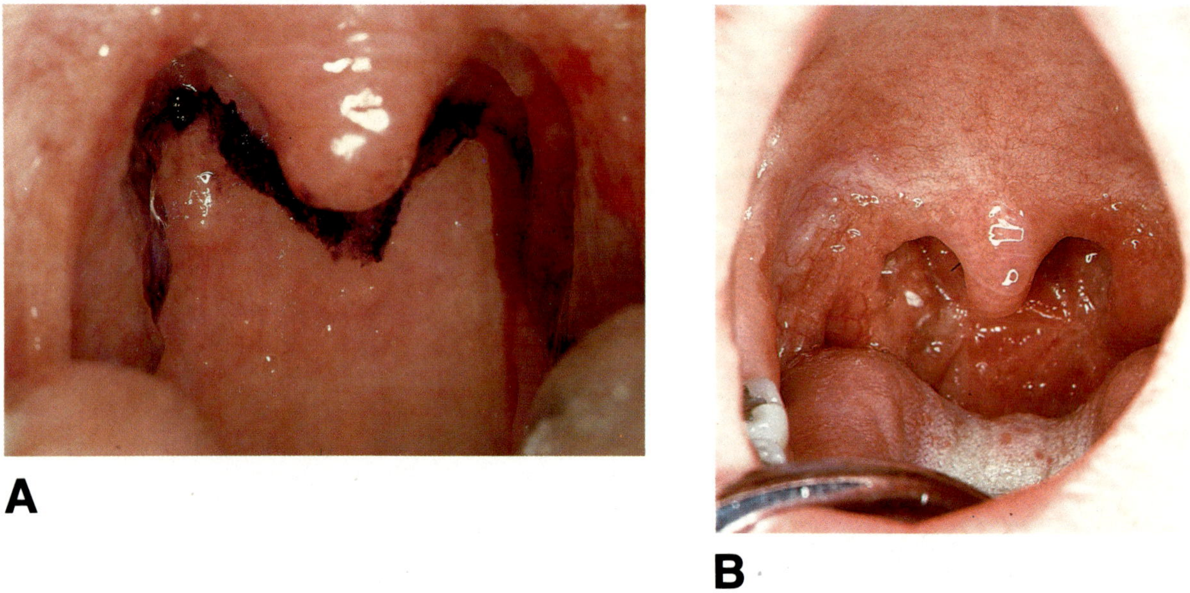

Fig. 249. Velopharyngoplast according to Fig. 247. (A and B) Pre- and postoperative view.

(1983) magnum procedure using longitudinal hemi-palatal mucosa flaps transferred into a transverse position.

SNORING AND SLEEP APNEA

The incidence of snoring in the general population is quoted by several large series as being approximately 45 percent for occasional snoring and 25 percent for the general population for snoring nightly, with loudness being measured up to 80 decibel. According to Moran snoring has been shown to be the primary sign of a potentially serious medical condition, i.e., obstructive sleep apnea (OSA). Traditionally, the otolaryngologist has been the primary medical resource for patients with snoring problems. Until recently, however, little was known about the now acknowledged potentially serious complications of this phenomenon.

Sleep apnea is diagnosed by polysomnography, monitoring evaluations of air flow, diaphragm movements, EEG, and ECG. OSA is defined as oxygen saturation of less than 85 percent during polysomnograph sleep monitoring.

An analysis of the snoring phenomenon shows that the situation is not desperate for all. Three parts of the upper airway may be the origin of the noise. Starting at the lowest point: the base of the tongue, together with the epiglottis, by excessive muscular relaxation, may slip backwards partially blocking the airstream. In the middle area the soft palate may vibrate into the airstream as does a vessel's sail under the wind. Finally, breathing problems such as obstruction causing turbulence may produce unwanted noise. Sometimes noise-producing mechanisms may exist simultaneously.

The two groups of patients that present with snoring are children and adults. In children sleep apnea is usually anatomically-related secondary to hypertrophy of the lymphoid tissues of Waldeyer's ring. Tonsillectomy and or adenoidectomy are usually curative.

Of the primary treatments of this condition, those most commonly utilized to date involve surgical procedures routinely performed by an otolaryngologist, i.e., tracheostomy and uvulopalatopharyngoplasty.

Adults with sleep apnea or snoring can present with a variety of complaints including observed loud snoring punctuated by periods of silence, followed by the classic resusitative snort. Patients may also complain of daytime hypersomnolescence and up to 70 percent in some series complain of nasal stuffiness.

Causative anatomic abnormalities in adults include nasoseptal deformity, turbinate hypertrophy, large tonsils, bulky, boggy thickened uvula with transverse ridges, and a long floppy soft palate that droops below its muscular layers into the pharynx posteriorly and inferiorly, narrowing the anterioposterior dimension of the nasopharyngeal space often to a slit-like opening. The pharynx and hypopharynx are often seen to be flabby with surface mucosal rugae or ridges. The posterior tonsillar pillars lay in a more medial position with an abnormally low insertion into the uvula. The classic body habitus is that of patient with gross obesity, short stocky neck, and receding chin. This is only occasionally seen. Respiratory monitoring during sleep is used to assess the severity of the condition (Hess, 1985).

After successful restoration to physiologic breathing, snoring often disappears. Conservative treatment includes daily exercise for weight loss and restoration of muscle tone, abstinence from alcohol, tranquilizers, sleeping pills, and antihistamines before bedtime; sleeping on one's side and not on the back; and elevation of the head on the bed. In some series this provided improvement of symptoms in 47 percent of cases but cure in only 5 percent of cases. The long-term use of a nocturnal nasal-airway pressure mask as recommended by Hess (1985) can also be effective.

A vibrating soft palate can be stiffened with a very cautiously applied injection of a vein-sclerosing material, as recommended by Langraf-Favre (1983), who injects 01–04 ml of acetoxysclerol 2% into the vibrating uvula 5 times with a delay of 20 days between injections.

Surgery can provide the cure and is the initial treatment of choice for patients whose oxygen saturation drops below 50 percent on polysomnography and who evidence any serious pulmonary or cardiac complications. Approximately 25 percent of patients will require this. Surgical options include nasal surgery and/or uvulopalatopharyngoplasty with pulling of the posterior tonsilar pillar and shortening of the palate.

The possible complication of velopharyngeal incompetence has been found in several large series to be only temporary. The most serious complications relate to the severity of disease in many of these patients and the concomitant anesthetic, airway, and potential catastrophic cardiopulmonary complications.

In 1976, Guilleminault et al described the sleep apnea syndrome and in 1981 Fujita et al published their first good results with reduction operation of the uvula and pharynx, which they called uvulopalatopharyngoplasty (UPPP). One year later, Hernandez recommended a palatopharyngoplasty as the treatment of choice for severe snoring with apnea. This is controversial among many authors advocating UPPP for snoring and tracheostomy for severe sleep apnea. The tonsils have to be removed if they have not already been so and the incisions are further extended along the border of the soft palate. Lozenge-shaped mucosal resections are added in the soft palate at the base of the uvula and at the posterior pharyngeal wall.

18

The Aging Nose

Any surgery of the aging nose, both primary and secondary, should always take into consideration any functional disturbance, because in the course of aging the nose undergoes changes in its shape that are usually associated with increasing disorders in function. Thus, in an aging patient we are sometimes confronted with either a primary or a secondary functional problem that was not manifested at a younger age, even after an uncomplicated primary operation.

As an exclusively rejuvenative procedure, the corrective rhinoplasty is sometimes combined with a rhytidoplasty or with other ancillary procedures in the aging face. In our experience, though, the most frequent indication for septorhinoplasty, primary or secondary, in aging patients is functional. Practically every rhinoplasty in the adult and aging patient is rejuvenative, but rarely do we perform a rhinoplasty solely for the purpose of rejuvenation. Usually, the functional aspect of the operation is more important.

The typical aging nose shows a flaccidity of the skin, a sagging of the tip, elongation of the dorsum, and a reduced nasolabial angle of less than 90 degrees. A big nose usually gives the illusion of advanced age to a patient, especially in a female patient.

The signs of aging are usually more manifest in the nose and face than in other parts of the body, and in many older individuals the correction of a droopy nose can have a more rejuvenative effect than other age-diminishing procedures such as rhytidectomy. The whole correcting procedure is then regarded by many patients as a therapy for their "age disease" (aetas ipse morbus).

Flaccidity of the soft tissues that lead to sagging and wrinkling of the teguments is the etiology of the aging nose. These changes in form and infrastructure of the nose have been particularly studied by Krmpotic-Nemanic et al (1972), Patterson (1977), and by Kaye (1984). The most significant changes occur in the cartilages. The upper lateral and lower lateral cartilages are held together by a firm connective tissue that becomes flaccid. Their attachments loosen and their curved edges flatten and fragment under the force of gravity. Thus, the soft part of the nose becomes ptotic.

In performing a rhinoplasty in the aging patient one has to pay special attention to the skin elevation at the dorsum. When accomplishing the osteotomies and bone mobilization, the approximation of the nasal bones in the midline has to be perfect because with the dorsal skin being so thin the danger of complications such as an open roof, or of visible osteotomy borders, is greater. If this happens, the secondary correction should include new osteotomies and, eventually, an interposition of dermis or fascia between the bony pyramid and the skin.

In older patients, the nasal tip skin adapts less readily to the underlying septal and nasal cartilages, so many surgeons position these structures lower than anticipated to compensate for this lack of elasticity.

The dissection of the skin over the nasal pyramid in the aging nose has its limits. With the removal of a large hump in an older patient with thick skin, the covering cutaneous layer does not possess the ability to sufficiently adapt to the newly reduced underlying bony and cartilaginous structures, and thus leaves folds and furrows.

Unlike younger patients, the older person frequently has more difficulties adjusting to a new nose and often is impatient with the prolonged period required for edema and connective tissue hyperplasia to subside.

When insufficient nasal shortening is performed in an older patient, the resultant effect may be that of a dropping tip because of the inelasticity of the aged skin. Such a dropping tip can be corrected with the helmet visor upward rotation technique, as described by Fomon (1953).

When lifting the tip one has to avoid a plicating of the skin and causing a bulging of the soft tissue in the supra-tip area. This requires undermining the entire skin envelope of the glabella dorsally and the side walls of the nose over to the frontal process of the maxilla.

Fritz (1981) advocated a lifting procedure of the nasal skin with a transverse skin resection at the glabella (Fig. 250) The skin excision in the form of a transverse ellipse is tailored to accommodate the looseness of the skin, the extent of which is dependent on the extent to which the tip of the nose has dropped. On average, the

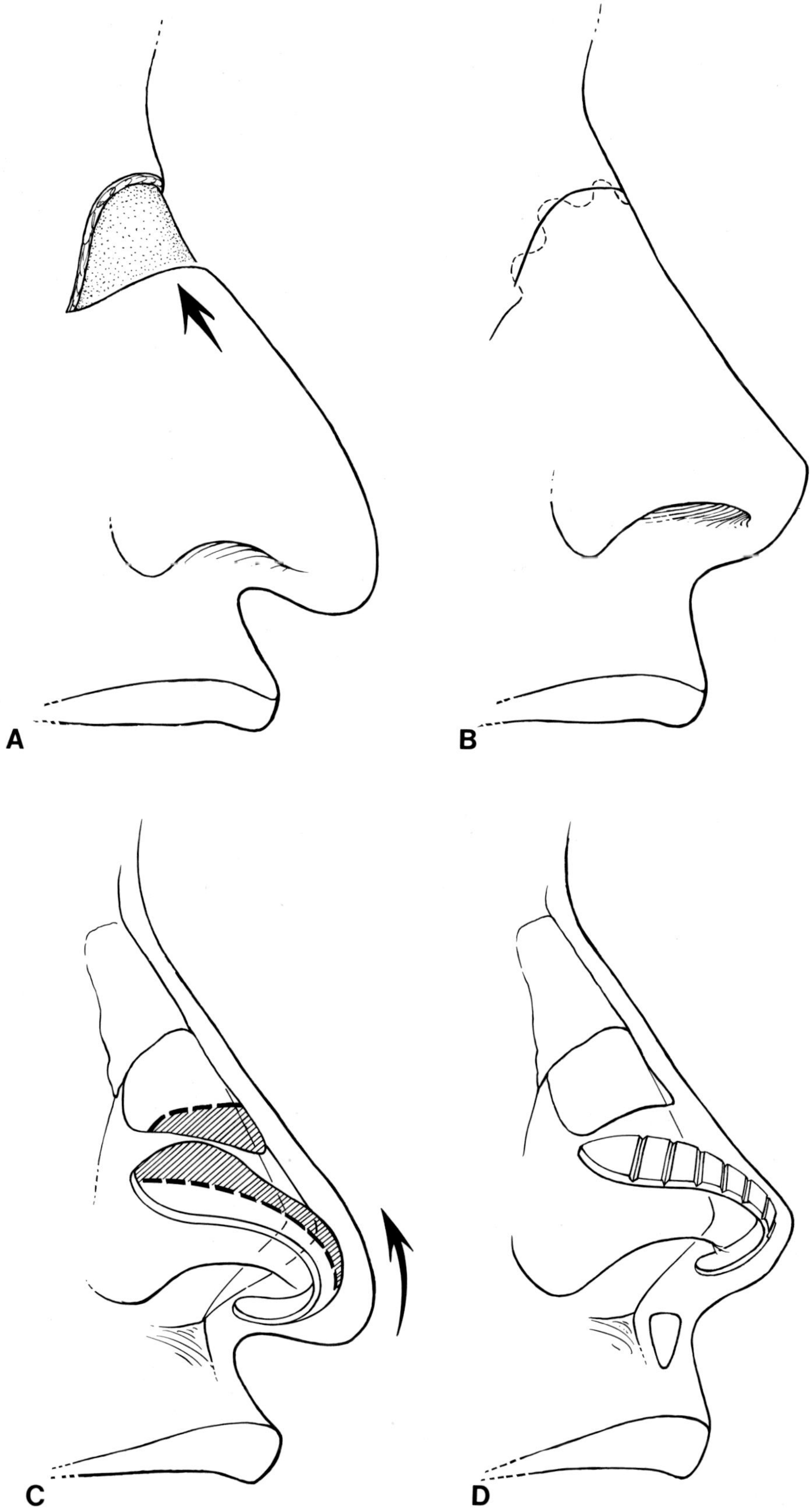

Fig. 250. Exceptional external excision used in the aging nose. Correction of the sagging tip by fusiform skin resection in the superior part according to Fritz (A and B). This excision can be combined with corresponding inner resections of mucosa, reduction of upper and lower lateral cartilages, and nasolabial onlay (C and D).

craniocaudal diameter reaches 15 mm, with the lateral extent of the wound approximating the medial canthus bilaterally. Through this incision the nasal skin is mobilized down to the middle of the upper lateral cartilages and the prominent nasal bridge can be rasped. After upward dissection into the forehead, the corrugator muscles can be totally or partially resected, and the glabellar and frontal skin tightened. The wound is closed in two layers. With more extensive resections, the unequal lengths of the wound edges can be compensated for by small Burow's triangle excisions at both extremities of the ellipse. The scar located in a transverse fold at the root of the nose becomes imperceptible after 6 months. We have used this procedure, proposed by Fritz (1981), in only a few cases of excessively folded dorsal skin in elderly patients with dropping tip.

Bosse (1986) proposes a similar dorsal lifting by superior excision, which he demonstrates on his own nose. Peterson (1976) published the technique of an "open-flap rhinoplasty," with excision of a cutaneous strip of redundant skin at the intercanthal level after having lifted the flaccid dorsal skin through an upside-down U-shaped incision at the nasion (Fig. 251), extending downward in the nasofacial grooves. Kabaker reported on a similar procedure in 1979.

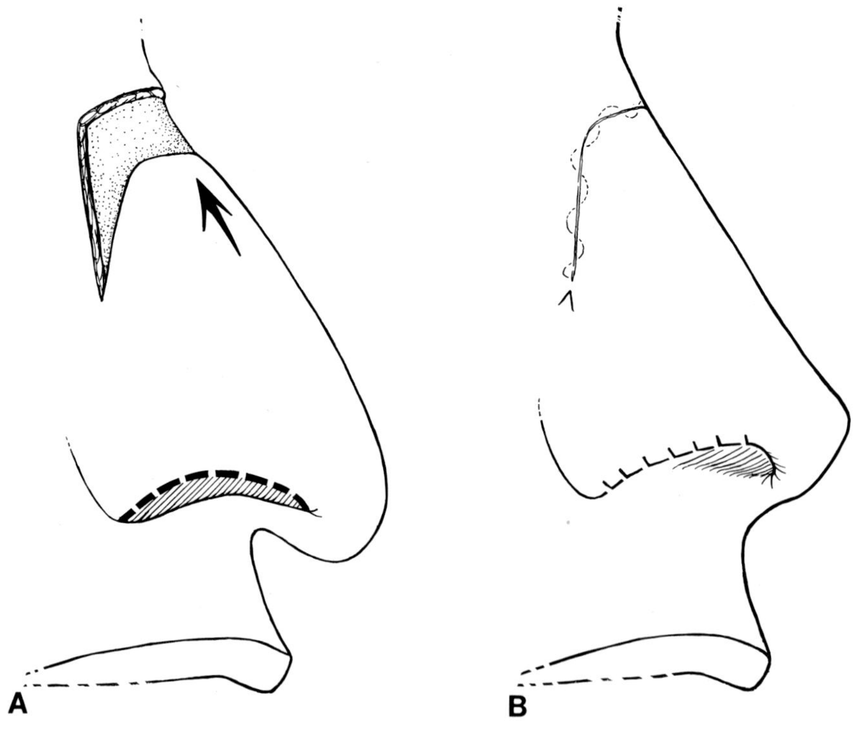

Fig. 251. Upper resection of Peterson for correction of the aging sagging nose, combined with marginal alar resection.

19

Rhinoplasty in Children

As in all phases of medicine and surgery, each case must necessarily be individualized, but the general dictum of waiting until the later teenage years to perform definite surgery remains a good one. There is wisdom in waiting for structural maturity to be reached with the purpose of not disturbing growth centers or interfering with the development as in this instance that of the nose as well as the entire face and allied structures. Nonetheless, in specific instances, particularly in deformities that severely disturb nasal function, some type of surgery, preferably conservative, is in order.

Nasal surgery in children should be done to restore nasal function and prevent the consequences of impeded function. However, care must be taken to preserve the continuity of the septal cartilage in order to prevent subsequent disturbances of nasal growth.

Until recently, the majority of surgeons did not dare operate on children for fear of impeding nasal growth. In most cases of trauma to the septum the correction of the septal deflection or defect is not sufficient to restore proper nasal function. Cases of Binders syndrome, consisting of a short columella with underdevelopment of the bony structures of the nose with a horizontal instead of a vertical slant to the nostrils, have to be operated on if the depression of the dorsum at the level of the valve causes a real obstruction of the airway. We described in 1969 (Meyer and Flemming) such a case involving a 7-year-old child in whom we had to straighten the septum to correct a saddle deformity and in whom we lengthened the columella by a V-Y plasty at the columellar base. The underdevelopment of the cartilaginous and bony structures was corrected by means of cartilage grafting to normalize the lumen of the vestibule. There is also a psychological reason to operate on such deformities even before school age. Similarly, after fresh nasal trauma the repair should be undertaken as early as possible. Children with severe congenital nasal deformities or after nasal trauma are generally operated on by us before the age of three.

Since development is generally completed earlier in girls and since slight underdevelopment of the nose is often pleasing in our culture, correction of pure cosmetic deformities may be performed earlier in girls than in boys. According to cephalometric investigations by Buck and Brown (1987), girls attain 87 percent of adult area at age 12, and boys attain 87 percent of adult area at age 15.

It is generally agreed that the purely aesthetic rhinoplasty should not be performed in children, but delayed until the nose is fully developed, which according to Flemming and Jazbi (1977) is not until the age of 16. If, however, there is a functional indication for septoplasty in a child, for instance the need to correct a septal subluxation with distortion of the columella, we can, during the same procedure, perform additional aesthetic correction such as modeling of the tip with or without cartilage resection.

In order to prevent or alleviate psychic trauma in childhood we correct marked nasal deformities such as those combined with hypertelorism, cysts, and naevi. Minimal removal of cartilaginous and bony structures and limited subperiosteal undermining is done. Supraperiosteal dissection along the dorsum when indicated is allowed in children below 12 years of age, as we stated in 1964 (Denecke-Meyer). Later, Farrior and Connolly (1970) as well as Ortiz-Monasterio and Olmedo (1981) expressed the same opinion. In a long-term follow-up of the last two authors concerning 44 patients between the ages of 8 and 12 years operated on for cleft deformities and trauma, no alterations were found in nasal growth. They concluded that the results were comparable to the results of the same operation when growth was completed.

Ortiz-Monasterio is also convinced that a complete conservative aesthetic rhinoplasty can be safely performed before puberty, when indicated. Rhinoplasty is less dangerous than septoplasty in the growing nose. Sometimes even surgery of the turbinates is necessary in children. In relation to nasal fractures in childhood, we agree with Safian (1936, 1986) who states that it is particularly important to minimize future deformity leading to psychological trauma by early corrective procedures attempted in the first or second decade of life. Studies concerning stages of growth of the septum are reported in the section on Septorhinoplasty (see Chapter 14).

Apart from a few investigations concerning the newborn's nose (Patrzek, 1890; Hillenbrand, 1930; Gray, 1965, 1972; and Krajina, 1969), histologic studies on the influence of trauma or surgery on the tissues of the growing human nose were not performed until 1974 (Pirsig and Kahl, 1974; Pirsig, 1975, 1986; Pirsig and Lehmann, 1975).

NASAL GROWTH

The septal cartilage is believed to be the key in maintaining nasal growth and projection. At the third fetal month the septum is represented by two midline mesenchymal condensations that gradually fuse. The sphenoid rostrum grows forward into the posterior septum. Chondrification of the nasal capsule begins by the third fetal month, and laterally, ingrowth partially separates the upper and lower lateral cartilages from the membranous septum.

In the first year of post-fetal life, ossification of the cephalic portion produces the perpendicular plates of the ethmoid. The vomer develops bilaterally, posterior, and inferior to the septum with an ossification center on each side, both of which usually become fused. A critical site for future growth and resulting projection is in the area of the vomeronasal organ of Jacobson and the paraseptal cartilages. The suture line between the vomer and the premaxilla (prevomerine bone) is an important area of growth potential and of important consideration in the management of the protruding premaxilla in cases of bilateral cleft lip.

A single cartilaginous capsule is the precursor of the nasal pyramid. The nasal bones develop as membranous bone from a single ossification center over this capsule and gradually absorb it. The exact site of this center is not known. Injury to the ossification center through trauma or early surgery can result in disturbances of bony growth. As the maxilla develops, the adjacent cartilages of the nasal capsule are incorporated, contributing to the lateral vault of the nose.

The maxillary contribution to the nasal framework forms the nasal process with its single ossification center and the maxillary crest, increasing the projection of the nose.

Nasal growth and development is an orderly process. The inherent growth pattern is influenced by many factors including enlargement of the sinuses, occlusion of the teeth, the facial musculature, and tongue placement. The rate of growth of the nose varies with age. After the first year of life the septum is surrounded by bone, except anteriorly and inferiorly, which is the direction of further growth. There is rapid growth up to 2 years of age, then a decreased rate until age 9 or 10. At puberty there is once again a spurt of nasal growth, which slows again into adult life. For practical purposes, growth is complete between the ages of 15 and 21, although many experienced clinicians consider that the nasal bones, and particularly the septum, continue to grow well into adult life. The exact influences on growth as a whole and the rate of growth of the individual anatomic components is not well documented, and our present conceptions are based largely on clinical impressions. Some of these observations are contradictory.

The infant nose is broad with a low bridge and a rounded elevated tip. The nostrils are circular and visible. During growth the lower lateral cartilages extend downward and the tip becomes more bulbous so that the external nares are no longer visible. This depression of the tip is further influenced by a lessening of fibrous tissue support with time. In adolescence, the lower lateral cartilages start to become more resilient and rigid, and thus easier to work with. Nasal cartilages continue their growth into adulthood, eventually producing a tip that sags in old age, a nasal dorsum that becomes higher, and minor deviations of the septum that may buckle and become symptomatic.

Concerning physiology of the nose, B. Mayer et al (1986) could demonstrate by active anterior rhinomanometry that the nasal air flow cycle is subject to a regulatory mechanism in children as young as 3 years of age.

STUFFY NOSE IN CHILDHOOD

Classification of nasal obstruction in the child's nose is as follows:

1. In the anatomically normal nose—soft tissue congestion or the "stuffy" nose.
2. Obstruction due to structural abnormalities.
3. Combination of congestion and abnormal structures.
4. Abnormal structure affecting the soft tissue adversely.
5. Chronic congestion affecting the hard tissue.

Factors that cause obstruction in the child's nose are similar to those affecting the adult. About 6 percent of all newborns start out with a nasal deformity due to injury while the head passes through the birth canal. Some of these improve spontaneously, some improve with septal reduction, and some remain deformed. Since the child's nose is wider in the turbinate area than the adult's, irritation and congestion of the turbinates are often followed by frequent infections. The child's septal cartilage is longer and thicker in relationship to the other parts of the nose than is the adult's. The mucoperichondrium covering the cartilage is also relatively thicker and more succulent than in the adult.

It is very easy for congestion to obstruct the child's nose. The child's immune system is not as developed as it becomes later in life, so infection occurs more frequently in the child.

20

Hare-Lip Nose

One of the most challenging rhinosurgical procedures is the functional and aesthetic correction of the cleft lip nasal deformity. Since this varies widely in its severity, it requires a great deal of individualization and special consideration as to the timing of surgery and in the selection of an appropriate surgical method, especially with concern for the lower lateral cartilages and the nasal base. In the newborn some repositioning of the alar structures, such as elevating the displaced lower lateral cartilage and fixing it with transalar mattress sutures, is often done at the time of the original cleft lip repair (McComb, 1986).

Despite the application of rhinoplastic techniques in primary cleft lip repair, the need for secondary nasal correction remains. The rationale for early secondary nasal surgery is based on the desire to reposition the structures as accurately as possible so that the distortions that are characteristic of this deformity do not tend to become aggravated during the major growth spurts.

In selected cases of vestibular stenosis it may be necessary to enlarge the vestibule and to correct the position of the caudal septum at the age of 3 years (Fig. 252). Tethering of the nasal tip by a short columella produces deformities that increase with age and should be released before rapid forward growth of the nose starts.

Most secondary hare lip nose corrections are performed between 10 and 15 years of age or in adults. One of the reasons for not operating on children is their inability to cooperate in the postoperative period. A fear of interfering with the continued development of the nose has caused many surgeons in the past to postpone surgery of these patients until after puberty (McComb, 1986). Children with facial abnormalities, however, become aware of the fact that they are different from other children quite early, and in many this can be a source of embarrassment and can cause problems in personality development. Thus, any procedure that favorably affects the child's psychological development, airway function, and soft tissue cosmesis should be considered in early childhood.

Most surgery on the base of the nose, done for both functional and cosmetic benefits such as columellar lengthening for the bilateral hare lip

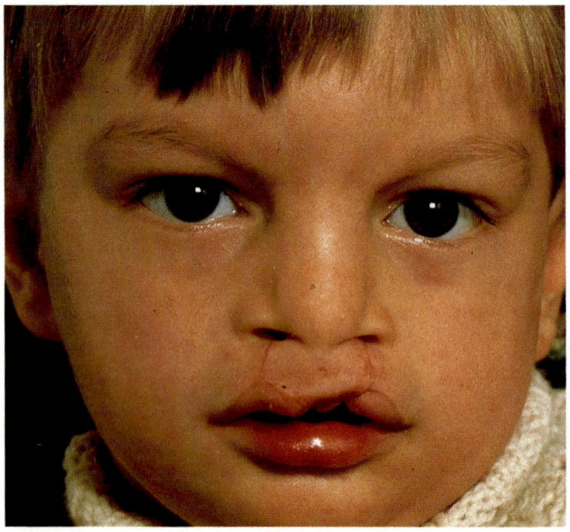

A

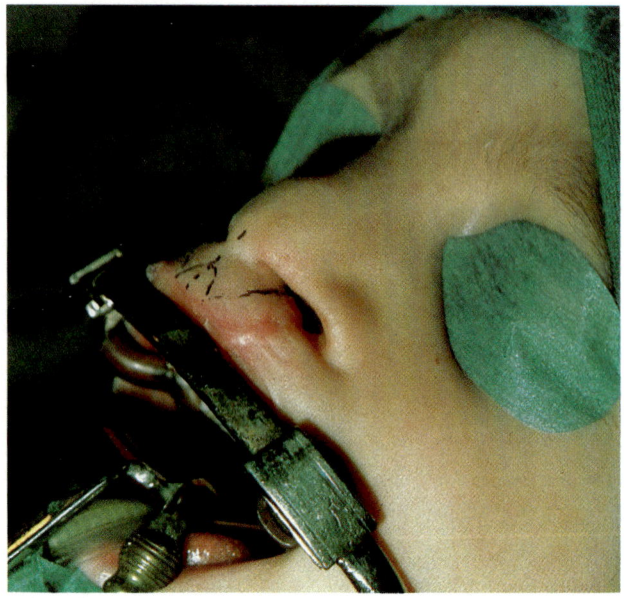

B

Fig. 252. Early repair of bilateral nose and lip with modified fork-flap (see p. 000). (A and B) Preoperative view and outline of the flap. (C) End of the operation. (D and E) Result.

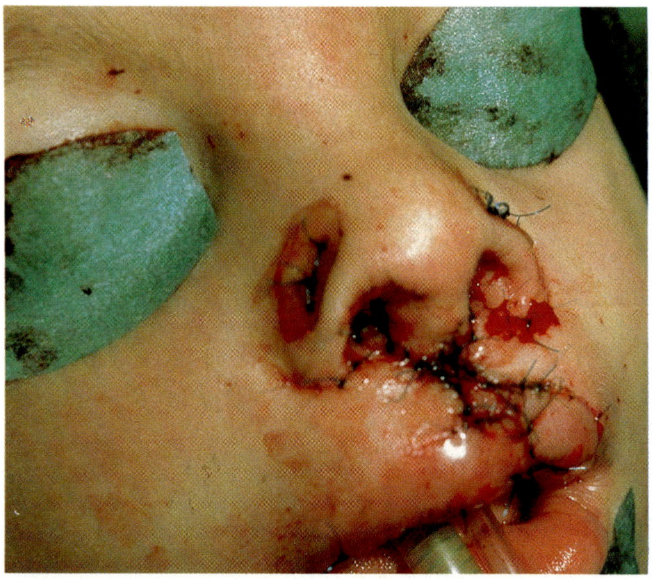

C

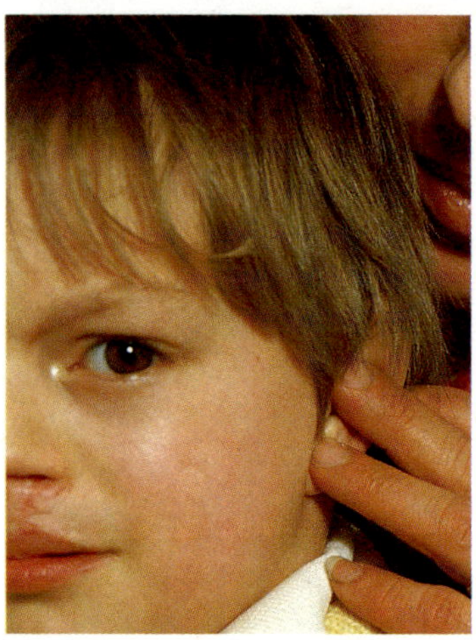

D

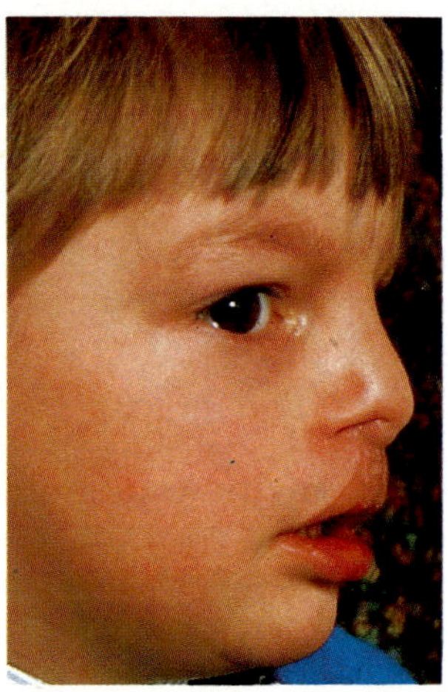

E

nose and columellar revision in unilateral clefts, is performed if possible during the preschool years. This will not be deleterious to either the future soft tissue growth or to further surgical intervention.

In the older patient with the cleft lip nose problem, a combination of the many techniques available may be required. Here it is important for the surgeon to be acquainted with as many methods as possible that have been practiced to date. The surgeon should also have the ability to adapt the methods to the conditions of the case at hand or, if necessary, to improvise modifications of them.

In bilateral hare lip nose a second correction is practically always necessary, in particular for lengthening the columella. In unilateral hare lip nose it is sometimes possible to correct the nose to such a considerable degree in the primary repair that in subsequent surgery only minimal or no alterations are required.

It is usual to begin with a conventional rhinoplasty, which consists of osteotomies, with or without hump reduction, dissection, repositioning of alar cartilages, septoplasty with centralization of the septum, which is usually deviated to the cleft side in unilateral cases, and fracture of the nasal spine.

For a very crooked septum, especially in its caudal and dorsal aspect, Davis (1983) recommends the in vivo slicing of the cartilage in a through-and-through manner to break its spring, complemented by the use of a straight onlay graft of auricular cartilage. This graft is placed alongside the "diced" septum to maintain the septum in a straight position. The graft is sutured in apposition to the septal cartilage with mattress sutures. In addition we place a dorsal graft harvested from the basal aspect of the quadrangular plate (see Chapter 14).

In cases of oronasal fistula, we choose the open procedure advocated by McIndoe (1938). For repair we cut the whole lip vertically to expose the fistula and close it again, after resection of the scar tissue, in three layers and with Z-plasties at the border of the vermilion and in the gingivolabial fold. Also, if a mismatch of the vermilion-cutaneous border is significant, the whole lip repair should be taken down and the entire repair redone. If there is too prominent an orbicularis muscle with puckering this can be reduced at the same time.

An upper lip deficient of tissue in a transverse direction is most unattractive. The flowing lines of the lip's graceful cupid's bow are transformed into a retracted scarred bow mostly at the expense of lip vermilion.

Loss of lip tissue at the alveolus can be repaired by grafting fascia, dermis, cartilage, or bone. In special cases of a poor vestibular floor with an oronasal fistula we advance the lip in its full thickness horizontally to the cleft side in order to close the dehiscence on the cleft side and to fill the lacking vestibular area with a paranasal appendix off the advancement flap (Fig. 253). At the same time, the angle of the mouth of the healthy non-cleft side has to be displaced laterally and modified. Using this technique, we can avoid the Abbe-Estlander flap, which is, however, necessary in extreme cases of retracted and thin upper lips.

Actually, we possibly avoid the use of the Abbe-Estlander flap as much as possible, trying to achieve protrusion of the upper lip and the base of the nose by bony or cartilaginous onlays or, if necessary, by advancement of the alveolar bone by means of a Le Fort I osteotomy procedure. In a few cases we have corrected the retrusion and retraction of the upper lip by filling it with temporal or parietal fascia (Fig. 254), sculpturing a new vermilion border, and tracing a new cupids bow.

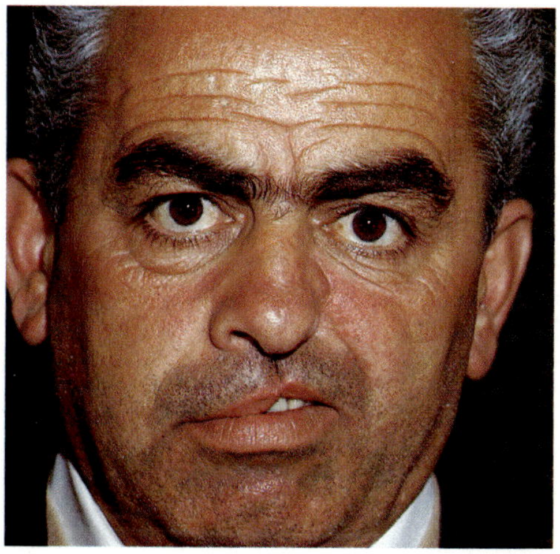

A

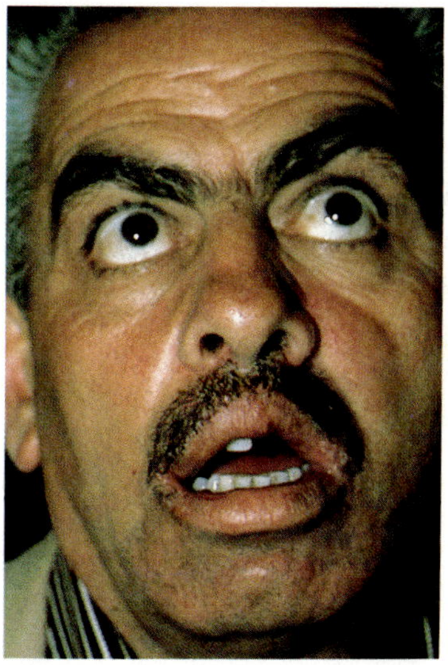

B

Fig. 253. Horizontal lip-advancement flap for partial reconstruction of vestibular floor in secondary unilateral cleft lip nose with oro-nasal fistula.

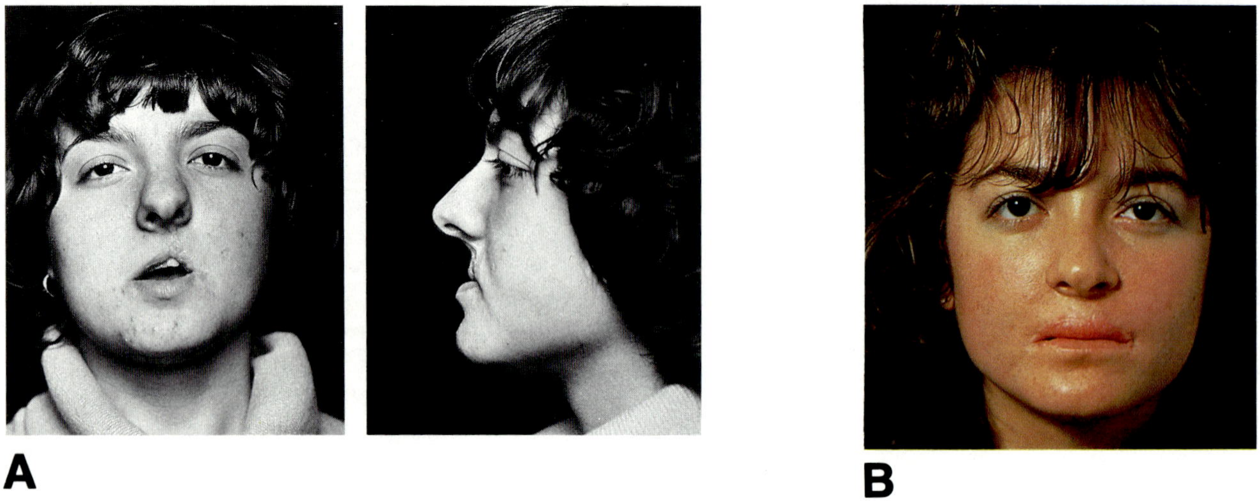

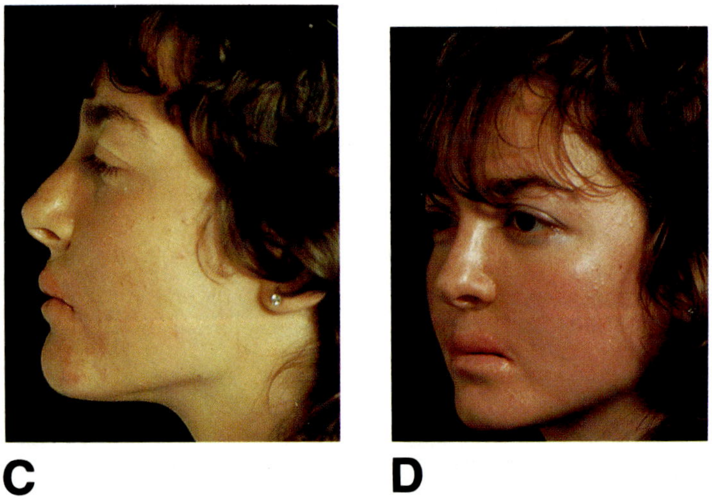

Fig. 254. Unilateral hare lip nose with protruding nasal tip and retruded lip. Correction of the nose with reduction of the bony skeleton, modeling of the tip, elevating of the left vest vestibular floor, and marginal resection. Augmentation of the lip with strips of parieto-temporal fascia. (A) Preoperative views. (B, C, and D) Late result.

The Abbe flap when used in an exceptionally deficient upper lip must be set into the midline and should be constructed so as not to override the breadth of the philtrum (Fig. 255). We outline the distal end of the flap in a fish tail shape with the bilateral extensions to the vestibular sill.

The choice of techniques we use in secondary hare lip repair is outside the scope of this book. It needs only be mentioned that the loss of tissue at the free border of the lip can be compensated through the use of local advancement flaps.

Thus, an excess of vermilion in the lateral aspects of the lip can be corrected with the paired pendulum flaps of Kapetanski (1971), swung to the midline where they drop down with a part of the orbicularis muscle giving an increased midline prominence.

We use bilateral island flaps joining in the midline for the same purpose, and in many cases we perfect the free border of the upper lip through marginal resections or by performing a vertical V-Y plasty in the center of the upper vermilion, everting as much of the mucosa as is necessary, carrying the dissection to the gingivolabial fold thereby releasing the adherence of gingivomucosa to the premaxilla.

For *unilateral hare lip nose* we correct the following points:

1. Deviation of the septum and columella toward the cleft side, with subluxation of the lamina quadrangularis at the vomer.
2. Flattening and caudal displacement of the cleft side ala with loss of protrusion of the dome when compared to the non-cleft side.

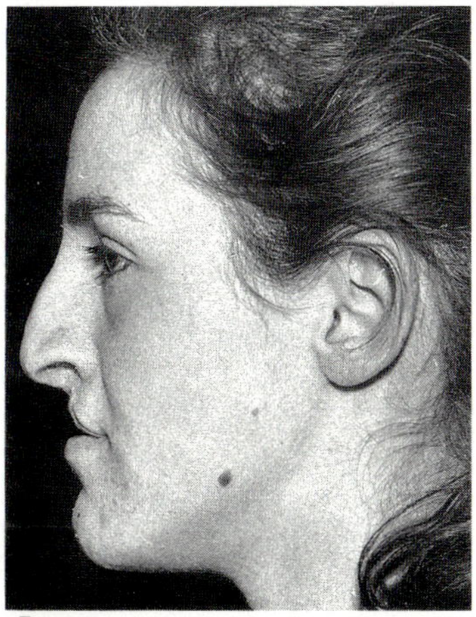

A

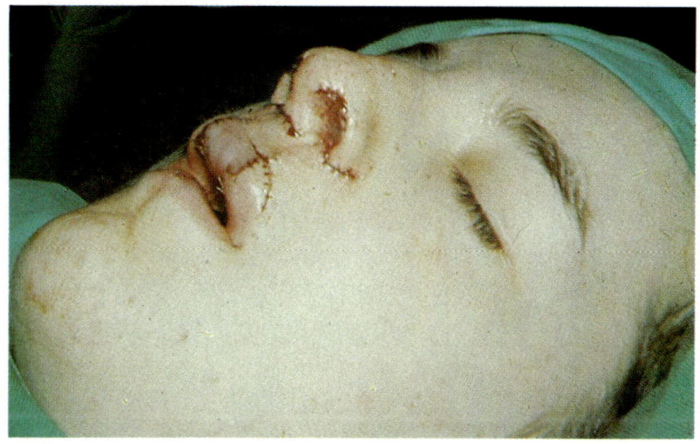

B

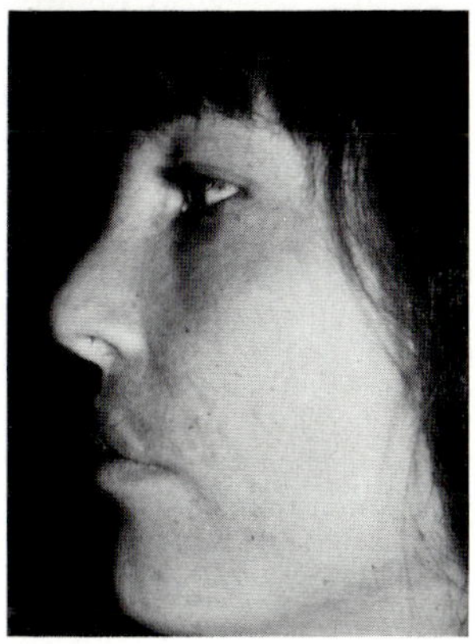

C

Fig. 255. Using the Abbé flap as in this young female, we sculp a vermilon border and a cupid's bow of attractive contour. (A) Preoperative profile. (B) End of the second stage. (C) Postoperative profile.

3. Advancement of the anterior commissure of the nares on the cleft side.
4. Shortness of the columellar border on the cleft side as compared to the other side.
5. Abnormal insertion of the cleft side ala in the nasolabial region.
6. Broadness of the floor of the nose which is held at a different level as compared to the other side.
7. Under development of the maxilla in the region of the insertion of the ala.
8. Caudal displacement with inward traction of the lateral crus of the ala.
9. Tendency to bifidity of the tip of the nose.
10. Asymmetry of the insertion of the upper lateral cartilages as seen in the crooked nose.
11. Asymmetry of the bony structures of the nose.

Of the multitude of methods in use for the correction of the unilateral hare lip nose, we want to consider here only a few. In the book by Denecke and Meyer (1964/1967), we described and mentioned more than 30 methods and we will now limit our report to a few with which we have had a good experience.

As the deformity of the columella often occurs in conjunction with an abnormal position of the rest of the nostril, many techniques have been developed to repair both of these deformities concomitantly. One of the most common techniques used is the Ivy (1932) modification of the Blair (1925) procedure. Here the constricted nostril is incorporated into a flap based on the lateral ala and advanced medially and superiorly. The apex of the nostril is advanced into a defect created by excision of a full-thickness wedge of tissue. This technique will also reposition an alar base that is located too far laterally on the maxilla.

Blair and Brown (1930) were the first to split the columella in the midline, the cut swinging outward along the line of the junction of the floor of the nostril with the lip. The whole nostril, with its broad ala, is rotated into a more normal position. Ivy in 1932 diagrammed the Blair rotation adapted for a primary nasal correction done at the same time as the lip closure.

A similar rotation of the hemi-columella was readvocated by Sheehan in 1936 and then modified by Young (1949), Wilkie (1969), and Millard (1976) in that the median incision is extended over and beyond the alar rim to the outer surface of the ala, which, in our opinion, should be avoided.

Further modifications of the method of Blair have been described by Gillies and Kilner (1932), Barsky (1950), Schjelderup (1955), and Meyer (1961). In all these procedures an inward rotation and medial repositioning of the lateral alar attachment takes place without the necessity for an additional labial flap to widen the vestibular floor.

In our hands, these procedures have proved to be quite effective. They can be used in children as young as 4 years and allow one to avoid marginal resections at the ala and columella that can interfere with growth at that age. Using our method, as also shown by Millard (1964), the median scar in the majority of cases is almost insignificant. The method of Gillies (1932) is characterized by a flap exchange on the vestibular floor.

In our method, the rotated hemi-columella is kept in place by a Z-plasty at the base of the columella (Figs. 256 and 257). We have also used this modification in children without observing any narrowing of the vestibule. If there is an important difference of circumference of the nares, an additional transposition flap can be brought from the opposite side to the cleft side floor (Fig. 258).

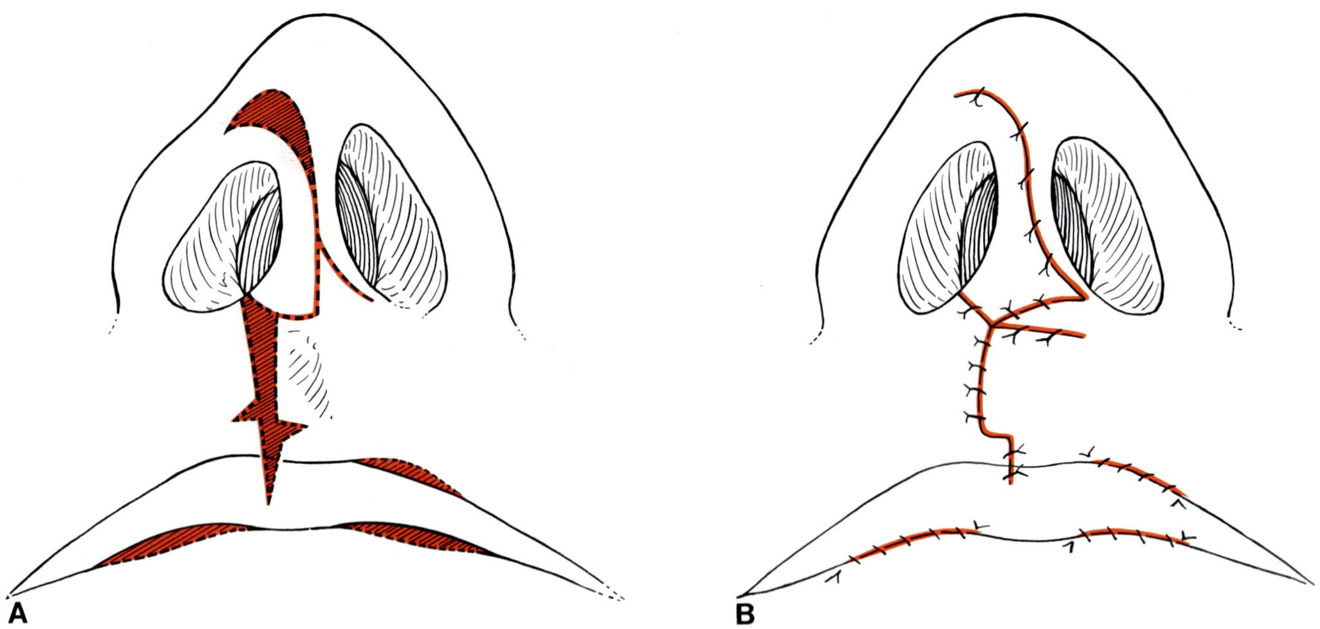

Fig. 256. Correction of unilateral hare lip nose by rotation of one half of the columella and a Z-plasty at the columellar base (Meyer). Lip correction according to Le Mesurier and refinement at the lip border and cupid's bow. (A) Incisions and excisions. (B) Sutures at the end of the operation.

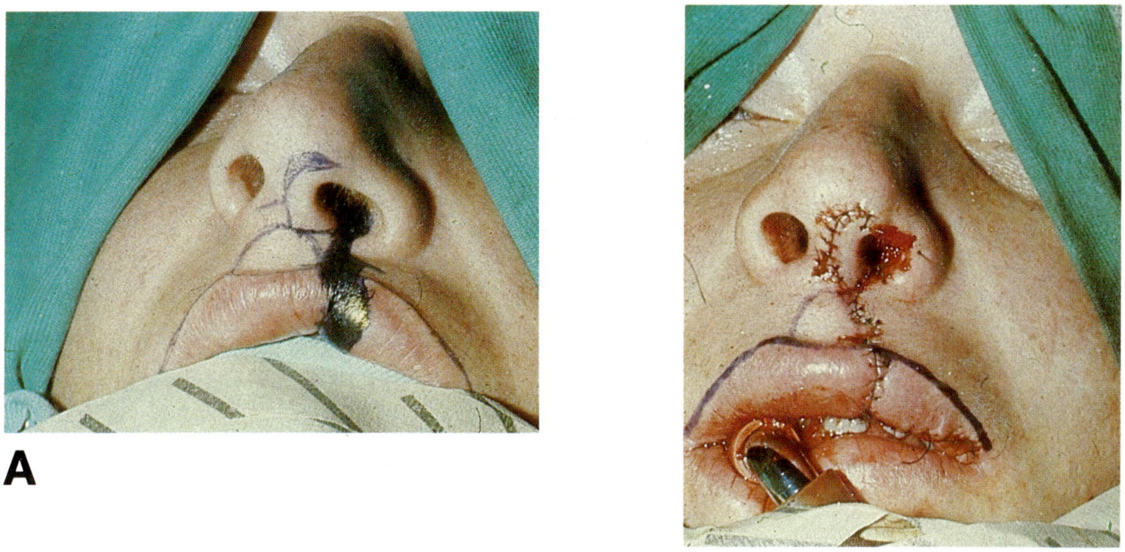

A

B

Fig. 257. Procedure of Figure 256 shown in a 4-year-old child at the beginning of the operation with the outline of the incision (A) and at the end (B).

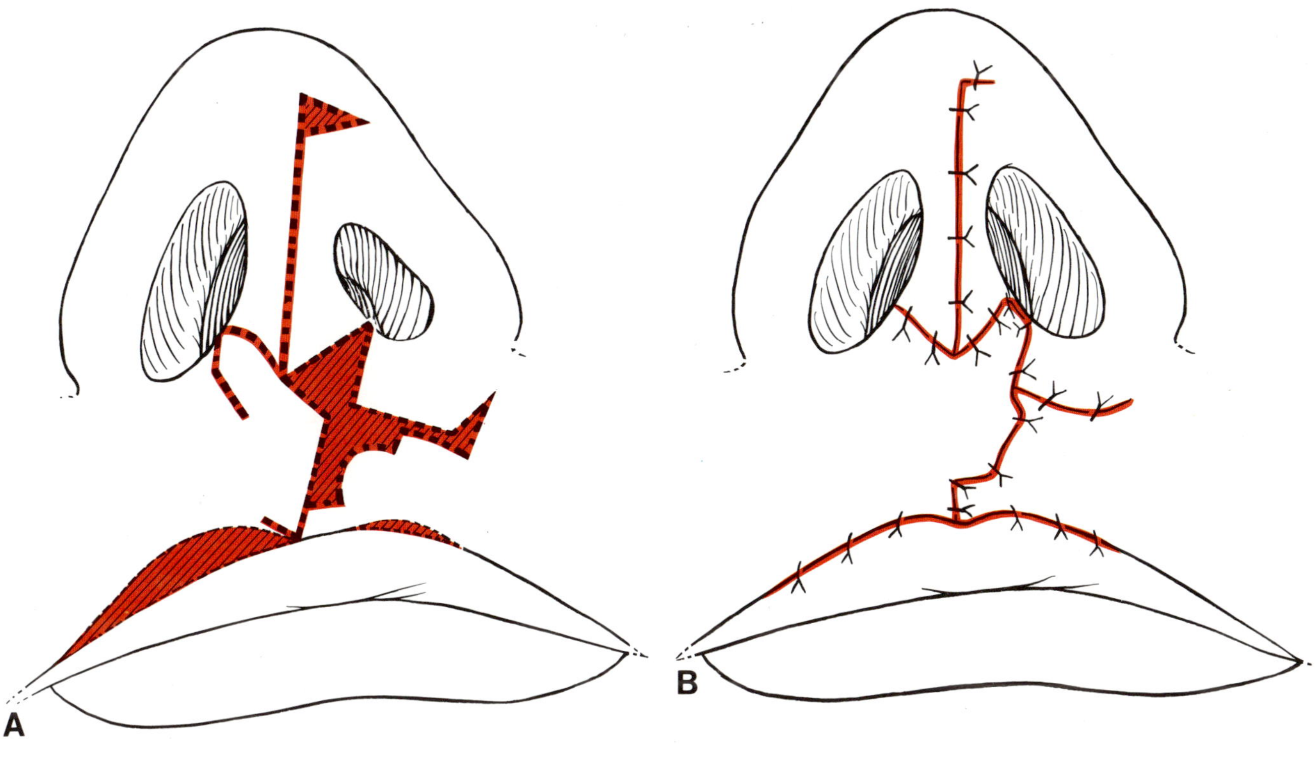

Fig. 258. Correction of unilateral hare lip nose with stenosis of the nostril on the affected side according to Meyer. The medial crus of the cleft side follows the rotation of the skin. A transposition flap at columellar base can be brought from the floor of the unaffected side to the floor of the cleft side thereby enlarging it. This procedure is combined with the lip correction of Le Mesurier and cupid's bow revision. (B) Closure of incisions.

Fig. 259. Rotation of alar base towards the columella, elevation of the vestibular floor combined with marginal resection of the lobular alar commissure. A 1 cm broad strip of skin from the vestibular floor and membranous septum is slid towards the tip. (A) Outline of the incisions. (B and C) Sliding flap sutured. Alar cartilage in new position after sectioning the medial crus on the cleft side.

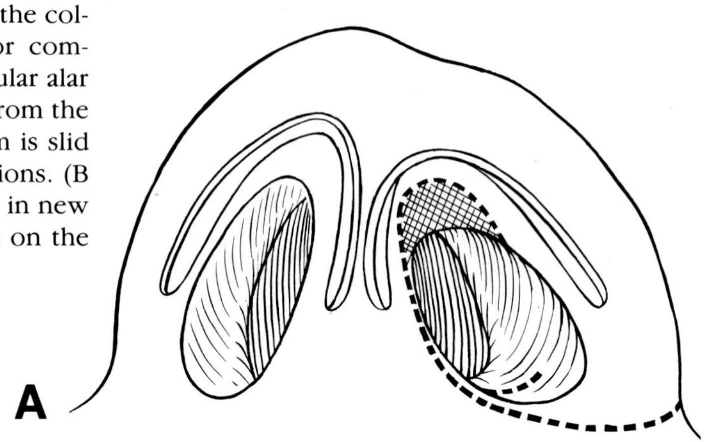

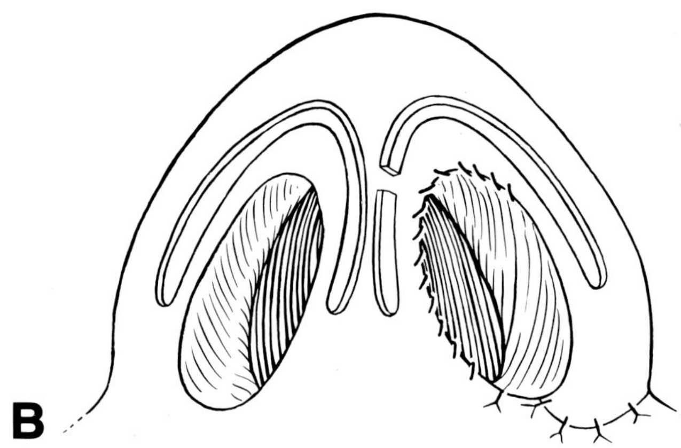

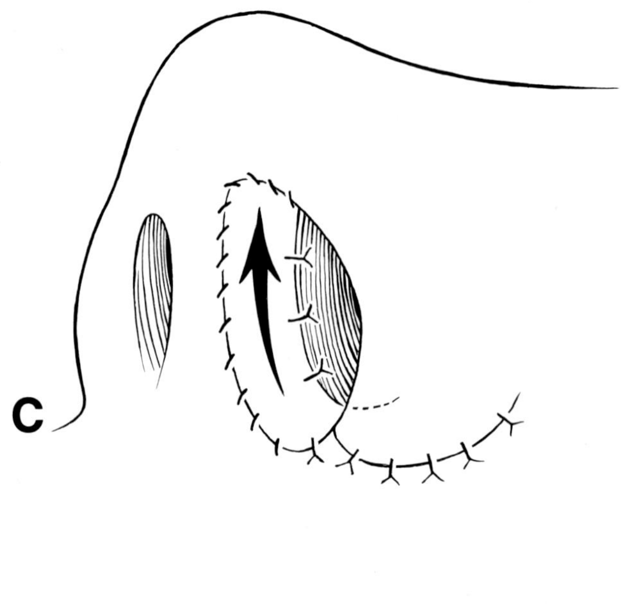

Another extension of the columella splitting method was used by us in adults with very satisfactory results and published in 1975. It concerns the concomitant rotation of the skin of the membraneous septum with the hemi-columella on the cleft side together with the medial crus of the alar cartilage. A 1 cm broad strip of skin from the floor of the vestibule is then advanced in a sliding manner toward the tip of the nose, like a carpet. The same sliding movement of a strip of skin can be performed with a marginal columella incision (this time not a mediocolumellar incision) (Figs. 259 and 260).

To achieve the same result there is an alternative to rotating vestibular skin. In elevating the anterior commissure at the soft triangle of the cleft side after a half-moon-shaped resection, we can provide the lining of the new border by inserting a composite graft. The composite graft is harvested from the inner aspect of the auricular crus helicis (Fig. 261). This procedure corresponds to that described for the correction of anterior vestibular stenoses after partial or total nose reconstruction (Fig. 220).

Using the decortication technique of Rethi, in which a horizontal incision through the anterior part of the columella is carried into the vestibule on both sides permitting an open exposure for the mobilization of the cartilaginous dome and its replacement in a symmetrical position, we have also obtained good results in secondary unilateral deformities in which scar tissue in the columella-tip complex had to be removed (Figs. 61 and 262).

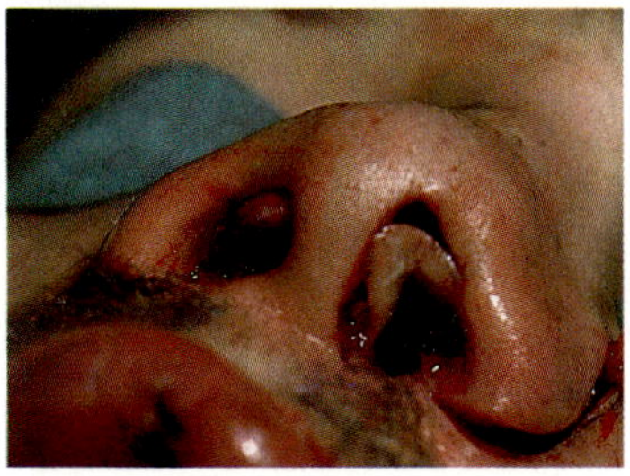

A

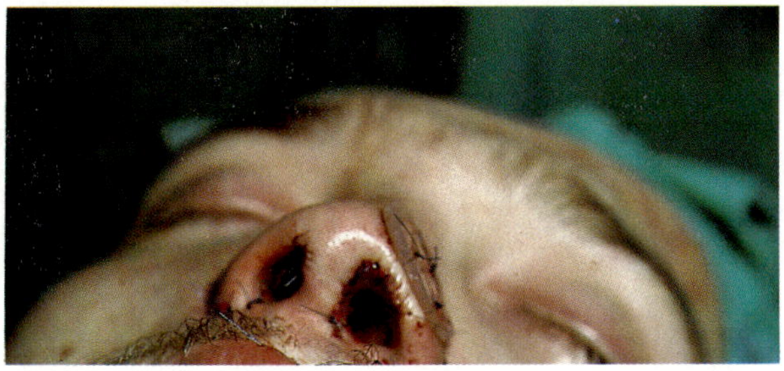

B

Fig. 260. Unilateral hare lip nose in young man operated with the technique of Figure 259. (A) Sliding flap dissected. (B) Flap sutured in advanced position.

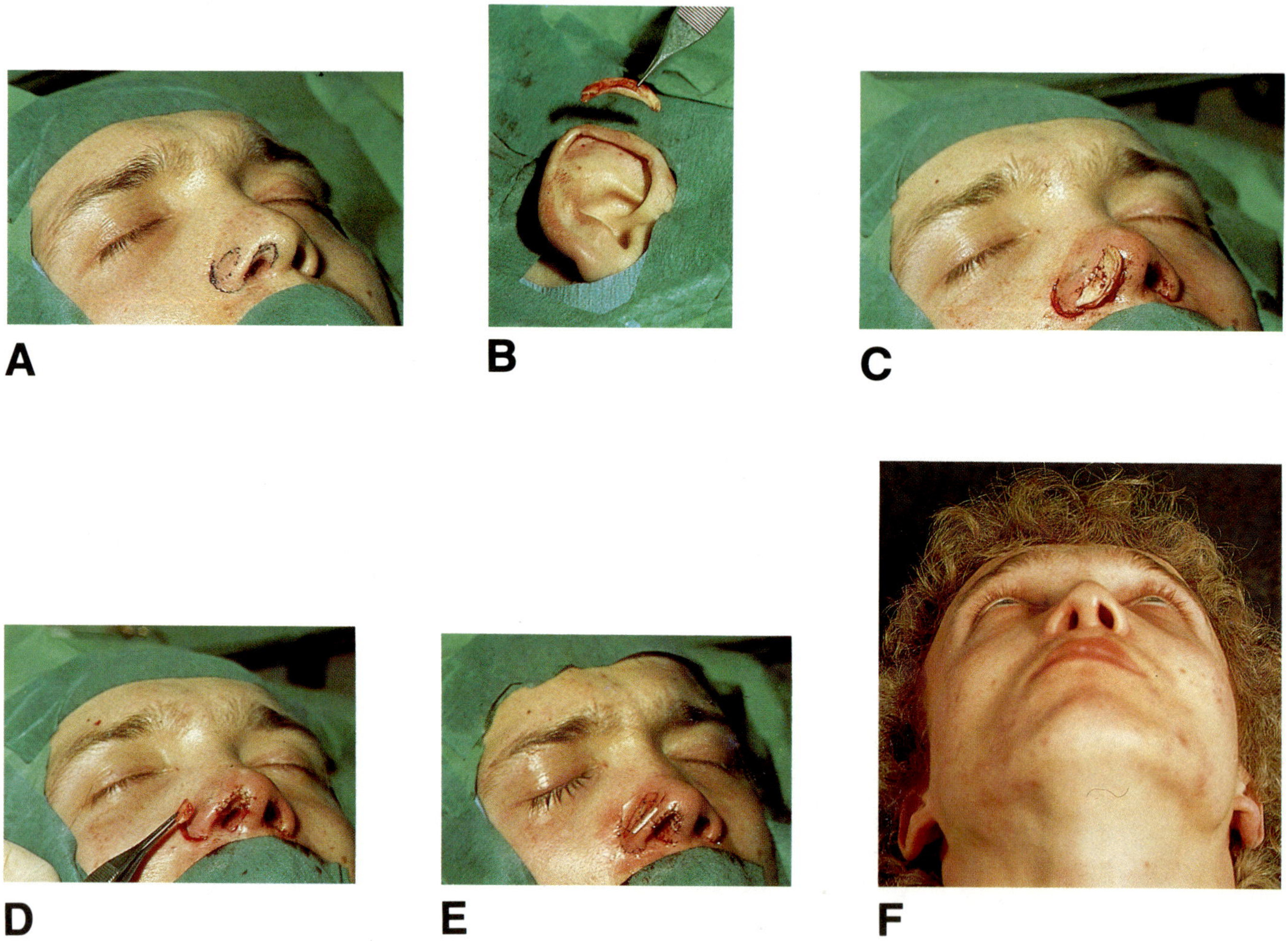

Fig. 261. Correction of unilateral hare lip nose with half-moon resection at the alar-columellar commissure of the cleft side and auricular composite graft for lining of the new border. An additional cartilage graft from the septum is placed into the ala as reinforcement. (A) Outline of resection. (B) Harvesting the auricular composite graft. (C) Transfer of the composite graft, which will be Flopped inside from the border. (D) Insertion of alar graft. (E) End of the operation with transalar mattress sutures. (F) Result.

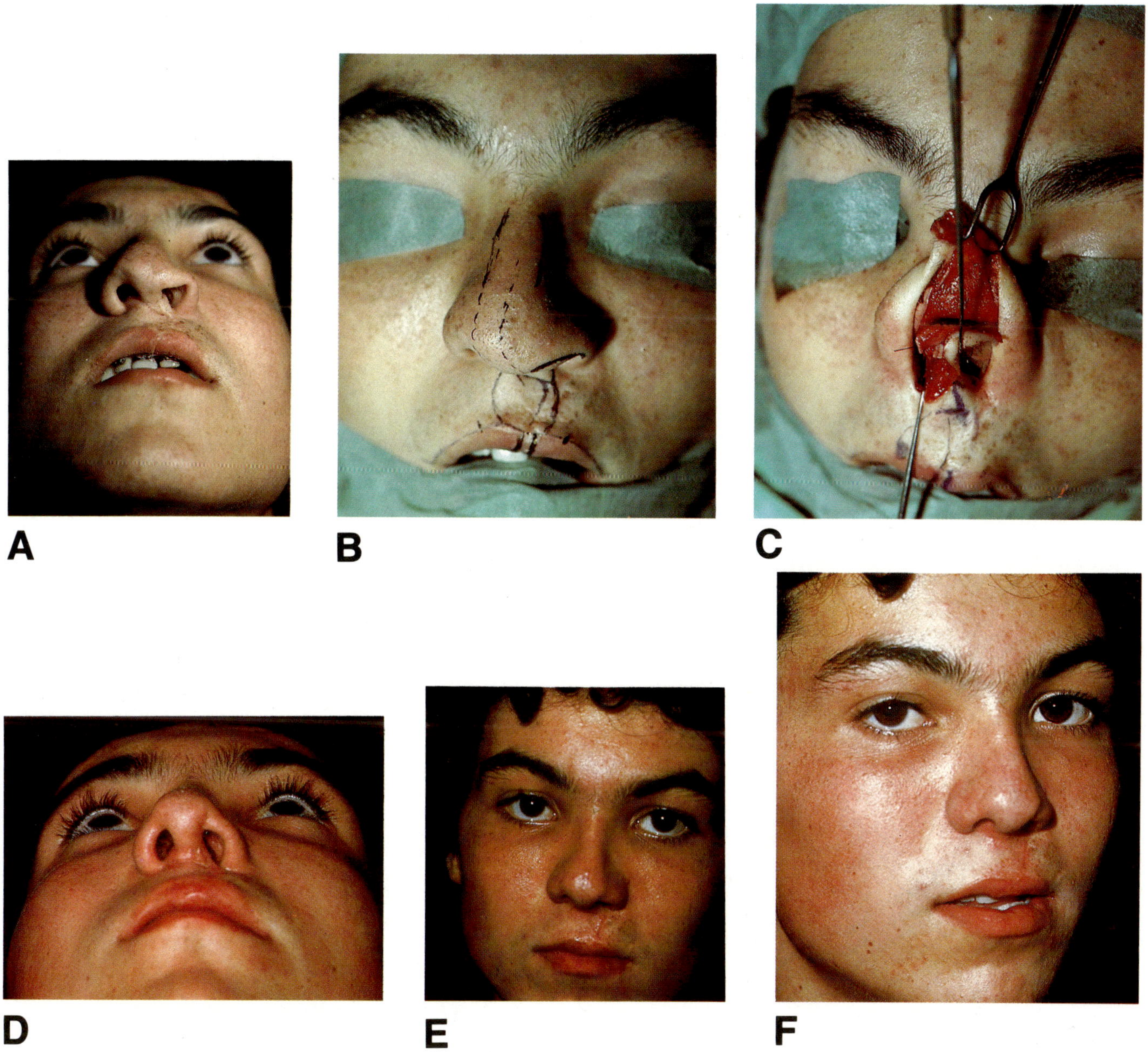

Fig. 262. Adolescent with unilateral hare lip nose corrected with Rethi incision (see Fig. 61), elevation of the dome on the affected side and interposition of a cartilage strut from the septum between the medial crura of the lower lateral cartilage. (A and B) Preoperative views. (C) Open access to the lower lateral cartilage. (D, E, and F) Result.

Another method for the direct exposure of the medial part of the upper lateral cartilages can be achieved by using the "listing sea gull" incision of Erich (1953) (Figs. 263 and 264). He also divided the medial crus of the cleft side alar cartilage and lifted it into balance with the opposite side and sutured it there. The excess alar rim skin on the cleft side is tailored, which levels the "list of the sea gull." A year prior to this, however, Figi designed an approach that never became popular: a flying baby bird incision across the upper columella with extension into the vestibule under the alar arches; this actually hid the scars better than the Erich (1953) design. It looks very similar to the recent modification of Rethi's incision by Goodman (1975) but with a downward instead of an upwardly directed median notch.

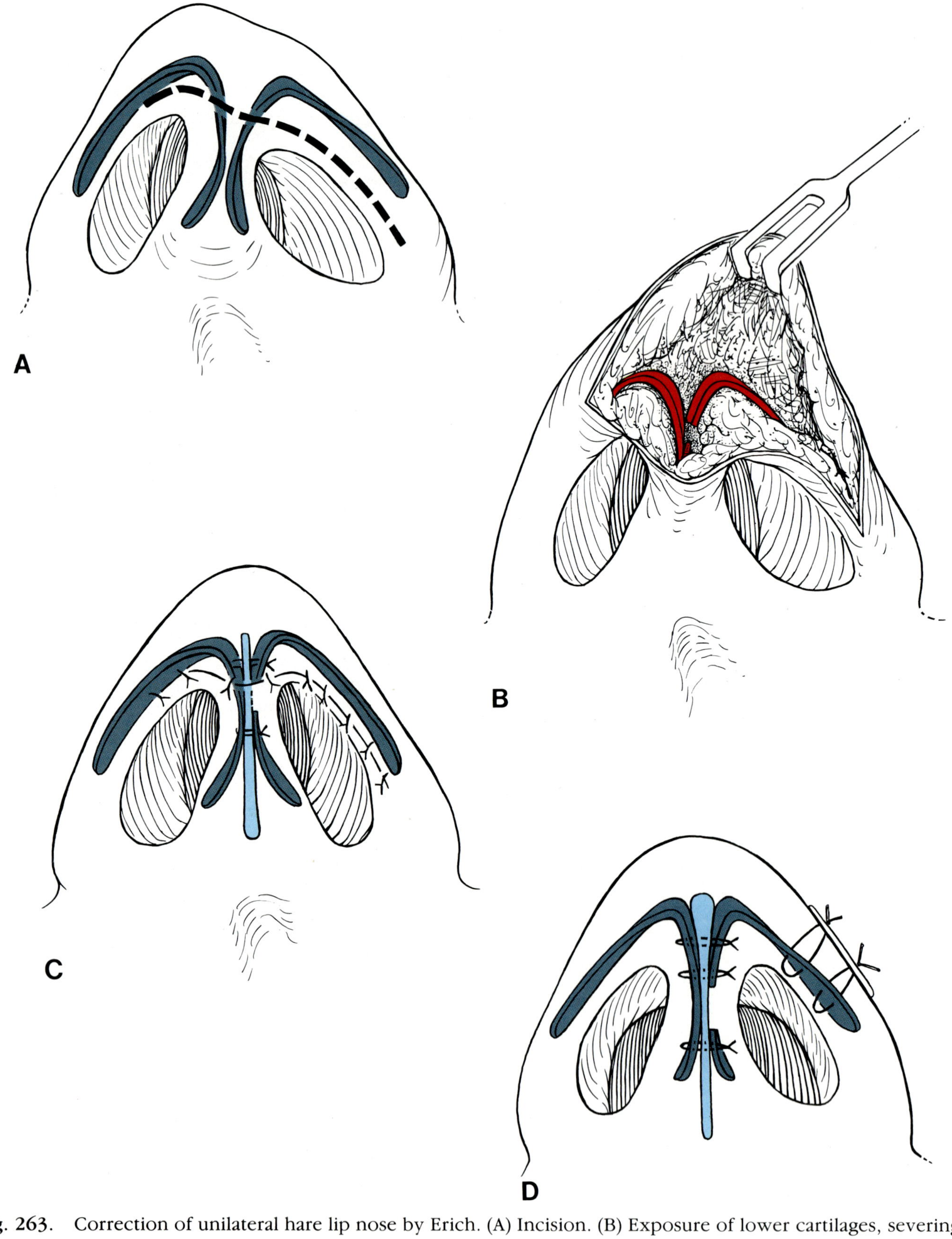

Fig. 263. Correction of unilateral hare lip nose by Erich. (A) Incision. (B) Exposure of lower cartilages, severing the medial crus on the cleft side and repositioning the cartilage arch at the level of the contralateral one. (C) Mattress sutures between the arches bilaterally and between the medial crura. Superimposed closure of wound. (D) Method of stabilizing repositioned lower lateral cartilage and an interposed batten with mattress sutures through the arch of cartilage, medial crura inferiorly and on nostril securing it to a plastic splint.

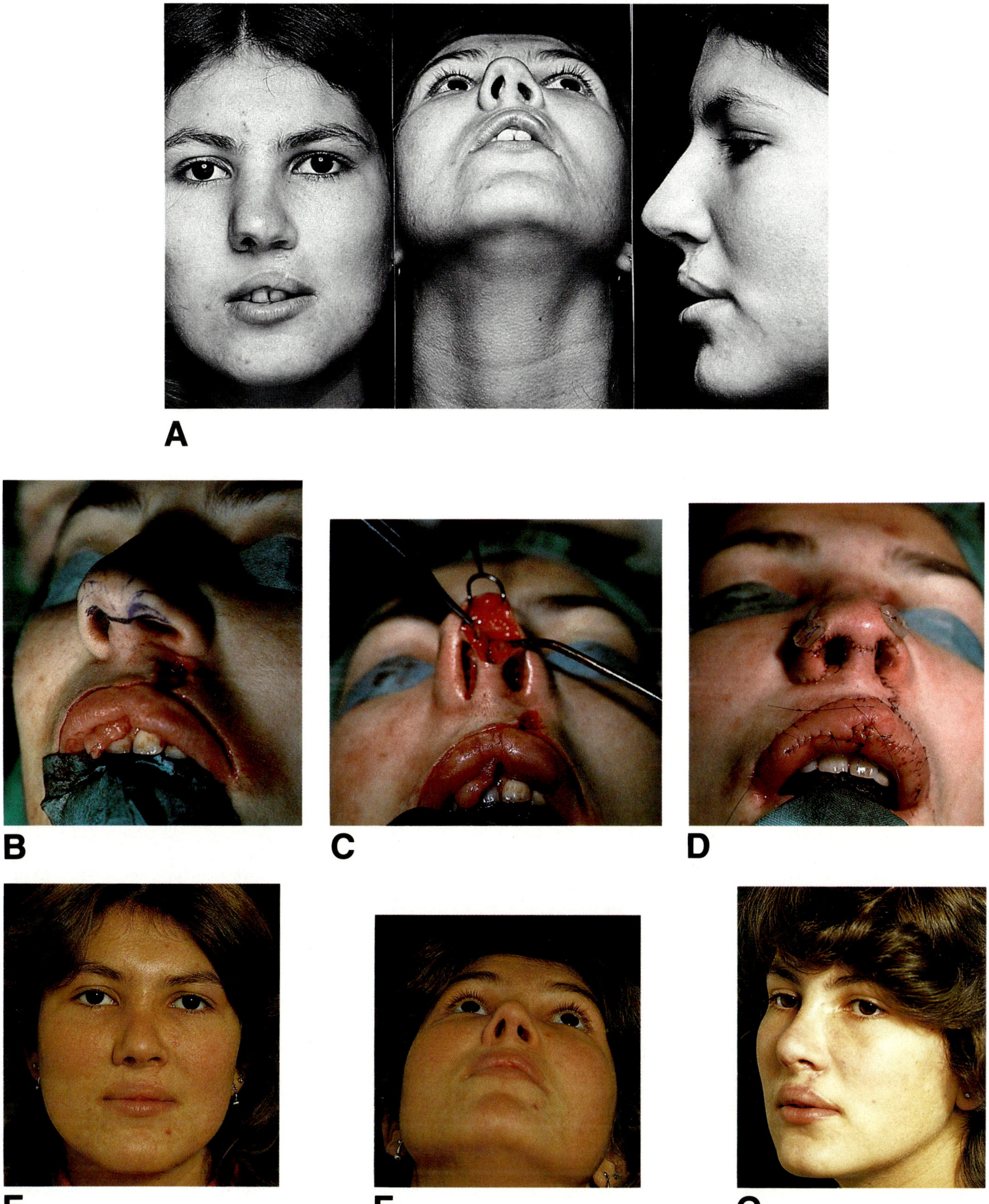

Fig. 264. Preoperative view of hare lip nose in a young female patient. (B) Outline of Erich's incisions intraoperatively with unilateral marginal lobular alar resection. (C) Open aspect of the tip. (D) End of the operation with transalar mattress sutures for holding the nostril in the new position. (E, F, and G) Late result.

For complete exposure of the lower lateral cartilages including the medial crura we incise around the columella according to the technique of Gensoul (1833), Lexer (1929), Cooghlin (1925), and Potter (1954) (Figs. 265 and 266), elevating the skin of the columella and extending the vestibular incisions to free the lateral crura.

With the method of Potter (1954), we can obtain an elongation of the columella through a V-Y plasty at its base, and an elevation of the dome of the cleft side alar cartilage by designing another V-Y plasty at the lateral wall of the vestibule—the skin flap is pushed forward together with the lateral crus, producing a protrusion of the dome. The dome of the cleft side has to be brought up at least to the level of the noncleft side or better to an overcorrected position. For this purpose we cut the medial crus on the cleft side into two pieces and mobilize the dome with the anterior part of the medial crus, pushing it forward, and fixing it in a new anterior position using mattress sutures to the opposite medial crus. We then interpose or appose a cartilaginous strut obtained from the contralateral alar cartilage or from the septum, which provides a stable support to the columella tip complex.

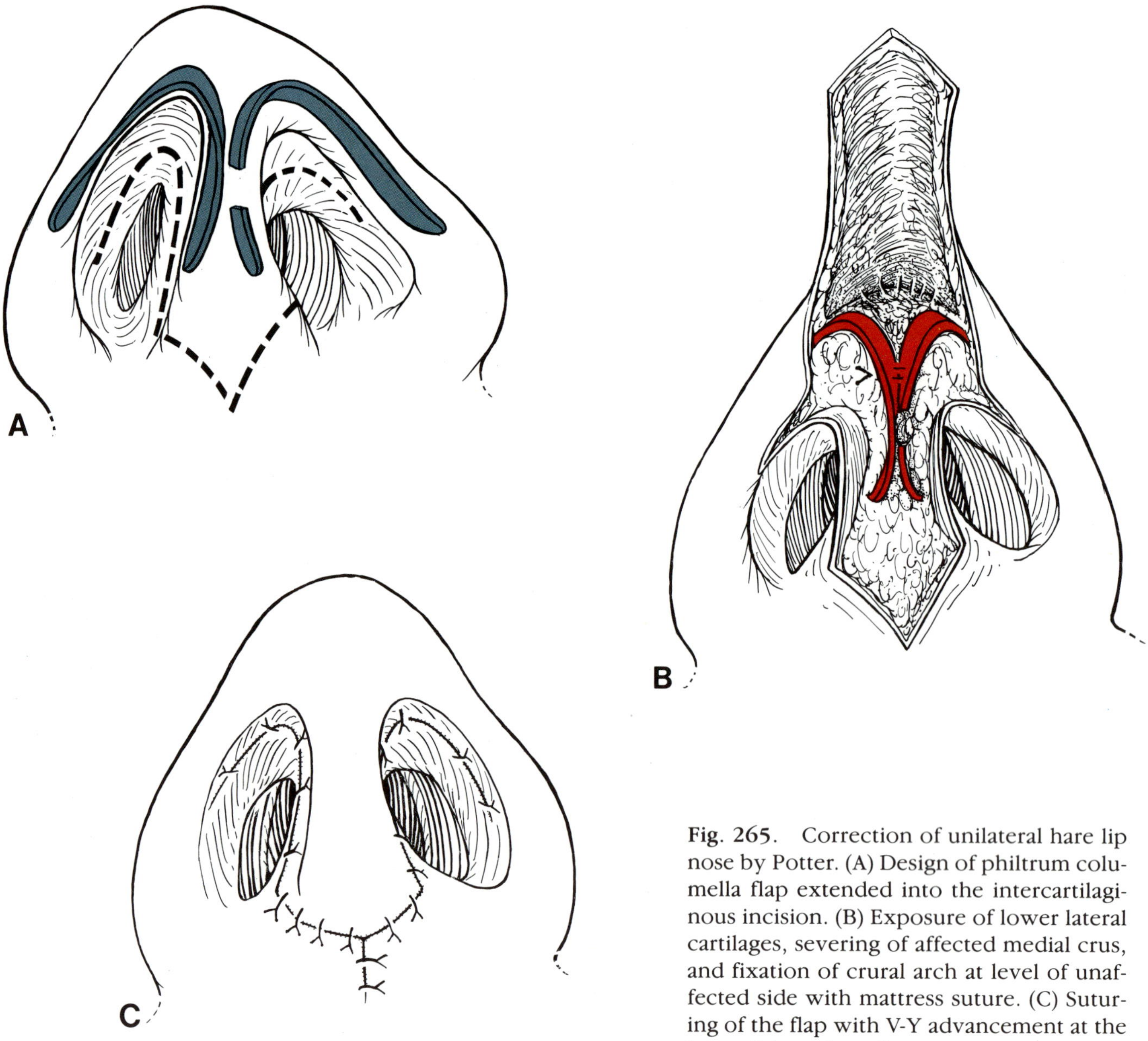

Fig. 265. Correction of unilateral hare lip nose by Potter. (A) Design of philtrum columella flap extended into the intercartilaginous incision. (B) Exposure of lower lateral cartilages, severing of affected medial crus, and fixation of crural arch at level of unaffected side with mattress suture. (C) Suturing of the flap with V-Y advancement at the base of the columella.

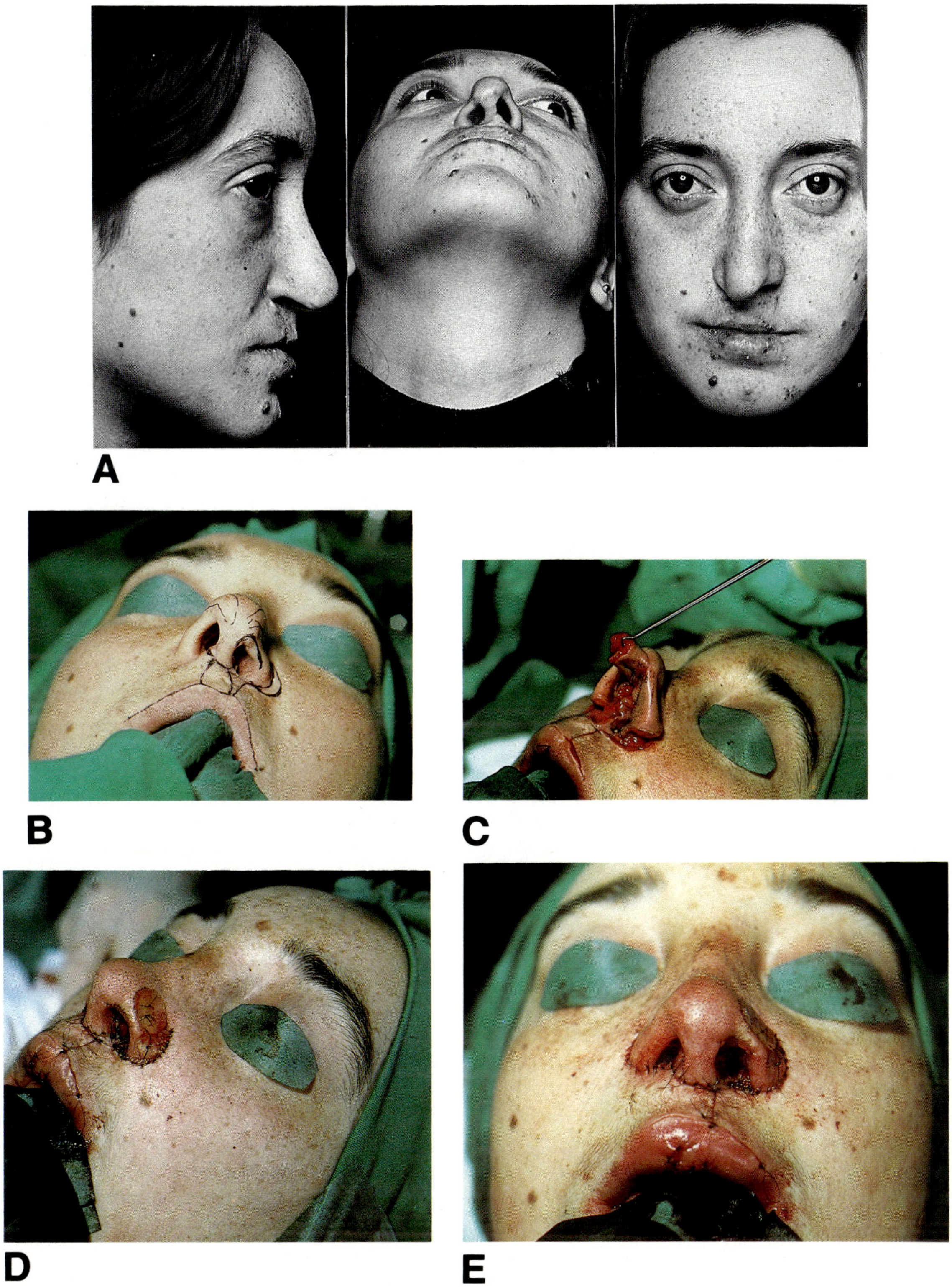

Fig. 266. Young female with unilateral hare lip nose. Correction with Potter technique. (A) Preoperative view. (B) Intraoperative design of incisions with lobular-alar marginal resection, paranasal island flap as shown in Figure 224 for enlargement of the vestibule. (C) Open aspect with island flap moving to the vestibular floor. (D and E) Closure of the wounds and suture of the island flap to the floor of the vestibule and transalar mattress suture. (F, G, and H) Late result. ***(Fig. 266. continues)***

Fig. 266. continued.

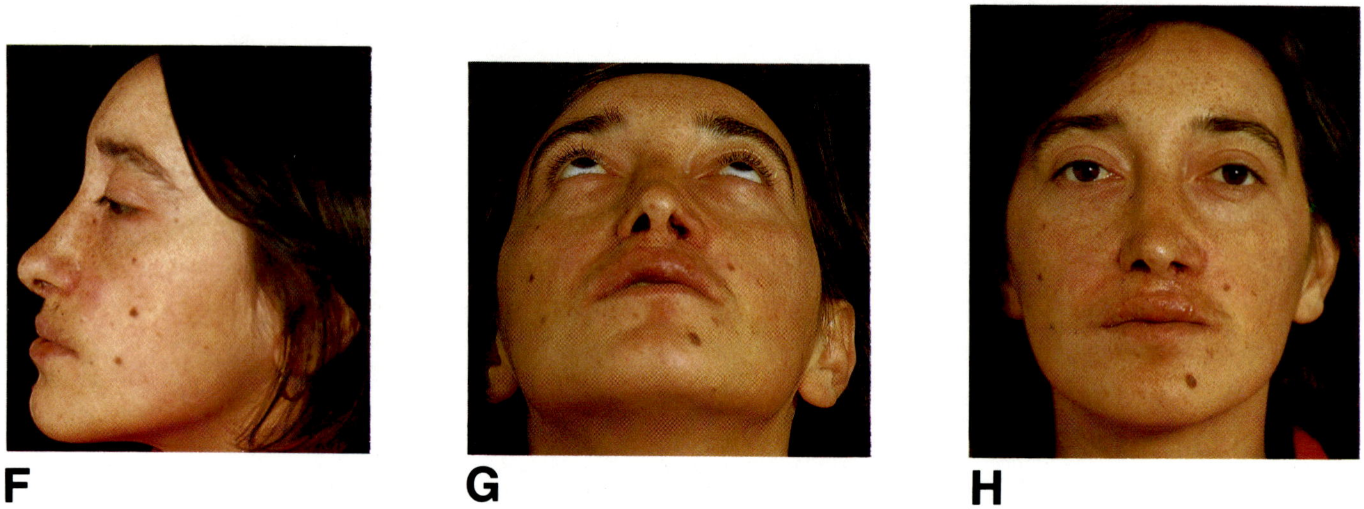

Augmentation of the tip can also be provided by a turn over of the cranial part of the alar cartilage from the nonaffected side.

Our modified technique of Potter includes the membranous part of the septum with the columella flap, which can thus be elevated like a proboscis together with the medial crura of the lower lateral cartilage (Figs. 265 and 266). The lateral crus is then everted and modeled by resections, scoring, and transalar fixation while the lateral intranasal defect is closed in a V-Y fashion.

A similar medial and superior advancement of the lateral crus with its attached vestibular skin into a more elevated position has been proposed by Rees (1977). The flattened dome is then sutured to the normal one so that their symmetric position is more likely to be assured postoperatively.

Holt (1986) sutures the mobilized lower lateral cartilage to the ipsilateral upper lateral cartilage. We prefer to free the upper lateral cartilages in an extramucosal fashion so that it cannot function anymore as a support for other structures. In our minds, the two cartilages (the upper and the lower lateral) have to be independent. Thus, we choose rather to suture the two domes together as an overcorrected position like Tolhurst (1983) also does, and, in addition, if necessary, we place a dome onlay or alar onlay on the flatter side. We believe that transalar mattress sutures looped over plastic sheets are quite important in stabilizing the new convex shape of the ala and to obliterate the potential dead space between the separated layers.

If, as in most cases of unilateral hare lip nose, the base of the ala has to be displaced or rotated, we insert a slightly convex cartilage graft from the septum or from the ear concha through the alotomy. The onlay alar graft is fixed by transcutaneous mattress sutures and the columella-tip complex is reinforced with a septal strut (Fig. 267). If necessary the naso-labial angle is protruded with cartilage onlay.

In the unilateral hare lip nose the affected side is almost always placed in a more caudal position and a simple inrolling of the nostril margin can produce symmetry. With a Z-plasty in the lateral vestibular wall we correct the level of the alar rim, as well as the collapsing alar fold. This can be combined with proper positioning of the domes after sectioning of the medial crus on the cleft side and fixation using transalar sutures (Fig. 268).

In particular cases of extreme caudal displacement of the cleft side ala with scar-like cicatricial rigidity, we perform an infolding of the alar and lobular skin in order to obtain a new alar border at the anterior commissure; i.e., in the soft triangle of Converse, extending to the columellar border. Instead of being resected, this skin is only folded into the vestibule after wide subcutaneous dissection and defatting. The new ala is kept in the new position by transcutaneous mattress sutures. The internal skin should never be rolled out. If necessary, any insufficient lining of the lateral vestibular wall can be restituted with a composite graft from the crus helicis of the external ear (see infolding technique in Chapter 17).

The infolding is a procedure that we actually

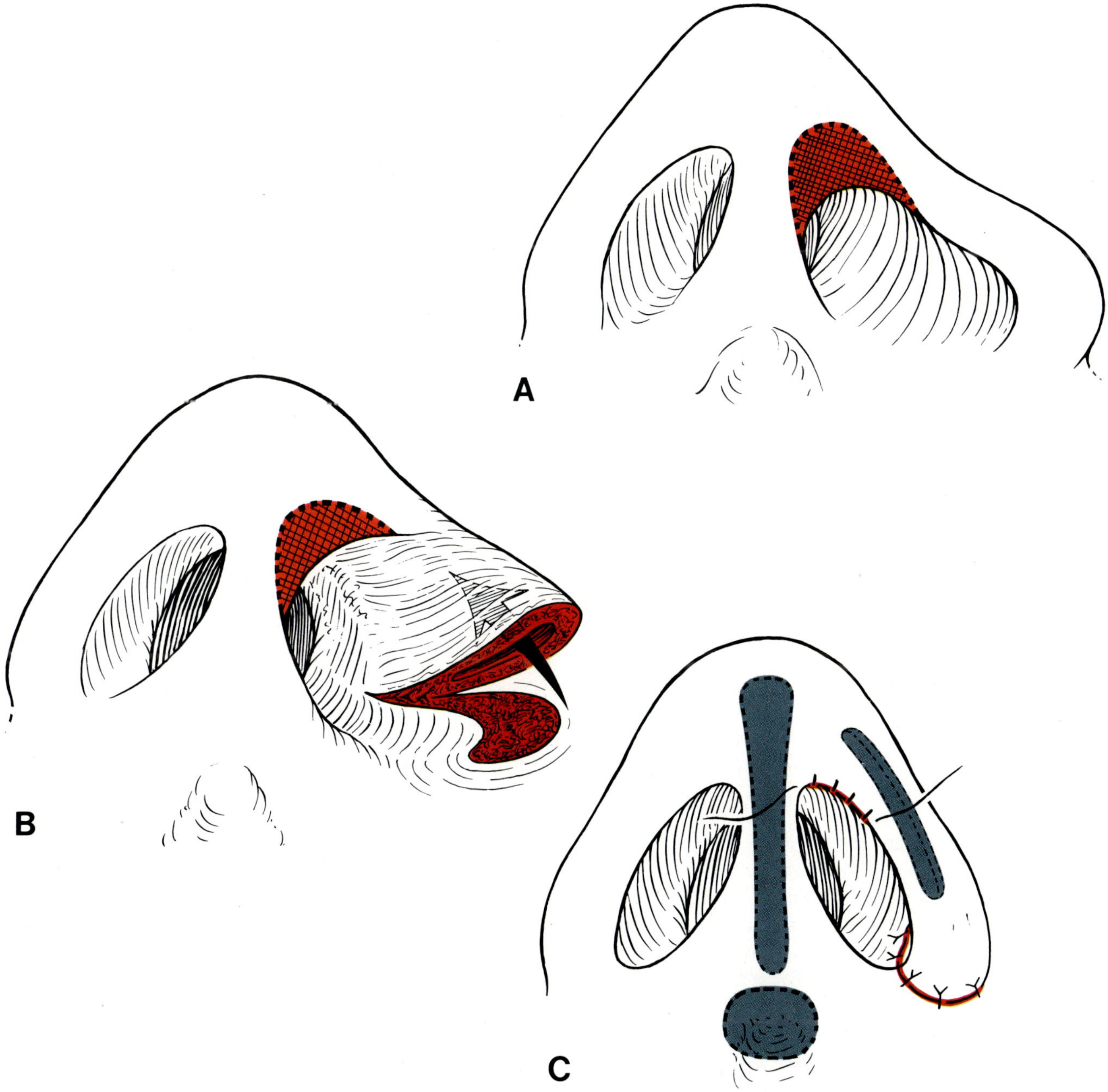

Fig. 267. Correction of unilateral hare lip nose by Fomon. (A) Marginal resection at the lobular-alar commissure outlined. (B) Through an alatomy the cleft side nostril is reinforced with cartilage graft from the septum slightly curved by scoring or morcelizing. (C) Cartilage strut from the septum is inserted into the columella-tip complex and cartilage onlay is placed in front of the spine.

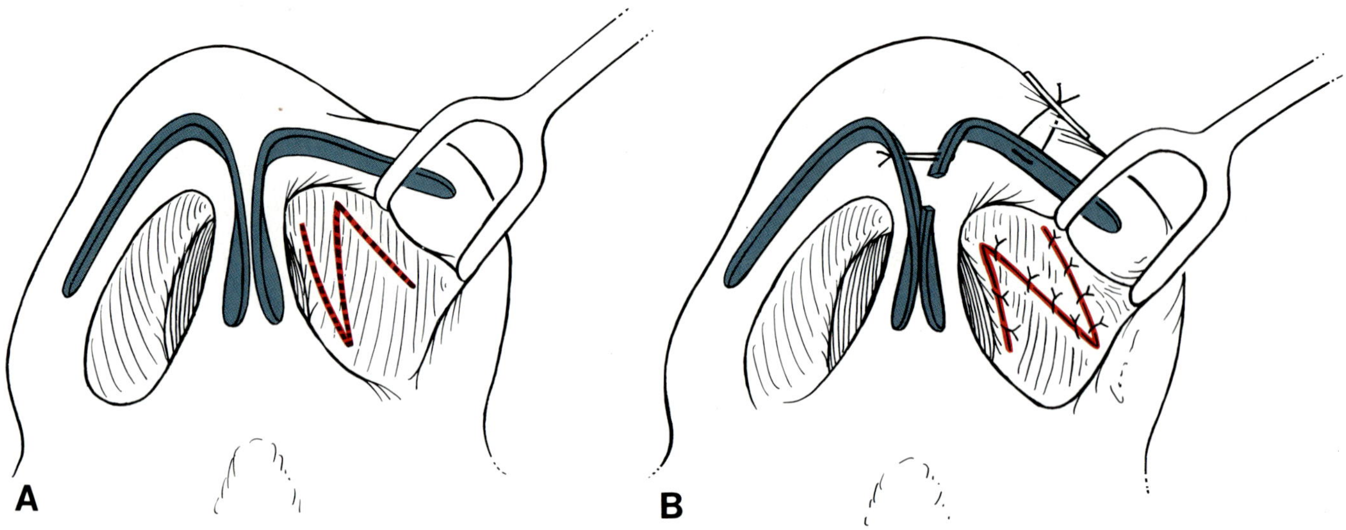

Fig. 268. Correction of collapsing alar folds with a Z-plasty on the inner surface of the ala. (A) The cleft side dome is elevated to the level of the contralateral by section of the medial crus and transalar suture. (B) Suturing of the vestibular skin flaps. The cartilage can be cross-hatched or morcelized.

use in secondary rhinoplasties with stenoses and in cleft noses. It was originally advocated by us for correction of unilateral hare lip nose at the Second Congress on Cleft Palate in Copenhagen in 1973. We presented an example of an extremely scarred unilateral cleft lip nose in a child in whom we undertook to infold the margin, adding an auricular composite graft for extra lining and to support the ala. That case was reproduced by Millard in 1976 in his book *Cleft Craft,* showing a degree of overcorrection as must be achieved, particularly in the growing nose.

Corrections of the alar base have been described by Fomon (1960) and Meyer (Denecke, Meyer, 1964/1967). Another simple and effective technique for shifting and rotating the alar base medially and correcting the nostril was diagrammed by Farrior (1962). To repair the constricted alar base Farrior mobilizes and moves it laterally while the membranous septal skin is advanced inferiorly. A V-Y closure of the floor of the vestibule widens the nostril. Another method to enlarge the vestibular floor in cases of constricted alar bases is to transpose a small paranasal flap into the floor (Meyer 1960, 1961; Farrior, 1962). This was reproduced by Denecke and Meyer (1964/1967). We abandoned this technique and actually prefer the myocutaneous island flap from the alar-facial junction (Fig. 266) (see Chapter 17).

This paranasal island flap, which is transferred into the vestibule through a tunnel under the alar footplate, or by means of an alotomy, can also be extended as a myocutaneous nasolabial flap as diagrammed by Conley, Sachs, and Donovan (1982).

Such a pedicle flap cut in the nasolabial sulcus and swung under the severed alar base into the vestibule has been already published as a two-stage procedure by Rethi in 1959 for treating cicatricial atresia in the nasal vestibule after scar excision. The raw surfaces of the interior of the ala and on the membranous septum are first covered with the skin flap. The latter is left pedicled laterally and is then severed from its pedicle after 3½–4 weeks. This method was reproduced in the book by Denecke-Meyer (1964/1967 and 1964). Subsequently we used this technique as a one-stage procedure with deepithelialization of the pedicle at the base. In 1977, Edgerton and Marsh readvocated the use of the nasolabial flap for fashioning a nasal sill, to restore an acute alar-facial angle, and to enlarge a stenotic nostril in unilateral cleft lip nasal deformities.

This procedure can be refined to create a missing vestibular-nostril sill. To provide vestibular lining in cases of stenosis of the nares we prefer the use of the above mentioned paranasal island flap combined with a composite graft from the auricle.

The depression of the alar base will cause asymmetry that has to be corrected by elevating the alar-facial junction to the level of the normal side through the use of bone or cartilage graft augmentation carried out at the same time as the secondary or tertiary hare lip nose revision.

The maxillary onlays may be taken from the bone or cartilage bank, or harvested from the iliac crest, the rib, and, if available, the nasal hump. It can be inserted through the alotomy, if combined with an extended transfixion incision, or through the gingivolabial sulcus depending on where one wishes to place the onlay and the degree of retraction.

For the correction of the *bilateral harelip nose,* we must take into account the fact that there are numerous patho-anatomic deformities present. We will take into consideration the analyses offered by Huffman and Lierle (1949, 1957) and by Denecke and Meyer (1964/1967). They list:

1. Excessive shortness of the columella.
2. Abnormally laterally displaced angles of the lower lateral cartilages, creating a sharp bend and producing an oblique oval position of both nares.
3. Broadness of the lobule with tendency of bifidity of the tip.

In children we employ the technique of Burian and Millard. Both authors described this flap independently in 1958 (Burian) and also in 1958 (Millard). Two lateral prongs of a fork on either side of the philtrum, rather than one central philtrum flap, are raised, leaving the shield-shaped philtrum intact so that a better cosmetic result is obtained on the lip. The two skin flaps are not turned, but left in their longitudinal position, advanced forward with the columellar skin in the manner of Gensoul (1833), and sutured as columellar skin. The forked flap columellar advancement also affords protrusion to the tip of the nose and offers the opportunity to remove undesirable scarring from the lip. Later on we may refine the lip, accentuating the philtral columns, the concavity of the philtrum, and the line of the cupid's bow.

We have modified this method, outlining a very broad fork in cases with a wide prolabium, thus providing the necessary amount of skin for the formation of a firm columellar base along with obtaining elongation of the columella (Fig. 252). When using Potter's procedure bilaterally, in both adolescents and adults, a philtral flap is cut in the same way as in the unilateral approach and the incision around the columella is extended on both sides into the nasal vestibule. A V-Y advancement is done on both lateral vestibular walls, which elevates the entire vestibular vault bilaterally. The lateral crus of the lower alar cartilage is included in the V-Y advancement bilaterally. We have modified the bilateral technique of Potter much as we did the unilateral technique. The membranous septum and the enclosed medial crura of the lower lateral cartilages are included in the columellar flap, which is to be swung upward (Figs. 269 and 270).

The infolding technique described for unilateral cleft nose is also valuable in bilateral cases. For lengthening the columella in adult cases of bilateral cleft lip nose there are three methods of choice: (1) the forked flap of Burian (1958) and Millard (1958) and modifications (Fig. 252), (2) the basal V-Y technique of Cronin (1983), which has been described in the chapter on nonCaucasian noses (Fig. 113), and (3) the reverse columella-lobule V-Y plasty of Brauer and Foerster (1966).

Cronin (1958) refined and popularized the ingenious principle of Carter (1917), shifting the nasal floor into the columella in a V-Y fashion.

In the procedure of Cronin (1958), bipedicle flaps that are based medially on the columella and laterally on the alae are formed. The two lateral incisions in the groove at the junction of the alae and upper lip join in the midline of the mid or upper part of the columella so that a triangle of skin is left attached to the lip. The inner incision in the vestibule is nearly parallel to the outer incision in order to separate the columella from the septum. The inner incision is continued laterally. This is not required in every case. Thus, the tip of the nose is elevated by advancement of the flaps, which are sutured medially. The columellar elevation also permits correction of the flaring nostrils commonly seen in bilateral clefts.

The reverse V-Y plasty of Brauer and Foerster (1966), which is an extension of the V-Y advancement of the nasal tip by Blair (1925), has been used by many surgeons. It is not a technique we have used in the correction of hare lip noses, but, instead, in cases following tumor excision in the tip region, in particular for cavernous hemangiomas, for which it can be very valuable (*see* Fig. 272). Using this technique, two tapered flaps based on the columella take up the excess skin of the tip-lobule complex along the medial and superior alar rim. The two flaps are

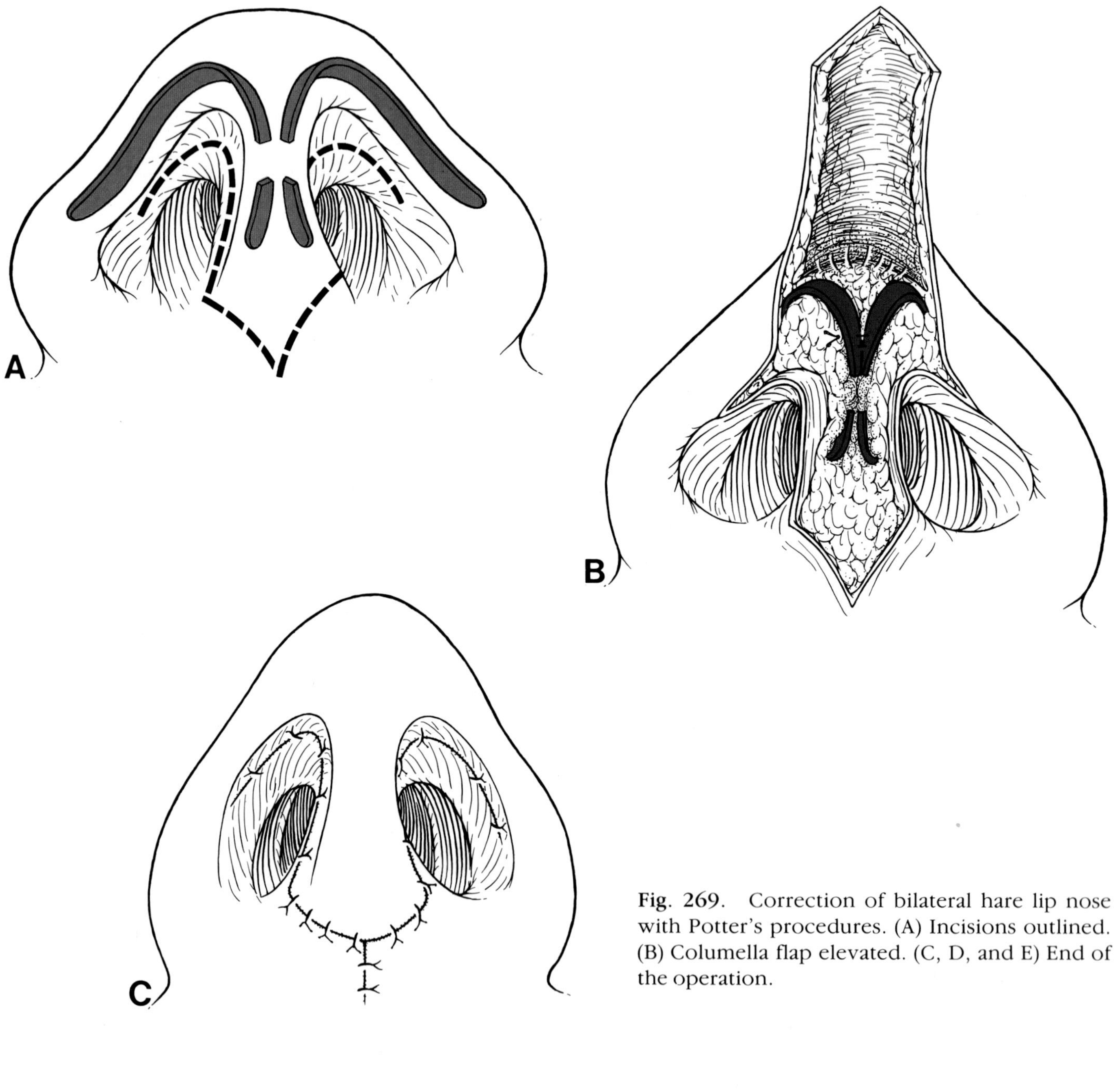

Fig. 269. Correction of bilateral hare lip nose with Potter's procedures. (A) Incisions outlined. (B) Columella flap elevated. (C, D, and E) End of the operation.

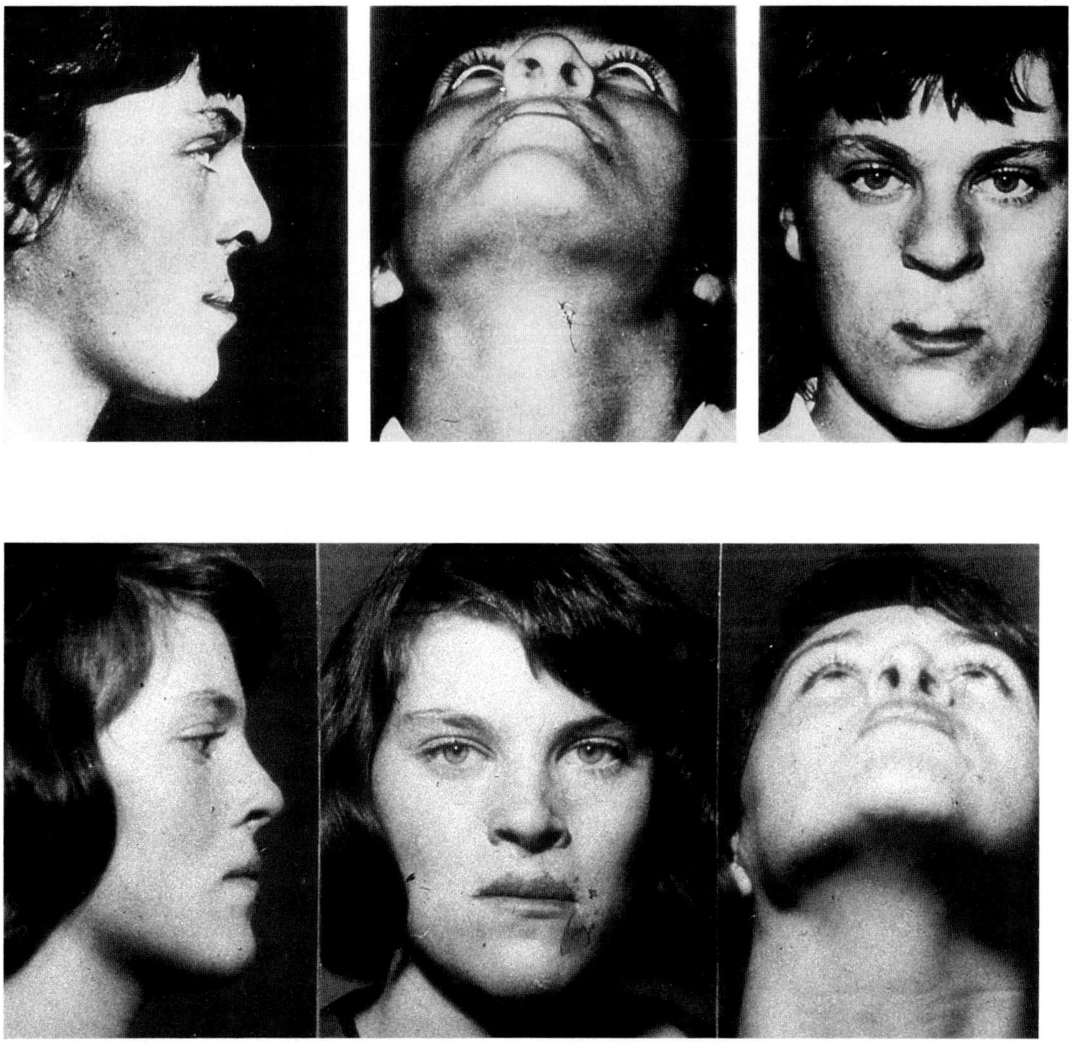

Fig. 270. Young female with bilateral hare-lip nose and excessively long upper lip operated with Potter's technique and reshaping of the vermillon.

brought together in an inverted V-Y suture and elongate the columella. The incision is made through the skin and subcutaneous tissue. Part of the inferior border of the lower lateral cartilage can be included in the flap to give more support.

The soft tissues of the tip are dissected over the upper lateral cartilages to release the tip from its tethered or sagging position. An inner resection at the columella membranous-septum level can reduce the lining, adapting it to the new external surface.

The lobular-columellar skin is closed in a Y-shape, extending into the nostrils, thus forming a longer columella and smaller lobule. Instead of using the excessively broad lobule to elongate the columella, we obtain additional length and simultaneous correction of the nasolabial angle in cases of moderate columellar discrepancy by using a procedure that we have advocated in the book by Denecke and Meyer (1964/1967). It consists of a wide bilateral marginal resection of the Converse soft triangle at the ala-columellar commissure, through-and-through triangular excision of the base of the membranous septum at the transfixion incision area, and cranial displacement of the columellar base in a V-Y fashion.

The overabundance of all these more or less complicated methods and variations on methods shows that the secondary corrective surgery of the cleft lip nose and the cleft lip is quite a difficult one and demands a large amount of experience on the part of the operator, who must be familiar with the many current procedures available. It is important that a combination of methods be applied in order to minimize, if not completely correct, the deformity. Today, in many cases we strive for an attractive appearance while 20 years ago the goal of this secondary surgery was just a normal look.

21

Plastic Procedures in Nasal Tumors

Since it is not within the scope of this work to deal with the reconstructive surgery of the nose, we have limited the topic of repair procedures to septocolumellar reconstruction shown in Chapter 14, dealing with the septum, as well as in Chapter 17, dealing with the reconstructive methods eliminating nasal stenoses often with composite grafts and island flaps for vestibular lining and for repair of alar rim. We showed in Figure 141 a case of septocolumellar tumor in which we repaired the loss of tissue reaching to the middle of the septum using the frontotemporal flap. This is in our opinion the only secure method for such extensive septocolumellar reconstruction achieving a most aesthetic result. For introduction of the compound three-layer flap we have to open the nose by median or lateral rhinotomy (Figs. 141 and 143). In Chapter 17 we have shown another preferred method for subtotal and total nose reconstruction, the Galvao flap (1981). For seven years we have repaired columellar tip defects using a prefabricated forehead island flap.

Procedures for total and partial reconstruction of the nose were only mentioned in cases in which the problem of stenosis had to be discussed. For more information we would refer you to the book by Denecke and Meyer (1964/1967) and to the chapter by Meyer and Kesselring in the book on reconstructive surgery of the nose, *Clinics in Plastic Surgery* (1981).

Concerning the access for the removal of intranasal tumors we want to mention and illustrate the rhinotomy of Bordley and Longmire (1949), which is reproduced in the Denecke and Meyer book. It is particularly effective for cases of ethmoidal tumors extending to the dura, as we have had occasion to deal with in a few cases (Fig. 271). In our extension of this opening procedure, we leave the nasal flap attached only at the lateral osteotomy and the alar facial fold on one side with skin and periosteum as hinge. While septocolumellar tumors are more frequently benign, malignant lesions involving only the nasal septum are an uncommon entity (Weimert, et al, 1978; Beatty, et al, 1982). It is

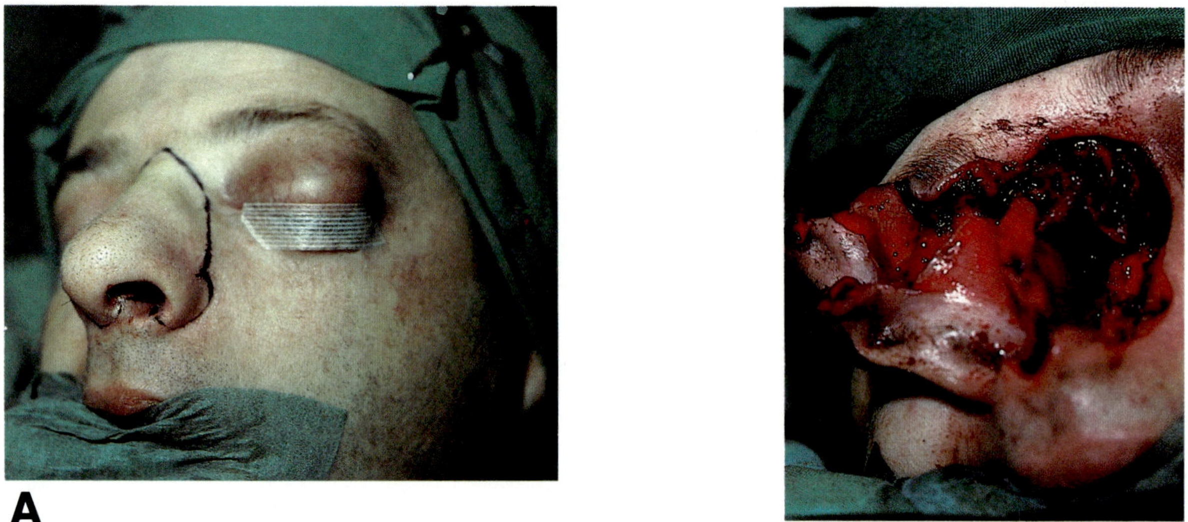

A

B

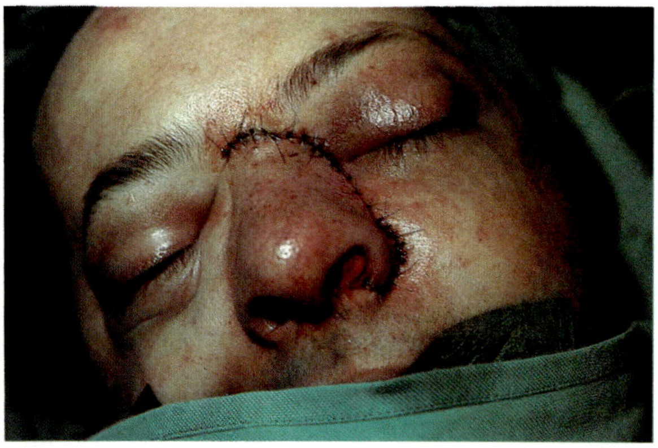

C

Fig. 271. Rhinotomy as maximally extended access for frontoethmoidal tumor surgery. (A) Perinasal incision outlined in a young man with ethmoid carcinoma. (B) Nasal cavities opened for tumor resection in the ethmoidal region. (C) Suture of the nasal flap.

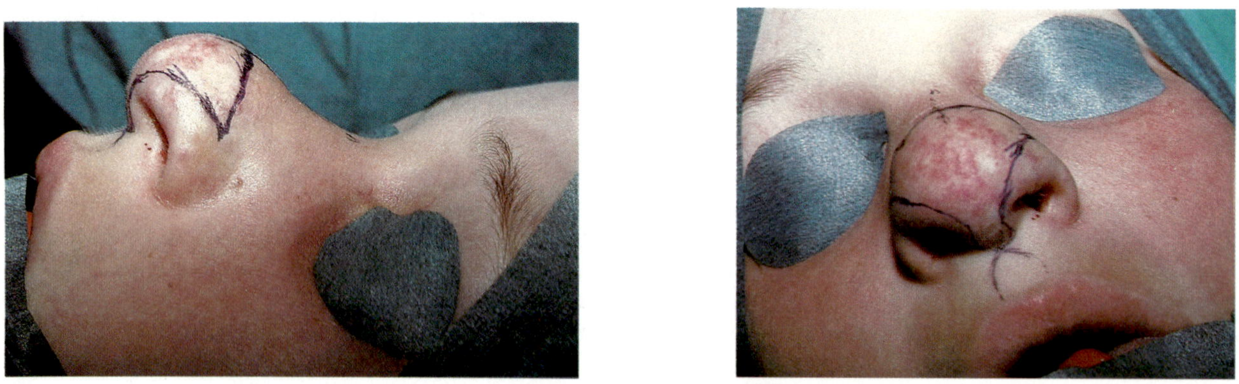

A

B

Fig. 272. Resection of cavernous hemangioma of the nasal tip in a boy. Incisions according to Brauer and Foerster technique. (A and B) Outline of the resection area. (C and D) Y-suture after resection. (E and F) Final result after 1 year.

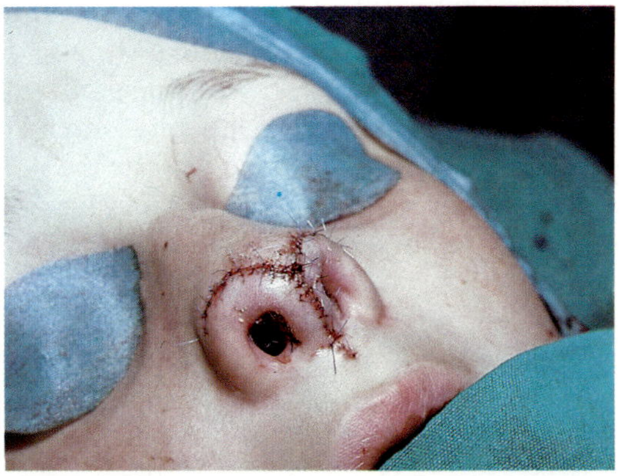

C

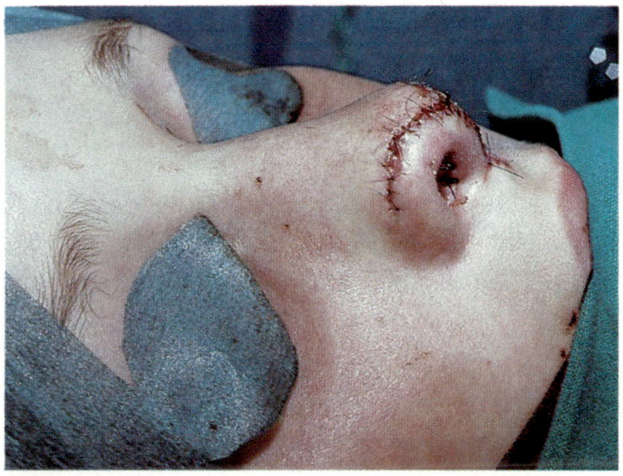

D

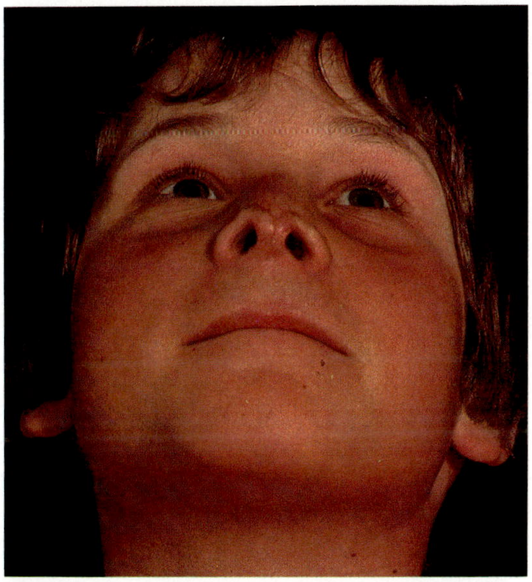

E

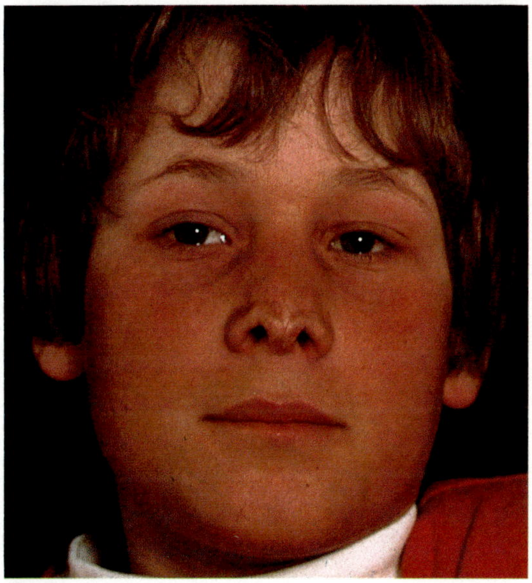

F

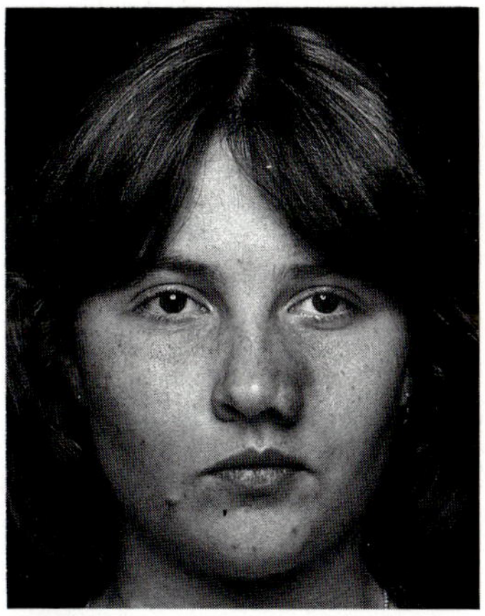

A

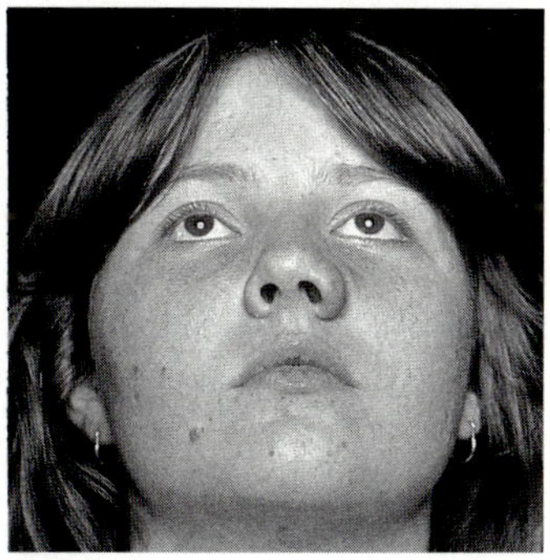

B

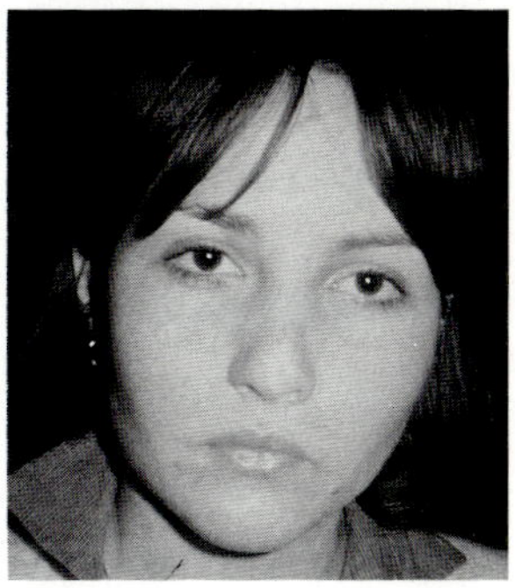

C

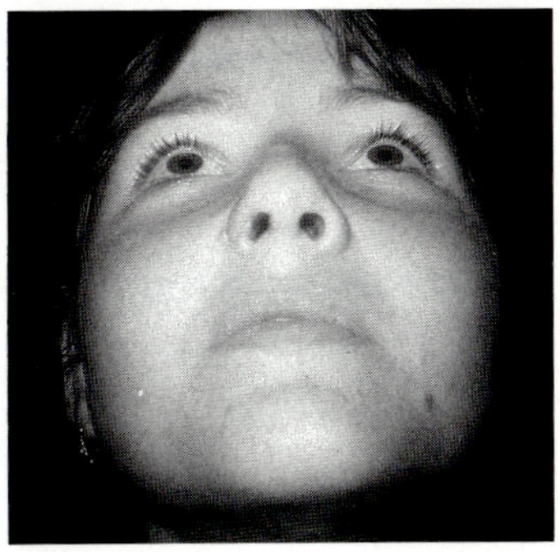

D

Fig. 273. Young girl with cavernous hemangioma of the left ala. (A and B) Preoperative views. (C and D) Result after resection of the hemangioma and remodeling of the nostril.

reported that the total number of cases published is probably no more than 300 (McGuirt and Thompson, 1984; Hasegawa, et al, 1987). Like Hasegawa et al., we performed a bilateral rhinotomy removing the posterior two-thirds of the septum on three of those cases. In two cases, basal cell carcinoma lesion extended to the base of the nasal cavity and the hard palate, which had to be perforated. It was closed by a dental prosthesis after surgery.

An alternative to the open access method to the nasal cavity is the "crossbow" incision and bilateral rhinotomy of Hassard and Holmess (1984), permitting the elevation of an inferiorly based nasal flap and giving a good exposure for tumors involving the nasal and paranasal cavities. For the surgical treatment of nasal hemangiomas, which are usually congenital and located on the nasal tip or in the region of the nasal root, we propose the already mentioned utilization of the method of Brauer and Foerster (1966) with invented V-Y plasty described in the chapter on hare-lip nose (Fig. 272). If the site of the hemangioma is in the nostril, which is very rare, the treatment may be a marginal resection with reduction of the alar width, after excising the layer involved (Fig. 273).

22

Deformities Concerning the Skin

THICK SKIN

Special attention should be given to the type and nature of the skin covering the nose. The thickest skin of the nose is located at the tip and alar regions. Nasal skin thickness varies with age, ethnic and racial characteristics, and sebaceous activity. Increased thickness of nasal skin is predominantly due to an increase in the size and numbers of sebaceous gland and skin appendages. Characteristics of thick nasal skin include an absence of tip definition and alar cartilages highlights, lack of definition of supporting skeletal structures, and a thick appearance with prominent pores or sebaceous glands. Reduced contractility of the skin is present.

The thick skin over the nasal dorsum and tip can also create problems. This skin does not always adapt readily to the newly modeled bony and cartilaginous structures. It just is not elastic enough to adapt completely to a new shape, especially in the tip region. Sometimes fat, spongy tissue adapts particularly poorly over the nasal tip.

Our experience with aesthetic rhinoplasty in these patients has been encouraging and has shown that a predictable and satisfying result can be achieved without calling on unusual external dorsal or supratip incisions. Marginal alar resections and alar base as well as columellar base and rim resections are all that are required. If one has to reduce a very large, thick, and long nose with spongy skin, one must clearly inform the patient that a later correction may be necessary.

Information regarding rhinoplasty in patients with thick nasal skin consists essentially of warnings that less dramatic and predictable results will be achieved or that unusual approaches may be necessary. With this type of skin one is advised to tell the patient that the reduction operation may have to be repeated or at least secondarily completed by refinement. This must be thoroughly explained to the patient. One may encounter conditions in the skin such as dilated nasal capillaries of which the patient is not aware.

Meticulous defatting and subcutaneous excision of excess soft tissue, combined with adequate skeletal reduction is very important. As mentioned, modification of the tip is facilitated by the use of alar base and nostril floor resections. In cases as these, one sometimes tries to press the nasal skin into a new shape and to retain it there by tightly packing the nasal vestibules, applying a firm adhesive tape dressing and plaster cast for 2 weeks (see Fig. 52). When this is done there is a danger of producing small ischemic ulcers caused by the external pressure of the dressing on the alae and nasal tip. These ulcers are usually not dangerous since they almost always disappear after a few weeks without leaving visible scars. Treatment with hydrocortisone ointment is required. A small circumscribed area of skin necrosis can also occur in the region of the medially repositioned nasal bones after correction of the wide and hump nose. The location of such an area of necrosis may remain visible for years because of a slight bluish discoloration. Thus, the excessive pressure exerted by dressings should be avoided, whether it is of plaster, metal, or stents.

The skin of a thick sebaceous nose makes it difficult for the surgeon to produce a neat profile with definition of the tip. For thinning the skin in such fat noses Gonzales-Ulloa (1984) proposes elimination of the excessively thick tissue through a bilateral vertical resection at the height of the redundant skin.

We try to perform the whole reduction subcutaneously from inside the nose and only in exceptional cases do we add a horizontal skin excision in the supratip area. The scarred, fibrous subcutaneous tissue encountered in secondary cases interferes with the elasticity of the skin and makes the remodeling of the dorsum, tip, and alar skin more difficult, especially when the nose has to be elongated.

A shiny dorsum following surgery is almost never improved by dermabrasion, as is erroneously thought. The patient complaining of a shiny nose usually has very thick overly sebaceous nasal skin that is best treated by a good dermatologist and through the skillful use of cosmetics.

Klatsky and Manson (1983) suggest a special preoperative skin preparation. All facial acne and sebaceous hyperactivity must be controlled preoperatively. Their program consists of cleansing the face several times daily with the hands and a mild soap. The use of abrasive soaps and wash cloths is avoided as they traumatize the skin and contribute to sebaceous plugging and infection. Cleansing is followed by hot and cold clear water rinses. Oral tetracycline may be helpful.

In all cases of thick skin we maintain splinting for 2 weeks. The first plaster of Paris remains in place for 1 week. A second one is then applied for 1 additional week. In many cases, a Xomed (Jacksonville, FL) external nasal splint is applied for 2 or 3 more weeks covering overlapping tapes until there are no signs of edema (see Chapter 23).

FURROWS AND DIMPLES

Unsupported soft tissues contract and then they thicken. Such contractions and uncontrolled soft-tissue changes are among the causes of the unpredictability and often unsatisfactory results obtained following secondary rhinoplasty. Such dimples, furrows, and contours are then encountered as tertiary deformities. They were addressed by Constantian (1984, 1985) in his work relating to the creation of nasal planes, and refinements in primary and secondary rhinoplasty.

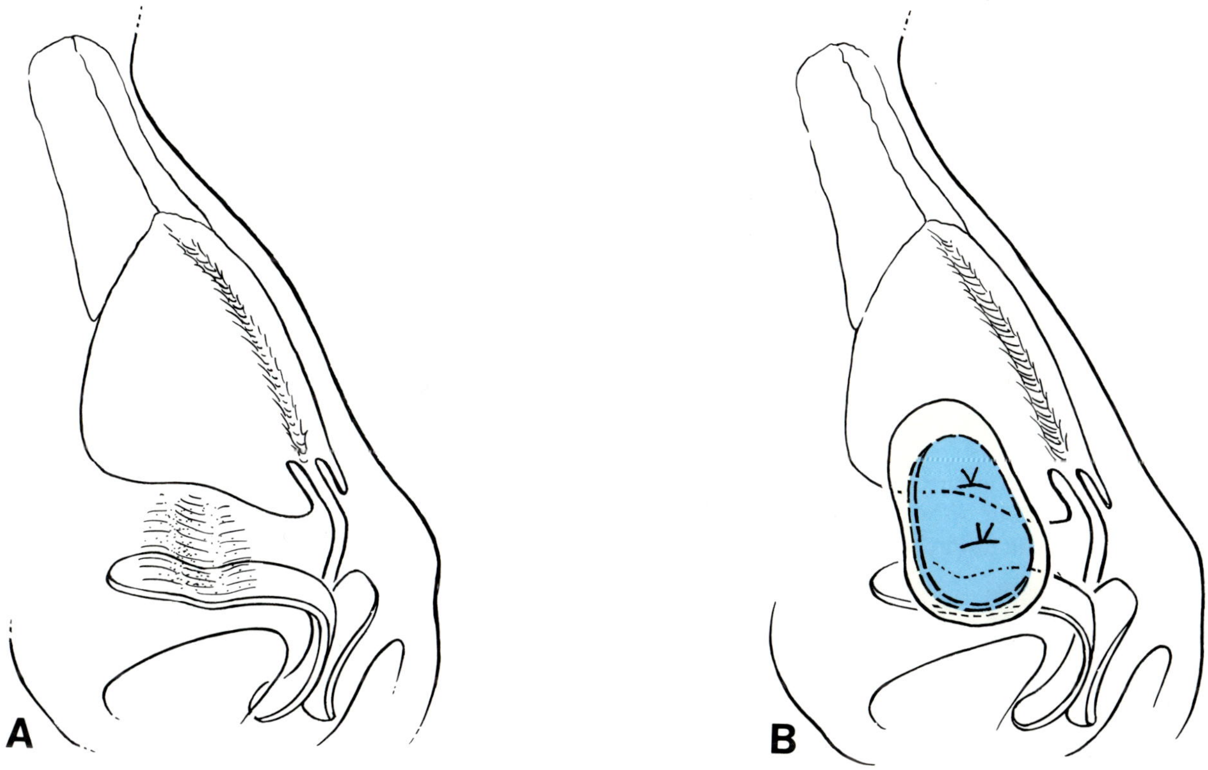

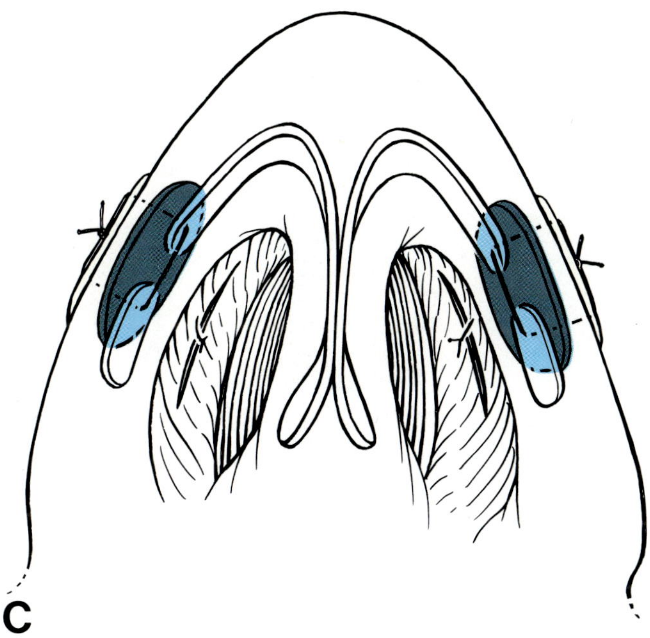

Fig. 274. Correction of iatrogenic furrow in the nasal skin. (A) Dorsal and alar area of furrow. (B and C) Subcutaneous placement of cartilage from the cephalic part of the lower lateral cartilage. Sutures tied over plastic sheets.

It is important for the surgeon to judge how the tissues will conform to a reduced skeletal framework. Sometimes the reduction of the skeleton must be limited because of the poor character of a skin sleeve, which tends to contract and distort the nose if the supporting bony and cartilaginous skeleton is over-reduced. In these cases it may be necessary to plan a two-stage reduction rhinoplasty. Furrows are treated by undermining the depression, filling out the loss of tissue with dermis, fascia, or a slice of cartilage, and by removing the excessive tissue in the immediate adjacent skin fold (Figs. 274–276). In a few cases we obtained satisfactory results with an adequate dermabrasion (Fig. 278) like Ortiz-Monasterio (1974). Similar solutions are provided for dimples and other contour imperfections occurring after excessive subcutaneous defatting in the alar and supratip areas (Figs. 278–280).

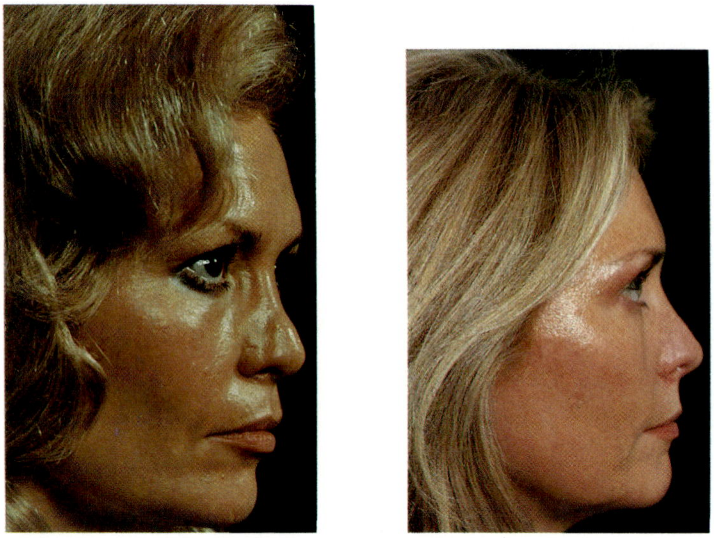

A B

Fig. 275. A furrow secondary to three rhinoplasties is corrected with the technique shown in Figure 276. (A) Preoperative aspect. (B) Result after revision.

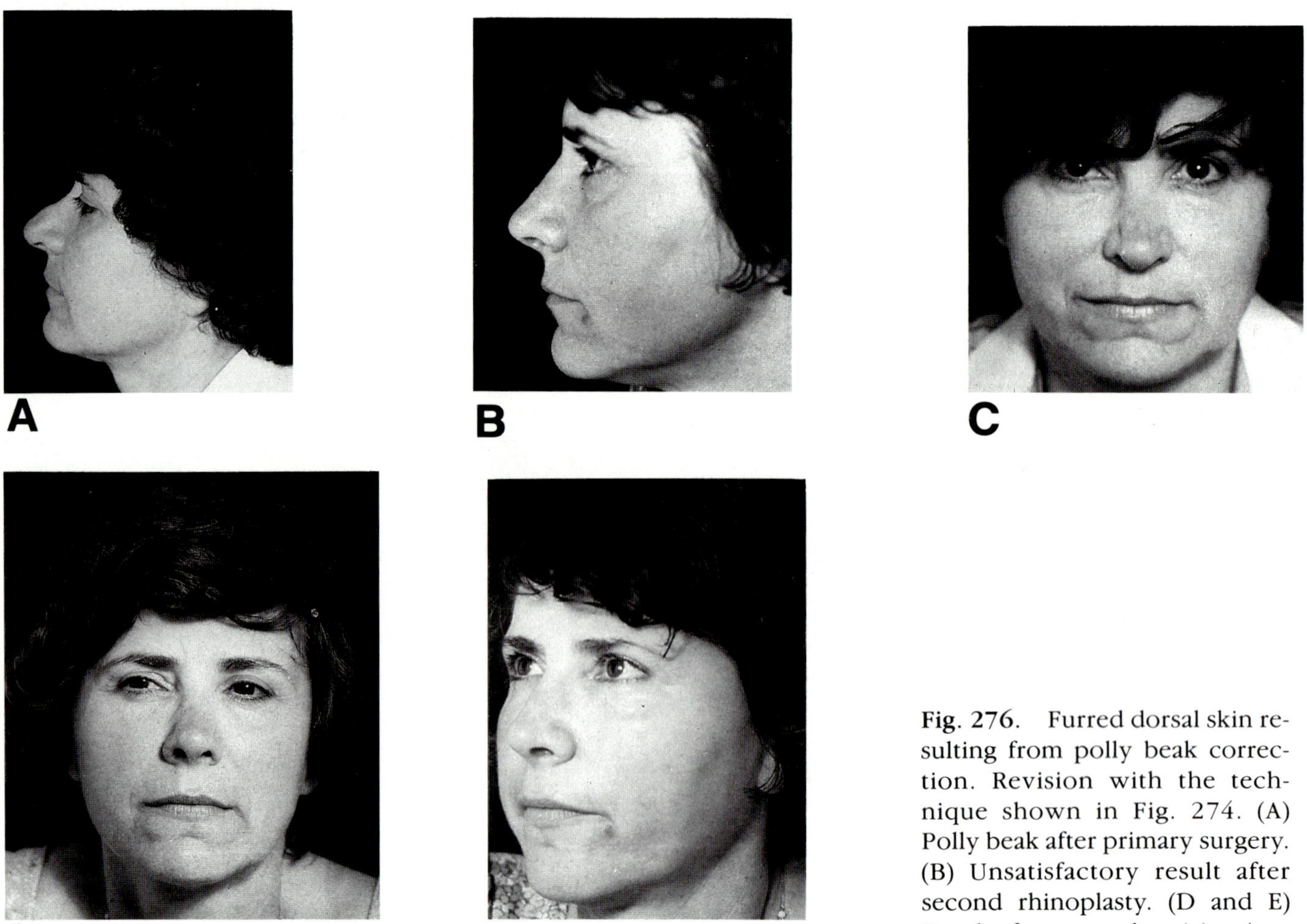

A B C D E

Fig. 276. Furred dorsal skin resulting from polly beak correction. Revision with the technique shown in Fig. 274. (A) Polly beak after primary surgery. (B) Unsatisfactory result after second rhinoplasty. (D and E) Result after second revision (tertiary rhinoplaty).

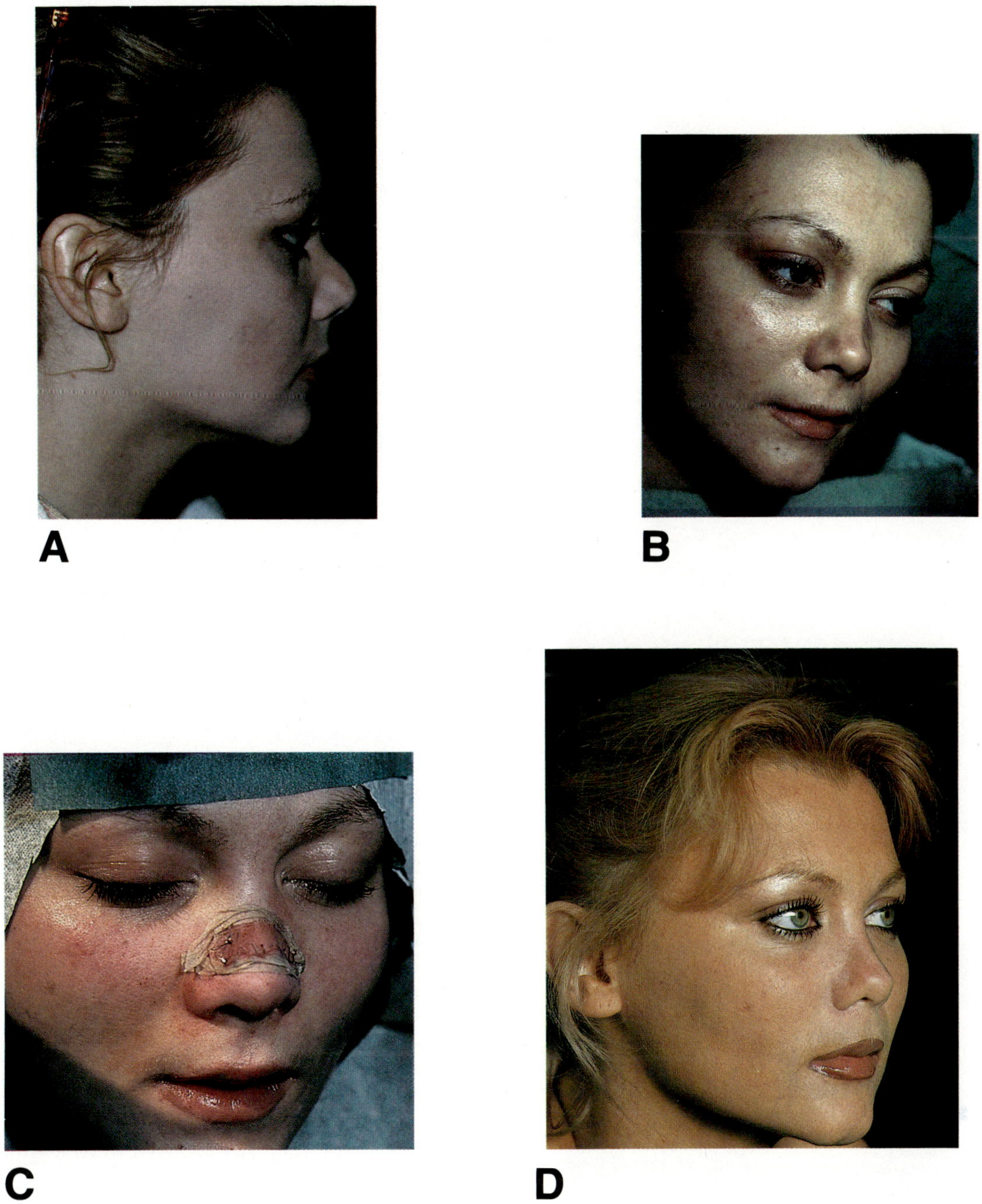

Fig. 277. After correction of a polly beak (A) two furrows occurred at the dorsum of the nose in a young girl. (B) Skin dissection and dermabrasion were sufficient for correcting the furrows. (C) Dermabrasion of the furrowed skin. (D) Final result.

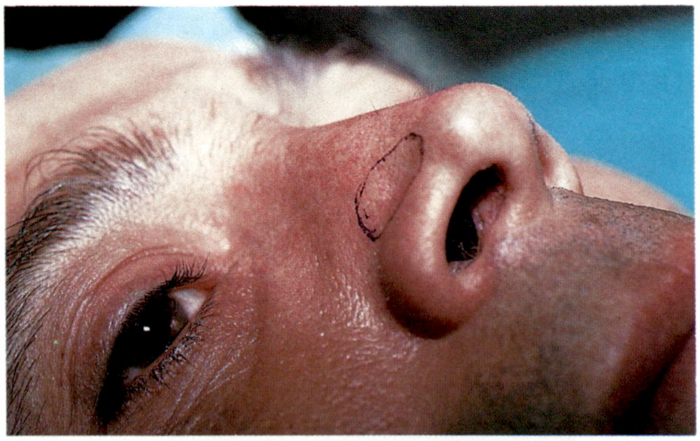

A

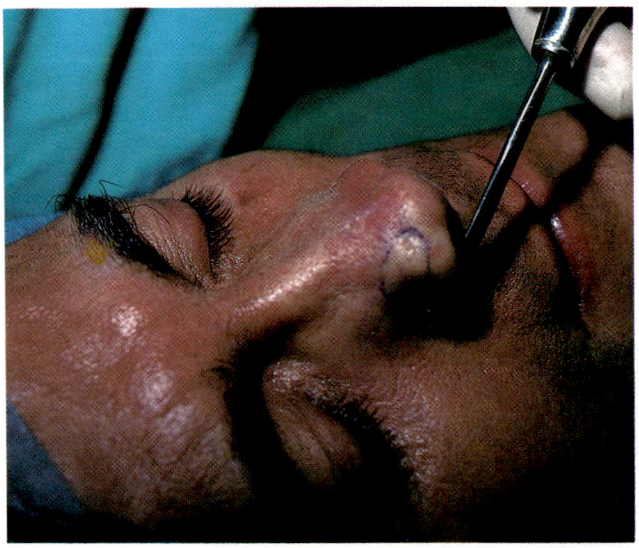

B

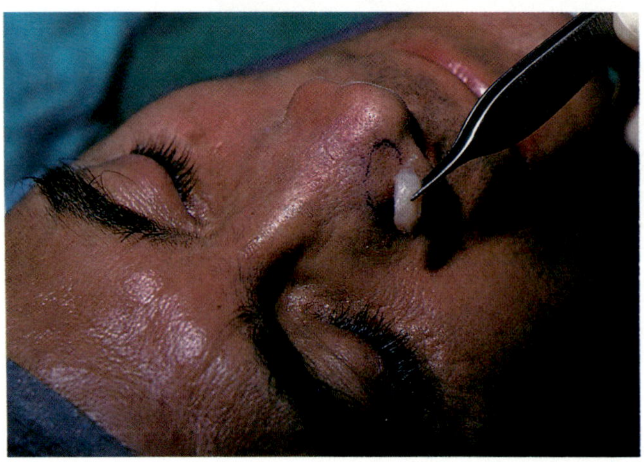

C

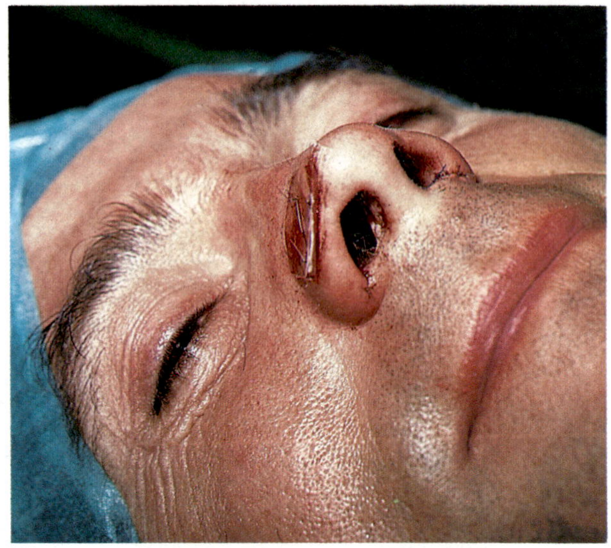

D

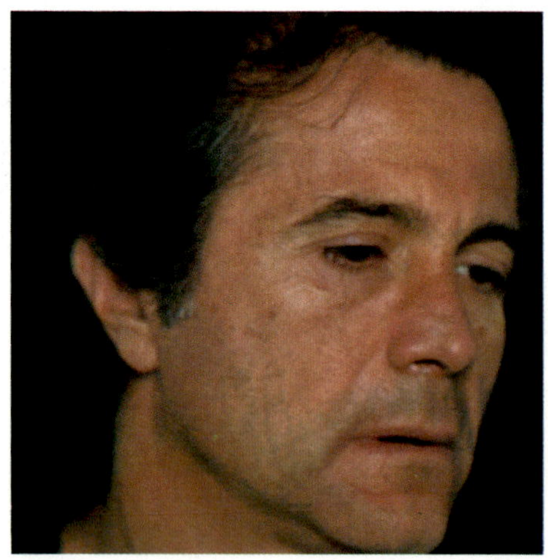

E

Fig. 278. Correction of deep dimple at the alar-nasal crease using cartilage graft. (A) Outline of the depression area. (B) Formation of a subcutaneous pocket from the intercartilaginous incision. (C) Convex cartilage graft from the septum to be inserted subcutaneously. (D) Transalar mattress suture for graft fixation. (E) Result.

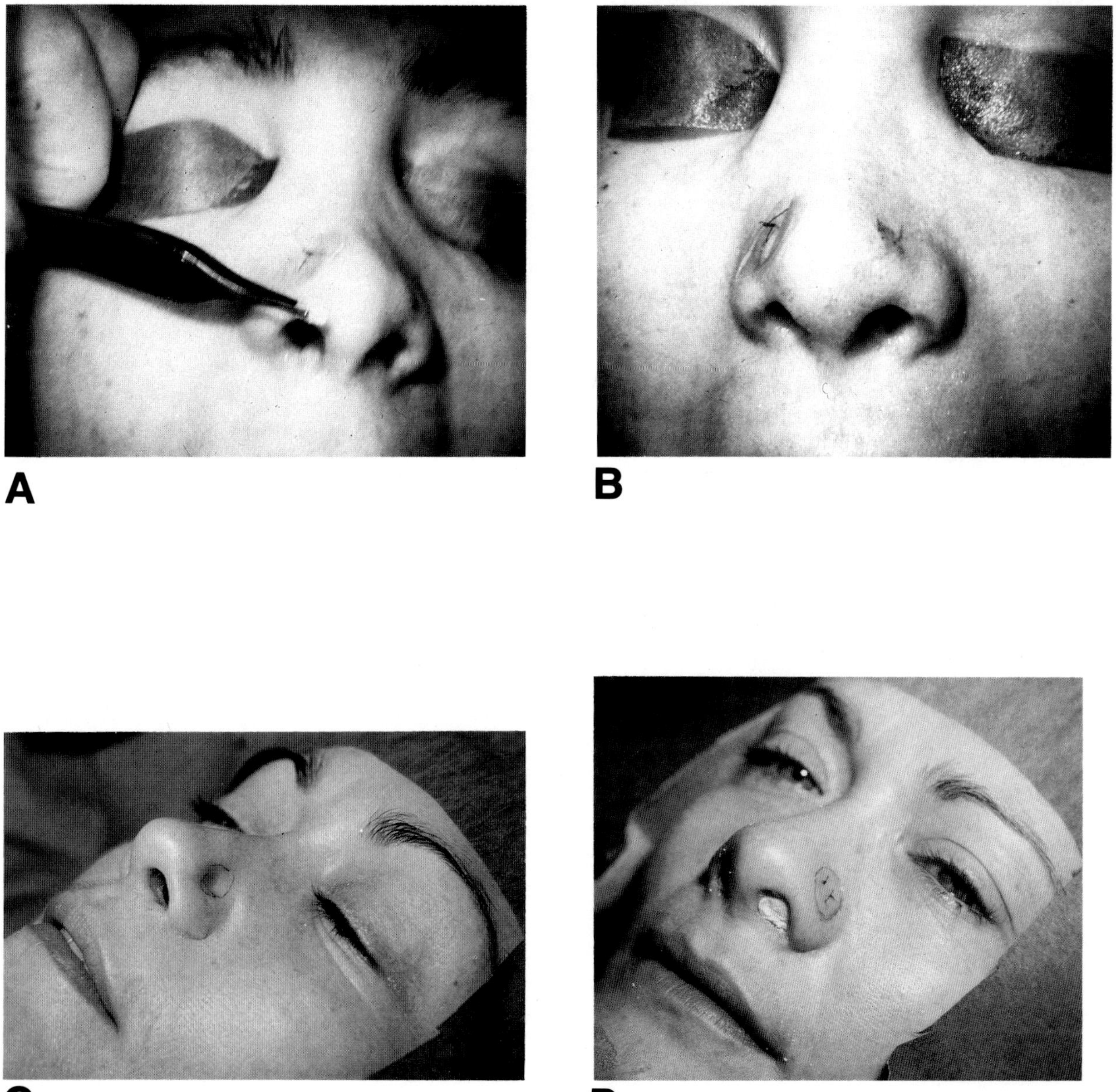

Fig. 279. Deep dimple in tip-alar complex requires filling of the subcutaneous loss of tissue with cartilage grafting. (A) Right side corrected with grafting and transalar mattress suture. A small cartilage graft carved from the septum is ready to be introduced to the left side. (B) Both sides. (C) Other patient presenting dimple in the supra-alar crease before being filled with graft. (D) Graft fixed with transalar mattress suture.

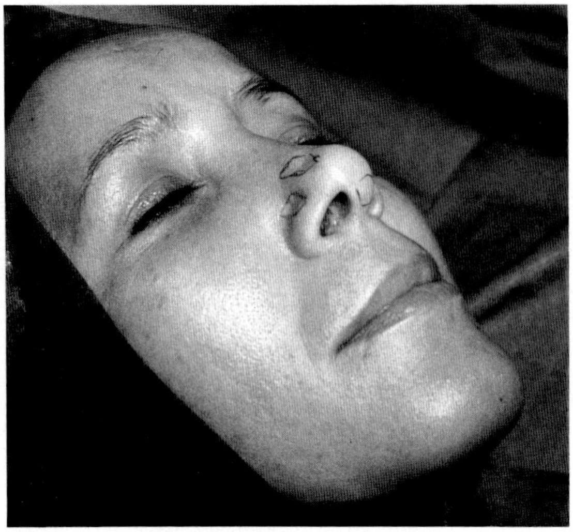

A

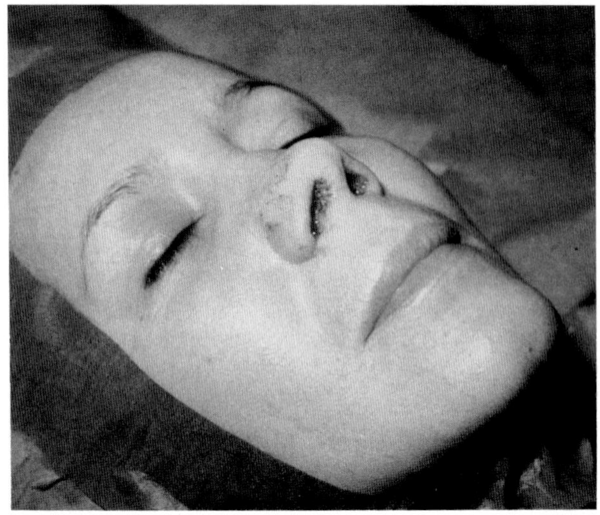

B

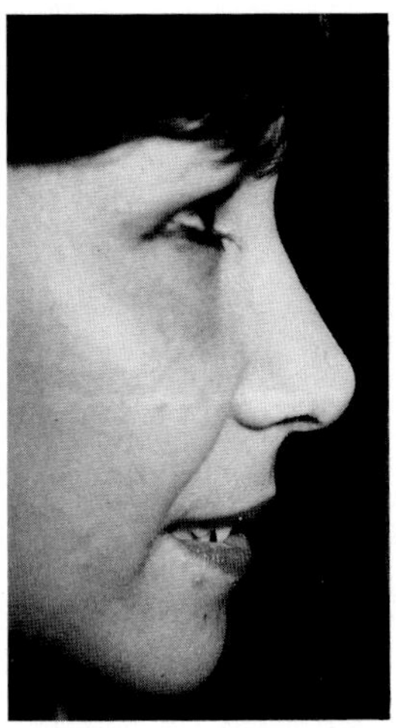

C

Fig. 280. Tip alar complex with irregular facets as result of polly beak correction. The facets have to be undermined again and eventually filled with dermis or fascia and corrected additionally with dermabrasion. In this young lady undermining and careful taping was sufficient. (A) Preoperative outline of the dimples. (B) End of the operation. (C) Late result.

RHINOPHYMA

Rhinophyma is a dermatosis, considered a complication of acne rosacea. This affliction strikes the central part of the face, particularly the nose. Depending on the most prominent tissue component, rhinophymic may be fibroangiomatose or glandullotuberous in nature (Kening and Braun-Falco, 1969).

The characteristic nasal deformity is a consequence of hypertrophy of the sebaceous glands and also of the adjacent fat and connective tissue, due to a chronic inflammation. In addition, we sometimes observe epithelial metaplasia, with an associated higher risk of carcinomatous degeneration, as well as intrafollicular abcesses due to Demodex folliculorum.

The development of rhinophyma occurs over a 5–20-year period under the influence of extrinsic factors, like alcoholism, and also of intrinsic ones such as hereditary factors and endocrine problems. The tuberous, erythroplastic appearance of the nose connotes the diagnosis. Sometimes rhinophyma has to be distinguished from rhinoscleroma, a condition which does not infiltrate the vestibule or the upper lip. Other congenital diseases (hemangioma, lymphangioma, hemartoma), or infections (for instance, leishmaniosis), or autoimmune phenomena (sarcoidosis) can also produce cutaneous nasal deformities.

The treatment of rhinophyma is surgical and consists of excising the pathologic tissue, which permits, in addition, histologic examination of the specimen. The first surgical treatment was performed by Sennert, but he did not describe his operation. Dieffenbach (1845) used elliptical excisions to treat the hypertrophy of the nose in older people. These were composed of a vertical ellipse over the dorsum and the nasal tip, and horizontal ones from each ala. This method was then recommended by von Bruns (1903) and later by Borges (1983).

Langenbeck (1951) and Trendelenburg (1886) preferred to dissect the proliferation from off the cartilaginous nasal structures. Strohmeyer described also the same kind of method, called "decortication du nez"by Ollier (1876) later on.

At the turn of the century another surgical procedure appeared: the extirpation of rhinophyma tissue by Weinlechner (1901), which consisted of the resection of the pathologic tissue using an inverted Y incision. This method was abandoned because of unsatisfactory scarring. This type of intervention was used by Joseph (1928) who described an endonasal method for excision of the rhinophyma, protecting the superficial skin layer and placing it on the intact cartilaginous structures after the excision. A further adaptation of Weinlechner's method was diagrammed by Berson (1948), but useful only for those rhinophymas of minor degree.

After the excision of a large rhinophyma, in order to minimize the skin defect, Joseph additionally reduced the cartilaginous nasal structures by means of horizontal wedge excision of the lower lateral cartilages and of the septal cartilage. To cover the skin defect he rotated a pedicled flap from the region of the glabella, the neighboring cheeks, or a forehead flap.

Ollier (1876) introduced the use of thermocautery, which unfortunately has an attendant high risk of cartilage necrosis. Some others, following Schreus (1955), proposed the reduction of rhinophyma through dermabrasion.

Our choice of treatment is the excision of the rhinophymatous tissue, which permits a histologic examination, followed by some final sculpturing using dermabrasion, followed by split skin grafting. Friedrich (1967) and Nolan (1973) also mentioned cryosurgery as possible treatment.

Recently, the CO_2 laser has completed the list of the instruments available for use. The CO_2 laser method is interesting because it allows for the excision of the pathologic tissue with less bleeding and without compromising the subsequent histologic examination. At the end of the operation using the CO_2 laser, dermabrasion can improve the aesthetic result. There is minimal risk of cartilage necrosis because of its low thermic radiation.

To cover the raw surface of the nose, we can choose from several methods. First, a thin layer of chorion and glandular tissue can be preserved so that reepithelialization may occur. In cases where the entire epithelium is removed, the covering can be provided by a split skin graft or full thickness skin graft. We, like other authors, recommend that to adhere the thin split skin grafts or the intermediate skin grafts, one uses fibrin glue, which works like a seal against bleeding and promotes healing. Staindl (1986) covers the raw surface with a thick layer of fibrin glue. Without skin grafting the viscoelastic fibrin film dries gradually and can be removed after some days like a graft. In most cases subjacent round surface reepithelialized spontaneously. Wound healing is complete within 5–10 days.

For any type of rhinophyma surgery, one must take care that the lower and upper lateral cartilages are not injured. Preserving the perichondrium prevents necrosis and ugly scar retraction in the nose. As a rule, we find no indication for the use of local flaps as propounded by Joseph (1928, 1932) or Sanvenero-Rosselli (1931).

In addition to the rhinophyma excision, we sometimes have had to perform a rhinoplasty. It can be a total one, but in most cases, it is a matter of tip reduction with modeling of the lower lateral cartilages, because of the frequent ptosis of these structures with lack of the tip support. These corrections can be performed through intracartilaginous, infracartilaginous, and transfixion type incisions to reshape the alar cartilages, as well as put a cartilage graft into the columella to improve the tip support, if necessary.

THIN SKIN

The characteristic of skin thickness varies over different areas of the nose and changes with age, which affects its ability to drape properly over a newly shaped framework in some cases. If the skin is very thin with little subcutaneous fat, it will drape itself over the underlying structures so closely after rhinoplasty that even minor irregularities will become evident.

The skin must be handled with care during

surgical interventions to avoid excessive scar tissue formation. Thus it is with thin skin, particularly in the older patient, that the stigmata of rhinoplasty are most conspicuous. If the outlines of the nasal bones and cartilages can be seen and palpated, great care must be taken to avoid too superficial a skin elevation and to ensure that symmetry is achieved in removal of the nasal bones and cartilages with no uneven edges remaining. It is also with thin skin that tethering and teleangiectasia may occur, especially with secondary procedures. As well it is necessary to make sure that no particles of bone or cartilage or foreign body are left under the skin. These may cause a foreign body reaction with concurrent inflammation and discharge.

The skin of the elderly is known to be reduced in elasticity. If, therefore, a large nasal hump is removed in the older patient, wider undermining is advisable otherwise the skin will not assume the new nasal contour. The elasticity of the skin almost invariably allows the skin to shrink, however large the bony or cartilaginous deformity that is removed. In the elderly, however, a transverse crease may remain as a stigma of rhinoplasty. Care must therefore be taken in making radical changes in the nose in those cases and the removal of bone and cartilage should be more conservative.

Postoperatively the very thin skin is likely to become even thinner, especially in the region of the nasal tip, and reveals every irregularity and asymmetry of the underlying structures.

In many secondary and tertiary cases the thinning is thus even more evident. In those cases we have to be careful in excising any segment from the arch of the lower lateral cartilage. If it is necessary, the excision should be done only very sparingly and in the region of the medial crura. The method of Lipsett (1959) is also to be recommended here. In some cases it is sometimes better to do the modeling of the lower lateral cartilage by means of the eversion method rather than with the luxation method, particularly in revision surgery. In this way the lower lateral cartilage remains intact along its caudal border if this is not visible. One must also be very careful when using subcutaneous cartilage grafts if the skin is thin.

As Lenz (1954) has also shown, the tip can change during the weeks following the operation, as well as after several years. Thus, on the basis of experience one must predict what extent of excision is compatible with the consistency of the skin. At the end of the operation the tip should be somewhat shorter than what one actually wants it to be, because postoperative thickening of tissue in the region of the dome is to be considered, this occurring more in secondary than in primary rhinoplasties.

23

Dressings

The favorable result of rhinoplasty depends on the meticulous care of the surgeon during all steps of the intervention, including the application of the nasal dressing. Dressing consists of packing the two nasal fossae and protecting the nasal pyramid with a cast. The endonasal packing essentially maintains the mucosal flap, coapted helping to avoid a hematoma. In addition, the bilateral packing acts through counter pressure to shape and model the nose. There are surgeons who do not use any packing. We utilize fat powder gauze packing, leaving it in the nose for 24 or 48 hours.

In most septorhinoplasties the packing is applied firmly only in the inferior part of the nasal cavities and loosely upward, to avoid moving the realigned bones apart. The nasal vestibule should be completely filled with the packing, so that the alae and nasal tip can be pressed against a relatively firm support by the external dressing in order to achieve the desired size.

Before packing we sometimes insert plastic tubes bilaterally along the nasal floor in order to permit nasal breathing. In cases involving the correction of vestibular and cavity stenoses as well as the repair of septal perforations, in addition to the packing we affix to the septomucosal flap a special silicone sheet, manufactured by Xomed (Jacksonville, FL), which incorporates a tube in its external surface to the septomucosal flap. This can be left in place for 10–14 days. Other manufactured nasal splints are the "Atkins" splint and the Shah splint (both Founton, Somerset, England). Some authors use complementary antibiotic ointment. This is particularly useful in case of mucosal grafting or composite graft application.

We sometimes glue the mucoperichondrial flap to the septum in primary and secondary septorhinoplasties (Meyer and Kesselring, 1981; Rheims, Meyer, and Daverio, 1986). By doing so, Wullstein (1979) even avoids any endonasal packing.

After having sculptured the nose we like to

protect the nose and maintain it in its new shape during the first healing period by using a plaster splint. Just before covering with the plaster, we apply a tight adhesive tape dressing directly to the skin of the nose in order to separate the skin from the plaster, but principally also to accentuate the new shape of the nose during modeling. The adhesive tape strips are placed on the dorsum like roof tiles (Fig. 47E). To those areas of the nasal dorsum lined with cartilage grafts, one wishes to maintain the increased height by means of pressure from the dressing. Then, one applies the strips loosely on the dorsum and tighter above and below the areas of desired prominence. It seems especially important to emphasize the slight supratip depression when applying adhesive tape strip. This is done by pulling the adhesive tape strip tighter at the supratip. A few other strips are applied laterally from one nasal wall to the alar attachment on the opposite side, so that they cross each other over the columella and somewhat depress the medial part of the ala against the resistance of the vestibular packing. In this way, we obtain and maintain the proper form of the nasal tip and can immobilize the second lower lateral cartilages in their new position and shape their curvature.

Like many surgeons, we use in most cases the plaster cast dressing. Others prefer metallic splints or thermo molding synthetic material, such as Aquaplast (WFR/Aquaplast, Ramsey, NJ). We have experimented with all kinds of materials. When using the custom-made Aquaplast splint we have found it somewhat bothersome to soften the material in hot water. A quick and clean way to achieve a desired degree of softness is by heating the splint with a hair dryer or an industrial hot air paint remover (Kesselring, 1986).

Plaster cast dressings adapt well to the new nasal shape, extending from the glabella over the dorsum to the nasal tip. It must be supported to the forehead and cover all the nasal pyramid. In the correction of a deflected nose, the pressure is held slightly more on one side to overcorrect it, while the plaster sets. When it is cool and firm, we fix it in place with adhesive tape strips. Removal of the entire plaster dressing after 1 week or 10 days is recommended, except in cases of a crooked nose or supratip revision, where we change the plaster after 1 week and apply a readjusted one for a second week of time. In the next weeks our external metal and foam splint (Xomed) can be used for reducing the late edema.

References

Abbe R: A new plastic operation for the relief on deformity due to double hare-lip. Med Reg 53:477, 1898

Abdalhady MR, B Ghannamb: Pathological changes of the nasal mucosa after surgical treatment of atrophic rhinitis. Rhinology 19:209, 1981

Abonsheled WH, Moustafa HM: Correction of nasal septal perforation through external rhinoplasty approach. Abstract 13 World Congress Otolaryngology, Miami, 1985, p 112

Aboulker T: La voie d'abord palatine dans les interventions sur les choanes, le cavum et éventuellement la sphénoide. Ann Otolaryng 68:255, 1951

Abramson M, Harker LA: Physiology of the nose. Otolaryngol Clin North Am 6:623, 1973

Aiach G: Intérêt d'une dissection extra-muqueuse dans le traitement de certaines sténoses vestibulaires. Ann Chir Plast Esthet 19:273, 1974

Aiach G: Modifications de l'angle naso-labial au cours des rhinoplasties. Ann Chir Plast Esthet 27:137, 1982

Aiach G, Gomulinski L: Resection contrôlée de la bosse nasale osseuse au niveau de l'angle naso-frontal. Ann Chir Plast Esthet 27:226, 1962

Ainoda N, Yamashita K, Tsukuda S: Velopharyngeal closure function and speech in the submucous cleft palate. Chir Plastica 7:1, 1983

Akyildiz AM: Septoplasty in perforations of the nasal septum. Int Rhinol 7:1, 1983

Almeida DA, Rebello C: Nariz negroide. Rev Bras Cir 63:355, 1973

Almeida Ramos JE, Barbosa VA, Brasil AG Jr: Myocutaneous flap of the nasalis muscle. Rev da Sociedade Brasileira de Cirurgia Plastica 1:1, 1986

Altamar Rios J: Various considerations on juvenile nasopharyngeal angiofibroma. Report of 3 cases. Ann Otorinolaringol Ibero Am 7:467, 1980

Amabile G, Pastorello E, Silva U, et al: Valutazione con rinomanometria anteriore attiva del ciclo nasale in soggetti normali. Otorinolaringologia 34:407, 1984

Anderson JR: Rhinoplasty and the Otolaryngologist. South Med J 53:321, 1960

Anderson JR: The dynamics of rhinoplasty. Proceedings of the Ninth International Congress in Otorhinolaryngology. Excerpta Medica, International Congress Series, Amsterdam: Excerpta Medica, 1969, p 206

Anderson JR: Philosophical considerations in revising cosmetic surgical operations. Otolaryngol Clin North Am 7:57, 1974

Anderson JR: On the selection of patients for rhinoplasty. Otolaryngol Clin North Am 8:685, 1975

Anderson JR: Symposium: The supra-tip in rhinoplasty: A dilemma. Laryngoscope 86:53, 1976

Anderson JR: A reasoned approach to nasal base surgery. Arch Otolaryngol 110:349, 1984

Anderson JR, Calvin M, Johnson JR: A self-administered history questionnaire for cosmetic facial surgery candidates. Arch Otolaryngol 104:89, 1978

Anderson JR, Dykes ER: Surgical treatment of rhinophyma. Plast Reconstr Surg 30:397, 1962

Anderson JR, Johnson CM, Adamson P: Open rhinoplasty: An assessment. Head Neck Surg 90:272, 1982

Anderson JR, Ries WR: Rhinoplasty the external approach. The American Academy of Facial Plastic and Reconstructive Surgery: Georg Thieme Verlag, New York, 1986

Anderson RG, Shanon DN, Schaefer SD, et al: A surgical alter-

native to internal maxillary artery ligation for posterior epistaxis. Otolaryngol Head Neck Surg 92:427, 1984
Anderson JR, Sprinkle PM, Bouquot J, et al: Complication of septorhinoplasty. Benign or malignant? Arch Otolaryngol 109:489, 1983
Anderson JR, Willett M: How to do it—Head and neck and plastic surgery. Laryngoscope 94:1115, 1984
Andra A, Hartel J, Stohring M: Einfluss von operationsverfahren beim verschluss einseitiger lippenspalten auf form und stellung der äussern nase. Zahn Mund Kieferheilkd 73:358, 1985
Andrews EB: Island flaps in facial reconstruction. Plast Reconstr Surg 44:49, 1969
Antia NH, Daver BH, Budi VI: Prefabricated silicone nasal implants. Plast Reconstr Surg 52:264, 1973
Arbour P, Bilgen E: Understanding airodynamic in the correction of the narrow nose. Rhinology 24:41, 1986
Arena S: The posterior scalping flap. Laryngoscope 87:98, 1977
Arons MJ: The application of the cantilever bridge principle to silastic nasal support: A preliminary report. Br J Plast Surg 33:404, 1980
Arons MJ: Dr. Frank McDowell on grafts to the nose. Plast Reconstr Surg 70:118, 1982
Asch M: A new operation for deviation of the nasal septum. Trans Am Laryngol Assoc New York, 1891
Ashley FC: Primary and secondary correction of the nasal tip, in Millard DR (ed): Symposium on Corrective Rhinoplasty, vol. 13. St. Louis, 1976
Aston SJ, Guy CL: The nasal spine. Clin Plast Surg 4:153, 1977
Aubone JC: Tratamiento immediato de las perforaciones quirurgicas del septum nasal. Rev Med Arg 10:669, 1937
Aubry M, Garez J: La chirurgie correctrice des perforations de cloison. Les Annales d'Otolaryngol 75:1, 1958
Aubry M, Giraud JC: Chirurgie fonctionnelle et restauratrice du nez. Paris, Arnette, 1956
Aubry M, Jost G: Malformation du squelette du nez. Encycl Med Chir, Paris, Flammarion, 20315 A. 1963, p 20
Aufricht G: Combined nasal plastic and chin plastic. Amer J Surg 25:292, 1934
Aufricht G: Dental moulding compound cast and adhesive strapping in rhinoplasty. Arch Otolaryngol 32:333, 1940
Aufricht G: A few hints and surgical details in rhinoplasty. Laryngoscope 53:317, 1943
Aufricht G: History of plastic surgery in U.S.A. Transactions of American Society of Plastic and Reconstructive Surgery, 13th annual meeting. New Orleans, 1944
Aufricht G: Surgery of the radix and the bony nose: Preliminary report of a new type of nasal clamp. Plast Reconstr Surg 22:315, 1958
Aufricht G: Symposium on corrective rhinoplasty. Plast Reconstr Surg 28:241, 1961
Aufricht G: Rhinoplasty and the face. Plast Reconstr Surg 43:219, 1969
Austin HW: The lip lift. Plast Reconstr Surg 77:990, 1986
Avelar JM: Personal contribution for the surgical treatment of negroid noses. Aesthetic Plast Surg 1:81, 1976
Avelar JM: The negroid nose. VIII Congress of the International Society of Aesthetic Plastic Surgery. Madrid, Spain, 1985
Avelar JM, Psillakis JM, Viterbo F: Use of large composite grafts in the reconstruction of deformities of the nose and ear. Br J Plast Surg 37:55, 1984
Baarsma EA: External septo-rhinoplasty. Arch Otorhinolaryngol 224:169, 1979
Bachmann W: The present status of rhinomanometry. Int Rhinology 14:5, 1976
Bachmann W: Die Funktionsdiagnostik der behinderten Nasenatmung. Springer-Verlag, Berlin, Heidelberg, New York, 1982
Bachmann W: Klinische Funktionsdiagnose der behinderten Nasenatmung. HNO Berlin 31:320, 1983
Baiocchi R, Biagioli M, Fimiani M, et al: La nostra esperienza nel trattamento del rinofima. Riv Ital Chir Plast 17:137, 1985
Bajaj PS, Bailey BN: Stenosis of the nostrils. B J Plast Surg 22:269, 1969
Baker DC: Chapter Physiology in Aesthetic Plastic Surgery. Philadelphia, W.B. Saunders, 1980
Baker DC, Strauss RB: Intranasal injections of long acting corticoids. Ann Otol Rhinol 71:525, 1962
Baker DG, Strauss RB: The physiologic treatment of nasal obstruction. Clin Plast Surg 4:121, 1977
Baker SR: Management of nasal cutaneous malignant neoplasms. An interdisciplinary approach. Arch Otolaryngol 109:473, 1983
Baker TJ: Patient selection and psychological evaluation. Plast Surg 5:3, 1978
Ballenger WL: The submucous resection of the septum. Laryngoscope 16:265, 1905
Ballenger WL: Diseases of the Nose, Throat and Ear. London, Kimpton, 1943
Bames HO: Elective rhinoplasty. Plast Reconstr Surg 8:113, 1951
Baraglia M, Ungari L, Ponti G: Utilizzazione di un lembo dorsale della mano nella ricostruzione della punta del naso. Valsalva 58:221, 1982
Barbosa JF: Surgical Treatment of Head and Neck Tumors. New York, Grune & Stratton, 1974
Bardenheuer 1892. Quoted by J Owsley, 1966
Barsky AJ: Moulded bone graft. Surgery 18:755, 1945
Barsky AJ: Principles and Practice of Plastic Surgery. Baltimore, Williams & Wilkins, 1950
Barton RT: Use of the Kazanjian rongeur in rhinoplastic surgery. Arch Otolaryngol 55:478, 1952
Baud CA: Harmonie der Gesichtszüge. Basel, Karger, 1982, p 263
Baumgartner P, Hippert F: Behandlungsmöglichkeiten der septumperforation. ORL (Basel) 34:28, 1972
Beatty CW, Pearson BW, Kern EB: Carcinoma of the nasal septum: Experience with 85 cases. Otolaryngol Head Neck Surg 90:90, 1982
Beck JC: Pathology and intramural electrocoagulation of inferior turbinate. Ann Otol Rhinol Laryngol 39:349, 1930
Becker OJ: Aids in rhinoplastic procedures. Ann Otolaryngol 55:562, 1946
Becker OJ: Problems of septum in rhinoplastic surgery. Arch Otolaryngol 53:622, 1951
Becker OJ: Principles of otolaryngologic plastic surgery. Am Acad Ophthalmol Otolaryngol 1952
Becker OJ, Converse JM, Peer LA: Implants in nasal plastic surgery: A panel discussion. Trans Am Acad Ophthalmol Otolaryngol 55:522, 1955
Becker OJ: La correction du tiers inférieur du nez dans la chirurgie rhinoplastique. Semin Hôp Ann Chir Plast 2:119, 1957
Becker OJ: Plastic surgery of the nose. Am J Med Sci 240:499, 1960

Beekhuis GJ: Silicone rubber implants in nasal reconstructive surgery. Laryngoscope 74:1405, 1964
Beekhuis GJ: Nasal septoplasty. Otolaryngol Clin North Am 6:693, 1973
Beekhuis GJ: Saddle nose deformity: Etiology, prevention and treatment; augmentation rhinoplasty with polyamide. Laryngoscope 84:2, 1974
Beekhuis GJ: Nasal obstruction after rhinoplasty: Etiology and techniques for correction. Laryngoscope 86:540, 1976
Beekhuis GJ: Silastic alar-columella prothesis in conjunction with rhinoplasty. Arch Otolaryngol 108:429, 1982
Beekhuis GJ: Augmentation mentoplasty with polyamide mesh. Arch Otolaryngol 110:364, 1984
Beekhuis GJ, Federson MS: Anesthesia for facial cosmetic surgery, in Bernstein L (ed): Plastic and Reconstructive Surgery of the Head and Neck, 1981, p 220
Beheri GE: Rhinoplasty in Egyptians. Aesthetic Plast Surg 8:145, 1984
Beinfield HH: Surgery for bilateral bony atresia of the posterior nares in the newborn. Arch Otolaryngol 70:1, 1959
Belifante LS: Total treatment planning for esthetic problems of the face: A team approach. J Oral Surg 37:178, 1979
Bell RC: A surgeon of Pompei. Br J Plast Surg 177:1960
Bennett JP: Sandwich pushback and lateral pharyngoplasty. Br J Plast Surg 26:16, 1973
Berdel D, et al: Comparison of active foreign flow rhinomanometric (oscillation method) and active personal flow rhinomanometry in 17 patients before and after correction of the nasal septum. Arch Otolaryngol 237:115, 1983
Berendes J: Kosmetisch schonendes Operationsverfahren bei angeborener Fistel des Nasenrückens. Arch Ohr Nas u Kehlk-Heilk 180:784, 1962
Berghaus A: Porous polyethylene in reconstructive head and neck surgery. Arch Otolaryngol 111:154, 1985
Berman WE: Surgery of the nasal tip. Otolaryngol Clin North Am 8:563, 1975
Berman WE: Rhinoplasty. Edited by the American Academy of Otolaryngology, 1980
Berndorfer A: Die Aesthetik der Nase. Vienna, Maudrich, 1949
Berndorfer A: Importance of physiognomy in esthetic rhinoplasty. Plast Reconstr Surg 6:242, 1950
Bernstein D: Homologous nasal hump implant. Arch Otolaryngol 98:385, 1973
Bernstein D: Homologous nasal hump implant: Follow-up studies. Plastic and Reconstructive Surgery of the Face and Neck. Proceedings of the Second International Symposium, vol. 1. New York, Grune & Stratton, 1977
Bernstein D: The present status of the homologous nasal hump graft. Ear Nose Throat J 62:37, 1983
Bernstein L: Submucous operations on the nasal septum. Otolaryngol Clin North Am 6:675, 1973
Bernstein L: Applied anatomy in corrective rhinoplasty. Arch Otolaryngol 99:67, 1974
Bernstein L: Rhinoplasty for the negroid nose. Otolaryngol Clin North Am 8:3, 1975(a)
Bernstein L: Surgical anatomy in rhinoplasty. Otolaryngol Clin North Am 8:549, 1975(b)
Bernstein L: Aesthetics in rhinoplasty. Otolaryngol Clin North Am 8:705, 1975(c)
Berson MI: Prevention of deformities in corrective rhinoplasty. Laryngoscope 53:276, 1943
Berson MI: Atlas of Plastic Surgery. London, William Heinemann, 1948
Berson MI: Rhinophyma. Plast Reconstr Surg 3:745, 1945
Betzel F, Schilling H: Über die biologie, konservierung und verpflanzung von knorpelgewebe. Zentralbl Chir 21:1170, 1960
Bianchi A, Galli S, Ferroni M: Eigene technik zur columellarekonstruktion (personal techniques for columella reconstruction). Laryngoscope 94:1613, 1984
Biasi R: Sulla rontgenterapia del rinofima. Gior Ital Mal Esot Trop 7:16, 1934
Bicknell PG: Gryosurgery for allergic and vasomotor rhinitis. J Laryngol Otol 83:143, 1979
Birrell J: Palatal disproportion in children. J Laryngol Otol 80:706, 1966
Biserni A, Raffaeli M, Filiaci F: Valutazione obiettiva mediante la rinomanometria degli effetti, della correzione chirurgica delle stenosi nasali. Valsalva 60:49, 1984
Bittle RM: Psychiatric evaluation of patients seeking rhinoplasty. Otolaryngol Clin North Am 8:689, 1975
Black PW, Hartrampf CR, Beegle P: Cleft lip type nasal deformity: Definitive repair. Ann Plast Surg 12:128, 1984
Blair VP: Nasal deformities associated with cleft of the lip. JAMA 84:185, 1925
Blair VP, Brown JB: Mirault operation for single hare-lip. Surg Gynecol Obstet 51:81, 1930
Blair VP: Congenital atresia: An obstruction of the nasal air passage. Ann Otol 40:1021, 1931
Bloom SM: The problem of implants in rhinoplasty. Including technique of obtaining iliac crest grafts. Arch Otolaryngol 71:778, 1960
Bloom SM: Rhinoplasty in adolescence. Arch Otolaryngol 92:66, 1970
Bobin S, Manach Y, Contencin P, et al: Imperforation choanale de l'enfant intérêt de la voie transpalatine. Ann Otolaryngol 100:371, 1983
Bockhoff E, Huffstadt AJC: Denonvillier's Z-plasty in reconstruction of alar defect, 1856. Chir Plast 1:192, 289, 1975
Boenninghaus G: Uber die beseitugung schwerer verbiegungen der knorpeligen und knöchnernen nasenscheidewand durch die resection. Archiv Laryngol Rhinol 9:269, 1899
Boenninghaus HG: Ueber mediane epidermoidfisteln undzysten der nase. Z Laryngol Rhinol 34:80, 1955
Boo-Chai K: Augmentation rhinoplasty in the oriental. Plast Reconstr Surg 34:87, 1964
Boo-Chai K: The management of ala ptosis in oriental rhinoplasty. Aesthetic Plast Surg 10:17, 1986
Bordley J, Longmire WP: Rhinotomy for exploration of the nasal passages and the accessory nasal sinuses. Ann Otol 58:1055, 1949
Borges AF: Palatal defect reconstruction with hinged nasal septum flap. Ann Plast Surg 10:167, 1983
Bosse JP: 1986 Personal communication.
Botnick E: Evaluation of surgical techniques on nasal tip projection. Laryngoscope 84:1316, 1974
Botnik E: Maintaining nasal tip projection, in Sisson GA, Tardy EE (eds): Plastic and Reconstructive Surgery of the Face and Neck. New York, Grune & Stratton, 1977
Bouchayer M, Rebattu JP, Escoubes B: Q̄uelques principes de base de la reposition de cloison. J.F.O.R.L. 16:347, 1967

Bozola AR, Cardozo de Oliveira M, Miura O, et al: Uso de retalho miomucoso de musculo buccinato na correçao de fissuras palatinas. Rev de Soc Bras Chir Plast 0:19, 1985

Bozzi E, La Ferla S, d'Alvino A: Chirurgia Funzionale e Ricostruttiva del Naso. Torino, Ed Capella, 1951

Bozzi E, La Ferla S, Meyer R: Trattamento chirurgico dell' ozena. Otorhinolaryngol Ital 28:1, 1959

Bradley SA: The use of silicones in plastic surgery: A retrospective review. Plast Reconstr Surg 51:280, 1973

Brain DJ: Septorhinoplasty: The closure of septal perforations. J Laryngol Otol 94:495, 1980

Brain DJ: The management of the deviated nose. Laryngol Otol 95:471, 1981

Brain DJ, Rock WP: The influence of nasal trauma during childhood on growth of the facial skeleton. J Laryngol 97:917, 1983

Brain DJ: The septum in functional rhinoplasty. Facial Plast Surg 3:4, 236, 1986

Brauer RO: Lengthening the columella. Symposium on management of cleft palate and associated deformities. 8:270, 1974

Brauer RO, Foerster DW: Another method to lengthen the columella in the double cleft patient. Plast Reconstr Surg 38:27, 1966

Breadon GE, Kern EB, Neel HB: Autografts of uncrushed and crushed bone and cartilage. Arch Otolaryngol 105:75, 1979

Brennan HG: Dome-splitting technique in rhinoplasty with overlay of lateral crura. Arch Otolaryngol 109:586, 1983

Brent B: The versatile cartilage autograft: Current trends in clinical transplantation. Clin Plast Surg 6:163, 1979

Brent B, Ott R: Perichondro-cutaneous graft. Plast Reconstr Surg 62:1, 1978

Bridger GP: Physiology of the nasal valve. Trans Am Acad Ophthalmol Otolaryngol 70:183, 1970

Bridger GP: Physiology of the nasal valve. Arch Otolaryngol 107:110, 1981(a)

Bridger GP: Split rib graft for alar collapse. Arch Otolaryngol 107:110, 1981(b)

Broadbent RT, Woolf RM: Anatomy of a rhinoplasty-saw technique. Symp. Aest. Surg. Nose, Ears, Chin. St. Louis, Mosby Comp, 1973

Broadbent RT, Woolf RM: Anatomy of a rhinoplasty-saw technique. Ann Plast Surg 13:67, 1984(a)

Broadbent RT, Woolf RM: Basic Anatomy: Clinical application in rhinoplasty. Ann Plast Surg 13:1, 1984(b)

Broadbent RT, Woolf RM: Cleft lip nasal deformity. Ann Plast Surg 12:216, 1984(c)

Brohms P: Rhinomanometry. Procedures and criteria for distinction between skeletal stenosis and mucosal swelling. Acta Otolaryngol 94:361, 1982

Brohms P, Johnson B, Lamm CJ: Rhinomanometry. A system for numerical description of the nasal airway resistance. Acta Otolaryngol 94:157, 1982

Brown BL, Kern EB: Implants of supramid, proplast, plastipore, and silastic. Arch Otolaryngol 105:605, 1979

Brown JB: Preserved and fresh homotransplants of cartilage. Surg Gynecol Obstet 70:1079, 1940

Brown JB: Preserved and fresh homotransplants of cartilage and isolated chondrocytes. An experimental study in rabbits. J Bone Joint Surg 50:184, 1968

Brown JB, Cannon B: Composite free grafts of skin and cartilage from ear. Surg Gynecol Obstet 82:253, 1946

Brown JB, Demere FM: Establishing a preserved cartilage bank. Plast Reconstr Surg 3:283, 1948

Brown JB, McDowell F: Plastic Surgery of the Nose. St. Louis, C.V. Mosby, 1951

Brown JB, McDowell F: Plastic Surgery of the Nose. London, Kimpton, 1952

Brown JB, McDowell F: Plastic Surgery of the Nose. Springfield, Charles C. Thomas, 1965(a), p 63

Brown JB, McDowell F: Secondary nasal operations. Plastic Surgery of the Nose (ed 2). Springfield, Charles C. Thomas, 1965(b)

Brown JB, McDowell F: Plastic Surgery of the Nose (ed 2). St. Louis, C. V. Mosby, 1967

Bruck HG: Special techniques for problems in rhinoplasty, in Bernstein L (ed): Plastic and Reconstructive Surgery, vol. 1. Aesth Surg, 1981, p 28

Brunk A: Ein neuer fall von einseitigen knöchernen choanalverschluss. Operationsversuch vom gaumen aus. Z Ohrenheilk 59:221, 1909

Brunner H: Fate of autogenous rib cartilage transplanted into nose. Plast Reconstr Surg 4:439, 1949

Buck DL, Brown CM: A longitudinal study of nose growth from ages 6 to 18. Ann Plast Surg 18:310, 1987

Bull TR: Stigmata of rhinoplasty, in Bernstein L (ed): Plastic and Reconstructive Surgery, vol. 1. Aesth Surg, 1981, p 66

Bull TR: Operation on the saddle nose. Laryngol Rhinol Otol 62:201, 1983

Bull TR, Mackay IS: Augmentation rhinoplasty. Facial Plast Surg 1:125, 1984

Bull TR, Mackay IS: Alar Collapse. Facial Plast Surg 3:4, 268, 1986

Burian F: Chirurgie der Lippen-und Gaumenspalten. Berlin, Verlag Volk und Gesundheit, 1963

Burian S: Median clefts of the nose. Indian Med Rec 78:71, 1958

Burke J: Closure of large septal perforations with a labial buccal flap. Plast Reconstr Surg 46:514, 1970

Busca GP, Bussi M, Amasio ME: Possibilitá e limiti delle tecniche di lussazione delle cartilagini alari nella chirurgia della punta del naso. Acta ORL Ital 3:649, 1983

Busca GP, Bussi M, de Vicariis A: L'osteotomia basale secondo il metodo continentale ed anglo-americano. Indicazioni e limiti nella nostra esperienza. Min Stomatol 31:487, 1982

Busca GP, Lambertoni G, Pia F, et al: Ricerche di rinomanmetria elettronica in casi di insufficienza respiratoria nasale. Nuov Arch Ital Otolaryngol 6:435, 1978

Cabouli JL, Guerissi JO, Mileto A, et al: Local infection following aesthetic rhinoplasty. Ann Plast Surg 17:4, 1986

Cabrera Trigo JS, Iapalucci L: Tratamiento de la perforacion del septum nasal por abordaje vestibulo-oral. La Prensa Med Arg 47–31:2152, 1960

Caliceti G: La chirurgia del setto e la sua importanza nelle rinoplastiche. ORL Ital 24:113, 1956

Caliceti P: Trattato di patologia e clinica otorinolaringologica. Bologna, Capelli, 1948

Calnan JS: Permanent nasal escape in speech after adenoidectomy. Br J Plast Surg 24:197, 1971

Cannoni M, Pech A, Tomassin JM, et al: Le traitement chirurgical de l'ensellure nasale. JF Otorhinolaryngol 32:199, 1983

Cantrell RW, Defebre BK: Silicone implants in head and neck reconstructive surgery, in Sisson GA, Tardy EE (eds):

Plastic and Reconstructive Surgery of the Face and Neck. Second International Symposium, vol. 2. New York, Grune & Stratton, 1977

Cardoso AD: Reconstruction of cicatricial nasal retraction after leishmaniasis. Plast Reconstr Surg 7:309, 1951

Cardoso AD: Loss of columella after leishmaniosis reconstruction with subcutaneous tissue pedicle flap. Plast Reconstr Surg 21:117, 1958

Caronni E: Correzione dell'angolo nasolabiale. Riv Ital Chir Plast 4:275, 1972 (a)

Caronni E: A new method to correct the nasolabial angle in rhinoplasty. Plast Reconstr Surg 50:338, 1972 (b)

Carter WW: Transplantation of bone for correction of depressed deformities of the nose with report of cases. Laryngoscope 21:95, 1911

Carter WW: Cases of nasal deformity corrected by transplantation of bone. Med Rec 85:237, 1914

Carter WW: Ann Surg 162, 1917

Carter WW: The value and ultimate fate of bone and cartilage transplants in the correction of nasal deformities. Laryngoscope 33:196, 1923

Cash TF, Horton CE: Aesthetic surgery: Effects of rhinoplasty on the social perception of patients by others. Plast Reconstr Surg 72:349, 543, 1983

Casserius J: Pentaestheseion, p 112. N. Miserinum Venise 1609. Cited by Courtiss, Goldwyn and O'Brien, 1978

Causabon JN, Dion MA, Labrisseau A: Septic cavernous sinus throbosis after rhinoplasty. Plast Reconstr Surg 59:119, 1977

Chalaye JCJM, Levignac J: La réparation des perforations du septum nasal provoquées par la cocaïne (ou le lambeau muqueux en aile de planeur). Ann Chir Plast Esthét 30:229, 1985

Champion R: Reconstruction of the columella. Brit J Plast Surg 12:253, 1959

Champion R: Anosmia associated with corrective rhinoplasty. Br J Plast Surg 19:182, 1966

Champion 1966. Quoted by Rogers, 1976.

Chapnik JS: Current thoughts on implants in rhinoplasty. J Otolaryngol 7:67, 1978

Chen HS: The ozena problem: Clinical analysis of atrophic rhinitis in 100 cases. Acta Otolaryngol 93:461, 1982

Cherpillod J, Dutoit-Marco ML: Bilan fonctionnel de l'insuffisance vélaire. Méd et Hyg 40:3736, 1982

Chessen J, Philpott I: Some rhinologic syndromes and vasomotor rhinitis. Laryngoscope 65:85, 1955

Chouard CH, Senechal G: Rhinites chroniques: Rhinites atrophiques et ozène. Oto-Rhino-Laryngol, (ed 2). Masson, 1965

Cinelli AA: Collapse of the nares. Arch Otolaryngol 33:683, 1941

Cinella JA: Correction of combined elongated nose and recessed naso-labial angle. Plast Reconstr Surg 21:139, 1958

Cinella JA: Rhinoplastic principles: Complications and solutions. Eye, Ear, Nose Throat Monthly 45:102, 1966

Clark GM: Specially processed heterogenous bone and cartilage transplants in nasal surgery. J Laryngol Otol 83:27, 1969

Clark JL, Neel HB, Kern EB: Preservation of homograft cartilage and bone, in Bernstein L (ed). Plastic and Reconstructive Surgery, vol. 1. Aesth Surg 1981, p 86

Clement PAR: Committee report on standardization of rhinomanometry. Rhinology 22:151, 1984

Clement PAR, Hirsch C: Rhinomanometry. A review. ORL (Basel) 46:173, 1984

Clement PAR, Kaufmann L, Rousseau P: Active anterior rhinomanometry in pre- and postoperative evaluation, use of Brom's mathematical model. Rhinology 21:121, 1983

Climo MS: The surgical closure of a large anterior perforation of the nasal septum. Plast Reconstr Surg 17:410, 1956

Climo MS: Nasolabial flap for alar defect. Plast Reconstr Surg 44:303, 1969

Cochran JH, Kurtz JA, Ewanowsky SJ, et al: The Magnum procedure: Surgical salvage of end-stage velopharyngeal incompetence. Plast Reconstr Surg 71:473, 1983

Cohen A: Advantage of mixed bone and cartilage grafts in correction of saddle nose. Trans Am Laryngol Rhinol Otolaryngol Soc 33:233, 1927

Cohen L: Corrective rhinoplasty: Some reasons for faulty results. Ann Otol 33:342, 1924

Cohen S: Complications following rhinoplasty. Plast Reconstr Surg 18:213, 1956

Coiffman F: External incisions on the nose. Aesthetic Plast Surg 1:363, 1978

Cole P: Upper respiratory airflow, in Proctor DF, Andersen IB (eds): The Nose: Upper Airway Physiology and the Atmospheric Environment. New York, Elsevier Biomedical Press, 1982, p 163

Cole P, Haight JSJ: Contrôle de la résistence nasale. European Rhinologic Society, Nancy, 1984

Collom 1968 quoted by Fairbanks BJ: Plast Surg 24:382, 1971

Coman WB, Reilly PF: General anesthesia for cosmetic rhinoplasty, in Bernstein L (ed): Plastic Reconstructive Surgery of the Head and Neck. vol. 1. Aesth Surg 1981, p 224

Conley J: Intranasal composite grafts for dorsal support. Arch Otolaryngol 111:241, 1985

Conley JJ, Sachs ME, Donovan DT: The mini alar base myocutaneous flap. Meeting, American Academy Head and Neck, New Orleans, 1982

Conrad K: Correction of crooked noses by external rhinoplasty. J Laryngol 7(1):32, 1978

Conroy WC: Simple nasal tip setback. Plast Reconstr Surg 33:564, 1964

Constantian MB: Toward refinement in rhinoplasty. Plast Reconstr Surg 74:19, 1984

Constantian MB: Grafting the projecting nasal tip. Ann Plast Surg 14:391, 1985

Constantian MB: A model for planning rhinoplasty. Plast Reconstr Surg 79:3, 1987

Converse JM: Corrective surgery of nasal deviations. Arch Otolaryngol 52:671, 1950

Converse JM: The cartilaginous structures of the nose. Ann Otolaryngol 64:220, 1955

Converse JM: Reconstructive Plastic Surgery: Head and Neck, vol. 2. Philadelphia, W.B. Saunders, 1964(a)

Converse JM: Deformities of the nose. Reconstruction Plastic Surgery, Vol 2. Philadelphia and London, W.B. Saunders, 1964(b), p 695

Converse JM: Technique of bone-grafting in contour restoration of the face. Plast Reconstr Surg 14:332, 1970

Converse JM: Surgical elongation of the traumatically foreshortened nose. Plast Reconstr Surg 47:539, 1971

Converse JM: Corrective plastic surgery of the nose, in Paparella, Shumrick (eds): Otolaryngology. Philadelphia, W.B. Saunders, 1973

Converse JM: Deformities of the nose, in Kazanjian VH, Converse JM (eds): Surgical Treatment of Facial Injuries, (ed 3). Baltimore, William and Wilkins, 1974
Converse JM: The deviated nose, in Millard D Jr (ed): Symposium on Corrective Rhinoplasty. St. Louis, 1976
Converse JM, Campbell RM: Bone grafts in surgery of the face. Surg Clin North Am 375:1954
Converse, JM, Horowitz SL, Valauri AJ, et al: The treatment of nasomaxillary hypoplasia. A new pyramidial naso-orbital maxillary osteotomy. Plast Reconstr Surg 45: 527, 1970
Conway H: The surgery of benign and malignant tumors of the skin and of the head and neck. Rocky Mtn Med J 49:673, 1952
Conway H, Goulian D: Experiences with the pharyngeal flap in cleft palate surgery. Plast Reconstr Surg 26:590, 1960
Conway H, Stark RB: Pharyngeal flap procedure in management of complicated cases of cleft palate. Ann Surg 142:114, 1955
Cook TA: Butophanol tartrate: An intravenous analgesic for outpatient surgery. Otolaryngol Head Neck Surg 91:251, 1953
Corgiolu E, Marconi P: Studio rinomanometrico su un gruppo di bambini affetti da rinopatia ostruttiva subcronica. 70 Cong Naz Soc Ital ORL, Bologna, 1983
Corgiolu E, Marconi P, Alpini D, et al: Studio rinomanometrico su un gruppo di bambini affetti da rinopatia ostruttiva subcronica. Otorinolaringologia Ital 34:395, 1984
Corradini C, Calabrese V, Mormile F, et al: La dispnea nasale: Basi fisiopatologiche del suo persistere o recidivare dopo correzione dell'ostruzione nàsale. Valsalva 59:322, 1983
Cottle MH: Nasal septum surgery in children. Rev Illinois Med J 161; 1939
Cottle MH: Nasal roof repair and hump removal. Arch Otolaryngol 60:408, 1954
Cottle MH: Nasal atrophy. Atrophie rhinitis, ozena; medical and surgical treatment; repair of septal perforations. J Int Coll Surg 29:472, 1958
Cottle MH, Concepts of nasal physiology as related to corrective nasal surgery. Arch Otolaryngol 72:11, 1960 (a)
Cottle MH: Surgical corrections of the septal deformities. Ann Rhinol Soc 7:14, 1960 (b)
Cottle MH: Rhino-sphygmo-manometry an aid in physical diagnosis. Int Rhinol 6:7, 1968
Cottle MH, Loring RM: Corrective surgery of the external nasal pyramid and the nasal septum for restoration of normal physiology. Eye, Ear, Nose Throat Monthly 26:207, 1947
Cottle MH, Loring RM, Fischer G, et al: The maxilla-premaxilla approach to extensive, nasal septum surgery. Arch Otolaryngol 68:301, 1958
Cottle MH, Quitly TJ, Buckingham RA: Nasal implants in children and in adults, with preliminary note on the use of ox cartilage. Ann Otol Rhinol 62:169, 1953
Cotton RJ: Uvulopharyngopalatoplasty. Arch Otolaryngol 109:502, 1983
Coughlin WT: New procedure for relief of facies scaphoidea (dishfaces) Surg Gynec Obstet 40:109, 1925
Coursey DL: Staphylococcal endocarditis following septorhinoplasty. Arch Otolaryngol 99:454, 1974
Courtiss, EH, Gargan TJ, Courtiss GB: Nasal physiology. Ann Plast Surg 1984
Courtiss EH, Goldwyn RM: The effects of nasal surgery on airflow. Plast Reconstr Surg 72:9, 1983(a)
Courtiss EH, Goldwyn RM: Update resection of obstructing inferior turbinates: A 6-year follow-up. Plast Reconstr Surg 72:913, 1983 (b)
Courtiss EH, Goldwyn RM, O'Brien JJ: Resection of obstructing inferior nasal turbinates. Plast Reconstr Surg 62:249, 1978
Crestinu J: New data in the correction of twisted noses. Aesthetic Plast Surg 10:231, 1986
Crikelair GF: Reduction rhinoplasty. Plast Reconstr Surg 36:626, 1960
Crikelair GJ: Rhinophyma skin grafts. Plast Reconstr Surg 49:98, 1972
Cronin TD: Lengthening columella by use of skin from nasal floor and alae. Plast Reconstr Surg 21:417, 1958
Cronin TD: The V-Y rotational flap for nasal tip defects. Plast Reconst Surg 11:282, 1983
Cronkite EP, Lozner EL, Deaver JM: Use of thrombin and fibrinogen in skin grafting. JAMA 124: 976, 1944
Crysdale WS, Tatham B: External septorhinoplasty in children. Laryngoscope 95:12, 1985
Culf NK, Chong JK, Cramer LM: Different surgical approach to secondary velopharyngeal incompetence, in Georgiade N, Hegerty RF (eds): Proceedings Symposium on Management of Cleft Lip and Palate and Associated Deformities. St. Louis, Mosby, 1974, p 178
Czerny V: Drei plastische operationen. Deutsche ges chir 14:211, 1895 (translated by U. Schmidt-Tintemann in Plast Reconstr Surg 60:595, 1970)
D'Alessio E: La rinoplastica. Il problema tecnico. Giornale Ital di Chirurgia 10:632, 1954
Daley J: Retaining a correct septo-labial angle in rhinoplasty. Arch Otolaryngol 39:348, 1944
Daley J: Role of columellar and septocolumellar suture in rhinoplasty. Arch Otolaryngol 45:178, 1947
Dankmeijer J: Some remarks on the development and anatomy of the septum nasi. Int Rhinol 7:1, 1968
Da Silva G: A new method of reconstructing the columella with a nasolabial flap. Plast Reconstr Surg 34:63, 1964
Davidson TM: Photography in facial plastic and reconstructive surgery. J Biol Photogr 47:59, 1979
Davidson TM, et al: Tip suspension suture for superior tip rotation in rhinoplasty. Laryngoscope 93:1076, 1983
Davidson TM, Webster R: High septal transfixion incision in septal, sinus and nasal surgery. Laryngoscope 89:1008, 1979
Davis CL: Psychiatric screening of patients for cosmetic surgery, in Bernstein L (ed): Plastic and Reconstructive Surgery, vol. 1. Aesth Surg 1981, p 227
Davis PKB: Chin augmentation with rhinoplasty: A tutorial dissertation. Br J Plast Surg 36:204, 1983
Davis PKB, Jones SM: The complications of ilastic implants. Br J Plast Surg 24:405, 1971
Davis WB: External nasal deformities and methods used in their repair. Arch Otolaryngol 36:619, 1942
Davis WB, Gibson T: Absorption of autogenous cartilage grafts in man. Br J Plast Surg 9:177, 1956
Dawson RLG: Nasal bone grafts—the correction of acquired deformities, in Millard RD Jr (ed): Symposium on Corrective Rhinoplasty, vol. 13. St. Louis, Mosby Co, 1976, p 242
Dehan F, Clement PAR: Endonasal surgical treatment of bilateral choanal atresia under optic control in the infant. J Otolaryngol 14:95, 1985
Del Bene M, Petrolati M, Delaria G, et al: L'innesto osseo di

olecrano nel trattamento del naso a sella. Atti del Congresso Italiano di Chirurgia Plastica. Bari, 1985

Denecke HJ, Ey W: Die Operationen an der Nase und im Nasopharynx. Berlin, Springer-Verlag, 1984

Denecke HJ, Meyer R: Plastische Operationen an Kopf und Hals. Korrigierende und Rekonstruktive Nasenplastik. Berlin, Springer-Verlag, 1964

Denecke HJ, Meyer R: Plastic Surgery of Head and Neck. Berlin and New York, Springer, 1967

Denny WR, Wilson CP: Nasopharyngeal stenosis. J Laryngol 71:645, 1957

Denonvilliers M: Ablation et cheiloplasty cancroide de la lèvre supérieure. Quoted by Nélaton CP and Ombredanne L. La rhinoplastie Steinheil. Paris 1904. Bull Gén Thér 65:257, 1863

Dent 1890. Quoted by Freer, 1902

Desprez JD, Kiehn CL: Valvular obstruction of the nasal airway. Plast Reconstr Surg 56:306, 1975

Devgan BK, Leach W: Submucosal diathermy of inferior turbinates. Eye Ear Nose Throat Monthly 55:156, 1976

De Vido G: La deviazione patologica del setto nasale nell'etá infantile. Atti Soc Med Chir Padova, 1953

De Vincentiis I: Esplorazione dell'olfatto mediante metodiche obiettive. Cah d'ORL 13:943, 1978

De Wit G, Kappeyn TS, Van Bochove VWM: Some remarks on the physiology, the anatomy and the radiology of the vestibulum and the isthmus nasi. Int Rhinology 8:56, 1970

De Wit G, Kappeyn TS, Van Bochove W: Some remarks on the physiology, the anatomy and the radiology of the vestibulum and the isthmus nasi. Rhinology 3:37, 1965

Diamond HP: La tecnica della rinoplastica. Clin Chir North Am 4:332, 1971

Diamond HP: Rhinoplasty. Ann Plast Surg 1:582, 1978

Dibbel DG: Cleft lip nasal reconstruction. Correcting the classic unilateral defect. Plast Reconstr Surg 69:264, 1982

Dicker RL, Syracuse VS: Epistaxis after rhinoplasty. It's prevention, in Sisson GA, Tardy ME (eds): Plastic and Reconstructive Surgery of the Face and Neck. New York, Grune & Stratton, 1977

Dieffenbach JF: Die nasenbehandlung in: Operative Chirurgie. Fa, Leipzig, Brockhaus, 1845

Di Giunta ED, Conticello S: La settorino-plastica e la pervientà funzionale del naso. La Clin ORL 20:575, 1968

Di Giuseppe A, Bertani A: Gli innesti d'osso per la correzione dei difetti estetici della piramide nasale. Atti del Congresso Italiano di Chirurgia Plastica. Bari, 1985

Dillinger A: Funktionelle ergebnisse nach septumplastik. Aktuelle probl der otorhinolaryngol 9:26, 1985

Dingman N: Surgical anatomy in aesthetic and corrective rhinoplasty. Clin Plast Surg 4:111, 1977

Dingman RO: The use of illiac bone in the repair of facial and cranial defects. Plast Reconstr Surg 6:179, 1950

Dingman RO: Corrections of nasal deformities due to defects of the septum. Plast Reconstr Surg 18:291, 1956

Dingman RO: Follow-up on costal cartilage homografts preserved by irradiation. Plast Reconstr Surg 50:516, 1972

Dingman RO, Grabb WC: Costal cartilage homografts preserved by irradiation. Plast Reconstr Surg 28:562, 1961

Dingman RO, Natvig P: The infracartilaginous incision for rhinoplasty. Plast Reconstr Surg 69:134, 1982

Dingman RO, Walter C: Use of composit ear graft in correction of the short nose. Plast Reconstr Surg 43:117, 1969

Dingman RP: Local anesthesia for rhinoplasty and the nasal septum in rhinoplastic surgery. Plast Reconstr Surg 28:251, 1961

Dion MD: The anatomy of the nose. Arch Otolaryngol 104:145, 1978

Dionis M: Cours d'opération de chirurgie demonstrés au jardin royal. Paris, L. D'Houry, 1716

Dirlewanger A, Meyer R: Plastik und Rekonstruktion des Nasenseptums. Schweiz ORL. Congress Délémont. 1968

Diwan VS: The depressed nose in leprosy. Brit J Plast Surg 21:295, 1968

Dixon FW: The nasal turbinates. Trans Am Acad Ophthalmol Otolaryngol 54:107, 1949

Dolezal R, Schultz RC: Rhynophyma. Ann Plast Surg 11:5, 1883

Donders FC: Thesis, quoted by Kortekangas

Donelan 1899. Quoted by O Freer, 1902

D'Orans: Arch Oto laryngol 14:7, 1931. Quoted by Réthi, 1932

Dorrance GM: Arch Otolaryngol. 14:731, 1936. Quoted by Réthi

Douglas B: The relief of vestibular nasal obstruction by partial resection of the nasal process of the superior maxilla. Plast Reconstr Surg 9:42, 1952

Douglas-Snell GE: History of external rhinoplasty. J Laryngol 7:6, 1978

Doyle DE, Stoller KP: Intranasal airway pack: Description of a new device. Laryngoscope 93:808, 1983

Draf W: Erfahrungen mit der technik der fibrinklebung in der hals-nasen-ohren-chirurgie. Laryngol Rhinology 59:99, 1980

Drettner B: Vascular reactions of the human mucosa on exposure to cold. Acta Otolaryngol 166:supp 1, 1961

Drettner B: A review of the relationship between upper and lower respiratory airways. Int Rhinology 8:12, 1970

Dufourmentel C, Mouly R: Chirurgie plastique. Paris, Flammarion, 1959

Dufourmentel C: Le greffon osseux en auvent pour reconstruction de l'arête nasale. Ann Chir Plast 15(4):348, 1970

Dufourmentel C: Les greffes auriculaires cómposées dans la reconstruction de l'étage infirieux de la pyramide nasale—apropos de 43 greffes. Chir Plast 18:199, 1973

Dufourmentel, L: Chirurgie Correctrice Du Nez. Paris, Masson & Cie, 1926

Dufourmentel L: Difficultés et dangers de la chirurgie corrective nasale. Congr Franc d'ORL, Paris, 1953. Presse Méd 62:152, 1954

Dufourmentel L, Ginested: Acrylic inclusions for deformities; two cases of elimination of prothesis. Mem Acad Chir 74:201, 1948

Dumbach J, Steinhäuser EW: Zeitpunkt und technik des restlochverschlusses bei spaltpatienten unter besonderer berücksichtigung der zungenlappentechnik. Öst Z Stomat 80:182, 1983

Dupertuis SM: Free ear lobe grafts of skin and fat: Value in reconstruction about nostrils. Plast Reconstr Surg 1:135, 1946

Dupont C, Cloutier GE, Prevost Y: Autogenous vomer bone graft for permanent correction of the cartilagenous septal deviations. Plast Reconstr Surg 38:243, 1966

Dupuis A, Hainsdorf F: Traitement des ensellures nasales à l'aide d'un lambeau naso-frontal médian en étoile à cinq branches. Rev Stomatol Chir Maxillo-fac 5:289, 1983

Dutoit-Marco ML, Brandt E: Troubles orthodontiques majeurs en phoniatrie. Méd et Hyg 40:3741, 1982
Earley MJ, Lendrum J: The alar swing technique in the correction of the saddle nose deformity. Brit J Plast Surgery 37:307, 1984
Ecker HA: A direct approach to the more severely deformed cleft lips nose. Plast Reconstr Surg 67:369, 1981
Eckert-Moebius A: Implantation von macerierten spongiösen rinderknochen zur behandlung der ozaena: Rhinitis atrophicans. Z Hals-Nas-und Ohrenheilkd 7:108, 1923
Eckert-Moebius A: Grundsätzliches zum problem der operativen nasenverengung bei ozaena. HNO (Berlin) 13:350, 1965
Edgerton MT, Lewis C, McKnelly LO: Lengthening of the short columella. Plast Reconstr Surg 40:343, 1967
Edgerton MT, Marsch JL: Uses of the nasolabial flap in the correction of cleft lip nasal deformities. Plast Reconstr Surg 60:56, 1977
Egyedi P: Degloving the nose. J Max Fac Surg 2:101, 1974
Eichhorn T, Schroeder HG, Kleinsasser O: Nachuntersuchungen von patienten mit isolierten frakturen des knöchernen nasenskelettes. Rhinol Otolaryngol 62:112, 1983
Eichner H, Behlbehani AA, Hochstrasser K: Nasensekretsdiagnostik, aktueller stand normalwerte. Laryngol Rhinol Otol 62:561, 1983
Eicken CV: Zur behandlung der choanalatresie z ohrenheilk 63:295, 1911
Eisenstodt LW: Management of septal deformities in rhinoplastic correction. Arch Otolaryngol 45:77, 1947
Eitner E: Ueber Unterpolsterung der gesichtshaut. Med Klin 16:93, 1920
Eitner E: Kosmetische Operationen. Wien, Springer, 1932
Eitner E: Kosmetische korrekturen im bereiche der nasenspitze und ihrer umgebung. Z Laryngol Rhinology 26: 46, 1935
Eitner E, Karpelis E: Kosmetische Therapie. Wien, Urban & Schwarzenberg, 1932
Eitschberger E, Merklein C, Masing H, et al: Das histologische verhalten plangeschlagenen septum-knorpels nach retransplantationen zur versteifung der hinteren septumregion. HNO 28:158, 1968
El Ghazali AM: Chondrosarcoma of the paranasal sinuses and nasal septum. J Laryngol Otolaryngol 97:543, 1983
Ellenbogen R: Alar rim lowering. Plast Reconstr Surg 79:1, 1987
Ellenbogen R, Swara N: The improvement of the gummy smile using the implant spacer technique. Ann Plast Surg 12:16, 1984
Ellenbogen R, Zwahra N: A technique for the closure of septal perforation. Ann Plast Surg 11:390, 1983
Ellis DAF, Le Liever WC: The nose-check flap in total columellar reconstruction, in Bernstein L (ed): Plastic and Reconstructive Surgery of the Head and Neck. Third Internat Symp, vol. 2, 1981, p 26
Ellis DAF, McDonald GA: Narrowing of the wide nasal tip. J Otolaryngol 13:55, 1984
Emmert 1853. Quoted by Bobin S, et al, 1983
Enzmann H: Vergleich rhinomanometrischer verfahren. HNO (Berlin) 31:327, 1983
Erich JB: A technique for correcting a flat nostril in cases of repaired harelip. Plast Reconstr Surg 12:320, 1953
Erich JB: Plastic correction of the crooked nose. Proc Mayo Clin 34: 397, 1959
Ersek RA, Hart WG, Greer D: Processed bovine cartilage: An improved bio-synthetic implant for contour defects. Ann Plast Surg 12:397, 1984
Ersek RA, Rothenberg PB, Denton DR: Clinical use of an improved processed bovin cartilage for contour defects. Ann Plast Surg 13(1):44, 1984
Ersner M: Reconstruction of the deformed nasal septum. Arch Otolaryngol 39:476, 1944
Ersner MS: Rhinoplastic procedures to establish normal physiologic nasal function. Pa Med J 51:749, 1948
Ersner MS: Physiological principles in rhinoplasty. Arch Utolaryngol 53:256, 1951
Escoubes B: Le problème septal dans la rhinoplastie. Ann Chir Plast 13:289, 1968
Escoubes B: La largeur de la racine du nez en rhinoplastie. Cah d'ORL 7:659, 1972
Ey W: Fehler und gefahren bei operativer behandlung anatomischer und funktioneller veränderungen am vorderen septum. Z Laryng Rhinol 48:38, 1969
Ey W: Fehler und gefahren bei der verwendung von composite graft. HNO (Berlin) 30:133, 1982
Ey W: Potentials of reconstructive plastic surgery in the area of the nose. Laryngol Rhinol Otol 62:1, 1983
Ey W: Die operationen an der nase und im nasopharynx, in Denecke HJ, Ey W (eds): Berlin, Heidelberg, New York, Tokyo, Springer-Verlag, 1984
Ey W: Die verwendung von autogenetischen knorpeltransplantaten in der plastischen rhinochirurgie. HNO Plast Chirurgie an Kopf und Hals 133:11, 1987
Eyries C: Rhinites atrophiques et ozène. Otorhinolaryngol 1:28, 1951
Facer GW, Kern EB: Non-surgical closure of nasal septum perforations. Arch Otolaryngol 105:6, 1979
Fairbanks DNF: Closure of nasal septal perforations. Arch Otolaryngol 106:509, 1980
Fairbanks DNF: Surgical management of large nasoseptal perforations, in L. Bernstein (ed): Plastic and Reconstructive Surgery, vol. 1. Aesth Surg 1981, p 86
Fairbanks DNF, Chen SC: Closure of large septum perforations. Arch Otolarynogol 91:403, 1970
Fairbanks DNF, Fairbanks GR: Surgical management of large nasal septum perforations. Br J Plast Surg 24:382, 1971
Fairbanks, DNF, Fairbanks GR: Nasal septal perforation: Prevention and management. Ann Plast Surg 5:452, 1980
Faivre J: Surgical treatment of the flat nose: African and oriental subjects, in Bernstein L (ed): Plastic and Reconstructive Surgery, vol. 1. Aesth Surg 1981, p 73
Faivre J, Carissimo A: Les cartilages alaires et la chirurgie de la pointe du nez. Chirurgie Esthétique 1983-1984, Paris, Maloine, 1984
Faivre J, Simeoni CM: Chirurgie de la pointe du nez et de la narine. Rev Chir Esth Langue Franç 1:5, 1975
Falces E: Cosmetic surgery of the non-caucasian nose. Plast Reconstr Surg 45:317, 1970
Falces E, Gorney M: Use of ear cartilage grafts for nasal tip reconstruction. Plast Reconstr Surg 50:147, 1972
Falces E, Wesser D, Gorney M: Cosmetic surgery of the non-caucasian nose. Plast Reconstr Surg 45:317, 1970
Fanous N: The "light reflex" tip-plasty: A new theory in tip aesthetics and tip correction. J Otolarynogol 10:162, 1981
Fanous N: The light reflex tip-plasty: Surgical application of a new theory in the tip aesthetics. Laryngoscope 92:310, 1982

Fanous N: Expression plasty: A new approach to esthetic surgery. Head Neck Surg 5:306, 1983
Fanous N: Correction of thin lips: "Lip Lift." Plast Reconstr Surg 74:33, 1984
Fara M: Rhinophym erfahrungen an 65 operierten patienten. Acta Chir Orthop Traum Cech 29:523, 1962
Fara M: Experience with eight operated rinophyma patients. Acta Chir Plast 13:254, 1971
Fara M: The anatomy of cleft lip. Clin Plast Surg 2:205, 1975
Faria V, Sandall V: Nariz negroide. Boll Centro Est Hosp Serv Estado 22(2):61, 1970
Farina R: Rinofima. Decorticaçao electrocirùrgica simples. Rev Hosp Clin 4:107, 1949
Farina R: Deformity of nasal dorsum through loss of substance. Plast Reconstr Surg 8:320, 1951
Farina R: Loss of substance from the nasal alae and tip. Plast Reconstr Surg 9:52, 1952
Farina R: Deformidade de dorso do nariz por perda de substancia osteocartilaginea. An Paulist Med e Circ 65:339, 1953
Farina R: Nose tip collapse through loss of chondromucous substance (repair of nasal lining). Plast Reconstr Surg 13:137, 1954
Farina R: Cirurgia Plàstica e Reparadora. Sao Jose, Sao Paulo, 1965
Farina R, Cury E, Ackel IA: Shaped nasal wings: Rhinopteroplasty. Case reports. Aesth Plast Surg 7:177, 1983(a)
Farina R, Cury E, Ackel IA: Saddle and boxer's nose. Aesth Plast Surg 7:171, 1983(b)
Farina R, Cury E, Ackel IA: The prominent nasal tip. Aesth Plast Surg 8:141, 1984
Farina R, Dias JV, Castro O: Development of bone integration as established by x-ray follow-up in correction of deformity of nasal dorsum. Plast Reconstr Surg 20:297, 1957
Farina R, Mion D, Baroudi R, et al: Avantages comparés des lambeaux frontaux et des lambeaux nasogéniens dans la substitution de l'étoffe nasale. Ann Chir Plast 5:279, 1960
Farina R, Villano JB: Follow-up of bone graft to the nose. Plast Reconstr Surg 48:25, 1971
Farkas LG, Deutsch GK, Hreczko TA: Asymmetries in nostrils and the surrounding tissues of the soft nose: A morphometric study. Ann Plast Surg 12:10, 1984
Farkas LG, Hreczko TA, Deutsch CK: Objective assessment of standard nostril types: A morphometric study. Ann Plast Surg 11:5, 1983
Farkas LG, Hreczko TA, Kolar JC, et al: Vertical and horizontal proportion of the face in young adult North American caucasians: Revision of neoclassical canons. Plast Reconstr Surg 75:328, 1985
Farkas LG, Kolar JC, Munro IR: Geography of the nose: A morphometric study. Aesth Plast Surg 10:191, 1986
Farkas LG, Lindsay WK: The columella in cleft lip and palate anomaly, in Hueston JT (ed): Transactions of the Fifth International Congress of Plastic and Reconstructive Surgery, 1971, Melbourne, Australia, Butterworths, 1971, p 373
Farlan S: Correction of saddle nose deformities by costal cartilage grafts. Ann Plast Surg 9:32, 1982
Farrior RT: The problem of the unilateral cleft lip nose. A composite operation for revision of secondary deformity. Laryngoscope 72:289, 1962
Farrior RT: Synthetics in head and neck surgery (with particular reference to silicone) Arch Otolaryngol 84:82, 1966
Farrior RT: The cleft lip nose (septo-rhinoplasty and combined lip repair). International Congr Cleft Palate, Houston, 1969
Farrior RT, Connolly ME: Septorhinoplastic in children. Otolaryngol Clin North Am 3:345, 1970
Farrior RT: Korrigierende and rekonstruktive plastische chirurgie der äusseren nase. H.H. Naumann Kopf-u. Halschir. Bd 2,5, G. Theime, Verlag, 1974
Farrior RT: The cleft-lip nose septo-rhinoplasty and combined lip repair, in Sisson GA, Tard ME (eds): Plastic and Reconstructive Surgery of the Face and Neck. New York, Grune and Stratton, 1977
Favoino B, Pascone M, Brienza E: Comportamento Dell'-idrossiprolina nel Connetivo Inglobante L'impianto di una Protesi Solida al Silicone nel Coniglio. Del Bari, 1985
Fearon B, Dickson J: Bilateral choanal atresia in newborn: Plan of action. Laryngoscope 78:1487, 1968
Femenic B: Über die chirurgie der doggennase. Mschr Ohrenheilk 89:109, 1955
Fenton RS: Surgery of the nasal dorsum. J Laryngol 7:24, 1978(a)
Fenton RS: External septorhinoplasty: Why the fuss? J Laryngol 7:3, 1978(b)
Ferrari F, Pomatto E, Lavagnino G et al: Rinoplastica: Osteotomia laterale transcutanea. Riv Ital Di Chir Plast 18:373, 1986
Ferrari-Parabita G, Derada-Troletti G, Vinci R, et al: Impiego Della Idrossiapatite di Calcio nel Trattamento Delle Deformitá della Piramide Nasale. Del Bari, 1985
Ferraro G, Di Girolamo A, Lusi G: Il ruolo della valvola di mink nell' insufficienza respiratoria nasale. Considerazoni clinico-terapeutiche. Ann Laryngol Otol Rinol Faringol 77:241, 1979
Feuerstein: 1985 Personal communication
Feuerstein SS: Intraoral augmentation mentoplasty with a hinged silastic implant. Arch Otolaryngol 104:343, 1978
Fiebach A: The place of rhinomanometry in septum surgery. Laryngol Rhinol Otol 62:264, 1983
Figi FA: Cicatricial stenosis of the nasopharynx corrected by skin graft. Plast Reconstr Surg 2:97, 1947
Figi FA: The repair of secondary cleft lip and nasal deformities. J Int Coll Surg 17:297, 1952
Filiberti AT: Plastic closure of a septal perforations. Ann Clin Otol (Cordoba) 96:1, 1965
Filippi B, Fruttero F: Chirurgia Plastica del Naso. Savona, Italy, Sabatelli Ed, 1967
Filippi B, Lovo GF, Ponti L: La chirurgia corretiva delle strutture osteocartilaginee del naso nei suoi indirizzi funzionali. Minerva ORL 9:451, 1959
Filippi B, Moretto G: Considerazioni sulla chirurgia riparatrice delle perforazioni del setto. Minerva ORL 9:89, 1959
Filippi B, Teich-Alasia: Correzioni plastiche delle deviazioni della parte anteroinferiore cartilaginea del naso. Minerva ORL 8:411, 1958
Finzi NA: Radium Therapeutics. London, Hodder and Sloughton, 1913
Fischer 1957. Quoted by JP Reidy
Fischer G: Fischer's nasal "hump shaver". Bolletino International Academy of Cosmetic Surgery. 1:68, 1982
Fischer R: Die Messung and graphische auswertung des stromungswiderstandes der nase. Arch Klin Exp 197:72, 1970
Fisher WJ: Rhinophyma: Its surgical treatment. Plast Reconstr Surg 45:466, 1970

Fissette J: Preoperative planning of the profile in aesthetic surgery: Apropos of a method and experience with 500 rhinoplasties. Ann Chir Plast Esthet 28:33, 1983

Fittipaldi L: Conocimiento y pensamiento creativo en la correcion logica de una nariz. Plastica Ibero-Latinoamericana 8:511, 1982

Flageul G, Grignon JL: Reconstruction nasale par autogreffe osseuse mortaisée. Ann Chir Plast 27:152, 1982

Flake G, Ferguson CF: Congenital choanal atresia in infant children. Ann Otol Laryngol 73:1, 1964

Flemming I: Fehler und gefahren bei der korrektur der knöchernen nase. Arch HNO 325:223, 1979

Flemming I: Rhinoplasty in children. Aesth Plast Surg 5:145, 1981

Flemming I, Jazbi B: Rhinoplasty in children. Otolaryngology Clinic North America. Philadelphia, W.B. Saunders, 1977

Flowers RS, Anderson R: Injury to the lacrimal apparatus during rhinoplasty. Plas Reconstr Surg 42:6, 1968

Fomon S: The Surgery of Injury and Plastic Repair. Baltimore, Williams & Wilkins, 1939

Fomon S: Reimplantation of the septal cartilage. Arch Otolaryingol, 47:7, 1948

Fomon S: Corrective Surgery: Principles and Practice. Philadelphia, Lippincott, 1960(a)

Fomon S: Deformities of lower cartilaginous vault. Otolaryngol 26:117, 1960(b)

Fomon S, Bell J: Rhinoplasty: New concepts. Thermos publ, 1953

Fomon S, Bell JW: Silicones in facial surgery. Arch Otolaryngol 84:514, 1966

Fomon S, Bell J: Rhinoplasty New Concepts. Evaluation and Application. Springfield, Thomas, 1970

Fomon S, Sayad WY, Schattner, A et al: Physiological principles in rhinoplasty. Arch Otolaryngol 53:356, 1951

Fontana AM, Muti E: The nasofrontal angle and profile in rhinoplasty: Case Presentations. Aesth Plast Surg 7:169, 1983

Ford CN, Battaglia DG, Gentry LR: Preservation of periosteal attachment in lateral osteotomy. Ann Plast Surg 13:107, 1984

Forster H: The submucous rectification of the nasal septum. Proc Roy Soc Med 42:283, 1949

Fournier P, Otteni F: Les ostéotomies dans la rhinoplastie de reduction: Technique et tactique. Chirurgie esthétique 1983-1984, Paris, Maloine, 1984

Francesconi G, Donati L, Fittipaldi L: Osservazioni sul comportamento dell'innesto osseo autoplastivo in sede nasale. Minerva Chir 22(17):979, 1967

Francesconi G, Fenili O: Treatment of deflection of the anterocaudal portion of the nasal septum. Plast Reconstr Surg 51:342, 1973

Francesconi G, Grassi C: Considerazioni sulle cisti e fistole dermoidi del naso. Riv Ital Chir Plast 15:81, 1983

Franke G: Experimentelle untersuchungen über luftdruck, luftbewegung und luftwechsel in der nase und ihren nebenhöhlen. Arch Laryngol Rhinol 1:260, 1894

Fred GB: Nasal tip in rhinoplasty; Invaginating technique to prevent secondary dropping. Ann Otol Rhinol Laryngol 59:215, 1950

Fred GB: Role of depressor septi nasi muscle in rhinoplasty. Arch Otolaryngol 62:37, 1955

Fredricks S: Tripod resection for "Pinocchio nose." Plast Reconstr Surg 53:531, 1974

Freeman BS: Reconstructive rhinoplasty for rhinophyma. Plast Reconstr Surg 45:265, 1970

Freeman BS: Rhinophyma, in: Converse JM (ed): Reconstr Plast Surg Vol. 2. Philadelphia, W.B. Saunders, 1977

Freer O: The correction of deflections of the nasal septum with minimum of traumatism. JAMA 38:636–692, 1902

Freer O: Deflection of the nasal septum. Ann ORL 14:214, 1905

Frey H, Weinaug P: Zur häufigkeit und ätiologie der nasenseptum-perforation. HNO (Berlin) 16:33, 1968

Friederich HC: Zur therapie des rhinophyms. Aesth Med 16:196, 1967

Freidman WH: Evaluation of nasal tip surgery: The intracartilaginous and rim approaches. Plastic Reconstructive Surgery of the Face and Neck. Second International Symposium, New York, Grune & Stratton, 1977

Friedmann WH, Oliver M, Biller HF: Evaluation of nasal tip surgery. Laryngoscope 85:1539, 1975

Friedmann WH, Rosenblum BN, Krebs FJ: The Goldman tip in secondary rhinoplasty. Plast Reconstr Surg 79:3, 1987

Friedrich JP, Terrier G: Chirurgie endoscopique de la sinusite par voie endonasale. Méd et Hyg 41:3722, 1983

Frileck SP: The nasal vestibule. Ann Plast Surg 17:320, 1986

Fritz K: Funktionelle Methoden der Ästhetischen Gesichtschirurgie. München, Urban & Schwarzenberg, 1981

Fruehwald V: Korrektive Chirurgie der Nase, der Uhren und des Gesichtes. Wien, W Maudrich, 1952

Fry H: Interlocked stresses in human nasal septal cartilage. Br J Plast Surg 19:276, 1966

Fry H: Cartilage and cartilage grafts: The basic properties of the tissue and the components responsible for them. Plast Reconstr Surg 40:426, 1967(a)

Fry H: Nasal skeletal trauma and the interlocked stresses of the nasal septal cartilage. Br J Plast Surg 20:146, 1967(b)

Fry H: The importance of the septal cartilage in nasal trauma. Br J Plast Surg 20:392, 1967(c)

Fry H: The distorted residual cartilage strut after submucous resection of the nasal septum. Br J Plast Surg 21:170, 1968

Fry H: Judicious turbinectomy for nasal obstruction. Austr NZ J Surg 42:291, 1973

Fuchs J: A rapid approach to the deviated septum in rhinoplasty. Plast Reconstr Surg 18:133, 1956

Fujita S, Conway W, Zorick F, et al: Surgical correction of anatomic abnormalities in obstructive sleep apnea syndrome. Uvulopalatopharyngoplasty. Otolaryngol Head Neck Surg 89:923, 1981

Furlan S: Correction of saddle nose deformities by costal cartilage grafts: A technique. Ann Plast Surg 9:32, 1982

Furukawa M: Management of m depressor septi nasi in rhinoplasty. Proceedings of the IV Congress of Plastic Surgery, Excerpta Medica Foundation, Amsterdam, 1967, p 1081

Furukawa M: Oriental rhinoplasty. Clin Plast Surg 1:129, 1974

Furukawa M: Recent methods of rhinoplasty for orientals. Aesth Plast Surg 4:325, 1980

Furukawa M: Proportions of the nose and changes with age in Oriental. VIIIth Congress of the International Society of Aesthetic Plastic Surgery. Madrid, 1985

Furukawa M, Furukawa H: A method of correcting the alar base in Oriental rhinoplasty. Transactions of the VIII international Congress Plastic and Reconstructive Surgery. Montreal, 1983, p 492

Gabka HJ: Hasenscharten and Wolfsrachen. Berlin, Walter de Gruyter, 1962

Galassi A: Chirurgia Plastica. Bologna, Capelli Ed, 1950

Gallanti S: Tecnica di JB Goldman per la cura delle deviazioni anteriori del setto nasale mediante rinoplastica. Valsalva 30:27, 1954

Galtier M: Chirurgie esthétique nasale. Paris, G Doin, 1950

Galvao MSL: A postauricular flap based on the contralateral superficial temporal vessels. Plast Reconstr Surg 68:891, 1981

Gammert C: Erste erfahrugen mit tricalciumphosphat als implantationsmaterial in der rekonstrucktiven chirurgie im kopfbereich. Acktuelle probleme der otorhinolaryngologie. Toronto, Huber Berne Stuttgart, 1984, p 131

Gammert C, Masing H: Langzeiterfahrungen mit konserviertem knorpel in der wiederherstellungschirrurgie der nase. Laryngol Rhinology 56:650, 1977

Ganz H: Die Septumperforation und ihre behandlung, in Schretzenmayr A (ed): Almanach für Ohren-, Nasen-, Rachen-, und Kehlkopfkrankheiten. Munchen, JF Lehmann, 1976, p 130

Ganz H: Septumplastik oder Killiansche Resektion. Eine kritische Betrachtung aus der Praxis, in Ganz HNO (ed): Praxis heute. Berlin, Springer, 1982

Ganzer H: Verschluss grosser gaumendefekte. Klin Wschr 54:1095, 1917(a)

Ganzer H: Weichteilplastik des gesichts bei kieferschussverletzungen. Dzsch Mschr Zahnheilk 35:348, 1917(b)

Garcia-Velasco J, Rivera JF, Garcia-Velasco M: A conservative approach to rhinoplasty. Aesth Plast Surg 3:119, 1979

Garcia-Velasco J, Garcia-Velasco M: Tip graft the cartilaginous dorsum in rhinoplasty. Aesth Plast Surg 10:21, 1986

Gastpar H, Kastenbauer, ER, Behbehani, AA: Erfahrungen mit einem humanen fibrinkleber bei operativen eingriffen im kopf-hals-bereich. Laryngol Rhinology 58:389, 1979

Gaynon JE: The maxilla, premaxilla approach to extensive nasal septum surgery. Arch Otolaryngol 68:301, 1958

Gelb J: Lateral osteotomy through existing alar base incision. Ann Plast Surg 8:269, 1982

Gelbke H: Zur plastischen operation der sog doggennase. Chir 24:209, 1953

Gensoul J: J Hebd Med Chir Pratique, 1933. Quoted by DR Millard, Cleft Craft, vol. 2, 1977

Georgi W: Der doppelmeissel, ein neues osteotom zur medianen osteotomie. HNO (Berlin) 25:401, 1977

Georgi W: Eine modifizierte operationstechnik beim nasenflügelkollaps. HNO (Berlin) 30:213, 1982

Georgi W: Application of chondromucosal transposition flaps for closure of septal perforation. Chir Plast 7:29, 1983

Georgiade NC, Hagerty RF: Secondary procedures in the treatment of cleft lip and palate patients. Symposium on Management of Cleft Lip and Palate and Associated Deformities. 8:265, 1974

Georgiade NC, Mladik R, Thorne F: The nasolabial tunnel flap. Plast Reconstr Surg 43:463, 1969

Gerhardt HJ: Zum plastischen verschluss von septumperforationen. Z Laryngol Rhinology 47:392, 1968

Gerow FJ Stahl S: Keystone graft correction of the deviated nasal tip. Ann Plast Surg 11:319, 1983

Gerow JF, Stahl S, Spira M: The totem pole rib graft reconstruction of the nose. Ann Plast Surg 11:273, 1983

Giachero E: Implicanze psicologiche in tema di rinoplastica estetica. Riv Ital Chir Plast 15:305, 1983(a)

Giachero E: La ricostruzione del "Dome" nella chirugia estetica del lobulo nasale. Riv Ital Chir Plast 15:103, 1983(b)

Gibb AG: Hypernasality (rhinolalia aperta) following tonsil and adenoid removal. J Laryngol Orol 72:433, 1956

Gibson T: Cartilage grafts. Bull Soc Int Chir 18:553, 1959

Gibson T: Cartilage grafts. Brit Med Bull 21:153, 1965

Gibson T: Bone and cartilage transplantation, in Rapaport FT (ed): New York, Grune & Stratton

Gibson T, Davis WB: The distortion of autogenous cartilage grafts: Its cause and prevention. Br J Plast Surg 4:257, 1958

Gibson T, Davis WB, Curran RC: The long term survival of cartilage homografts in man. Br J Plast Surg 11:177, 1958

Gierek T: Fibrosarcoma of the nasal cavity and paranasal sinuses. Otolaryngol Pol 36:373, 1982

Giguere P: Les homogreffes de cartilage costal irradié. Rev Stomatolog 83:284, 1983

Gilden MH, Miller EM, Johnson WG: Central nervous system histoplasmosis after rhinoplasty. Neurology 24:874, 1974

Gillies, HD: Plastic Surgery of the Face. London, Oxford University Press, 1920

Gillies H: New free graft (of skin and ear cartilage) applied to reconstruction of nostril. Br J Surg 30:305, 1943

Gillies HD, Kilner TP: Hare-lip. Operation for the correction of secondary deformities Lancet 2:1369, 1932

Gillies HD, Millard R: The Principles and Art of Plastic Surgery, vol. I and II. Boston-Toronto, Little, Brown and Co., 1957

Ginsel A, Illum P: Nasal mucociliary clearance in patients with septal deviation. Rhinology 18:177, 1980

Giunta SX: Nasal tip surgery: A simple technique to aid in symmetry. Laryngoscope 94:974, 1984

Gliosci A, Sabbache, Hipps CJ: Reconstruction of ala of the nose by local pedicle flap. Plast Reconstr Surg 43:149, 1968

Goin J, Goin MK: Changing the Body: Psychological Effects of Plastic Surgery. Baltimore, Williams and Wilkins, 1981

Goin MK, Goin J: Dissatisfaction, in Kaye, B Gradinger, GP (eds): Symposium on Problems and Complications in Aesthetic Plastic Surgery of the Face, 1984

Goldman IB: The Goldman nose. Plastic and Reconstructive Surgery of the Face and Neck, Proceedings of The First International Symposium, New York, Grune & Stratton, 1920(a)

Goldman IB: The rim incision. Plastic and Reconstructive Surgery of the Face and Neck, Proceedings of The First International Symposium, New York, Grune & Stratton, 1920(b)

Goldman IB: The maxillo-facial triad and its correction. J Int Coll Surg 17:167–180, 1952

Goldman IB: Direct vision bone-cutting forceps for rhinoplasty. Trans Am Acad Ophthalmology Otolaryngol 57:628, 1953(a)

Goldman IB: New technique for corrective surgery of nasal tip. Arch Otolaryngol 53:183, 1953(b)

Goldman IB: New techniques in surgery of deviated nasal septum. Arch Otolaryngol 64:183, 1956

Goldman IB: The importance of the medial crura in nasal tip reconstruction. Arch Otolaryngol 65:143, 1957

Goldman IB: Rhinoplastic sequelae causing nasal obstruction. Arch Otolaryngol 83:151, 1966

Goldmann J: Nasal plastic surgery in children. EENT Monthly, 42:58–67, 1963

Goldwyn RM: The consultant and the unfavorable result, in Goldwyn RM (ed): The Unfavorable Result in Plastic Surgery: Avoidance and Treatment. Boston, Little, Brown, and Co, 1972

Goldwyn, Shore: The effect of submucus disection in rhinolasty and the sense of smell. Plast Reconstr Surg 41:427, 1968

Gollom, J: Perforation of nasal septum: The reverse flap technique. Arch Otolaryngol 88:518, 1968

Gomez AD: Rhinomanometry. Simplified technique of recording and evaluation II. Quantitative results in septal deviations. Objective evaluation of functional results of septoplasty. Ann Otorrinolaringol Ibero Am 7:493, 1980

Gomulinski L: La traduction morphologique des deformations septales. Leur correction au cours des rhinoplasties complexes. Ann Chir Plast 27:343, 1982

Gonzales A: Occlusion quirugica de las perforaciones septales con hueso costal de la mastoides. Abstracts 13 World Congress of Otolaryngology, Miami, 1985

Gonzales-Ulloa M: Plastic surgery of nose. Vida Nueva 58:65, 1946

Gonzales-Ulloa M: Correction of a wide nose with a pinch. Plast Reconstr Surg 10:31, 1952

Gonzales-Ulloa M: An articulated acrylic prosthetic structure for the repair of flat nose. J Int Coll Surg 27:359, 1957

Gonzales-Ulloa M: Planning the integral correction the human profile. J Int Coll Surg 36:364, 1962(a)

Gonzales-Ulloa M: Quantitative principles in cosmetic surgery of the face (profileplasty). Plast Reconstr Surg 29:186, 1962(b)

Gonzales-Ulloa M: The fat nose. Aesthetic Plast Surg 8:135, 1984

Gonzales-Ulloa M, Stevens E: Implants in the face. A review on experience in the subcutaneous use of methylmethacrylate. Plast Reconstr Surg 33(6):532, 1964

Gonzales-Ulloa M, Stevens E: Syndrome of retraction of the middle third of the face: Its importance in profileplasty. Int Surg 51:345, 1969

Goodale R: The correction of old lateral deplacement of the nasal bone. Med Surg J, 1901

Goode RI: Diagnosis and treatment of turbinate dysfunction. Am Acad of Otolaryngol 41–51, 1977

Goode RI, Ross J: Columellar advancement for nasal tip elevation. Laryngoscope 83:1123, 1973

Goodman WA, Charles D: Why external rhinoplasty? J Otolaryngol 7:9, 1978

Goodman WS: External approach to rhinoplasty. Can J Otolaryngol 2:3, 1973

Goodman WS: Recent advances in external rhinoplasty. J Otolaryngol 10:433, 1981(a)

Goodman WS: The rotating burr in rhinoplasty. Arch Otolaryngol 107:436, 1981(b)

Goodman WS: The surgical closure of nasoseptal perforations. Laryngoscope 92:121, 1982

Goodman WS, Charbonneau PA: External approach to rhinoplasty. Laryngoscope 84:2195, 1974

Goodman WS, Charles DA: Technique of external rhinoplasty. Otolaryngol 7:13, 1978

Goodman WS, Miller R: Surgery of the nasal tip by external rhinoplasty. ENT J (Toronto) 61:436, 1982

Gorman JB, Curtiss EH: Another nasal pack. Plast Reconstr Surg 70:233, 1982

Gorney M: The septum in rhinoplasty form and function, in Millard D Jr (ed): Symposium on Corrective Rhinoplasty, vol. 13. St. Louis, 1976

Gorney M: Correction of the deviated nose. Ann Plast Surg 8:201, 1984(a)

Gorney M: Medical-legal criteria, in Kaye B, Gradinger GP (eds): Symposium on problems and complications in Aesthetic Plastic Surgery of the Face, 1984(b)

Gorney M: Patient selection criteria: An ounce of prevention, in Kaye B, Gradinger GP (eds): Symposium on Problems and Complication in Aesthetic Plastic Surgery of the Face, 1984(c)

Gosepath J: Frequent mistakes in corrective rhinoplasty. Laryngol Rhinol Otol 62:196, 1983(a)

Gosepath J: Haüfige fehler bei korrektiven rhinoplastiken. Laryngol Rhinol Otol 62:196, 1983(b)

Gosepath J: Korrektive rhinoplastik bei neugeborenen, kindern und erwachsenen mit LKG-spalten. HNO Plastische Chirurgie an Kopf and Hals 133:11, 1987

Gotzfried MF, Masing M: On the improvement of nasal breathing following mid-face osteotomies, and possible reasons for the phenomenon. J Maxillofac Surg 12:29, 1984

Graamans K: Does septal surgery influence submucous congestion. Rhinology 21:21, 1983

Grabb W, Myers MB: Skin Flaps. Boston, Little, Brown & Co, 1975

Gray LP: The deviated nasal septum. J Laryngol Otolaryngol 79:567, 1965

Gray LP: Early treatment of septal deformity and associated abnormalities, in Modern Trends in Disease of Ear, Nose and Throat. London, Butterworth, 1972, p 219

Gray LP: Deviated nasal septum: Incidence and ethology. Ann Otol 87 Suppl 50:3, 1987

Gray LP, Brogan WF: Septal deformity, malocclusion and rapid maxillary expansion. Orthod 4:2, 1972

Gray VD: Physiologic returning of the upper lateral cartilage. Int Rhinology. 8:56, 1970

Greer DM: Secondary cleft lip repair. Facial Plast Surg 3:155, 1986

Griesman BL: Base of the nose: Anatomy and plastic repair. Arch Otolaryngol 52:541, 1950

Grignon L: Les échecs des rhinoplasties. Ann Otolaryngol (Paris) 80:51, 1963

Gubisch W, Reichert H, Widmaier W: Die grosse nase, Pfeifer G (ed): Ein Äesthetisches und Funktionnelles Problem. Die Ästhetik von Form und Funktion in der Plastischen u. Wiederherstellungschirurgie. Springer-Verlag, 1985, p132

Guerreros-Santos J: Cosmetic repair of acute columellar lip angle. Plast Reconstr Surg, 52(3):246, 1973

Guerrero-Santos J: Temporoparietal free fascia grafts in rhinoplasty. Plast Reconstr Surg 74:465, 1984

Guillen G: Essai de systemation des septo-rhinoplasties. Supp. 1967, Rev. Laryng. Otol. Rhigol. 2nd. Congr. Europ. Rhinopl. 1966, Internat. Rhinol. Vol. V, N.3, 1967

Guilleminault C, Tikian-Dement W: The sleep apnea syndrome. Ann Rev Med 27:465–484, 1976

Gunter JP Bell WH: Rhinoplasty and ortognathic surgery. Plastic Reconstructive Face and Neck, Proceedings of the Second International Symposium, vol. 1, New York, Grune & Stratton, 1977

Gurdin M Pangman WJ: A simple electrosurgical treatment of rhinophyma. Calif Med 73:171, 1950

Haas E: Fehler und gefahren bei der korrektiven rhinoplastik. Z Laryngol Rhinology Otol 40:224, 1961

Haas E: Materialbedingte gefahren bei der sattelnasenkorrektur. Z Laryngol Rhinology 48:28, 1969

Haas E, Meyer R: Konstruktive und rekonstruktive chirurgie

der Nase, in Gohrbrandt E, Gabka J, Berndorfer A (Eds): Handbuch der Plastischen Chirurgie. Berlin, De Gruyter, 1968

Habermann G: Der hauchfleck des stabsarzt glatzel. Ein Berliner Beitrag zur Geschichte der Rhinologie. Ordentliche Sitzung der Oto-laryngologischen Gesellschaft. Berlin, 1986

Hadjean E, Ferran F: Le recul de la pointe du nez. Ann Chir Plast 27:3, 286, 1982

Hady MR: The effect of nasal packing on arterial blood gases and acid-base balance and its clinical importance. J Laryngol Otol 97:599, 1983

Hage J: Surgical approach of the external and internal nose. Brit J Plast Surg 12:4, 1960

Hage J: The butterfly cartilage graft for correction of inadequate alae. In Transactions of the 3rd International Congress of Plastic Surgeons, Amsterdam, Excerpta Medica Foundation, 1964

Hage J: Collapsed alae strengthened by conchal cartilage. Br J Plast Surg 18:92, 1969

Hagege JC: L'enroulement—avancement narinaire au cours des rhinoplasties. Ann Otolaryngol 99:423, 1982

Hagege JC, Pollet J: Le dogme du dome. Ann Chir Plast 21:215, 1976

Haight JSJ, Cole P: Lage und funktion der nasenklappe (the site and function of the nasal valve). Laryngoscope 93:49, 1983

Hall WJ, Wanabe T: Transseptal repair of unilateral choanal atresia. Arch Otolaryngol 108:659, 1982

Halle M: ZBL Halls-Nas u Ohrenheilk 4:222, 1924

Hallock GG, Trier WC: Cerebrospinal fluid rhinorrhea following rhinoplasty. Plast Reconstr Surg 71:109, 1983

Hartman A: Partielle resection der nasenscheidewand bei hochgradiger verkrümmung derselben. Dtsch Med Wochenschr 8:691, 1882

Hasegawa M, Ishikawa N, Teramura K, et al: Surgical approach to tumors arising from the posterior third of the nasal septum. ORL 49:157, 1987

Hasegawa M, Kern EB, O'Brien PC: Dynamic changes of nasal resistance. Ann Otol 88:66, 1979

Hassard AD, Holmess RO: The crossbow incision and the nasal flap, its blood supply and clinical applications. Head and Neck Surg 7:135, 1984

Hauben DJ: The history of rhinoplasty. Laryngol Rhinol Otol 62:53, 1983(a)

Hauben DJ: Jacques Joseph. Laryngol Rhinol Otol 62:56, 1983(b)

Hauberg G, Brucksehen E: Über eine einfache methode der knochenkonservierung. Chir 25:249, 1954

Hauberisser E: Zur operationstechnik missgestalteter und verlagerter nasenknorpel. J Med Kosmet 4:37, 1956

Haynes 1956. Quoted by Orticochea 1969

Hayton 1916. Quoted by JP Reidy 1968

Hayward PJ, Mackay IS: Fibrin glue in nasal septal surgery. J Laryngol Otol 101:133, 1987

Healy GB: An approach to the nasal septum in children. Laryngscope 96:1239, 1986

Healy GB, McGill T, Jako G, et al: Management of choanal atresia with the carbon dioxide lather. Ann Otol Rhino Laryngol 658, 1978

Healy MJ: Indications for rhinoplasty in children. Eye Ear Nose Throat Monthly 42:58, 1963

Heanley C: The subcutaneous tissue pedicle in columella and Other Nasal Reconstruction. Br J Plast Surg 8:60, 1955

Heerderks, Stockstead 1969. Quoted by H Masing 1977

Heermann, J: Behandlung grosser septumperforationen mit ohrmuschel-haut-knorpel-transplantaten, 2-wochen-tamponade, hautabstanzung. Laryngol Rhinology, 53:935, 1974

Heimer D, et al: Sleep apnea syndrome treated by repair of deviated nasal septum. Chest 1983: 184–185, 1984

Heinberg CE, Kern EB: The Cottle sign and aid in the physical diagnosis of nasal airflow disturbance. Int Rhinol 11:89, 1973

Heir F 1983. Quoted by Rettinger et al, 1986

Helder AH, Huizing EH: Transplantation terminology in nasal surgery. Rhinology 24:235, 1986

Hellmich S: Moderne technik der plastischen septumkorrektur. HNO (Berlin) 17:223, 1969

Hellmich S: Die Verträglichkeit konservierter homoioplastischer knorpelimplantate in der nase. Z Laryngol Rhinol Otol 49:742, 1970(a)

Hellmich S: Homogenous cartilage implants in rhinosurgery. First International Symposium on Plastic and Reconstructive Surgery of the Face and Neck. New York, 1970(b)

Hellmich S: Cartilage implants in rhinoplasty—problems and prospects. Rhinology 10:1, 1972(a)

Hellmich S: Operativ wesentliche gesichtspunkte bei spanimplantationen der nase. Z Laryngol Rhinol 51:298, 1972(b)

Hellmich S: Präoperative risikobilanz bei spanimplantationen der nase. HNO 20:218, 1972(c)

Hellmich S: Strahlenkonservierung von bankknorpel mit kobalt-60. Archiv Klin Exp Ohren Nasen und Kehlkopfheilk 202:671, 1972(d)

Hellmich S: Das problem der knorpelverbiegung in der nasenchirurgie (experimentelle und praktische aspekte) HNO 21:223, 1973(a)

Hellmich S: Reconstruction of the destroyed cartilaginous septum: Unity of functional and cosmetic surgery of the nose. Otorhinolaryngology 337:719, 1973(b)

Hellmich S: Der einfluss unterschiedlicher konservierungsmethoden auf die biologische qualität von knorpel implantaten. Z Laryngol Rhinol 53:711, 1974

Hellmich S: Die bedeutung unterschiedlicher Lager für Knorpelimplantate in klinischen und experimentellen Untersuchungen. Jahrestagung der Deutschen Gesellsch. Für Plast und Wiederherstellungschirurgie, Sonderdruck, 1978

Hellmich S: Die therapie des frischen septumabszesses. HNO (Springer) 22:278, 1979(a)

Hellmich S: Materialbedingte gefahren der korrektiven rhinoplastik. Archiv für Ohren-, Nasen-, und Kehlkopfheilkunde 223:336,1979(b)

Hellmich S: Die Bedeutung unterschiedlicher Lager für Knorpelimplantate in klinischen und experimentellen Untersuchungen. 16th Congress German Society of Plastic Reconstructive Surgery 1978, Düsseldorf, Berlin, Springer, 1980

Hellmich S: Nasal grafts. Proceedings Internat Meet Joseph Spc London, Birmingham, R Evans, 1981

Hellmich S: Fehler und gefahren bei der freien knorpeltransplantation im gesichtsbereich. HNO 30:140, 1982

Hellmich S: Die verwendung von kunststoff bei nasenplastiken. Laryngol Rhinology Otol 62:321, 1983

Herbert DC, Harrison RG: Nasolabial subcutaneous pedicle flaps. Br J Plast Surg 28:85, 1975

Herfert O: Zur technik der pharynxplastik. Fortschr. Kiefer Ges Chir I:82, 1955

Hernandez SF: Palatopharyngoplasty for the obstructive sleep apnea syndrome: Technique and preliminary report of results on ten patients. Am J Otolaryngol 3:229–234, 1982

Herrmann IF: Die behandlung der beidseitigen, kompletten choanalatresie beim neugeborenen. Ben Ges Plast Wiederherstellungschir 31:1983

Hertig P: Traitement chirurgical des atrophies nasales et leurs résultats. Aktuelle Probleme der Otolaryngologie, Toronto, Huber Berne, 1984.

Hertig P, Meyer R: Closure of septal defects and septocolumellar reconstruction. Excerpta Medica, International Congress Series No. 206, Oto-Rhino-Laryngology: Proceedings of the Ninth International Congress, Mexico, August, 1969, p 714

Hertig P, Meyer R: Closure of Septal Defects and Septocolumellar Reconstruction. In Proceedings of the Ninth International Congress of Oto-Rhino-Laryngology. Amsterdam: Excerpta Medica Foundation, 1970

Herzon FS: Bacteremia and local infection with nasal packing. Arch Otolaryngol 94:317, 1971

Hess CW: Das schlaf-apnoe-syndrom. Wie gefährlich ist schnarchen. Gazette Médical 13:35, 1985

Hewell TS, Tardy E: Nasal tip refinement. Fac Plast Surg 1:87, 1984

Heybroeck G: Some application of the nasolabial flap in reconstruction of the nose and lips. Br J Plast Surg 23:26, 1970

Heylen: Déviation et longueur trop considérable du cartilage de la cloison du nez. Gaz Mèd de Paris 13:810, 1847

Heymann P: Über korrektion der nasenscheidewand. Münchner Med Wochensch 13:231, 1886

Hiebert AE, Brooks HW: Sublabial approach for the insertion of L-shaped bone strut for the correction of saddle nose. Plast Reconstr Surg 29:608, 1962

Hildebrand 1930. Quoted by Pirsig, 1975

Hilger JA: The internal osteotomy in rhinoplasty. Arch Otolaryngol 88:211, 1968

Hill G, Silver AG: Psychodynamic and aesthetic motivations for plastic surgery. Psychosom Med 12:345, 1950

Hinderer KH: Diagnosis of anatomic obstructions of the airways. Arch Otolaryngol 78:660, 1963

Hinderer KH: Surgery of the valve. Int Rhinol 8:60, 1970

Hinderer KH: Fundamentals of Anatomy and Surgery of the Nose. Birmingham, Aesculapius Publishing Company, 1971

Hinderer KH: Correction of deformities of the base of the nose. Plastic and Reconstructive Surgery of the Head and Neck, Proceedings Second International Symposium, vol. 1. New York, Grune & Stratton, 1977(a)

Hinderer KH: Correction of deformities of the base of the nose, in Sisson GA, (ed): Plastic and Reconstructive Surgery of the Face and Neck, New York, Grune & Stratton, 1977(b)

Hinderer UT: Profileplasty. Int Micro J Aesth Plast Surg 1:1, 1971

Hinderer UT: Nuevo tratamiento de las perforaciones del tabique nasal mediante colgajos vertibulo-labiales compuestos. Rev Esp Cirg Plast 6:2, 1973

Hinderer UT: La rinoplastia y technicas adicionales de perfiloplastia. Cir Plast Ibero-Latinoam 1:49, 1975

Hinderer UT: Das verhältnis zwischen projektion der nasenspitze und des nasenrückens bei rhinoplastischen eingriffen. Aesthetic Plast Surg 8:201, 1984(a)

Hinderer UT: Relationship between the protrusion of the nasal tip and the dorsum in the rhinoplasty. Aesth Plast Surg 8:201, 1984(b)

Hinsberg V: Operative behandlung der ozaena. Mschr Ohrenheilk 55:1969, 1921

Hirschowitz B, Moscona R, Eliachar I: Closure of septal perforation in Osler-Weber-Rendu's disease by bilateral labial-buccal flaps. Plast Reconstr Surg 62:296, 1978

Holcomb H: Primary correction of unilateral cleft lip nasal deformity: A 10-year review. Plast Reconstr Surg 75:791, 1985

Holmes CR: Hypertrophy of the turbinated bodies. NY Med J 72:529, 1900

Holmes M: The correction of nasal skeletal defects. 63 Annual Session of the Am Acad Opht and Otol, Chicago, 1958

Holt GR: Management of cleft lip nasal deformity. Fac Plast Surg 3:161, 1986

Holt JAB, Lloyd RS: Rhinoplasty: Use of methyl methacrylate implants. Arch Otolaryngol 47:406, 1948

Horn H: The treatment of intumescent rhinitis by a submucous method. Ann Otol Rhinol Laryngol 17:490, 1908

Horton CE: Combined septoplasty and rhinoplasty, in Masters FW, Lewis JR Jr (eds): Symposium on Aesthetic Surgery of the nose, ears and chin. St. Louis, The C.V. Mosby Co, 1973

House HP: Submucous resection of the inferior turbinal bone. Laryngoscope 61:637, 1951

Hueston JT: The silver wishbone in nasal tip surgery. Aesthetic Plast Surg 6:153, 1982

Huffman W, Lierle DM: Progress in septal surgery. Plast Reconstr Surg 20:185–198, 1957

Huffman WC, Lierle DM: Studies on the pathological anatomy of the unilateral harelip nose. Plast Reconstr Surg 4:225, 1949

Huizing EH: Septumchirurgie bij kinderen. Ned Tijdschr Geneeskd 110:1293–1296, 1966

Huizing EH: Experience on the use of homologous cartilage in nasal surgery. Acta Otorhinolaryngol 24:194, 1970

Huizing EH: Implantation and transplantation in reconstructive nasal surgery. Rhinology 12 (93):106, 1974

Huizing EH: Septum surgery in children: Indications, surgical technique and long-term results. Rhinology 17:91, 1979

Huizing EH: Long term results of reconstruction of the septum in the acute phase of a septal abscess in children. Rhinology 22:55, 1984(a)

Huizing EH: Reconstruction of the septum skeleton after nasal removal or destruction. Proceedings of the 10th European Congress in Rhinology, France, Nancy, 1984(b)

Huizing EH: The management of septal abscesses. Fac Plast Surg 3:4, 1986

Huizing EH, Sedee GA, Wentges RTR: Correctieve Neuschirurgie. Rapport der 136. Versammlung der Neederlands Keel-Neus-Oorheelkunde Vereniging, Leiden, 1973

Hurd LM: Bipolar electrode for electrocoagulation of the inferior turbinate. Arch Otolaryngol 13:442, 1931

Hurman H: Large septal perforation treatment using free skin cartilage-skin grafts from the pinna. Laryngol Rhinology Otol 53:935, 1974

Hynes W: Pharyngoplasties by muscle transplantation. Br J Plast Surg 3:129, 1950

Illum P: Congenital choanal atresia treated by laser surgery. Rhinology 24:205, 1986

Ingals EF: Deflection of septum narium. Arch Laryngol 3:291, 1882

Ismail HK: Closure of septal perforations: A new technique. J Laryngol Otol 78:620, 1964

Ivy RH: Nelson's Loose Leaf Surgery. New York, Thomas Nelson & Sons, 1932

Jackson C, Coates GM: The Nose, Throat, and Ear and Their Diseases. Philadelphia, W.B. Saunders, 1929

Jackson IT: Discussion to Orticochea. A review of 236 cleft palate patients treated with dynamic muscle sphincter. Plast Reconstr Surg 71:187, 1983

Jackson IT, McGlynn MJ, Huskie CF, et al: Velopharyngeal incompetence in the absence of cleft palate results of treatment in 20 cases. Plast Reconstr Surg 66:211, 1980

Jackson IT,, Pellett CC, Smith JM: The skull as a bone graft donor site. Ann Plast Surg 11:527, 1983

Jackson IT, Smith J, Mixter RC: Nasal bone grafting using split skull grafts. Ann Plast Surg 11:533, 1983

Jacobs KF: Angeborene aplasie von nasensteg und knorpeligem septum. Laryngol Rhinol Otol 63:344, 1984

Jacobs SI, et al. Nasal abnormality and the carrier rate of staphylococcus aureus. J Clin Pathol 14:519, 1961

Jafek BW, Rhew K, Bryant KC, et al: Current concepts in the management of velopharyngeal incompetence, in Bernstein L (ed): Plastic and Reconstructive Surgery of the Head and Neck, vol. 2. Rehabilitative surgery. 1981, p 345

Jahnke V: Der gesichts und kopfschmerz aus der sicht des Otorhinolaryngol. 36:385, 1977

Janeke JB, Wright WK: Studies on the support of the nasal tip. Arch Otolaryngol 93:458, 1971

Janeke JB: Sphenopalatine ligation for epistaxis and postnasal drip (letter) S. Afr Med J 2:64, 1983

Jazby J: Nasal septum deformity in the newborn. Clin Pediatr 13:953, 1974

Jefferson S: History of rhinoplasty. An epitome of plastic surgery. J Flamed Ass 56:622, 1969

Jescheck J: Uber den versuch einer mundschleimhautplastik bei ozaena. Arch Ohr Nas u Kehlk Heilk 172:704, 1960

Jescheck J: Die oronasale schleimhautplastik bei ozaena. Mschr Ohrenheilk 95:282, 1961

Jeschek J: Methoden zur verhütung und behebung von postoperativen septumperforationen. Üsterr Otolaryngol 103:504, 1969

Jeschek J, Denecke HJ, Ey W: Die Operationen an der Nase und im Nasopharynx. Berlin, Springer-Verlag, 1984

Jennes ML: Corrective nasal surgery in children. EENT Monthly 33:583, 1954

Jennes ML: Corrective nasal surgery in children; long-term results. Arch Otolaryngol 79:145, 1964

Jessen M, Malm L: The importance of nasal airway resistance and nasal symptoms in the selection of patients for septoplasty. Rhinology 22:157, 1984

Jobe R: En bloc nasal shift rhinoplasty: An approach to the small crooked nose. Ann Plast Surg 7:120, 1981

John A: Management of the difficult septum. Arch Otolaryngol 78:652, 1963

Johnson NE: Septal surgery and rhinoplasty. Transaction of the A.A.O.O. 68:869, 1964

Johnson NE: Septal perforations and secondary septal surgery. Laryngoscope 78:586, 1968

Johnson NE: Secondary surgery of the septum. Otolaryngol Clin North Am 7:75, 1974

Johnsson JT, Sanders MH: Breathing during sleep immediately after uvulopalatopharyngoplasty. Laryngol 96:1236, 1986

Jones M: Turbinal hypertrophy. Lancet 2:879, 1895

Jones TC: Turbinotomy. Lancet 2:496, 1985

Jordan LW: The correction of the anterior deviations of the nasal septum. Trans Pacific Coast Otolaryngol Ophthalmol Soc 29:216, 1948

Jordan LW: External nasal pyramid and septum reconstruction. Arch Laryngol 67:521, 1958

Joseph G: Preliminary discussion on the thick septum problem. Supp. 1967. Rev Laryngol Otol Rhinol 2nd. Congr. Europ. Rhinol. 1966. Intern. Rhinol. Vol. V, Number 3, 1967

Joseph J: Uber die operative verkleinerung einer nase (rhinomiosis). Berl Klin Wochenschr 40:882, 1898

Joseph J: Über die intranasale höckerabtragung (ohne jede verletzung der äusseren haut.) Deutsche Med Wochensch 30:1095, 1904

Joseph J: Nasenplastik und sonstige gesichtsplastik (ein atlas und lehrbuch.) Leipzig, Curt Kabitzsch, 1932

Jost G: Correction du défaut de la pointe du nez. Ann Chir Plast 12:4, 1972

Jost G: Mode de surture au cours des rhinoplasties suivant la technique extra-muqueuse. Ann Chir Plast 18:271, 1973(a)

Jost G: Usage d'une cisaille au cours de la rhinoplastie. Ann Chir Plast 18:279, 1973(b)

Jost G: Atlas de Chirurgie Esthétique et Plastique, vol. 1. Paris, Masson éd., 1975

Jost G, Meresse B: Etude de la fonction entre les cartilages lateraux du nez. Ann Chir Plast 18:175, 1973

Jpvicevic B: Approccio semplificato alla chirurgia delle ptosi nell'infanzia. Atti del Congresso Italiano di Chirurgia Plastica, Bari 1985

Jugo SB, Padovan IF: A new method of total septal reconstruction in children. Abstracts, 13 World Congress Otolaryngology, 1985, p 112

Juri J: Secondary rhinoplasty. Transactions of the VII International Congress of Plastic Surgery, Montreal, Canada, 1983, p 731

Juri J, Juri C: Secondary rhinodeformity. Transactions of the VII International Congress of Plastic and Reconstructive Surgery, Rio de Janeiro, 1979, p 482

Juri J, Juri C, Belmont JA, et al: Neighboring flaps and cartilage grafts for correction of serious secondary nasal deformities. Plast Reconstr Surg 76:876, 1985

Juri J, Juri C, Colnago A: Implants and grafts in secondary rhinodeformities. Aesthetic Plast Surg 4:135, 1980

Juri J, Juri C, Elias JC: Ear cartilage grafts to the Nose. Plast Reconstr Surg 63:377, 1979

Juri J, Juri C, Grilli DA, et al: Correction of the secondary nasal Tip. Ann Plast Surg 15:4, 1984

Kabaker S: An approach to aesthetic rhinoplasty in the caucasian nose. Arch Otolaryngol 103:461, 1977

Kabaker SS: Personal communication, 1985

Kabaker SS: Rhytidorhinoplasty for the senile nose, in Bernstein L (ed): Plastic and Reconstructive Surgery, vol. 1, Aesth Surg 1981, p 118

Kalick SM: Toward an interdisciplinary psychology of appearances. Psychiatry 41:243, 1978

Kalick SM: Aesthetic surgery: How it affects the way patients are perceived by others. Ann Plast Surg 23:128, 1979

Kamer FM: Lengthening the short nose. Ann Plast Surg 4:281, 1980

Kamer FM, Binder WJ: Pseudomonas infection of the nose. Arch Otolaryngol 106:505, 1980

Kamer FM, Churukian MM: Chirurgie der nasenspitze (Surgery of the nasal tip). ENT 61:444, 1982

Kamer FM, Churukian MM: High septal hemitransfixion for the correction of caudal septal deformities. Laryngoscope 94:391, 1984(a)

Kamer FM, Churukian MM: Shield graft for the nasal tip. Arch Otolaryngol 110:608, 1984(b)

Kamer FM, Cohen A: Median horizontal split tip. Otolaryngol Head Neck Surg 93:35, 1985

Kamer FM, Parkes ML: An absorbent, non adherent nasal pack. Laryngoscope 85:384, 1975(a)

Kamer FM, Parkes ML: The conservative management of the negro nose. Laryngoscope 85:551, 1975(b)

Kamer FM, Parkes ML: Gelatin film: A useful adjunct in rhinoplastic surgery. Arch Otolaryngol 103:667, 1977

Kapetansky DI: Double pendulum flaps for whistling deformities in bilateral cleft lips. Plast Reconstr Surg 47:321, 1971

Kaplan EN, Falces E, Tolleth H: Clinical utilization of injectable collagen. Ann Plast Surg 10:437, 1983

Karlan MS, Madden M, Habal MB: Biostereometric analysis in plastic and reconstructive surgery. Plast Reconstr Surg 62:235, 1978

Karlan MS, Ossoff R, Christu P: Reconstruction for large septal perforations. Arch Otolaryngol 108:433, 1982

Kastenbauer ER: Nasenseptumersatz und dermoplastik bei der rendu-weber'schen erkrankung. Z Laryng Rhinol 56:890, 1977

Kastenbauer ER: Arbeitsgemeinschaft plastische chirurgie: Fehler und gefahren bei verwendung freier transplantate und implantate im gesichtsbereich. HNO30:131, 1982(a)

Kastenbauer ER: Fehler und gefahren bei der knochentransplantation. HNO 30:145, 1982(b)

Kastenbauer ER: Pedicle transplants in rhinoplasty. Laryngol Rhinol Otol, 62:19, 1983(a)

Kastenbauer ER: Konservierung und anwendungsmöglichkeiten allongener (homologer) transplantate im halsnasen-ohrenbereich. HNO 31:371, 1983(b)

Kawamoto HK, Jr: Treatment of the elongated lower face and gummy smile. Clin Plast Surg 9:479, 1982

Kaye BL: Rhinoplasty in the older patient. Aesthetic Plast Surg 3:57, 1979

Kaye BL: Rhinoplasty in the older patient, in Kaye B, Gradinger G (eds): Troubles and Complications, Symposium. St. Louis, CV Mosby, 1984, p 125

Kayser R: Die exacte messung der luftdurgängigkeit der nase. Arch Laryngol Rhinology, Berlin 3:101, 1895

Kazanjian H, Holmes EM: Stenosis of the nasopharynx and its correction. Arch Otolaryngol 44:261, 1946

Kazanjian VH, Converse JM: second edition. London, Baillière, Tindall & Cox, 1959

Kazanjian VH, Converse JM: Surgical Treatment of Facial Injuries. Baltimore, Williams and Wilkins Co, 1974

Kean H: Management of the columellar lip angle, in Bernstein L (ed): Plastic and Reconstructive Surgery, vol. 1. Aesth Surg, 1981

Keegan DF: Rhinoplastic Operations, with a Description of Recent Improvements in the Indian Method. Ballière, London, Tindall and Cox, 1900

Kening E, Braun-Falco O: Dermatology und Venerolgie, (ed 2). Münich, JF Lehmans, 1969

Kern EB: Rhinomanometry. Otolaryngol Clin North Am 6:863, 1973

Kern EB: Surgery of the nasal valve, in Sisson GA, Tardy EM (eds): Plastic and Reconstructive Surgery of the Face and Neck. Stuttgart, George Thieme, Ed., 1975

Kern EB: Standardization of rhinomanometry. Rhinology 15:115, 1977(a)

Kern EB: Surgery of the nasal valve. Plastic and Reconstructive Surgery of the Face and Neck. Proceedings of the Second International Symposium, vol 1, New York Grune & Stratton, 1977(b)

Kern EB: Surgical approaches to abnormalities of the nasal valve. Rhinology 16:165, 1978

Kern EB: Committee report on standardization of rhinomanometry. Int Rhinology 19:231, 1981

Kern EB: Rhinologic assessment of nasal obstruction. Otolaryngol Head Neck Surgery, 15(16), 1982

Kern EB: Applied physiology of the nasal cavities. Rhinology 22:91, 1984

Kern EB, Facer GW, McDonald TJ, et al: Closure of nasal septal perforations with a silastic button. ORL Dig 39:9, 1977

Kesselring UK: Hot air. Ann Plast Surg, 16:454, 1986

Killian G: Die submucöse fensterresektion der nasenscheidenwand. Arch Laryngol Rhinol (Berlin) 16:362, 1904

Killian G: The submucous window resection of the nasal septum. Ann Otol Rhinol Laryngol 14:363, 1905

Killian G: Beiträge zur submukösen fensterresektion der nasen-scheidewand. Passow u. Scaefer Beitr. etc, 1: 183–192, 1908

Kilner TP: The management of the patient with cleft lip and/or palate. Am J Surg 95:204, 1958

Kilner TP, Gillies H: Operations for corrections of secondary deformities. Lancet 1:1932

King ED, Ashley FL: Correction of the internally and externally deviated nose. Plast Reconstr Surg 10:116, 1952

Kitajiaha T: Repair of septal perforation with a pedunculated flap of mucous membrane from the maxillary sinus. Otolaryngol (Tokyo) 37:141, 1965

Klablunde EH, Falces E: Incidence of complications in cosmetic rhinoplasties. Plast Reconstr Surg 34:192, 1964

Klaff DD: The surgical anatomy of the anterocaudal portion of the nasal septum: A study of the area of the premaxilla. Laryngoscope 66:995, 1956

Klatsky SA, Manson PN: Aesthetic rhinoplasty in patients with thick nasal skin. Ann Plast Surg 11:10, 1983

Kleine EH: The chondrojet: Simplified method for handling of diced cartilage. Plast Reconstr Surg 3:95, 1948

Kleine EH: Nasal tip reconstruction through external incisions. Plast Reconstr Surg 15:502, 1955

Koburg E: Über ein einfaches verfahren zum verschluss grosser septumperforationen. Arch Klin Exp Ohr Nas u Kehlk Heilk. 205:289, 1973

Koechlin H: New instruments in rhinoplasty. Plast Reconstr Surg 8:132, 1951

Kortehangas AE: Funktion and Funktionsprüfung der Nase und der Nasennebenhöhlen. In: Berendes, Link u.Zöllner, HNO–Heilkunde in Praxis und Klinik, vol. I, 2nd Edit, Stuttgart, Thieme, 1977

Kosenko VF: Multiple teratoma of the nose. Vestn Otorinolaringol 74, 1983

Kosoy J: Nasal surgery and airway resistence. Laryngoscope 89:1655, 1979

Kovalenko PP, Yemelianov VA: Conservation and transplantation of cartilage. Acta Chir Plast (Praha) 9:304, 1967

Krajina 1969. Quoted by Pirsig, 1975

Kratz, RC: Repair of septal perforations with composite graft. Arch Otolaryngol (Chic) 98:380, 1973

Krause CJ: Augmentation rhinoplasty. Otolaryngol Clin North Am 743, 1975

Kressner A, Kornmesser, HJ: Operative treatment of rhinopathia vosomotoria. Rhinology 14:133, 1976

Krickoon LA: Contribution to surgical technique in operations on the septum nasi in outer nose disfigurement. Acta Chir Plast 6:124, 1964

Krieg R: Über die fensterresektion des septum narium zur heilung der skoliosis septi. Arch Laryngol 10:477–488, 1900

Krizek TJ: The normal body defends against foreign implants, in Rubin LR (ed): Biomaterials Reconstructive Surgery. St. Louis, C.V. Mosby, 1983, p 9

Krmpotic-Nemanic J, Kostivic J, Rudan P: Aging changes of the form and infrastructure of the external nose and its importance in rhinoplasty. Plast Reconstr Surg of the Face and Neck 1:84, 1972

Kubik CS, Adams RD: Subdural empyema. Brain 66:18, 1943

Kuderna H: Ergebnisse und erfahrungen in der klinischen anwendung des fibrin-klebers bei der wiederherstellung durchtrennter peripherer nerven, in Implantate und Transplantate in der Plastischen und Wiederherstellungschirurgie, Basal, Springer-Verlag, 1981, pp 96–100

Lacy GM, Conway H: Recovery after meningitis with convulsions and paralysis: Cause for pause. Plast Reconstr Surg 36:254, 1965

LaFerla S: Chirurgia combinata funzionale e cosmetica della platyrrina ozena tosa. Arch Otol 70:1103, 1955

LaFerla S: La correzione chirurgia dell'abnorme brievatà della columella nasale. Act Ital Otol 70:979, 1959(a)

LaFerla S: Settoplastica. Nuovi orientamenti nella correzione del setto nasale deviato. Arch Ital ORL 70:789, 1959(b)

Lafuente DJ: Personal Communication, Barcelona, 1987

Lagrot F: Drow bridge reconstructive rhinoplasty. Plast Reconstr Surg 42:37, 1968

Lamont E: Rhinoplasty: securing the graft. Ann Plast Surg 4:84, 1980

Lamont ES: Reconstructive surgery of the nose in congenital deformity: Injury and disease. Am J Surg 65:17, 1944

Landegham K: Closure of septal perforations. HNO 19:158, 1971

Langraf-Favre F: Veröden gegen schnarchen. Medical Tribune 6:53, 1983

Langraf-Favre F: Snoring: A problem for the rhinologist. Abstract 10 Congress European Society of Rhinology, Nancy, 1984

Langraf-Favre F: Schnarchen heute. Hospitalis 12:1986

Langraf-Favre F: The "common" snorrer in front of his doctor. Proceedings of the First International Congress of Chronic Rhoncopathy, Paris, 1987

Lapidot A: Construction of a neo-valve for nasal insufficiency. Rhinology 23:333, 1985

Lapins NA: Dermabrasion for telangiectasia. J Dermatol Surg Oncol 9:470, 1983

LaRossa DD, Rich JD, Zbylski JR: Correction of alar notches by rotation-advancement of a nostril rim segment. Plast Reconst Surg 60:267, 1977

Larrabee WF Jr, Maupin G, Sutton D: Profile analysis in facial plastic surgery. Arch Otolaryngol Head Neck Surg 111:682, 1985

Latham RA: Development and structure of the premaxillary deformity in bilateral cleft lip and palate. Br Plast Surg 26:1, 1973

Larentaci G, Dioguardi G, Pascone M, et al: Esperienze sulle proprietà antigeniche della cartilagine umana trattata o meno con glutaraldeide per l'impiego come impinato sostitutivo in chirurgia. Atti del Congresso Italiano di Chirurgia Plastica, Bari, 1985

Lautenschlager A: Die rhinitis atriphicans, in: Handbuch der Hals-Nasen-OHren-Heilkunde, vol. 2, 1952, p 604

Lautenschlager A: Die eingriffe am ohr und an der nase, in: Kirschnners Operationslehre, Berlin, 1934

Lavine DM, Lehman JA, Jackson I: Is the lacrimal apparatus injured following cosmetic rhinoplasty? Arch Otolaryngol 103:719, 1979

Lee T: Augmentation rhinoplasty with plasticene modelling design and the dynamic new nose. Proceedings of International Congress of Plastic Surgery, Montreal, 1983

Lemperle G, Spitanly HH: Long term experience with silicone implant in the face, in Caronni EP (Ed): Cranio Facial Surgery. Boston, Little, Brown, and Co., 1985, p 490

Lemoine J: Un cas de sténose narinaire traité par le procédé de la greffe en charnière et par diathermocoagulation linéaire. Ann Otolaryngol Chir Cervicofac 1:151, 1931

Lenz H: Endonasal laser surgery, in Koechlner HK (ed): Laser's in Medicine. Toronto, Wiley and Sons, 1980(a), p 63

Lenz H: Laserchirurgische behandlung des morbus rendu–osler–weber. Arch Otolaryngol 277:580, 1980(b)

Lenz H: Septumperforationsverschiuss durch composite graft aus der ohrmuschel. Arch Otorhinolaryngol (Suppl) 62, 1983

Lenz H: 8 jahre laser chirurgie and den unteren nasenmuscheln der rhinophathia vasomotoria in form der laserstichkarbonisation. HNO 33:422, 1985

Lenz H, Eicher J, Salk J, et al: Parameters for argolaser surgery of the lower human turbinates. Acta Otolaryngol 83:360, 1977

Lenz H, Sedee GA: Chirurgie der nase und der nasennebenhölen unter durchleuchtungkontrolle. HNO 19(7):281, 1971

Lenz LL: Praxis der Kosmetischen Chirurgie. Stuttgart, Hippocrates, 1954

Lenz H: Septumperforationsverschluss durch composite graft aus der ohrmuschel. Arch Otorhinolaryngol (Suppl) 62, 1983

Leperchey F, Cotin G, Bodard M, et al: Deux modalités dans le porcessus embryogénique des kystes et fistules fronto-nasaux. Ann Otolaryngol (Paris) 100:247, 1983

LePesteur JS, Sarazin A, Tristant H: La xérographie intérêt en rhinoplastie et en chirurgie maxillofaciale. Ann Chir Plast 21:2, 1976

Levet Y: Correction of defects in the projection of the tip of the nose after surgery. Ann Otolaryngol Chir Cervicofac 100:77, 1983

Levet Y, Ferran F: Correspondance. Plast Reconstr Surg 79:2, 1987

Levignac J: Des petits et des gros ennuis dans la rhinoplastie. Ann Otolaryngol 75:500, 1958

Levignac J: Greffes et implants, greffes ou implants, dans la réparation du soutien nasal après enfoncement. Ann Otolaryngol 76:758, 1959

Levignac J: A propos des anomalies nez-menton et de leurs corrections. Réflexions sur la morphologie et l'esthétique. Orthod Fr 47, 1977

Levine PA: Reconstruction of large nasal defects with a sub-

cutaneous pedicle nasolabial flap. Arch Otolaryngol 111(9):628–630, 1985
Lewin M, Argamaso RV, Friedman S: Localized cerbritis. Plast Reconstr Surg 64:720, 1979
Lewin ML: Prevention and correction of cicatricial intranasal adhesion in rhinoplastic surgery. Arch Otolaryngol 60:415, 1954
Lewin ML, Argamaso RV, Friedman S: Localized cerebritis following an esthetic rhinoplasty. Plast Reconstr Surg 64:720, 1979
Lewis JR: The nasal profile. Panminerva Med 2:170, 1969
Lewis JR: Atlas of Aesthetic Surgery. Boston, Little, Brown and Co., 1973
Lewis JR: The nasal profile, in Millard DR Jr (ed): Symposium on Corrective Rhinoplasty. St. Louis, Mosby, 1976, p 146
Lexer E: Der plastische ersatz des septum cutaneum. Dtsch Z Chir 81:560, 1906
Lexer E: Kosmetische Operationen der Nase. In der HNO-Heilkunde von Denker-Kahler. Bd.V.S., 1929, p 991
Libra G, Mezzoli G: Deformità del setto nasale e funzione tubo-timpanica: Studio rinomanometrico e impedenzometrico. 70 Cong. Naz. Soc. Ital. ORL Bologna, 1983
Liebermann T: HNO 30:562, 1932
Liebermann 1932. Quoted by McLaughlin, 1950
Link R: Zur plastik des knorpeligen-nasengerüstes. Z Laryngol Rhinology 30:84, 1951
Linn L, Goldman JB: Psychiatric observation concerning rhinoplasty. Psychosom Med 11:307, 1949
Lippi L, Porzio P, Ciabatti PG: Human fibrin sealant our experience on its use and limits in rhinology. ENT Clin 62:103, 1986
Lipset EM: A new approach to surgery of the lower cartilaginous vault. Arch Otolaryngol 70:42, 1959
Lipshutz H: Submucous resection. Symposium on Aesthetic Surgery of the Nose and Ears. St. Louis, Master & Lewis Ed, Mosby, 1973
Little SW: Management of enlarged turbinates. Va Med 90:484, 1963
Litton C, Fournier P: Simple surgical correction of the gummy smile. Plast Reconstr Surg 63:372, 1979
Lore JM: An Atlas of Head and Neck Surgery. Philadelphia, WB Saunders, 1962
LoRusso D: Techniques to repair nasal septal perforations. Boll Mal Orech Gola Naso 88:183, 1970
LoRusso D: La punta del naso considerazioni estetiche e techniche. Riv Ital Chir Plast 15:96, 1981
Lovas RM: Secondary rhinoplasties. Aesth Plast Surg 5:361–368, 1981
Lowenthal G: Secondary surgical treatment of intranasal deformities of the unilateral cleft palate nose. Laryngoscope 91:1641, 1981
Lupo G: Histoire de la rhinoplastie esthétique. Méd et Hyg (Genève) 40:777, 1982
Mabry RL: Surgery of the inferior turbinates; How much and when. Otolaryngol Head Neck Surg 92:574, 1984
Maceri DR, Makielski KH: Intraoral ligation of the maxillary artery for posterior epistaxis. Laryngoscope 94:737, 1984
MacKay IS, Bull TR: The fate of silastic in the management of saddle deformity in the nose. Procedings of the International Joseph Society, London, Birmingham, 1981
MacKay JS: Measurement of nasal, airflow and resistence. J R Soc Med 72:852, 1979
MacKenzie MRG: The anatomy of the external nose. Course in Septorhinoplasty, Toronto, 1975–76
Mahe E, et al: Transcartilaginous approach in surgery of the nasal tip. Ann Chir Plast 27(2):147, 1982
Mahe E, Gambling J: Le muscle dépresseur de la pointe. Ann Chir Plast 19(2):57, 1974
Mahe E, Gambling J: La voie transcartilagineuse dans la chirurgie de la pointe du nez. Ann Chir Plast 27:147, 1982
Mahe E, Gamblin J, Micheli-Pellegrini V: Traitement du bec corbain post-opératoire par injection itérative in situ d'acetonid de triumcinolone. Ann Chir Plast 20:79, 1975
Maher A: Treatment of choanal atresia by endonasal microsurgery. J Microsurg 3:231, 1982
Mahler D, Moses S, Last U: A measuring scale for objective evaluation of the nasal shape. Aesth Plast Surg 7:223, 1983
Mahler D, Tovi F, Zirkin H: Bilateral nasal glandular cysts: An occasional finding in rhinoplasty. Aesth Plast Surg 8:119, 1984
Majumdar B: Malignant neoplasms of the nose and paranasal sinuses: A survey of cases treated in a regional centre. Clin Otolaryngol 8:97, 1983
Malbec EF: Algunos errores cometidos en las rinoplastias. Prensa Méd Argent 40:2470, 1953
Malbec EF, Beaux AR: Reconstruction of columella. Br J Plast Surg 11:142, 1958
Maler L: Rinoplastias en la infancia. Chirurgia Plastica Ibero Latinoamericana. 13(1):54, 1987
Maliniac JW: Nasal deformities, their prevention and correction following submucous resection. Arch Otolaryngol 6:320, 1927
Maliniac JW: Rhinophyma Arch Otolaryngol 13:270, 1931
Maliniac JW: Correction of depressions by transposition lateral cartilaqes. Arch Otolaryngol 15:280, 1932
Maliniac JW: Prevention of late sequelae in corrective rhinoplasty. Am J Surg 50:84, 1940
Maliniac JW: Procedure for elevation of nasal dorsum by transposition of lateral cartilages. Arch Otolaryngol 41:214, 1945
Maliniac JW: Rhinoplasty and Restoration of Facial Contour. Philadelphia, F.A. Davis Co, 1947
Maliniac JW: Role of the septum in rhinoplasty. Arch Otolaryngol 48:189, 1948
Man A: Surgical reduction of the broad nose. Am J Otolaryngol 5:446, 1980
Man A: Molding the nasal tip: A modified lipsett technique for the wide lobule, in Bernstein L (ed): Plastic and Reconstructive Surgery, vol. 1. Aesth Surg 1981(a), p 53
Man A: A simplified technique of septal correction in the deflected nose, in Bernstein L (ed): Plastic and Reconstructive Surgery, vol. 1. Aesth Surg 1981(b), p 81
Mangoldt F: Die einpflanzung von rippenknorpel in dem kehlkopf, heilung schwerer stenosen and defekten, and heilung der sattelnase durch knorpelübertragung. Deutsche Ges Chir 29:460, 1900 (translated in English by McDowell F: Reconstruction of Saddle nose by cartilage overlay. Plast Reconstr Surg 46:498, 1970)
Marchac D, Toth B: The axial frontonasal flap revisited. Plast Reconstr Surg 76:686, 1985
Marcks KM, Trevaskis AE, Berg EM: Nasal defects associated with cleft-lip deformity. Plast Reconstr Surg 34:176, 1964
Marcus P: Psychological aspects of cosmetic rhinoplasty. Br J Plast Surg 37:313, 1984
Mariano A: Analysis and treatment of a case of nasal obstruction of complex etiology. Ann Chir Plast 27:384, 1982

Marinelli L, Tripodi D: Considerazioni anatomocliniche sulla rinoplastica. Il Valsalva 41:289, 1965
Marino A: Rhinophyma and its treatment. Scand MAJ 1948:58, 1969(a)
Marino A: Reconstructive plastic surgery in extensive perforations of the nasal septum: Personal technique. Acta Chir Plast (Prague) 11:1969(b)
Marino E: Contribuciòn a la reparaciòn de las alas nasales aperadas, gravemente collapsadas. Zeitschr HNO 96:498, 1968
Marino H: Adverse results and complications in rhinoplasty. Abstract book first, in the National Congress ISAPS, Rio de Janeiro, 1972, p 13
Marquet J: The fibrin seal in otorhinolaryngology. J Head Neck Pathol 3:71, 1982
Marquit B, GI Harrison: A new method of utilizing homografts. Arch Otolaryng 73:528, 1961
Marshall DR: Intracranial complications of rhinoplasty. Br J Plast Surg 36:342, 1983
Martin BC: Cancellous bone grafts for restoration of contour. Plast Reconstr Surg 3:202, 1948
Martin F: Treatment of snoring and some obstructive sleep apnea syndromes by combined nasal and palatopharyngeal surgery. Laryngol Rhinol Otol 65:(10)562, 1986
Martin F, Spitzer H, Gastpar H: Endolaryngeale eingriffe unter verwendung hochkonzentrierten humanen fibriogens als gewebekleber. Laryngol Rhinol 60:369, 1981
Martinez SA, Nissen AJ, Stock CR, et al: Nasal turbinate resection for relief of nasal obstruction. Laryngoscope 93:871, 1983
Martins LC: Rinoplastica corretiva (punta nasale). Riv Ital Chir Plast 8:1, 1976
Martins M: Ein beitrag zum operativen verschluss der septumperforation. HNO 26:183, 1978
Marvin J: Application of the cantilever bridge principle to silastic nasal support: A preliminary report. Br J Plast Surg 33:404, 1980
Masing H: Zur versorgung von nasenflügelverletzungen. Laryng Rhinol 42:370, 1963
Masing H: Zur plastisch-operativen versorgung von septumhämatomen und abscessen. HNO Wegweiser 13:235, 1965
Masing H: Experimentelle untersuchungen über die strömung im nasenmodell. Arch Ohr Nas Kehlk Heilk 189:59, 1967
Masing H: Die klinische bedeutung der nasalen widerstandsmessung. Arch Ohr Nas Kehlk Heilk 189:763, 1969
Masing H: Fortschritte auf dem gebiete der chirurgie der äusseren and inneren nase in den letzten 10 jahren. HNO (Berlin) 18:329, 1970
Masing H: Eingriffe an der Nase, in von Theissing G (ed): Kürze HNO-Operations lehre, Bd I, hrsg. Stuttgart, Thieme, 1971(a)
Masing H: Die chirurgie der äusseren nase und der nasenscheidewand, in Theissing G (ed): Kurze HNO-Operationslehre. Stuttgart, Thieme, 1971(b)
Masing H: Die behandlung der stenosen der nase. Arch Ohr Nas Kehlk Heilk 199:173, 1971(c)
Masing H: Operative behandlung von atresien and stenosen der nase, in Naumann HH (ed): Kopf-and-Hals-Chirurgie, Bd II/1. Stuttgart, Thieme, 1974(a)
Masing H: Versorgung frischer nasenverletzungen und chirurgie der inneren nase, in Naumann HH (ed): Kopf-and-Hals-Chirurgie, vol. 2(1). Stuttgart, Thieme, 1974(b), p 356
Masing H: Eingriffe an der nasenscheidewand, in HH Naumann (ed): Kopf-und-Hals-Chirurgie. Stuttgart, Thieme, 1974(c), p 341
Masing H, Feinberger R: Ein neues rhinomanometer für die. Prax Z Laryngol Rhinol Otol 53:717, 1974
Masing H, Gammert CH, Jaumann MP: Unser konzept zur operativen behandlung von septumperforationen. Laryngol Rhinol Otol 59:50, 1980
Masing H, Hellmich S: Erfahrungen mit konserviertem knorpel im wiederaufbau der nase. Z Laryng Rhinol 47:904, 1968
Masing H, Laacke R, Leykauf R: Nasal pressure flow studies in adults and children. Rhinology 12:137, 1974
Masing H, Lehmann W, Stadler J: Uber sekundäroperationen nach submuköser septumresektion. Laryngol Rhinol 57:931, 1978
Matory WE Jr, Falces E: Non caucasian rhinoplasty: A 16-year experience. Plast Reconstr Surg 77:239, 1986
Matras H: Fibrin sealant in maxillofacial surgery-development and indications: A review of the past 12 years. Fac Plast Surgery 2(4):297, 1985
Matras H, Dinges HP, Lassmann H: Zur nahtlosen interfaszikulären nerven-transplantation im tierexperiment. Wien Med Wischr 122:515, 1972
Matras H, Kuderna H: Glueing nerve anastomoses with clotting substances. Plast Reconstr Surg 134, 1975
Matschke RG, Fiebach A: Septum deviation and begleitsinusitis. HNO (Berlin) 33:541, 1985
Matten G, Beck H: Closure of a large nasal septal perforation with a lined nasolabial flap. Chir Plastica 93:61, 1985
Matton G: The surgical treatment of rhinophyma. Plast Reconstr Surg 30:403, 1962
Matthews D: The nose tip. J Plast Surg 21:160, 1968
May H: Plastic and Reconstructive Surgery, First edition. Davis and Co, 1947
May H: The Rethi incision in rhinoplasty. Plast Reconstr Surg 8:123, 1951
May H: Reconstructive and Reparative Surgery. Philadelphia, F.A. Davis, 1960
Mayer B, Hoth S, Haels J, et al: Regulation of the nasal resistance in children. Laryngol Rhinol Otol 65: 1986
Mayer E: The Asch operation for deviations of the cartilagineous nasal septum with a report of two hundred operations. Med Rec 53:190, 1898
Mayer E: Psychiatric aspect of plastic surgery, in Converse JM (ed): Reconstructive Plastic Surgery. Philadelphia, WB Saunders, 1964
Mazzola RF, Marcus S: History of total nasal reconstruction with particular emphasis in the folded forehead flap technique. Plast Reconstr Surg 72:408, 1983
McCaffrey TV, Kern EB: Clinical evaluation of nasal obstruction. Arch Otolaryngol 105:542, 1979
McCaffrey TV, Kern EB: Nasal reflexes. Audio-digest. Otolaryngol Head Neck Surg 15:16, 1982
McCaffrey TV, Kern EB: Rhinomanometry. Fac Plast Surg 3:4, 1986
McCollough EG: An approach to repair of septal perforations. ORL Dig 38:11, 1976
McCollough EG: An approach to repair of septal perforations. Plastic Reconstr Surgery Face and Neck. Proceedings of the Second International Symposium, vol. I, New York, Grune & Stratton, 1977
McCollough EG: Systematic approach to correction of the nasal tip in rhinoplasty. Arch Otolaryngol 107:12, 1981
McCollough EG, English JL: A new twist in nasal tip surgery:

An alternative to the Goldman tip for the wide or bulbous lobule. Arch Otolaryngol Head Neck Surg 111:524, 1985
McComb H: Primary correction of unilateral cleft-lip nasal deformity: A 10-year review. Plast Reconstr Surg 75:791, 1985
McComb H: Primary repair of the bilateral cleft lip nose: A 10-year review. Plast Reconstr Surg 77:714, 1986
McCurdy JA: Surgery of the nasal tip: Current concepts. Ear Nose Throat J 56:238, 1977
McDowell F: Kiel bone grafts. Plast Reconstr Surg 41:370, 1968
McDowell F: History of rhinoplasty. Aesthetic Plast Surg 1:321, 1978
McDowell F, Valone JA, Brown JB: Bibliography and historical note on plastic surgery of the nose. Plast Reconstr Surg 10:149, 1952
McGlynn MJ, Sharp DT: Cialit preserved homograft cartilage in nasal augmentation: A long-term review. Br J Plast Surg 34:53, 1981
McGovern FH, Fitz-Hugh GS: Surgical management of congenital choanal atresia. Arch Otolaryngol 73:267, 1961
McGregor FC: Selection of cosmetic surgery patients, social and psychological considerations. Surg Clin North Am 51:289, 1971
McGregor FC, Schaffner B: Screening patients for nasal plastic operations. Some sociologic and psychiatric considerations. Psychosom Med 12:277, 1950
McGregor MC, Vistnes LM: Unsatisfactory cosmetic rhinoplasty. Symposium on Aesthetic Surgery of the Nose, Ears, and Chin. Master & Lewis, Ed. St. Louis, C.V. Mosby, 1973.
McGregor MW, O'Connor GB, Saffier S: Complications of rhinoplasty, skin and subcutaneous tissues. J Int Coll Surg 30:179, 1958
McGuirt WF, Thompson JN: Surgical approaches to malignant tumors of the nasal septum. Laryngoscope 94:1045, 1984
McGuirt WF, Thompson JN: Surgical approaches to malignant tumors of the nasal septum. Laryngoscope 94:1045, 1984
McGuirt WF, Thompson JN 1984. Quoted by M Hasegawa, et al. ORL 49:157, 1987
McIndoe AH: Restoration of depressed nose by grafting of cartilage. Six cases. Proc R Soc Med 27:1278, 1934
McIndoe AH: Correction of alar deformity in cleft lip. Lancet 1:607, 1938
McIndoe AH, Langhlin: Advances in plastic surgery. Practitioner 169:427, 1951
McKinney P: Sandpaper for nasal cartilage grafts. Plast Reconstr Surg 69:565, 1982
McKinney P, Johnson P, Walloch J: Anatomy of the nasal hump. Plast Reconstr Surg 77:3, 1986
McKinney P, Shively R: Straightening the twisted nose. Plast Reconstr Surg 64:176, 1979
McKinney P, Stainecker ML: The hanging ala. Surg. Univ. School, Chicago, II. Plast Reconstr Surg 73:427, 1984
McKinney P, Stainecker ML: Surgery for the bulbous nasal tip. Ann Plast Surg 11:106, 1983
McLaughlin CR: Absence of septal cartilage with retarded nasal development. Br J Plast Surg 2:60, 1950
McNabb T, Goldwyn RM: Blood gas and hemodynamic effects of sedatives and analgesics when used as a supplement to local anesthesia in plastic surgery. Plast Reconstr Surg 58:37, 1976
McQuown SA: Intracranial extension of nasal dermoids. Neurosurgery 12:531, 1983
Meada RJ: Composite ear grafts for construction of columella. Plast Reconstr Surg 23:134, 1959
Meda P: Otorinolaringologia Pediatricà. Milano, Ambrosia, 1963
Meijer R: Secondary repair of the bilateral cleft lip deformity. Cleft Palate J 21:86, 1984
Melsen B: Hystological analysis of the postnatal development of the nasal septum. Angle Ortod 47:83, 1977
Metzenbaum M: Replacement of the lower end of the dislocated septal cartilage versus submucous resection of the dislocated end of the septal cartilage. Arch Otolaryngol 9:282, 1929
Metzenbaum M: Dislocation of lower end of nasal septal cartilage. Arch Otolaryngol 24:78–88, 1936
Metzenbaum M: Recent fractures of the nose. Arch Otolaryngol 34:723, 1941
Mertz JS, McCaffrey TV, Kern EB: Objective evaluation of anterior septal surgical reconstruction. Otolaryngol Head Neck Surg 92:308, 1984
Mertz JS, Pearson BW, Kern EB: Lateral rhinotomy. Arch Otolaryngol 109:235, 1983
Meyer R: Neuerungen in der nasenplastik. Pract Otorhinolaryngol 13:373, 1951
Meyer R: Nasenplastik mit dem zahnärztlichen bohrer. Kosmetikerinnen-Fachzeitung 26:1954
Meyer R: Ucber angeborene äussore nasendeformitäten. Practica Otorhinolaryng 18:399, 1956
Meyer R: Zur korrektur der hasenschartennase. Helvet Chir Acta 26:299, 1959
Meyer R: Sekundäre nasenplastik bei lippen-kiefer-gaumenspalten. Aesthetische Med 2:30–36, 1960
Meyer R: Aeussore und innere chirurgische dehandlung der ozaena-nase monatschr. Ohrenheilkunde 95:29, 1961(a)
Meyer R: Correzione secondaria delle deformazioni nasali del labbro leporino. Annali di Laring Otol Rinol Faringol 60:269, 1961(b)
Meyer R: Die korrektur der hasenschartennase. Arch Ohr Nas Kehik Heilk 2:537, 1962(a)
Meyer R: Rhinoplastik bei ozaena. Arch Ohr neilk Heilk, Hals Heilk Ed. 180(2):781, 1962(b)
Meyer R: Die partielle ersatzplastik der nase. Aesth Med Heft 1:1, 1963
Meyer R: 1964: in Denecke HJ and Meyer R (ed) 1964(a)/1967
Meyer R: Verschluss von septumperforationen, in Denecke HJ, Meyer R (Eds): Plastische Operationen an Kopf and Hals I Korrigierende Nasenplastik. Berlin, Springer-Verlag, 1964(b)
Meyer R: Dauerhaftigkeit: Gefahren and misserfolge kosmetischer eingriffe im gesichtsbereich. Aesth Mediz 13:273, 1964(c)
Meyer R: The frontal-temporal flap in facial repairs, in Proceedings of the first annual meeting of the Swiss Society of Plastic and Reconstructive Surgeons, Amsterdam, Excerpta Medica Foundation, 1965
Meyer R: Sekundarplastik nach verbrennungsschäden der nase und der Ohren. Chir Plast 135:1966(a)
Meyer R: The frontotemporal flap in facial repairs, in Plastic Surgery of Head and Neck Tumors. Excerpta Medica International Congress Series, No 98. 1966(b), p 34
Meyer R: Reconstructions orbito-palpebrales par lambeau frontotemporal. Ophthalmologica 154:328, 1967
Meyer R: La Chirurgie reconstructive de la face et du cou après ablation de tumeurs. Méd et Hyg 26:542, 1968(a)

Meyer R: Plastische chirurgie bei anomalien, defekten and narben. Aesth Medizin 17(10):229, 1968(b)
Meyer R: Les malformations de la teto. Med et Hyg 28:414, 1970
Meyer R: Traitement chirurgical reconstructif des sténoses narinaires. Otorhinolaryngol 33:140, 1971(a)
Meyer R: Correction of rhinoplasty complications, in Transactions of the Fifth International Congress Plastic & Reconstructive Surgery, Melbourne, Butterworth's, 1971(b), p 1153
Meyer R: Sonderdruck aus plastischer chirurgie, in Transacta III Tagung der Verein. Deutsch Plast Chir., (ed): Schrudde J, Pilgram, Hoffnungsthal, 1972(a)
Meyer R: Nasal-septal perforation and nostril stenosis, in Goldwyn RM (ed): The Unfavourable Result in Plastic Surgery. Boston, Little, Brown and Co., 1972(b), p 321
Meyer R: Der verschluss von grossen septumperforationen. Pract ORL (Basel) 34:371, 1972(c)
Meyer R: Total nasal reconstruction, in Conley J, Dickinson JT (eds): Plast and Reconstructive Surgery of the Face and Neck. New York, Grune and Stratton, 1972(d)
Meyer R: Secondary repair of the hare-lip nose. Abstracts of 2nd International Congress on cleft palate. Copenaghen, 1973(a), p 225
Meyer R: La fermeture des grandes perforations de la cloison. Pract Otorhinolaryngol (Basel) 34:371, 1973(b)
Meyer R: La rhinoplastie aujourd'hui. Rev Med Suisse Romande 94:12, 1974(a)
Meyer R: The International Microfilm Journal of Aesthetic Plastic Surgery, New York, 1974(b)
Meyer R: La chirurgie de la déformation secondaire du nez de bec-de-lièvre. Médec and Hygiene 35:817, 1977
Meyer R: Secondary rhinoplasty in secondary nose. Transactions of the Seventh International Congress of Plastic and Reconstructive Surgery, Rio de Janeiro, 1979
Meyer R: Complications tardives en rhinoplasties. Med et Hyg 39:742, 1981
Meyer R: Reconstruction de la columelle et de la cloison nasale. ORL (Paris) 192:1, 1982(a)
Meyer R: Single bilobed flap for head and neck reconstruction. Reply to Dr. Vilar Sancho (letter). Ann Plast Surg 9:524, 1982(b)
Meyer R: Our concepts in the operative closure of septal perforations. HNO 31:10, 1983
Meyer R., Berghaus A.: Closure of perforations of the septum including a single-session method for large defects. Head Neck Surg. 5:390, 1983
Meyer R, Bianchi A: La chiusura delle perforazioni del setto nasale. Otorhinolaring 33:73, 1983
Meyer R, Boheim K: Unsere konzepte für den operativen verschluss von septumperforationen. HNO 31:10, 1983
Meyer R, Flemming I: Die angeborene flachnase und ihre korrektur zeitschr. Laryngol Rhinol Otol Heft 17:807, 1969
Meyer R, Kesselring UK: Reconstructive surgery of the nose and orbit, in Sisson GA, Tardy EM (eds): Plastic and Reconstructive Surgery of the Face and Neck, vol. 2. New York, Grune and Stratton 1977
Meyer R, Kesselring UK: New trends in the treatment of ageing face. Abstracts 4th Congress of the European Section of the IPRS, Athens, 1981(a)
Meyer R, Kesselring UK: Fibrinogen tissue adhesive glue in aesthetic plastic surgery. Abstracts of the 6th Congress of ISAPS, Tokyo, 1981(b)
Meyer R, Kesselring UK: Reconstructive surgery of the nose. Clin Plast Surg 8:435, 1981(c)
Meyer R, Kesselring UK: Funktionelle plastische chirurgie der nase. Laryngol Rhinol Otol 62:179, 1983
Meyer R, Kesselring UK: Secondary rhinoplasty, in Regnault P, Daniel RK (eds): Aesthetic Plastic Surgery. Boston, Little, Brown and Co, 1984, p 201
Meyer R, Novoselac M: Neue aspekte der korrigierenden nasenplastik. HNO 22:154, 1974
Meyer R, Oppliger GC: Correction des deformations nasaies chez le porteur de bec de lièvre. Rev Med Suisse Rom 83:990, 1963
Meyer R, Oppliger GC: Die partielle ersatzplastik der nase. Helv Chir Acta 31:304, 1964
Meyer R, Zaoli G: La chirugia reparatrice delle perforazioni del setto nasale. Minerva Otorinolaring 14:33, 1964
Meysmann L, Speelman G, Van Rattinghe R: Gorlin syndrome with nasal fistula. Bel-Dermatologica 165(5):522, 1982
Micheli-Pellegrini V: Cause d'insuccesso nella chirurgia estetica del naso. Rivista Italiana di Chirurgia Plastica 7, 419, 1975(a)
Micheli-Pellegrini V: A proposito della rhinoplastica correttiva. Considerazioni sull'opportunità di normalizzare le tecniche. Nuovo Arch Ital Otol Rinol Laringol 3:220, 1975(b)
Micheli-Pellegrini V: Passato, presente e futuro dei materiali alloplastici in chirurgia estetica. Min Chir 38:871, 1983
Micheli-Pellegrini V: Regles générales à observer dans la pratique de la rhinoplastie. Chirurgie Esthétique 1983–1984. Paris, Maloine, 1984(a)
Micheli-Pellegrini V: Les étapes de la rhinoplastie. Chirurgie Esthétique 1983–1984. Paris, Maloine, 1984(b)
Micheli-Pellegrini V: La pointe du nez. Chirurgie Esthétique 1983–1984. Paris, Maloine, 1984(c)
Micheli-Pellegrini V: Chirurgie de la pointe du nez par rapport aux voies respiratoires. Chirurgie Esthétique 1983–1984, Paris, Maloine, 1984(d)
Micheli Peligrini V: Il Naso Torto. La Garangola, 1985
Micheli-Pellegrini V, Carpino-Boeri A, Gianfranchi M: La neuroleptoanalgesia nella chirurgia otorinolaringoiatrica e maxillofacciale. Boll Mal OGN 82:251, 1964
Micheli-Pellegrini V, Carpino-Boeri A: L'anestesia per la rinoplastica. L'Informatore Medico 22:3, 1967
Micheli-Pellegrini V, Manfrida GM: Rhinoplasty and its psychological implications: Applied psychology observation in aesthetic surgery. Aesthetic Plast Surg 3:299, 1979
Mikhelson NM: Homogenous cartilage in maxillofacial surgery. Acta Chir Plast (Prague) 4:192, 1962
Mill and Silver 1950. Quoted by J. Reich 1984
Millard DR: Plastic peregrinations. Plast Reconstr Surg 5:26, 1950
Millard DR: Columella lengthening by a forked flap. Plast Reconstr Surg 5:454, 1958
Millard DR: The thimble hook. Plast Reconstr Surg 26:555, 1960(a)
Millard DR: External excisions in rhinoplasty. Br J Plast Surg 12:340, 1960(b)
Millard DR: The triad of columella deformities. Plast Reconstr Surg 31:370, 1963
Millard DR: Adjuncts in augmentation mentoplasty and corrective rhinoplasty. Plast Reconstr Surg 36:48, 1965
Millard DR Jr: Total reconstructive rhinoplasty and a missing link. Plast Reconstr Surg 37:167, 1966

Millard DR: Alar margin sculpturing. Plast Reconstr Surg 40:337, 1967(a)

Millard DR Jr: Alar marginal resection. Plast Reconstr Surg 40:4, 1967(b)

Millard DR: Alar margin sculpturing. Plast Reconstr Surg 44:545, 1969(a)

Millard DR: Secondary corrective rhinoplasty. Plast Reconstr Surg 44:545, 1969(b)

Millard DR: The versatility of a chondromucosal flap in the nasal vestibule. Plast Reconstr Surg 50:580, 1972(a)

Millard DR: Congenital nasal tip retrusion and three little composite ear grafts. Case report. Plast Reconstr Surg 48:501, 1972(b)

Millard DR: Problem cases in rhinoplasty. Symposium on Aesthetic Surgery of the Nose, Ears, and Chin. Master & Lewis Ed., CV Mosby, St. Louis, 1973

Millard DR: Secondary rhinoplasty surgery, in Symposium on Corrective Rhinoplasty. St. Louis, The C.V. Mosby Co, 1976(a)

Millard DR: Cleft Craft. The evolution of its surgery. The unilateral deformity. Little, Brown and Co. 1976(b)

Millard DR: Symposium on Corrective Rhinoplasty, vol. 13. St. Louis, the C.V. Mosby 1976(c), p 312

Millard DR: Alar cinch in the flat, flaring nose. Plast Reconstr Surg 65:669, 1980(a)

Millard DR: Three very short noses and how they were lengthened. Plast Reconstr Surg 65:10, 1980(b)

Miller TA: Temporalis fascial grafts. Plast Reconstr Surg 65:236, 1980

Milward TM: The fate of silastic and vitrathene nasal implants. Br J Plast Surg 25:276, 1972

Mink PJ: Le nez comme voie réspiratoire. Presse Otolaryng (Belge) 21:481, 1903

Mink PJ: Physiologie der Oberen Luftwege. Leipzig, Vogel, 1920

Mir Y, Mir L: Deformidad nasal y labio leporino unilateral. Med Clin 26:427, 1956

Mir Y, Mir L: El periostio y la reconstrucción estética nasal. Cirugia Plastica Ibero-Latinoamericana. 9:4, 1983

Miskinjar SAS: A new method for correcting a gummy smile. Plast Reconstr Surg 72:397, 1983

Mittelmann H: Marginal incision tip rhinoplasty in selected cases, in Bernstein L (ed): Plastic and Reconstructive Surgery, vol. 1. Aesth Surg, 1981, p 57

Monks GH: Correction, by operation of some nasal deformities and disfigurements. (Classic Reprint 1898. Plast Reconstr Surg 48:485, 1971)

Monasterio F, Olmedo A: Corrective rhinoplasty before puberty: A long-term follow-up. Plast Reconstr Surg 68:381, 1981

Monserrat-Valadiu JM, Iglesias J, Midon G: Contribution à l'étude des difformites nasales. Supp. 1967 Rev. Laryng. Otol. Rhinol. 2nd. Congr. Europ. Rhinol. Internat. Rhinol. vol. V, Nr. 3, 1967

Montserrat JM: Rhinoplastia funcional y sus bases anatomofisiologicas, in VII Congreso Nacional de Otorrinolaringologia, Sevilla, 1969. Edited by Liade. Madrid, 1969

Moore GF, Freeman JT, Ogren FP, et al: Extended follow-up of total inferior turbinate resection for relief of chronic nasal obstruction. Laryngol 95:1095, 1985

Moore JRM, Bicknell PG: A comparision of cryosurgery and submucous diathermy in vasomotor rhinitis. J Laryngol Otol 94:1411, 1980

Moore PM: Intranasal encephalomeningocele. Report of case. Laryngoscope 62:659, 1952

Moraes de Avelar J: Personal contribution for the surgical treatment of the negroid nose. Aesth Plast Surg 1:81, 1975

Moricca G, Ponti L, Cavaliere RV: L'analgesia loco-regionale potenziata nella chirurgiy correttiva della stutture osteocartilaginee del naso. Min ORL 12:155, 1962

Mortiner SA, Nissen AJ, Stark CR, et al: Nasal turbinate resection for relief of nasal obstruction. Laryngoscope 93:871, 1983

Moss ALH, Pigott RW, Albery EH: Hynes pharyngoplasty revisited. Plast Reconstr Surg 79:3, 1987

Mouly R: Le kyste mucoide: Complication inhabituelle de la rhinoplastie. Ann Chir Plast 15:153, 1970

Mowlem R: Use and behavior of iliac bone grafts in restoration of nasal contour. Rev Chir Structive 8:23, 1938

Mowlem R: Iliac bone and cartilage transplants: Use and behavior. Br J Surg 29:182, 1941

Muenker R: The bilateral conchal cartilage graft. A new technique in augmentation rhinoplasty. Aesth Plast Surg 8:37, 1984(a)

Muenker R: Die spätrekonstruktion traumatischer formveränderungen der nase. Ges Plast u Wiederherstellungschir. 1984(b), p 78

Müller D: Long-term results of rhinoplasty in nose injuries in childhood. Laryngol Rhinol Otol 62:116, 1983

Mullin WR, Millard DR, Jr: Management of congenital bilateral cleft nose. Plast Reconstr Surg 75:253, 1985

Murray JAM, Maran AGD, Mackenzie JJ, et al: A more effective treatment of the fractured nose. Clin Otolaryngol 9:304, 1984(a)

Murray JAM, Maran AGD, Mackenzie JJ, et al: Open versus closed reduction of the fractured nose. Arch Otolaryngol 110(12):797, 1984(b)

Musgrave RH: Surgery of nasal deformities associated with cleft lip. Plast Reconstr Surg 28:261, 1961

Musgrave RH, Garrett WS Jr: Preoperative consultation. A different concept, in Millard DR Jr (ed): Symposium on Corrective Rhinoplasty. St Louis, Mosby, 1976, p 50

Mygind N: Nasal Allergy. Oxford, Blackwell, 1979

Mygind N: Measurement of nasal airway resistences. Is it only for article writers? Clin Otolaryngol 5:161, 1980

Nace T: Lighting a path to the future. MacWorld 3:100, 1986

Nagayama I, et al: Reconstruction of nasal dorsum with septal flap. ORL (Tokyo) 29:435, 1986

Nagel F: Probleme bei der korrektur der sattelnase. Z Laryng Rhinol 49:250, 1970

Nagel F: Die knorpelige sattelnase: Ihre verhütung bei eingriffen am septum and ihre korrektur. Z Laryng Rhinol 50:567, 1971(a)

Nagel F: Our experience in closing nasal septum perforations using pedicled oral vestibular flaps. Ann Otol Rhinol Laryngol 50:446, 1971(b)

Nagel F: Unsere erfahrungen mit den gestielten mundvorhoflappen zur deckung von nasenseptumperforationen. Z Laryng Rhinol 50:446, 1971(c)

Nagelschmidt F: Uber diathermie (transthemie, thermopenetration). Münch Med Wschr 56:2575, 1909

Natvig P: Anatomy of the nose, in Millard ed: Symposium on Corrective Rhinoplasty. St. Louis, Mosby Co., 1976, p 40

Natvig P, Sether LA, Gingrass RP, et al: Anatomical details of the osseous-cartilaginous framework of the nose. Plast Reconstr Surg 48:528, 1971

Natvig P, Sether L, Dingman RO: Skin about skin at the alar margins of the nose. Ann Plast Surg 2:428, 1979

Nauhahn HH: On the physiology of the nasal cavity, in Conley J, Dickinson JT (eds): Plastic and Reconstructive Surgery of the Face and Neck. Stuttgart, George Thieme, 1972

Naumann, HH: On the physiology of the nasal cavity, in Conley J, Dickinson JT (eds.): Plastic and Reconstructive Surgery of the Face and Neck. Proceeding of the International Symposium. New York, Grune & Stratton, 1972

Naumann, HH, Naumann WH: Kurze pathophysiologie der nase and ihrer nebenhöhlen. In: Berendes, Link u. Zöllner, HNO-Heilkunde in Praxis und Klinik, Bd.I.2. Aufl. Thieme, Stuttgart, 1977

Neidlinger WJ: Present scope of septal surgery. Supp. 1967 Rev. Laryng. Otol. Rhinol. 2nd. Congr. Europ. Rhinol. 1966 Internat. Rhinol. Vol V, N. 3 1967

Neiger M: Diagnostik und therapie der frontobasal and mittelgesichtsfrakturen. Swiss Med 6:43, 1984

Neivert H: Principles and mechanics in surgery of the bony wall. Arch Otolaryngol 61:585, 1955

Nelaton C, Ombredanne L: The Rhinoplasty. Paris, G. Steinheil C, 1904

Neves-Pinto RM: Rinoplastia: Uma Pinça Para osteotomias transversais. Rev Bras Cir 73:331, 1983

Neves-Pinto RM: Rhinoplasty: A forceps for transverse osteotomies. Varig Brazillian Airlines Medical dept.-Rio de Janeiro-Brazil. Abstracts, 10e Congrès de la Soc. Europ. de la Rhinologie 26–28.8, 1984

Neves-Pinto RM, Cadar A, J. Nogueira-Costa: Cirurgia do septo e da piramide nasal uma ficha de avaliaçao preoperatoria. Rinosseptoplastia funcional, Rev. Brasil. de Otorhinolaring 45:111, 1979

New GB, Austin GW: The chrondrotome-ejector for shredding and inserting cartilage. Plast Reconstr Surg 5:444, 1950

Newmark H: Orbital floor fracture: An unusual complication of trans-septal, trans-sphenoidal hypophysectomy. Neurosurgery 12:555, 1983

Nichols JEH: The sequelae of syphilis in the pharynx and their treatment. Tran Am Laryngol Assoc 18:161, 1896

Nicolai JPA: Reconstruction of the columella with nasolabial flaps. Head Neck Surg 4:374, 1982

Nicolle FV: Correction of the overshortened nose. Aesth Plast Surg 10:27, 1986(a)

Nicolle FV: Secondary rhinoplasty of the nasal tip and columella. Scand J Plast Rec Surg 20:67, 1986(b)

Nolan JO: Cryosurgical treatment of rhinophyma. Plast Reconstr Surg 52:437, 1973

Noodt A, Draf W: Zur differentialdiagnose der sattelnase und der ohrmuschelperichondritis: Das v. meyenburg-altherr-uehlinger-syndrom (Panchondritis). Laryngol Rhinol Otol 63:27, 1984

Nyberg PJ, Gammert C: Erfahrungen mit der Kryotherapie bei Rhinopathia vasomotoria. ORL-Aktuelle Probleme der Otorhinoloaryngologie 1983, Huber-Bern, Stuttgart, Wien, p 149

New GB, Austin GW: The chrondrotome-ejector for shredding and inserting cartilage. Plast Reconstr Surg 5:444, 1950

O'Brien: Current concepts of nasal septal surgery. J Laryngol Otol 82:987, 1968

O'Connor GB, McGregor MW: Secondary rhinoplasties. Plast Rreconstr Surg 15:404, 1955

O'Connor GB, McGregor MW, Shapiro L, et al: The bulbous nose. Plast Reconstr Surg 27:19, 1974

O'Connor GB, McGregor MW, Tolleth H: Alar Collapse. Plast Reconstr Surg 40:49, 1967

O'Connor GB, Pierce GW: Refrigerated cartilage isografts. Surg Gynec Obstet 67:796, 1938

Odeneal TH: Submucous turbinectomy. Arch Otolaryngol 11:215, 1930

Ogura JH, Nelson JR, Dammkoehler R, et al: Experimental observations of the relationships between upper airway obstruction and pulmonary function. Ann Otol Rhinol Laryngol 73:38, 1964

Ogura JH, Togawa K, Dammloerley K: Nasal obstruction and the mechanics of breathing. Physiologic relationship and effects of nasal surgery. Arch Otolaryngol 83:135, 1966

Ogura JH, Unno T, Nelson JR: Nasal surgery. Physiological considerations of nasal obstruction. Arch Otolaryngol 88:288, 1968

Ohura T: Reconstructive surgery of the nose non-caucasians. Clin Plast Surg 1:93, 1971

Ojeda FX: Personal communication

Olley PC: Psychiatric Aspects of Cosmetic Surgery. Basingstoke, Macmillan, 1976, p 491

Olsen KD, Carpenter RJ, Kern EB: Nasal septal injury in children. Arch Otolaryngol 106:317, 1980

Ombredanne M: Les déviations traumatique de la cloison chèz l'enfant avec obstruction nasale. Traitement chirurgical et résultats éloignés. Arch Fr Pédiatr 1:20–26, 1942

Onizuka T: Procedures for repair of the cleft lip nose. Aesth Plast Surg 7:179, 1983

Orr WC, Marint RY: Obstructive sleep apnea associated with tonsillar hypertrophy in adults. Arch Intern Med 141:990–992, 1981

Orticochea M: Construction of a dynamic muscle sphincter in cleft palates. Plast Reconstr Surg 41:323, 1968

Orticochea M: A new method for repair of total or partial cleft lips. Transactions of the Fourth International Congress of Plastic and Reconstructive Surgery. Amsterdam, Excerpta Medica, 1969, p 337–348

Orticochea M: Results of the dynamic muscle sphincter in cleft palates. Abstracts of 2nd International Congress on cleft palate, Copenhaghen, 1973, p 233

Orticochea M: A review of 236 cleft palate patients treated with dynamic muscle sphincter. Plast Reconstr Surg 71:2, 180, 1983

Ortiz-Monasterio F, Lopez-Mas J, Araico J: Rhinoplasty in the thick-skinned nose. Br J Plast Surg 27:19, 1974

Ortiz-Monasterio F, Olmedo A: Rhinoplasty on the Mestizo Nose. Clin Plast Surg 4:89, 1977

Ortiz-Monasterio F, Olmedo A: Corrective rhinoplasty before puberty. A long term follow-up. Plast Reconstr Surg 68:381, 1981(a)

Ortiz-Monasterio F, Olmedo A: Reconstruction of major nasal defects. Clin Plast Surg 8:565, 1981(b)

Ortiz-Monasterio F, Olmedo A, Ortiz-Oscoy L: The use of cartilage grafts in primary aesthetic rhinoplasty. Plast Reconstr Surg 67:597, 1981

Ortiz-Monasterio S: Rhinoplasty in the thick skin nose. Abstract book first in the National Congress ISAPS. Rio de Janeiro, 1972, p 14

Orton CI: Loss of columella and septum from an unusual form of child abuse. Plast Reconstr Surg 56:345, 1975

Ossof RH, Karlan MS, Sisson GA: A compendium of intranasal flaps. Laryngoscope 92:774, 1982

Ossof RH, Weingarten CZ: Minimal requirements for intravenous sedation and anesthesia, in Bernstein L (ed): Plastic and Reconstructive Surgery, vol. 1. Aesth Surg, 1981, p 217

Osterwald L: Ein beitrag zum verschluss von septumperforationen. HNO (Berlin) 21:63, 1973
Oulié J: Le problème de la racine du nez dans les rhinoplasties de réduction. Ann Chir Plast 7:725, 1963
Oulié J: Correction des narines trop saillantes au cours des plasties nasales. Technique et résultats. 61 Congress ORL (Paris) 1964
Oulié J: The high radix of the nose. Trans. Internat. Congr. VI Paris. Plast. Rec. Surg., Masson, Paris, 1976
Owens A: Observations in treating 25 cases of choanal atresia by the transpalantine approach. Laryngoscope 75:84, 1965
Owsley JQ, Chierca G, Miller ER, et al: Cephalometric evaluation of palatal dysfunction in patients without cleft palate. Plast Reconstr Surg 39:562, 1967
Owsley JQ, Lawson LI, Miller ER, et al: Experience with the high attached pharyngeal flap. Plast Reconstr Surg 38:232, 1966
Ozenberger JM: Cryosurgery in chronic rhinitis. Laryngoscope 80:723, 1970
Ozenberger JM: Cryosurgery for the treatment of chronic rhinitis. Laryngoscope 83:508, 1973
Padovan I: External approach in rhinoplasty. Surg ORL Lug 3–4:354–360, 1966
Palange J, Facer G, Kern EB, et al: Prosthetic closure of nasal septal perforations. Otolaryngol Head Neck Surg 90:448, 1982
Paletta FX, Van Norman RT: Total reconstruction of the columella. Plast Reconstr Surg 23:134, 1959
Paludetti GT, Todisco F, Damiani M, et al: La clearance mucociliare nasale e l'ultrastruttura ciliare nel normale. Otorinolaringologia 34:317, 1984
Papangelou L: Closure of the nasal septum perforation. Arch Otolaryngol 90:528–530, 1969
Parcansky MJ, Corujo MR, Cabrera VN: Colgajo condrocutaneo alar controlateral procedimento original. Cir Plast Argent 2:17, 1978
Pardina AJ, Frontera J: Evaluation of the different methods used in the treatment of rhinoplastic sequelae. Aesthetic Plast Surg 7:237, 1983
Parell G, McCollough EG, Beeson WB: The tension nose anatomy and surgical repair. Otolaryngol Head Neck Surg 90:177, 1982
Parkes J, Tresley W: Surgery of the nasal tip. A new technique. Procedures of the Ninth International Congress. Otorhino-laryngol, Mexico, Excer Med Internat Cong Series n. 206, 1969
Parkes M: Avoiding bone resorption under plastic chin implants. Arch Otolaryngol 98:100, 1973(a)
Parkes M, et al: Rhinoplasty dressings. EENT Monthly 52:166, 1973(b)
Parkes M: Avulsion of the upper lateral cartilage: Etiology, diagnosis, surgical anatomy and management. Laryngoscope 91:758, 1981
Parkes M, Bassilios MI: Nasal deformity and harelip. Laryngoscope 88:1215, 1978
Parkes M, Binder WJ: Iceberg of the nose. Ann Plast Surg 5:146, 1980
Parkes M, Borowiecki B, Binder W: Functional sequelae of rhinoplasty. Ann Plast Surg 4:116, 1980
Parkes MI, Brennan HG: High septal transfixion to shorten the nose. Plast Reconstr Surg 45:487, 1970
Parkes ML: Current concepts in rhinoplasty. Plastic and Reconstruction Surgery of the Head and Neck, vol. 1. New York, Grune & Stratton, 1972
Parkes ML, Berman MG: High septal transfixion to shorten the nose. Plast Reconstr Surg 43:487, 1970
Parkes ML, Kamer FM: The mature nose. Laryngoscope 83:157, 1973
Parkhouse N, Evans D: Reconstruction of the ala of the nose using a composite free flap from the pinna. Brit J Plast Surg 38:306, 1985
Pascone M, De Robertis M, Petruzzelli G, et al: Utilizzazione della cartilagine bovina irradiata (chondroplast) nella chirurgia estetica del volto. Atti del Congresso Italiano di Chirurgia Plastica, Bari, 1985
Pasiries SC: Correction of deviated nose. Arch Otolaryngol 92:60, 1970
Passali D, De Seta E, Bellussi L: Studio del tempo di trasporto muco-ciliare nasale un campione di bambini normali. Acta Otorhino Ital 2:297, 1982
Patrzek 1890. Quoted by Pirsig 1975
Patow CA, Kaliner M: Corticosteroid treatment of rhinologic diseases. ENT J 62:14, 1983
Patrzek 1890. Quoted by Pirsig 1975
Patterson CN: The rhinologic septoplasty correction of internal and external nasal deformities. NC Med J 14:29, 1952
Patterson CN: Reconstructive septonasoplasty. Arch Otolaryngol 84:457, 1966
Patterson CN: Siliconized dacron implants in septal orbital surgery. Arch Otolaryngol 89:71, 1969
Patterson CN: Surgery of the aging nose, in Sisson GA, Tardy ME Jr (eds): Plastic and Reconstructive Surgery of the Face and Neck, Proceedings of the Second International Symposium, vol. I. Aesthetic Surgery, New York, Grune & Stratton, 1977
Patterson CN: Surgery of the crooked nose. Laryngoscope 91:939, 1981
Patterson CN, Durham MS: Physiologic septoplasty and rhinoplasty. NC Med J 27:2, 1966
Patterson CN, Durham NC: Reconstructive septonasoplasty. Arch Otolaryngol 84:457, 1966
Patterson CN, Powell DG: Facial analysis in patient evaluation for physiologic and cosmetic surgery. Plastic and Reconstructive Surgery of the Face and Neck, Proceedings of the Second International Symposium, vol. I. New York, Grune & Stratton, 1977(a)
Patterson CN, Powell DG: Surgery of the aging nose. Plastic and Reconstructive Surgery of the Face and Neck, Proceedings of the Second International Symposium, vol. I. New York, Grune & Stratton, 1977(b)
Patterson ME, Lockwood RW, Sheehy JL: Temporalis fascia in tympanic membrane grafting. Arch Otolaryngol 85:287, 1967
Paulsen 1882. Quoted by Masing 1977
Peacock MR: Sub-mucosa resection of the nasal septum. J Laryngol Otol 95:341, 1981
Pearson BW, Goodman WS: S.M.R., septoplasty, and the surgical relief of nasal obstruction. Can Otolaryngol 2:238, 1973
Pech A, Cannoni M: Anatomy chirurgicale du nez. La chirurgie corrective de la pointe du nez. Cah ORL 4:63, 1969
Pech A, Cannoni M, Abdul S, et al: External rhinoplasty: Technique and indications. Ann Chir Plast 26:380, 1981(a)
Pech A, Cannoni M, Abdul S, et al: La rhinoplastie par voie externe. Ann Chir Plast 26:263, 1981(b)
Pech A, Cannoni M, Borrot Y, et al: Technique de la chirurgie correctrice du nez. Tours: La Simarre, 1974
Pech A, Cannoni M, Gitenet: Difficultés et échecs de la

chirurgie de la pointe du nez dans la rhinoplastie correctrice. Ann Otolaryngol 693:621, 1976

Pech A, Jausseran: Une enquête sur les implants dans le traitement des ensellures nasales. Ann Chir Plast 15:38, 1970

Peck GC: Study session in corrective rhinoplasty. Presented at the 39th Annual Meeting of the American Society of Plastic and Reconstructive Surgeons, Los Angeles, 1970

Peck GC: Surgery of the nasal tip, in Master FW, Lewis JR (eds): Symposium on Aesthetic Surgery of the Nose, Ears and Chin. St. Louis, Mosby, 1973

Peck GC: The difficult nasal tip. Clin Plast Surg 4:1, 1977

Peck GC: Aesthetic rhinoplasty, in Grabb WC, Smith JW (eds): Plastic Surgery, (ed3). Boston, Little, Brown and Co. 1979, p 427

Peck GC: Onlay graft for nasal tip projection. Plast Reconstr Surg 71:27, 1983

Peck GC: Technique in aesthetic rhinoplasty. Aesthetic Plast Surg 8:196, 1984(a)

Peck GC: Techniques in Aesthetic Rhinoplasty. New York, Thieme-Stratton Inc, 1984(b)

Peer LA: Operation to repair lateral displacement of lower border of septal cartilage. Arch Otolaryngol 25:475, 1937

Peer LA: Cartilage grafting. Surg Clin North Am 24:404, 1944

Peer LA: Neglected cartilage graft (with experimental observation on growth on human cartilage grafts). Arch Otolaryngol 42:384, 1945

Peer LA: Cartilage grafting. Br J Plast Surg 7:250, 1954

Peer LA: Behaviour of grafts and implants. Observations on materials used for structural support of an external ear. Arch Otolaryngol 77:34, 1963

Peer LA: A method to correct saddle nose associated with retracted columella. Plast Reconstr Surg 38:477, 1966

Pelliciari DD: Columella and tip reconstruction. Plast Reconstr Surg 4:98, 1949

Penn J: The reconstruction of the nose. Br J Plast Surg 20:369, 1967

Penn J: Kiel bone implants to the chin and nose. Plast Reconstr Surg 42:203–206, 1968

Penn J, Jankowitz J, Bruwer A: Grated cadaver cartilage. Plast Reconstr Surg 3:228, 1948

Perpere C, Forli V: Plaidoyer pour un conservatisme éclairé dans les rhinoplasies. Ann Chir Plast Esthét 28:248, 1983

Perret P: Correction chirurgicale des nez déviés. Practica ORL 20:115, 1958

Perret P: Aspects de la rhinoplastie correctrice. Practica ORL 24:151, 1961

Pers M: Cheek flaps in partial rhinoplasty. Scand J Plast Reconstr Surg 1:37, 1967

Pers M: An operation for elongation of a short nose. Abstract book, Second Congress of the European Section of the IPRS, 80, 1973

Peska-Luskowska 1967. Quoted by Masing 1974

Peterson RA: Open-flap rhinoplasty, in Millard R (ed): Symposium on Corrective Rhinoplasty. Mosby Co, 1976, p 83

Petruson B, Goteborg: Reconstruction of the anterior nasal septum by transplantation. Rhinology 24:147, 1986

Piechotta FU, Flemming I: Fibrinogen adhesive in plastic surgery, in Bernstein L (ed): Plastic and Reconstructive Surgery, vol. 1. Aesth Surg 1981, p 195

Pieyre JM: Nouvelles adaptations de la greffe osseuse à la rhinoplastie.

Pieyre JM: Rhinoplasties: Greffe osseuse ou implant de silastic. Méd Hyg 40:3754, 1982

Pieyre JM: Le traitement chirurgical du ronflement. Méd Hyg 41:3752–3754, 1983

Pieyre JM: Le ronflement. Méd Hyg 42:769, 1984(a)

Pieyre JM: Le traitement du ronflenent. Med Hyg 42:769, 1984(b)

Pigott RW, Millard DR: Correction of the bilateral cleft lip nasal deformity, in Grabb WC (ed): Cleft Lip and Palate. Little Brown & Co, Boston, 1971

Piotti F: Secondary rhinoplasty. Aesthetic Plast Surg 5:259, 1981

Piotti F, Mascetti M, Gambaro G, et al: La deformazione postraumatica della piramide nasale. Min Otorhinol 29:93, 1979

Piquet JJ, Burny A, Ton Van J, et al: Le traitement chirurgicale des imperforations choanales. Acta Otolaryngol Belg 38:1, 5, 1984

Piragine F: La funzionalità ciliare dopo interventi chirurgici endonasali. Rilievi sperimentali sulla mucosa nasale umana. Boll Mal OGN 96:451, 1979

Pirsig W: Reduction of the middle turbinate. Rhinology 10:103, 1972

Pirsig W: Die regeneration des kindlichen septumknorpels nach septumplastiken. Acta Oto-laryng 79:451, 1975

Pirsig W: Operative Eingriffe an der kindlichen Nase. In Hals-Nasen-Ohren-Heilkunde in Praxis und Klinik. Ed. Berendes, Link, Zöllner, vol. 2:28.1, 39, Thieme Stuttgart, 1977(a)

Pirsig W: Septal plasty in children, influence on nasal growth. Rhinology 15:193, 1977(b)

Pirsig W: Morpholigic aspects of the injured nasal septum in children. Rhinology 17:65, 1979

Pirsig W: Septum deviation 1882: Beginning of systematic submucous septum surgery. Rhinol Otol 61:547, 1982

Pirsig W: Clinical aspects of the fractured growing nose. Rhinology 21:107, 1983(a)

Pirsig W: Die Wachstumszonen der Nase: Heutiger Stand des klinischen und experimentellen Wissens. Dtsch Ges Plast Wiederherstellungschirurgie, 1983(b)

Pirsig W: Historical notes and actual observations on the nasal septal abscess especially in children. Int J Ped Otorhinolaryngol 8:43, 1984(a)

Pirsig W: Zur chirurgie der nase im kindesalter. Wachstum und spätergebnisse. Laryngol Rhinol Otol 63:170, 1984(b)

Pirsig W: Die Chirurgie der kindlichen nase. Ordentliche Sitzung der Oto-laryngologischen Gesellschaft. Berlin, 1986(a)

Pirsig W: Rhinoplasty and the airway in children. Fac Plast Surg 3:4, 1986(b)

Pirsig W, Lehmann I: The influence of trauma on the growing septal cartilage. Rhinology 13:39, 1975

Pirsig W, Rohrs M: Ergebnisse der Septumplastik zur Verbesserung der Nasenfunktion bei Kindern mit Lippen-Kiefer-Gaumeh-Spalten.

Pitanguy I: Surgical importance of a dermocartilaginous ligament in bulbous noses. Plast Reconstr Surg 36:247, 1965

Pitanguy I, Caldeira A, Trevino MN: Rinofima consideraçoes clinic-cirurgicas. Rev Bras Cir 74(2):101, 1984

Pitanguy I, Ceravolo MP: Nasal polyposis after secondary rhinoplasty: A case report. Aesthetic Plast Surg 6:2, 1982(a)

Pitanguy I, Ceravolo MP: Secondary rhinoplasty. Aesthetic Plast Surg 6:47, 1982(b)

Planas J: Total extirpation of the septum, in Transactions of the Third International Congress of Plastic Surgeons, Washington, 1963. Amsterdam Excerpta Medica 1964

Planas J: The twisted nose. Clin Plast Surg 4:55, 1977

Planas J: The tile graft: A method of building the roof of the nose using preserved homograft septal cartilage. Eur J Plast Surg 9:140, 1987

Planas J, Brancati V: Concetti generali in rinoplastica estetica. Riv Italiana Chirur Plast 15:2, 1983

Plot S: Les ostéotomies dans les rhinoplasties. Chirurgie Esthétique 1983–1984, Paris, Maloine, 1984

Podvinec S, Maksimovic D: Traitement chirurgical dans l'inversion des ailes du nez. J Franc Oto-rhino-laryngol 15:69, 1966

Poget M: Plastic Surgery at La Source Clinic. Rev Med Suisse Romande 103:223, 1983

Pollet J: Le point de vue du plasticien. Cah d'ORL 6:197, 1971

Pollet J: L'utilisation des exerèses osteo-cartilagineuses au cours de la rhinoseptoplastie. Ann Chir Plast 17:90, 1972

Pollet J: Use of osteocartilaginous fragments removes during rhinoplasty. Yearbook of Plastic and reconstructive Surgery. Chicago Yearbook, 1974, p 73

Pollet J: Revision rhinoplasty. Clin Plast Surg 4:1, 1977

Pollet J, Baudelot S: Séquelles de la chirurgie esthétique de la base du nez. Ann Chir Plast 12:185, 1967

Pollet J, Baudelot S: Greffe composée pour refection de l'aile d'un nez. Prélèvement avec débord de cartilage. Ann Chir Plast 15:67, 1970(a)

Pollet J, Baudelot S: La rhinoplastie extra-muqueuse. Ses indications. Ann Chir Plast 15:61, 1970(b)

Pollet J, Gehanno P, Hagege JC: Cutaneous problems in rhinoplasty. Transactions of the Sixth International Congress Plastic Reconstructive Surgery, Paris, Masson, 1976

Pollet J, Weikel AM: Some technical considerations in primary rhinoplasty. Aesthetic Plast Surg 1:25, 1976

Polli G, Dal Maso U: La metodica rinoreomanometrica nella valutazione dei resultati della chirurgia funzionale del naso. Riv Ital Otorinolaryngol 3:105, 1983

Pollock RA: Surgery of the nasal septum. International Correspondence Society of Ophthalmologists and Otolaryngologists, 27:10, 1982

Pollock RA: Surgical approaches to the nasal dermoid cyst. Ann Plast Surg 10:498, 1983

Pollock RA, Rohrich RJ: Inferior turbinate surgery: An adjunct to successful treatment of nasal obstruction in 408 patients. Plast Reconstr Surg 74:233, 235, 1984

Ponti L: La chirurgia correttiva del setto nasale nei bambini. Valsalva 33:97, 104, 1957

Ponti L: Etiopatogenesi e diagnostica nei nasi deviati (note di tecnica operativa). Clin Otorinolaringoiatrica 13:83, 1961

Ponti L: Surgery of the nasal tip. A modification of the Goldman technique. Excerpta Medica International Congress Series N 206, 1969

Ponti L: Aesthetic problems in surgical technique of the nasal tip. Plastic and Reconstructive Surgery of the Face and Neck, Proceedings of the Second International Symposium, vol. 1. New York, Grune & Stratton, 1977(a)

Ponti L: Revision of rhinoplasty. Plastic and Reconstructive Surgery of the Face and Neck, Proceedings of the Second International Symposium, vol. 1. New York, Grune & Stratton, 1977(b)

Pool R: Surgery of the alar wings and base, in Master FW, Lewis JR (eds): Aesthetic Surgery of the Nose, Ears and Chin. St. Louis, Mosby, 1973

Postema CA: The lateralization percentage as a measure of nasal flow asymmetry in active anterior rhinomanometry. Clin Otolaryngol 5:165, 1980

Potter J: Some nasal tip deformities due to altar cartilage deformities. Plast Reconstr Surg 13:358, 1954

Potter J: Some nasal deformities due to alar cartilage abnormalities. Plast Reconstr Surg 15:502, 1955

Potter J: Secondary repair of flattened alae in the cleft lip deformity. Chir Plastica 7:273, 1984

Powers WE Jr: A plea to teach septal surgery to plastic surgical residents (letter). Plast Reconstr Surg 71:285, 1983

Prado FA, Di Geronimo EM: Correction of the deformed alae secondary to cleft lip. Plast Reconstr Surg 69:541, 1982

Pratt JA: Conservation of turbinates. Trans Am Acad Ophthalmol Otolaryngol 20:136, 1915

Presecott CAJ: Experience with bilateral congenital atresia of the posterior nasal choanae. J Laryngol Otol 100:11, 1255, 1986

Principato JJ: Chronic vasomotor rhinitis: Cryogenic and other surgical modes of treatment. Laryngoscope 89:619, 1979

Proetz AW: Applied Physiology of the Nose. St. Louis, Annals Publishing Co, 1941

Proetz AW: Physiology of the nose from the standpoint of the plastic surgeon. Arch Otolaryngol 39:514, 1944

Proetz AW: Respiratory air currents and their clinical aspects. J Laryngol Otol 67:1, 1953

Protasevich GS: The management of nasal septum deformation combined with hypertrophic turbinated bones. Vestn ORL (Moscow) 4:46, 1983

Puhakka H, Rantanen T: Cryotherapy as a method of treatment in allergic and vasomotor rhinitis. J Laryngol 91:535, 1977

Quisling RA: Advantages of shatter-fracture lateral osteotomy. Arch Otolaryngol 78:693, 1963

Rakstang G: The effect of partial resection of the cartilaginous nasal septum on the osteogenic cells of the facial bones in rats. Eur J Orthod 5:67, 1983

Ramadier JA, Eyries C: Le traitement chirurgical de l'ozène. Rapport au Congrès de la Soc J Franc Oto-rhino-laryngol 55:107, 1948

Ramos J, Sanches A, Gonzalez E: Fistulas congenitas del dorso de la nariz y quistes dermoides. Caso de difficil diagnostico. Acta otorinolaringol 34:225, 1983

Randall P: Direct approach to the hanging columella. Plast Reconstr Surg 53:544, 1974

Randall P, Bakes EP, Kennedy C: Cleft palate type speech in the absence of cleft palate. Plast Reconstr Surg 25:484, 1960

Ranzolin G: La condro-riposizione nella settoplastica per deviaz deviazioni anteriori. Min Otorin 21:345, 1963

Ranzolin G, Jost G: La condroriposizione nella settoplastica per deviazioni anteriori. Min Otorin 11:245, 1961

Rasi HB: The fate of preserved human cartilage. Plast Reconstr Surg 24:24, 1959

Reed GF: Nasal obstruction: Causes and treatment. Postgrad Med 34:464, 1963

Rees TD: Basal cell carcinoma in association with rhinophyma. Plast Reconstr Surg 16:282, 1955

Rees TD: Nasal plastic surgery in the Negro. Plast Reconstr Surg 43:13, 1969

Rees TD, Krupp S, Wood-Smith D: Secondary rhinoplasty. Plast Reconstr Surg 46:332, 1970

Rees TD: An aid to the treatment of supratip swelling after rhinoplasty. Laryngoscope 81:308, 1971

Rees TD: Cosmetic Facial Surgery. Philadelphia, W.B. Saunders, 1973(a)
Rees TD: Secondary rhinoplasty. Symposium on Aesthetic Surgery of the Nose, Ears and Chin. Saint Louis, Mosby, 1973(b)
Rees TD: Current concepts of rhinoplasty. Chir Plast Surg 4:1977
Rees Th D, Anderson JR, Sheen JH: Colloquium rhinoplasty. Ann Plast Surg 1:6, 597, 1978
Rees TD: Aesthetic Plastic Surgery. Philadelphia, W.B. Saunders, 1980(a)
Rees TD: Secondary Rhinoplasty in Aesthetic Plastic Surgery. Philadelphia, W.B. Saunders, 1980(b), p 388
Rees TD: Surgical correction of the severely deviated nose by extramucosal excision of the osseocartilaginous septum and replacement at the free graft. Plast Reconstr Surg 78:320, 1986
Rees TD, Guy CL, Converse JM: Repair of the cleft lip nose. Plast Reconstr Surg 37:47, 1966
Rees TD, Wood-Smith D: Cosmetic Facial Surgery. W.B. Saunders, Philadelphia, 1973
Rees TD, Wood-Smith D: Aesthetic Plastic Surgery. W.B. Saunders, Philadelphia, 1980
Regnault PCL: Reconstructive rhinoplasty with nasal implants. Aesthetic Plast Surg 4:79, 1980
Regnault P, Alfaro A: The Skoog rhinoplasty. A modified technique. Plast Reconstr Surg 66:578, 1980
Regnault P, Daniel RK: Aesthetic Plastic Surgery. Boston, Little Brown, 1984, p 114
Rehrmann A: A new method of nasal reconstruction. Trans. International Congressional Society Plastic Surgery. Stockholm, Williams and Wilkins, 277, 1956
Rehrmann A: Plastische Operationen im Gesicht-Kieferbereich. HNO (Berlin) 6:139, 1957
Reich J: The surgery of appearance. Psychological and related aspects. Med J Austr 2:5, 1969
Reich J: Factors influencing patient satisfaction with the results of esthetic plastic surgery. Plast Reconstr Surg 55:5, 1975
Reich J: Aesthetic judgement in the surgery of appearance. Transactions of the Sixth International Congress on Plastic and Reconstructive Surgery. Paris, Masson, 1976
Reich J: The application of dermis grafts in deformities of the nose. Plast Reconstr Surg 71:772, 1983
Reich J: Problems in management of the aesthetic surgery patient, in Kaye B, Gradinger GP, (eds): Symposium on Problems and Complications in Aesthetic Plastic Surgery of the Face, 1984
Reichert H: Plastic surgery of the nose in children. Plast Reconstr Surg 31:51, 1963
Reichert H: The lateral velopharyngoplasty: A new method for the correction of open nasality. J Max Fac Surg 2:95, 1974
Reidy JP: Homogenous bone graft. Brit J Plast Surg 9:89, 1956
Reidy JP: The nasal septum. Ann R Coll Surg 43:141, 1968
Reiger, RA: A local flap for repair of the nasal tip. Plast Reconstr Surg 40:147, 1967
Reker U: Leistung der propriozeptoren der halswirbelsäule beim zerviko-okulären reflex. HNO 33:426, 1985
Rethi A: Plastische neubildung der nase. Chir 1:695, 1929(a)
Rethi A: Über die korrektiven operationen der nasendeformitäten Chir 1:1103, 1929(b)
Rethi A: Operation to shorten an excessively long nose. Rev Chir Plast 2:85–87, 1934
Rethi A: Operative treatment of ozaena. J Laryngol 62:139, 1948(a)
Rethi A: Right and wrong in rhinoplastic operation. Plast Reconstr Surg 3:361, 1948(b)
Rethi A: Chirurgie der verengungen der oberen luftwege. Stuttgart, Georg Thieme Verlag, 1959(a)
Rethi A: Le traitement chirurgical de l'ozène. Ann Otolaryngol 76:413, 1959(b)
Rettinger G, Deleye L: Knochenverstärkted knorpelstransplantat zur rekonstruktion der nasenscheidwand. HNO 133:11, 1987
Rettinger G, Masing H: Rotation of the air cartilage in collapsed ala. Internat Rhinol 19:81, 1981
Rettinger G, Masing H: Behinderte Nasenatmung durch altersbedingte Veränderungen der Flügelknorpel. Plastische u. Wiederherstellungschirurgie des Alters. Hrsg: H. Neubauer. Springer-Verlag, Berlin Heidelberg, 1986
Rettinger G, Masing H, Heinl W: Surgical closure of septal perforations with a septal mucosa rotation flap. HNO 34:461, 1986
Reynolds JR, Horton CE: An alar lift procedure in cleft lip rhinoplasty. Plast Reconstr Surg 35:377, 1965
Rheims D, Meyer R, Daverio P: Application de la colle fibrine en chirurgie plastique: Reconstruction et esthétique cervico-faciale. Ann Chir Plast Esthét 31:4, 384, 1986
Richardson JR: Turbinate treatment in vasomotor rhinitis. Laryngoscope 58:834, 1948
Riefkohl R: Rhinophyma: A thirty-five year experience. Aesthetic Plast Surg 7:131, 1983
Rieger RA: Local flap for repair of nasal tip. Plast Reconstr Surg 40:147, 1967
Riggs R: The relation of septum reconstruction to external deformities of the nose. Laryngoscope 63:293, 1953
Riggs, R: Physiological surgery of nasal septum and associated structure. J Arkansas Med Soc 51:62, 1954
Riggs R: The maxillary-premaxillary approach to septal surgery. Eye Ear Nose Thr Mouth 39:157, 1960
Riggs R: Nasal dysfunction in children. J La Med Soc, 113:257, 1961
Riggs R: Pediatric nasal surgery. J La State Med Soc, 115:329, 1963
Rish BB: Combined defects of the cosmetic profile. Corrective rhinoplasty with simultaneous repair of simple retruded. Chin Laryngoscope 65:9, 1955
Rish RH: Profile-plasty. Report on plastic chin implants. Laryngoscope 74:144, 1964
Riski JE, Serafin D, Riefkohl R, et al: A rationale for modifying the site of insertion of the orticochea pharyngoplasty. Plast Reconstr Surg 73:891, 1984
Ritter FN: Vasculature of the nose. Ann Otol 79:468, 1970
Robin JL: Transplantation d'os mastoïdien. Ann Chir Plast 3:55–59, 1958
Robin JL: Considérations techniques sur la chirurgie réductrice des arêtes nasales. Acta Otorhinolaryngol Belg 22:704, 1968
Robin JL: La rhinoplastie extramuqueuse. Communiqué Soc Franc Chir Plast Reconstr 23 1970
Robin JL: Rhinoplasty extra-muqueuse controlée avec mesure pré-opératoire de la modification du profil. Ann Chir Plast 18:2, 119, 1973
Robin JL: Extramucosal method in rhinoplasty. Aesthetic Plast Surg 3:171, 1979(a)
Robin JL: The preplanned rhinoplasty. Aesthetic Plast Surg 3:179, 1979(b)

Robin JL: Extramucosal method in rhinoplasty. Ann Chir Plast 25:27, 1980
Rode C: Zur tecknik des gipsverbandes in der behandlung der nasenbein—Frakturen und deformitäten. Z Halsnas Ohrenheilk 43:294, 1938
Roe JO: The deformity termed pug nose and its correction by a simple operation. Med Rec 31:621, 1887. Reprinted in Plast Reconstr Surg 45:78, 1970(a)
Roe JO: The correction of angular deformities of the nose by a subcutaneous operation. Med Rec 40:57, 1891. Reprinted in Plast Reconstr Surg 45:283, 1970(b)
Roe R: Zit von fomon caron, und bill. Arch Otolaryngol 62:409, 1955
Rogers BO: The importance of delay in timing secondary and tertiary corrections of post-rhinoplastic deformities, in transactions of the Fourth International Congress of Plastic and Reconstructive Surgeons, Amsterdam, Excerpta Medica, 1967
Rogers BO: Rhinoplasty, in Goldwyn RM (ed): Unfavorable Results in Plastic Surgery. Boston, Little, Brown and Co., 1972, p 283
Rogers BO: The roles of physical anthropology in plastic surgery today. Clin Plast Surg 1:439, 1974
Rogers BO: Secondary and tertiary corrections of postrhinoplastic deformities: Some dos and don'ts, in Millard DR (ed): Symposium on Corrective Rhinoplasty. St. Louis, C.V. Mosby Co., 1976(a)
Rogers BO: The development of aesthetic plastic surgery: A history. Aesthetic Plast Surg 1:3, 1976(b)
Rogers BO: Nasal reconstruction 150 years ago. Aesthetic and other problems. Aesthetic Plast Surg 5:283, 1981
Rollason WN: Hypotensive anaesthesia for operations on the ear, nose and parotid gland. Use of intravenous metoprolol as an adjunct to sodium nitroprusside and halothane. Anaesthesia 38:590, 1983
Romashov SS: Case of successful treatment of extensive esthesioneuroblastoma of the nasal cavity invading the ethmoid labyrinth, maxillary and frontal sinuses and the orbit. Vestn Otorinolaringol 79, 1983
Rosen Z: Nasal deformities in the Bible. Int Rhinol 9:26, 1971
Rotkitski VM: Free bony, cartilaginous, and cutaneous rhinoplastic surgery. Khir Arkh Velyaminova 30:431, 1914
Roward A: Rhinoplasty applications to submucous resection of the nasal septum (surgical anatomy: technique of a modified procedure). Otolaryngol 59:739, 1954
Rowe NL, Killey HC: Fractures of the Facial skeleton. Edinburg, Livinstone, 1955
Rozner L: Nasal obstruction due to restriction of the bony nasal inlet. Br J Plast Surg 17:287, 1964
Rozner L: Augmentation Rhinoplasty. Br J Plast Surg 33:377, 1980
Rozner L, Isaacs GW: Nasal obstruction after rhinoplasty. Aesthetic Plast Surg 3:89, 1979
Rubin FF: Permanent change in shape of cartilage by morselization. Arch Otolaryngol 89:602, 1969
Rubin FF: Improved reconstruction of the nasal pyramid, in Bernstein L (ed): Plastic and Reconstructive Surgery, vol. 1. Aesth Surg 1981
Rubin FF: Tip projection, ptosis and supratip thickening. ENT J 61: 460, 1982
Rubin FF: Controlled tip sculpturing with the morselizer. Arch Otolaryngol 109:160, 1983
Rubin LR: New rhinoplastic instruments. Plast Reconstr Surg 3:86, 1948
Rubin LR: Polyethelene—Three year study. Plast Reconstr Surg 7:131, 1951
Ruddy LW: A transpalatine operation for congenital atresia of the choana in the small child or the infant. Arch Otolaryngol 41:432, 1945
Rudert H: Von der submukösen septumresektion killians über cottles septumplastik zur modernen plastischen septumkorrektur und funktionellen septo-rhinplastik. HNO 32:230, 1984
Rudolph R: Pseudomonas infection in the postoperative nasal septum. Plast Reconstr Surg 70:87, 1982
Ruskin SL: A differential diagnosis and therapy of atrophic rhinitis and ozena. Arch Otolaryngol 15:222, 1932
Ryan RE, Ryan RE Jr: Headache of nasal origin. Headache 19:173, 1979
Saad MN, Barron JN: Reconstruction of the columella with alar margin flaps. Br J Plast Surg 33:427, 1980
Sachs ME: Enbucrilate as cartilage adhesive in augmentation rhinoplasty. Arch Otolaryngol Head Neck Surg 111:389, 1985
Safian J: Corrective Rhinoplastic Surgery. New York, Paul Hoeber Co, 1935
Safian J: Failures in rhinoplastic surgery; Cause and prevention. Am J Surg 50:274, 1940
Safian J: The uncontrollable factors in rhinoplasty. Plast Reconstr Surg 12:24, 1953
Safian J: Deceptive concepts of rhinoplasty. Plast Reconstr Surg 18:127, 1956
Safian J: Fact and fallacy in rhinoplastic surgery. Brit J Plast Surg 11:45, 1958
Safian J: Progress in nasal and chin augmentation. Plast Reconstr Surg 37:446, 1965
Safian J: Personal recollections of professor Jacques Joseph. Plast Reconstr Surg 46:175, 1970(a)
Safian J: The split-cartilage tip technique of rhinoplasty. Plast Reconstr Surg 45:217, 1970(b)
Safian J: A new anatomical concept of postoperative complications in aesthetic rhinoplasty. Plast Reconstr Surg 51:162, 1973
Safian J, Tamerin J: Recent fractures of the nose. Ann J Surg 31:10, 1936
Safian LS: Potentialities and limitations of corrective rhinoplasty. NY State J Med 48:2160, 1948
Safian LS: Cosmetic rhinoplasty: Radiological features. Head Neck Surg 7:2, 1984
Salasche SJ: Curettage and electrodesiccation in the treatment of midfacial basal cell epithelioma. Am Acad Dermatol 8:496, 1983
Salinger S: Deviation of the septum in relation of twisted nose. Arch Otolaryngol 29:520, 1939
Salinger S: Injuries to nose in children. Arch Otolaryngol 34:936, 1941
Salinger S: Cartilage homografts in rhinoplasty. Ann Otol 61:533, 1952(a)
Salinger S: The nasal septum: Some observations on its relationship to palatal deformities. Br J Plast Surg 5:129, 1952(b)
Salinger S: Correction of deformities involving the septum and external nose. Ann ORL 3:62, 1953
Salinger 1941. Quoted by Salinger and Cohen, 1955
Salinger S, Cohen BM: Surgery of the difficult septum. Arch Otolaryngol 61:419, 1955
Salis B, Ottoboni A: Chirurgie correttive del naso. Considerazioni clinico chirurgiche sugli interventi di settoplastica e rinoplastica. Min Otorinolaringol 17:99, 1967

Salked CR: A case of chianal atresia with Asherson's tubes. J Laryngol Otol 82:927, 1968
Sanchez AE: Rhinoplasty in the "chata" nose of Carribean. Aesthetic Plast Surg 4:169, 1980
Sandon RP: The bridge of the nose: A tutorial dissertation. Br J Plast Surg 36:210, 1983
Sanvenero Rosseli G: Chirurgia Plastica del Naso. Roma, Pozzi, 1931
Sarnat BG: Postnasal growth of the nose and face after resection of septal cartilage in the rabbit. Oral Surg 26:712, 1968
Sarnoff J: Pitfalls and safeguards in plastic surgery. Plast Reconstr Surg 5:168, 1950
Saunders G: Correction of deviation of the anterior nasal septum cartilage. Trans Pa Coast Opthalmol Soc 21:40, 1949
Saunders WH: Septal dermoplasty for control of nosebleeds caused by hereditary hemorrhagic telangiectasia or septal perforations. Tr Am Acad Opthalmol 64:500, 1960
Sayler KE: Primary correction of the unilateral cleft lip nose, a 15 year experience. Plast Reconstr Surg 77:558, 1986
Schafenegger J, Gubisch W: La reconstruction fonctionnelle et esthétique de la pyramide nasale antérieure par implants cartilagineux septo-columellaires. Abstracts, European Rhinology Society Tenth Congress, Nancy, 1984, p 95
Schell JJ: Polytef injection for nasal deformity. Arch Otolaryngol 92:554, 1970
Scherer H: Behandlungsmöglichkeiten des malignen melanoms des gaumens, der nasenhöle ind der nasennebenhölen. Laryngol Rhinol Otol 63:9, 1984
Schjelderup H: Treatment of severe nasal deformity in secondary harelips. Plastic Congress, Stockholm, 1955
Schmelzle R: Konservierte Transplantate in der Kiefer-und-Gesichtschirurgiw. München, Hanser, 1978
Schmid E: Über neue wege in der plastischen chirurgie der nase. Brun's Beitr Klin Chir 184:385, 1952
Schmid E: Partielle und totale nasenplastik. Fortschr Kiefer Gesichtschir 7:80, 1961
Schmid E: The nose, the mini flap in regional flaps of the Head and Neck, in Conley (ed): Stuttgart, Thieme, 1976
Schmid E: Rehabilitationsergebnisse nach nasenaplastik-und-hypoplasie. Ges Plast Wiederherstellungschir 24, 1983
Schmid RE, Widmajer WI: Über die haut-knorpel-transplantationen aus der ohrmuschel und ihre funktionelle und ästhetische bedeutung bei der deckung von gesichtsdefekten. Fortschr Kiefer Gesichtschir 7:48, 1961
Schmid W, Markmiller U: Rhinomanometrische ergebnisse nach operativen eingriffen an der nase. HNO (Berlin) 31:31, 1983
Schönborn: Zur operationstechnik der cheilognath-palatoschisis. Med 42, 1954
Schönfeld AL: A preliminary report on the use of preserved homogenous cartilage implants. Br J Plast Surg 6:26, 1953
Schönfeld R: Fibrinkleber zur verhinderung von hämatomen nach rhinochirurgischen eingriffen. HNO (Springer) 33:156, 1985
Schonsted-Madsen U, Stocksted P: Septal contact headache. Abstracts, European Rhinology Society Tenth Congress, Nancy, 1984
Schoofs M, Hamoir M: Correction chirurgicale de la sténose narinaire. Acta Otorhinolaryngol (Belg) 37:873, 1983
Schreus H Th: Schleifen und fräsen der haut. Aesth Méd (Heidelberg) 2, 1955
Schrudde J: La østeotomia subperiostica total en el estrechamiento de la nariz. Rev Esp Cir Plast 3:41, 1970
Schrudde J: Subperiostel osteotomy for narrowing the nose. Abstract book first in the National Congress ISAPS, Rio de Janeiro, 14, 1972
Schuffenecker J, Gubisch W: La reconstruction fonctionnelle et esthétique de la pyramide nasale antérieure par implants cartilagineux septocolumellaires. Abstracts Tenth Congrès de la Societé Européenne Rhinologie. Nancy, 1984
Schuller DE, Bardach J, Krause CJ: Irradiated homologous costal cartilage for facial contour restoration. Arch Otolaryngol 103:12, 1977
Schultz AH: The development of the external nose in whites and negroes. Contrib Embryol 9:173, 1920
Schultz-Coulon HJ: Die korrektur ausgeprägter deformitäten des ventro-caudalen septumabschnitts beim kind. HNO (Berlin) 31:6, 1983(a)
Schultz-Coulon HJ: The repair of extensive deformities of the ventrocaudal septu, segment in children. HNO 31:6, 1983 (b)
Schultz-Coulon HJ, Eckermeier L: Zum postnatalen wachstum der nasenscheidewand. Acta Otolaryngol (Stock) 82:131, 1976
Schurter M, Letterman G: Suggested anatomical nomenclature for the nose. Plast Reconstr Surg 57:4, 1976
Schweckendiek H: Transpalatine behandlung angeborener choanalatresien. Z Hals-Nas, Ohrenheilk 42:367, 1937
Seda HJ: Closure of nasal septal perforation with composite flaps. Laryngoscope 87:1942, 1977
Sedee G, Willemot J: La résection sous-muqueuse de la cloison qu'en reste-t-il? Acta Otorhinolaryngol (Belg) 27:539, 1973
Seeley RC: Repair a septal perforation, a rhinologic problem: A rhinoplastic approach. Laryngoscope 59:130, 1949
Seiferth LB: Verletzungen der Nase, der Nasennebenhöhlen und die frontobasalen Verletzungen. In: HNO-Heilkunde, Bd. I, hrsg. von J. Berendes, R. Link u.F. Zöllner. Stuttgart: Thieme 1964
Seiffert A: Perseptale naht bei ozaenaoperation. Z Hals-Nas und Ohrenheilk 17, 1922
Seiffert A: Die Operationen an Nase, Mund und Hals (ed 4). Leipzig, Barth, 1955
Selkin SG: Laser turbinectomy as an adjunct to rhinoseptoplasty. Arch Otolaryngol Head Neck Surg 111:446, 1985
Seltzer A: Characteristics peculiar to the cartilaginous septum of the nose. Ann ORL 65:198, 1956
Seltzer A: A new instrument for correcting the obstructing deviated septum. J Natl Med Assoc 55:409, 1963
Seltzer AP: On a hereditary factor in rhinophyma. M World 61:310, 1943
Seltzer AP: The nasal septum: Plastic repair of the deviated septum associated with a deflected tip. Arch Otolaryngol 40:433, 1944
Seltzer AP: Plastic Surgery of the Nose. Philadelphia, J.B. Lippincott Co, 1949
Seltzer AP: The Seltzer circular rhinoplastic saw. Plast Reconstr Surg 5:261, 1950
Seltzer AP: Cautions in rhinoplastic surgery. Eye, Ear, Nose Throat 32:350, 1953
Seltzer RC: Improved method for narrowing the nose. Ann Otol Rhinol Laryngol 52:640, 1943

Senechal G: Problèmes posés par la racine du nez au cours de la rhinoplastie. Ann Otolaryngol 79:12, 1962
Senechal G: Fractures du nez. Encycl Med Chir. Paris, Flammaron, 1963
Senechal G: Complications et échecs des rhinoplasties. Problèmes actuels d'ORL. 131; Libraire Maloine, 1967
Senechal G, Firmin F: La rhinoplastie chez l'homme. Ann Chir Plast 15:34, 1970
Senechal G: Séance consacrée aux difficultés et échecs au cours des rhinoplasties. Ann Oto-Laryngol 93:9, 589, 1976(a)
Sénéchal G: Principales complications et facteurs d'échecs des rhinoplasties. Ann Oto-Laryngol 93:40, 1976(b)
Senechal G, Neveu M: Les nez ensellés. Ann Otolaryngol 12:829, 1967
Senechal G, Neveu M: Perforations septales et rhinoplastie. Ann Chir Plast 17:83, 1972
Senechal G, Senechal B, Mamelle G: A rare and late complication in rhinoplasty. Ann Otolaryngol 98:385, 1981 (in short: Plast Reconstr Surg 70:777, 1982)
Sercer A: Dekortikation der nase. Chir Maxillofac Plast 1:149, 1958
Sercer A: Plastische Operationen an der Nase. Plastische Operationen an der Nase und an der Ohrmuschel. Stuttgart, Thieme, 1962
Sercer A: Plastische Operationen an der Nase und an der Ohrmuschel, in Sercer A, Mundrich K (eds): Thieme Verlag, Stuttgart, 1972
Sercer A, Munduich K: Plastic Operationen and der Ohr Muschal. Stuttgart, G. Rhienne Verlag, 1962
Serson-Neto D: Rhinoplasties esthétique. Ann Chir Plast 18:307, 1973
Sessions RB: Nasal hemorrhage. Otolaryngol Clin North Am, 1973
Sessions RB: Complications of rhinoplasty. Laryngol Rhinol Otol 62:185, 1983
Shahinian L: Chronic vasomotor rhinitis treatment by submucous diathermic coagulation. Arch Otolaryngol 57:475, 1953
Shapshay SM: Removal of rhinophyma with the carbon dioxide laser. Arch Otolaryngol 106:225, 1980
Shaw MH, Fell SR: Columella reconstruction. Br J Plast Surg 31:370, 1963
Sheehan JE: Gillies new method on giving support to the depressed nasal bridge and columella. J Med 16, 1921
Sheehan JE: Plastic surgery of the syphilitic nose. Laryngoscope 35:22, 1925
Sheehan JE: Plastic surgery of the nose. New York, Hoeber, 1936
Sheehan JE, Swanker WA: Surgical repair of congenital choanal atresia. Laryngoscope 59:1320, 1949
Sheen JH: Achieving more nasal tip projection by the use of small autogenous vomer or septal cartilage graft. Plast Reconstr Surg 56:211, 1975(a)
Sheen JH: Achieving more nasal tip projection by the use of a small autogenous bone or cartilage graft. Plast Reconstr Surg 56:35, 1975(b)
Sheen JH: Secondary rhinoplasty. Plast Reconstr Surg 56:211, 1975(c)
Sheen JH: Secondary rhinoplasty surgery, In Millard DR (ed): Symposium on Corrective Rhinoplasty, St-Louis, Mosby, 1976, p 133
Sheen JH: Aesthetic Rhinoplasty. St. Louis, CV Mosby, 1978 (a)
Sheen JH: Finesse in Rhinoplasty. Aesthetic Rhinoplasty. St. Louis, Mosby, 1978(b), p 267
Sheen JH: A new look at supratip deformity. Ann Plast Surg 3:498, 1979
Sheen JH: Spreader Graft: A method of reconstructing the roof of the middle nasal vault following rhinoplasty. Plast Reconstr Surg 73:230, 1984
Sheen JH: Secondary rhinoplasty, in Grabb WC, Smith JN (eds): Plastic Surgery: A Concise Guide to Clinical Practice, ed 3. Boston, Little, Brown & Co, (in press)
Sherlock EC: Anatomy of the nose and septum in Master FW, Lewis JR, (eds): Symposium on Aesthetic Surgery of the Nose and Chin. St. Louis, Mosby, 1973
Shidnia H, Hornback NB, Saghafi N, et al: The role of radiation therapy in treatment of malignant tumors of the paranasal sinuses. Laryngol 94:102, 1984
Shioya 1984. Quoted by Shirakabe, 1985
Ship AG: Alar base reconstruction for wide flaring nostrils. Br J Plast Surg 28:77, 1975
Shirakabe Y, Shirakabe T, Kishimoto T: The classification of complications after augmentation rhinoplasty. Aesthetic Plast Surg 9:185, 1985
Shirakabe Y, Shirakabe Y, Takayanagi S: A new type of prostheses for augmentation rhinoplasty: Our experience in 1600 cases. Br J Plast Surg 34:353, 1981
Shook FM: Submucous resection of the septum. Laryngoscope 88:750, 1981
Shtil' AA: Principles of surgical treatment of malignant tumors of nasal cavity and paranasal sinuses. Vestn Otorinolaringol 25, 1983
Shulman BH: Psychiatric assessment of the candidate for cosmetic surgery. Presented at the meeting of the American Academy of Facial Plastic and Reconstructive Surgery. St. Louis, 1973
Shulman J: A simple technique to straighten the slightly deviated nose in rhinoplasty. Ann Plast Surg 8:229, 1982
Shulman Y, Westrecih M: Postrhinoplasty Mucous Cyst of the Nose. Plast Reconstr Surg 421:71, 1983
Siegel RK: Cocaine: Recreational use and intoxication, in Peterson RC, Stillman RC (eds): Cocaine: 1977. N.I.D.A. Research Monograph No 13, Washington, 1977
Sigg O et al: Ornipressin as vasoconstrictor in rhinosurgery. Rhinology 2:21, 159, 1983
Silver AG: Pitfalls in rhinoplastic surgery. Eye, Ear, Nose, Throat 31:556, 1952
Silver WE: The use of aloplastie material in contouring the face. Facial Plast Surg 3:81, 1986
Simons RL: Adjunctive measures in rhinoplasty. Otolaryngol Clin North Am 8:717, 1975
Simons RL: Adjunctive offering in rhinoplasty. Plastic Reconstructive Surgery of the Face and Neck, Proceedings of the Second International Symposium, vol I. New York, Grune and Stratton, 1977
Simons RL: Nasal tip projection, ptosis and supratip thickening. ENT J 61:452, 1982
Simons RL, Fine IJ: Evaluation of the Goldman tip in rhinoplasty. Plastic and Reconstructive Surgery of the Face and Neck, Proceedings of the Second International Symposium, vol. I. New York, Grune and Stratton, 1977
Simmons FB, Guilleminault C, Miles LE: A surgical treatment for snoring and obstructive sleep apnea. West J Med 140:43, 1984
Simmons MW: Intranasal injection of corticosteroids in nasal disorders: Further observations. Trans Pacif Coast Oto-Ophthal Soc 45:95, 1964

Thornton JW: A reduction rhinoplasty technique and its applications, in Bernstein (ed): Plastic and Reconstructive Surgery vol. 1. 1981, p 49

Thumfart W: Electromyography in rhinoplasty. Rhinology 21:115, 1983

Tipton JB: Closure of large septal perforation with a labial-buccal flap. Plast Reconstr Surg 46:514, 1970

Tipton JB: Dislocation of upper lateral cartilages as a cause for nasal deformities. Plast Reconstr Surg 47:459, 1971

Tisserant J, Gehin P, Brichet B, et al: Interest of the Dilatator Naris Muscles Electromyography in Some Nasal. Congress European Rhinology Society. Nancy, 1984

Toback J: Toxic shock syndrome following septorhinoplasty Implications for the head and neck surgeon. Arch Otolaryngol 109:627, 1983

Tolhurst DE: Secondary correction of the unilateral cleft lip nose deformity. Br J Plast Surg 36:449, 1983

Tolsdorf T: Eingriff an den nasenmuscheln unter besonderer berücksichtigung der subperiostalen conchaltomie. Laryngol Rhinol 60:615, 1981

Tolsdorff P: Die osteomyelitis des os conchale und ihre bedeutung bei der chronischen sinusitis. HNO 31:314, 1983

Tong L: Augmentation rhinoplasty with plasticene modelling design and the dynamic new nose. International Congress of Plastic Surgery Montréal, 1983

Tonndorf J: Der weg der atemluft in der menschlichen nase. Arch Ohr Nas Kehlk Heilk 146:41, 1939

Tonndorf J: A note on measurement of nasal flow resistance. Ann Otol 67:984, 1958

Tremble GE: Methods of shrinking the inferior turbinates to improve the airway. Laryngoscope 70:175, 1960

Trendelenburg F: Verletzungen und chirurgische Krankheiten des Gesichtes, 1, S. 153, Stuttgart, Ferdinand Enke, 1886

Tschopp CF, Morrow RC: Transnasal correction of choanal atresia, microsurgery in newborn. Arch Otolaryngol 83:607, 1966

Tucker CA: Management of early nasal injuries with long term follow-up. Rhinology 22:45, 1984

Tucker LA: Rhinologic diagnosis correlated with structural changes of the nose. Otolaryngol Head Neck Surg 15:16, 1982

Uchida Y: Nasal function in relation to chronic nasal infection. Symposium Rhinology 22:91, 1984

Uffenorde W: Ein fall von choanalatresie mit demonstration. Z Laryngol Rhinol Otol 1:475, 1909

Uffenorde J, Georgi W: Einseitige erbindung nach intranasaler aethoxysklerol-injektion. HNO Berlin 31:236, 1983

Unger RM: Architecture of the nasal septum. How deviations are formed. Laryngoscope 75:322, 2965

Van Canwenberg C: Variations in nasal resistance in young children. Acta ORL (Belgium) 34:145, 1980

Van Cauwenberge PB, Deleye L: Nasal cycle in children. Arch Otolaryngol 110:108, 1984

Van Der Borg RS, Siemens BWL: Submucous septum corrections. Pract ORL 19(4):316, 1957

Van Dishoeck HAE: Inspiratory nasal resistance. Acta Otolaryngol 30:431, 1942

Van Dishoeck HAE: Some remarks on nasal physiology inspired by Sercer on nasal reduction. Acta Otolaryngol 36:467, 1948

Van Dishoeck HAE: Quelques remarques sur les bases phisiologiques de la chirurgie de la valve nasale. Suppl. 1967 Rev. Laryng. Otol. Rhinol. 2nd. Congr. Europ. Rhinol. 1966, Internat. Rhinol. Vol V, 3, 1967

Van Dishoeck EA, Lashley FON: Closure of septal perforation by means of an obturator. Rhinology 13:33–37, 1975

Van Lendeghem K: Zum verschluss von septumperforation. HNO 19:5, 1971

Vase P, Johannessen J,: Homograft cartilage in the treatment of an abscess in the nasal septum. J Laryngol Otol 95:357, 1981

Vaughan HS: Nasopharyngeal atresia. Plast Reconstr Surg 1:309, 1946

Vaughan HS: Secondary operations for cleft lip and associated nasal deformities, in Congenita Cleft Lip, Cleft Palate, and Associated Nasal Deformities. Philadelphia, Lea and Febiger, 1970, p 102

Vecchione TR: Columella reconstruction using internal nasal vestibular flaps. Br J Plast Surg 33:399, 1980

Vecchione TR: Repair of the unilateral cleft lip nose using contralateral alar crease grafts. Ann Plast Surg 14:148, 1985

Verwoerd CDA, Urbanus NAM, Nijdam DC: The effects of septal surgery on the growth of nose and maxilla. Rhinology, 17:53, 1979

Vetter U, Gammert C, Pirsig W, et al: Growth activities of the nasal septal cartilage in acromegaly. Rhinology 22:125, 1984

Vetter U, Heit W, Helbing G, et al: Growth of the human septal cartilage: Cell density and colony formation of septal chondrocytes. Laryngoscope 94:1226, 1984

Vetter U, Helbing W, Pirsig W, et al: Human septal cartilage: Local distribution of different enzyme activities in healthy adults and acromegalic patients. Laryngoscope 95:469, 1985

Vetter U, Pirsig W, Heinze E: Growth activity in human septal cartilage: Age-dependent incorporation of labeled sulfate in different anatomic locations. Plast Reconstr Surg 71:177, 1983

Vetter U, Pirsig W, Heinze E: Postnatal growth of the human septal cartilage. Acta Otolaryngol 97:131, 1984

Vetter U, Pirsig W, Helbing G, et al: Patterns of growth in human septal cartilage: A review of new approaches. Int J Pediatr Otorhinolaryngol 7:63, 1984

Vilar-Sancho B: Secondary rhinoplasty for correction of unfavorable surgical results due to the nasal septum. I Congr Brazil Cir Estet 1979

Vilar-Sancho B: Rhinoseptoplasty. Aesthetic Plast Surg 8:61, 1984

Vinas JC, Jager E: The push forward in velopharyngeal incompetence transactions of the 5th International Congress Plastic Surgery, Melbourne, 1971, p 252

Vitiello F: Tecniche chirurgiche di correzione per deviazione del setto nasale. Min Stom 23:180, 1974

Vogt T: Tip rhinoplastic operations using a transverse columellar incision. Aesthetic Plast Surg 7:13, 1983

Von Haacke NP, Hardcastle PF: Submucosal diathermy of the inferior ORL 47:189, 1985

Walter, C: Die plastische korrektur knöcherner und knorpeliger nasendeformitäten nach der methode von Goldman. Ärztl Kosmetik 4:146, 1957

Walter C: Aesthetische Chirurgie, Handbook der Plastischen Chirurgie. Berlin, Verlag de Gruyter, 1966(a)

Walter C: Komplikationen bei rhinoplastischen Eingriffen. In: Hanbuch der Plast. Chir. Bd. II. Beitrag 34, Gruyter Berlin 1966(b)

Walter C: Plastisch chirurgische gesichtspunkte bei der behandlung der medianen nasenfistel. Arch Ohr Nas Kehlk Heilk 191:803, 1968

Walter C: Composite grafts in nasal surgery. Arch Otolaryngol. 90:6, 1969(a)

Walter C: Fehlermöglichkeiten bei nasenplastiken. Arch Ohr Nas Kehlk Heilk 194:594, 1969(b)

Walter C: Composite grafts in nasal surgery. Arch Otolaryngol 90:662, 1969(c)

Walter C: Survey of the use of composite graft in the head and neck region. Otolaryngol Clin North Am 5:571, 1972

Walter C: The nasal septum, in Paparella MM, Shumrick DA (eds): Otolaryngology. WB Saunders, Philadelphia, 1973, p113

Walter C: Nasal reconstruction. Laryngoscope 85:1227, 1975

Walter C: Zum Thema: Nasenflüglekollaps. Laryngol Rhinol Otol (Stuttgart) 55:447, 1976

Walter C: Aesthetische Nasenchirurgie. Arch Otorhinolaryngol 216, 1977

Walter C: Secondary Nasal Revisions after Rhinoplasties. Aesthetic Plast Surg 2:317, 1978

Walter C, Mang WL: Künstlicher knochen (tricalciumphosphat) in der gesichtschirurgie. Laryngol Rhinol Otol 61:354, 1982

Walter C: Die Septo Rhinoplastik im Kindesalter. Ges Plast u Wiederherstellungschir. 1983, p 139

Wardill WEM, Wenay J: Bovine cartilage in plastic surgery: Preliminary communication. Lancet 2:389, 1947

Wardill 1930. Quoted by HJ Gabka 1962

Watanabe I: Surgical approach to tumors arising from the posterior two thirds of the nasal septum. J Otorhinolaryngol 49:157, 1987

Webber WB: Rhinoplasty: The importance of consistent documentation and significant long-term follow-up. Plast and Reconstr Surg 79:640, 1987

Webster GV: Rhinoplasty: The saw technique. Plast Reconstr Surg 28:249, 1961

Webster GV: Skin excisions in reduction rhinoplasty. Plast Reconstr Surg 51:289, 1973

Webster GV: Skin excisions in reduction rhinoplasty. Plast Reconstr Surg 54:289, 1978

Webster JP, Deming EG: Surgical treatment of bifid nose. Plast Reconstr Surg 6:1, 1950

Webster RC: Advances in surgery of the tip: Intact rim cartilage techniques and the tip-columella-lip esthetic complex. Otolaryngol Clin North Am 8:615, 1975(a)

Webster RC: Revisional rhinoplasty. Otolaryngol Clin 8(3):1975(b)

Webster RC: Progressi nella chirurgia della punta. Tecniche della cartilagine intatta del bordo e complesso estetico punta-columella-labbro. Otorinolaringol Clinica 1:78, 1976(a)

Webster RC: Rinoplastica de revisione. Otorinolaryngol Clinica I:222, 1976(b)

Webster RC, Davidson TM, Rubin FF, et al: Practical suggestions on facial plastic surgery. How I do it. Recording projection of nasal landmarks in rhinoplasty. Laryngoscope. 87:7, 1207, 1977

Webster RC, Davidson TM, Rubin FF, et al: Nasal tip projection changes. Related to cheeks and lip. Arch Otolaryngol 104:16, 1978

Webster RC, Davidson TM, Smith RC: Practical suggestion on facial plastic surgery. How I do it. External marking in rhinoplasty planning. Laryngoscope 86:126, 1976

Webster RC, Davidson TM, Smith RC: Curved lateral osteotomy for airway protection in Rhinoplasty Arch Otolaryngol 103:454, 1977(a)

Webster RC, Davidson TM, Smith RC: External marking in rhinoplasty planning. Laryngoscope 87:126, 1977(b)

Webster RC, Davidson TM, Smith RC: Browplasty as an adjunct to rhinoplasty. Head Neck Surg 1978, p 112

Webster RC, Davidson T, Smith R: Importance of the columellar labial junction in rhinoplasty. Head Neck Surg 1:423, 1979

Webster RC, Hopping B, Hall B, et al: Intraoral insertion of grafts in projecting the nasal tip. Arch Otolaryng 108:187, 1982

Webster, RC, Kattner MD, Smith RC: Injectable collagen for augmentation in facial areas. Arch Otolaryngol 110:652, 1984

Webster RC, Smith RC: Lateral crural retrodisplacement for supereior rotation of the tip in rhinoplasty. Aesthetic Plast Surg 3:65, 1979

Webster RC, Smith RC, Kazda G: Columella-labial changes in solution of rhinoplastic problems. Laryngoscope 95:629, 1985

Webster RC, White MF, Courtiss EH: Nasal tip correction in rhinoplasty. Plast Reconstr Surg 51:384–396, 1973

Wedig K: Operative behandlung des ansaugens der nasenflügel. HNO (Berlin) 13:183, 1965

Weerda H: Die rekonstruktion er ohrmuschel mit knorpeltransplantaten. HNO Plastischen Chirurgie an Kopf und Hals 133:11, 1987

Weikel A, Pollet J: Revision rhinoplasty. Clin Plast Surg 4:1, 1977

Weimert TA, Batsakis JG, Rice DH: Carcinomas of the nasal septum. J Laryngol Otol 92:209, 1978

Weinlechner 1901. Quoted by Joseph 1932

Weir RF: On restoring sunken noses without scarring the face. New York Med J 56:443, 1882 (In Plast Reconstr Surg 45:382, 1970)

Wepner FK, Hollmann F: Midface anthropometry on the cephalometric radiograph in cleft lip and palate cases. J Max Fac Surg 3:188, 1975

Wespi HH: Kopfschmerzen bei septumdeviation und muschelproblemen. Aktuelle Probleme der Otorhinolaryngologie. Stuttgart, Hans Huber Verlag Bern, 1983, p 143

Wespi HH: Kopfschmerzen bei septumdeviation und muschelproblemen. HNO 32:481, 1984

Wesser DR, Burt GB: Nasolabial flap for losses of the nasal ala and columella. Plast Reconstr Surg 44:300, 1969

Wexler AM: Post rhinoplastic complications. Eye, Ear, Nose & Throat Month 31:553, 1952

Wexler MR: Submucous resection of nasal septum in children. JAMA 157(4):333, 1955

Wexler MR: Septum surgery-general considerations. Int Rhinol 1; 123, 1963

Wexler MR: Nasal septum: Experimental and clinical correction of surgery or injury. Laryngoscope 71:1409, 1971

Wexler MR: Reconstructive surgery of the injured nose. Otolaryngol Clin North Am 88:663, 1975

Wexler MR: Chirurgia recostruttiva del naso lesionato. Otorinolaringol Clinica 1:128, 1976

Wheeler ES, Kawamoto HK, Zarem HA: Bone grafts for nasal reconstruction. Plast Reconstr Surg 69:9, 1982

White 1930. Quoted by JP Reidy 1968
Wilkie TF: The "alar shift" revisted. Br J Plast Surg 22:70, 1969
Willemot J: Histoire de la chirurgie plastique du nez. Acta Chir Belg 61:204, 1962
Willemot J: Corrective rhinoplasty and the nasal septum. Rev Laryngol 83:947, 1967
Willemot J: Cosmetic rhinoplasty and the nasal septum. Acta ORL Belg 22:725, 1968
Willemot J: Correction of old nasal deviations. Plast Reconstr Surg 43:430, 1969(a)
Willemot J: La septoplastie chez l'enfant. Acta ORL Belg 23:409, 1969(b)
Willemot J: Les relations de la pyramide nasale et de la cloison dans les rhinoplasties correctrices. Proceedings of the Ninth International Congress, Mexico, 1969(c)
Willemot J: Réflexes neuraux des cornets des fosses nasales. Proceedings of the Ninth International Congress, Mexico. 1969(d), p 211
Willemot J: La muqueuse olafactive chez l'homme. Premier résultats. Acta Otorhinolaryngol Belg 24:726, 1970(a)
Willemot J: Le rôle de la cloison dans la chirurgie correctrice du nez. Int Rhinol 8:133, 1970(b)
Willemot J: La muqueuse olfactive chez l'homme vivant. Acta Otolaryngol 71:197, 1971
Willemot J: La fracture du nez chez l'enfant. Acta Otorhinolaryngol Belg 28:991, 1974
Willemot J: Rhinomanométrie clinique et septorhinoplastie. J Fr ORL 24:681, 1975
Willemot J: Echecs et complications des rhinoplasties faites avec la méthode de Cottle. Ann Oto Rhinol Laryngol 93:637, 1976
Willemot J: Anatomie et traumatisme du nez—septo-rhinoplastie—nez et esthétique. Acta ORL Belg 35(2):201, 1981
Willemot J, Sedee GA: The indications for a septal approach in corrective rhinoplasty. Internat Rhinol 9:158, 1971
Willemot J, Pirsig W: Indications, technique and long term results of surgery of the nasal septum in children. Abstracts: European Rhinologic Society 10th Congress. Nancy, France, 1984
Williams HL: A consideration of the relation of the mechanism of nasal airflow to the function of the nose in respiration. Rhinology 10:145, 1972
Williams HR: A reconsideration of the mechanics of nasal airflow to the function of the nose in respiration. Rhinology 10:145, 1972
Williams R: Functions of the nasal septum as related to septal reconstruction surgery. Laryngoscope 63:212, 1953
Williams RI: Nasal index: Anthropological and clinical. Ann Otolrhinolaryngol 65:171, 1956
Wilson CP: Treatment of choanal atresia. J Laryngol Otol (London) 71:616, 1957
With FW: Submucous resection of the nasal septum. Ann ORL 331:520, 1924
Witwicka Z: Corrections of saddle nose by means of various transplants. Otolaryngol Pol 22:579, 1968
Woakes. Quoted by Pitanguy Y and MP Ceravolo. Aesth Plast Surg 6:93, 1982
Wolf G: Fibrin glue in otorhinolaryngology. Arch Otolaryngol 233:49, 1981
Wolf G: The concentrated autogenous tissue glue. Arch Otolaryngol 237:279, 1983
Wolf G, Stammberger H: Erster berichte über die anwendung eines autogenen gewebeklebers in der Hals-nasen-ohrenheilkunde. HNO (Springer) 33:152, 1985
Wolf RM, Snow J, Walker MD, et al: Correction of saddle nose deformity with upper-lateral turnover procedure. Plast Reconstr Surg 35:310, 1965
Wood JC: Rhinophyma. Surg Gynecol Obstet 15:622, 1912
Wright MR: Management of patient dissatisfaction with results of cosmetic procedures. Arch Otolaryngol 106:466, 1980(a)
Wright MR: Self-perception of the elective surgeon and some perception correlates. Arch Otolaryngol 108:460, 1980(b)
Wright MR: How to recognize and control the problem patient. J Dermatol Surg Oncol 10:5, 1984(a)
Wright MR: The elective surgeon's reaction to change and conflict. Arch Otolaryngol 110, 1984(b)
Wright WK: Lateral osteotomy in rhinoplasty. Arch Otolaryngol 78:680, 1963
Wright WK: Closure of large nasal septum perforations. Arch Otolaryngol 85:287, 1967
Wright WK: The relationship of the columella and nasal septum, in Conley J, Dickinson JT (eds): Plastic and Reconstructive Surgery of the Face and Neck. New York, Grune & Stratton, 1972, p 125
Wright WK: Photographic documentation of cosmetic surgery. Aesthetic Plast Surg 2:3, 1975
Wright WK: Chirurgia del dorso osseo e cartilagineo. Otorinolaringol Clinica 1:34, 1976
Wright WK: External septorhinoplasty. A tool for teaching and for improved results. Laryngoscope 91:945, 1981
Wright WK, Shambaugh GE, Green L: Congenital choanal atresia. A new surgical approach. Ann Otol (St. Louis) 56:120, 1947
Wullstein, SR: Die septumplastik bzw submuköse septumresektion ohne postoperative nasentamponade. HNO 27:322, 1979
Wüthrich B: Pollinose: Ursachen und therapeutische möglichkeiten. Medita 5: 1984
Yanai A, Nagata S, Yanaka H: Reconstruction of the columella with bilateral nasolabial flaps. Plast Reconstr Surg 77:129, 1986
Yankaur E: The technique of the submucous resection of the septum. Laryngoscope 16:294, 1906
Young A: Closure of the nostrils in atrophic rhinitis. J Laryngol 80:524, 1967
Young F: Principles to be considered in transplanting costal cartilage for repairing deficiencies of nasal skeleton. Ann Surg 108:670, 1946
Young F: The surgical repair of nasal deformities. Plast Reconstr Surg 4:59, 1949
Zarbo RJ: Nasopharyngeal hamartoma: Report of a case and review of the literature. Laryngoscope 93:494, 1983
Zelnik J, Gingrass RP: Anatomy of the alar cartilage. Plast Reconstr Surg 64:650, 1979
Zide BM: Nasal anatomy: The muscles and tip sensation. Aesthetic Plast Surg 9:193, 1985
Zloto R: Cartilages Alaires. Anatomie et Physiologie. Chirurgie Esthétique 1983–1984. Paris, Maloine, 1984
Zorzoli E: Sull'influenza dei fenomeni di collaborazione architettonica nel meccanismo delle deformazioni non non traumatiche del setto nasale. Boll Mal OGN 68:459, 1950(a)
Zorzoli E: I reinnesti de cartilagine nella correzione

chirurgica delle formazioni del setto nasale. Arch Ital Laryngol 58:334, 1950(b)

Zorzoli E: Presentazione di un procedimento per la correzione delle deviazioni della porzioni columellare del setto nasale. Valsalva 30:135, 1954

Zorzoli E: Il reinnesto subtotale della cartilagine del setto nella correzione dei difetti dell'estremità distale del naso. Minerva Chir 14:329, 1959

Zorzoli E: Le correzioni chirugiche del setto nasale nell'età pubere. Minerva Chir 15:1025, 1960

Zwaardemaker H: Ademaanslag als diagnosticum der nasale stenose. Ned Tijdschr Geneeskd 25:297, 1889

Index